Psychopathology in Women

80€

PPN

16

Margarita Sáenz-Herrero
Editor

Psychopathology in Women

Incorporating Gender Perspective into Descriptive Psychopathology

Springer

Editor
Margarita Sáenz-Herrero
Dept. of Psychiatry
Hospital Universitario de Alava
Victoria, Spain

ISBN 978-3-319-05869-6 ISBN 978-3-319-05870-2 (eBook)
DOI 10.1007/978-3-319-05870-2
Springer Cham Heidelberg New York Dordrecht London

Library of Congress Control Number: 2014952223

Printed on acid-free paper

Springer is part of Springer Science+Business Media (www.springer.com)

Foreword

Women suffer from depression and anxiety more often—much more often—than men and this has been attributed to nature and nurture, depending on the ideology of the author. The facts are that women use mental health services more than men and that depression is the most frequent ailment of women. In a globalized world, where information means power, we need to explore the roots of this phenomenon: this book is a much-needed tool toward a better understanding of the mental processes that give rise to mental health illnesses in women.

Women have been able to gain a place in the world. As we advance further in the society of "talentism," where wealth and resources are allocated to those showing more talent, we are faced with the need to look at the reasons that prevent countless women from developing their talents more fully and contributing their share to the development of their communities. Interest in the peculiarities of women's mental health is, however, new. Whatever happens in women's minds has for centuries been considered mysterious, sinful or whimsical. The existence of a male paradigm, from which the female body and mind were considered "deviant," rendered many experiences, thoughts, and feelings of women "abnormal" [1]. The supposed "neutrality" of research and theory that ignores gender differences does nothing but increase this "abnormalization" of the experience of women.

Several attempts have been made to explain the differential prevalence of depression, anxiety, alcoholism, and conduct disorders in men and women. Truly, differences in brain structure and function must be involved, the weight and relative volume of certain structures, and the different activities and effects of neurotransmitters and hormones must have an effect on the manifestation of lesions to the central nervous system; however, what these differences mean in terms of differential psychopathology is still, mostly, speculative.

It is tempting, of course, to consider that reproductive events, gonadal hormones and their relationship to the acute stress response, variations in cortisol-releasing hormone activity or serotonin transporter mRNA expression and epigenetic influences on glucocorticoid receptors can explain why women get depressed more often, or why they attempt suicide with more frequency. This reductionist approach prevents us from looking at other issues, which are probably more important: the weight of gender disparities as a cause of unspecified emotional distress in women (according to Burin [2]) and eventually as the root cause of the excess of depressive and anxious symptoms.

Gender identity and roles are constructed in the context of society, they are relational, the woman building her gender roles vis-à-vis those of men, and they have to do with power, resources, and opportunities. Gender is a powerful engine for stratification: it determines the distribution of wealth, power, and risks, including risks concerning mental health [3].

Consider exposure to violence. Women have a higher chance of being hurt by someone in their household than men. Many women have grown up in environments where it was not safe to go to the toilet. Almost a quarter of women in some countries initiate their sexual lives in the context of violence [4]. This disproportionate exposure of women to violence has to do with multiple factors, as recognized in the ecological model proposed by Heise [5]. However, understanding that the man's prerogative to control his woman is basic to integrating how educational level or unemployment interact with alcohol use and lack of implementation of the law to result in a woman—and not a man—being beaten up.

At the same time, we know that a sizable portion of the excess depression of women is linked to violence, particularly chronic physical and psychological violence. The force behind the disparity in exposure to violence is, clearly, gender relations of power. Looking at gender disparities in a violent context allows us to understand some of the excess depression in women.

Gender relations of power, then, must be considered a social determinant of health. Sex and gender, nature, and society interact in several ways to determine who is ill or well, who is treated or not, who is exposed to vulnerable or ill-health or not and whose health needs are acknowledged or dismissed. The Knowledge Network on Women, Gender Equity and Health of the WHO Commission for Social Determinants concluded that only focusing on economic inequalities does not give a full picture of the social gradient of health and may distort our understanding of how inequality works and who actually bears much of its burden [3].

This book, under the editorial leadership of Dr. Margarita Sáenz-Herrero, should provide us, the providers of mental health care to women, with a useful tool to understand the complex relationships of sex and gender, clarifying certain aspects and, hopefully, raising more questions for future research.

Lima, Peru Marta B. Rondon

References

1. Comesaña Santalices GM. Mujer, psicopatología y derechos humanos. Espacio Abierto, vol. 9 (1), enero-marzo. 2000. pp. 99–130.
2. Burin M. El malestar de las mujeres. La tranquilidad recetada. Buenos Aires Paidos. 1991. p. 35.

3. Sen G, Ostlin P. Unequal, unfair, ineffective and inefficient gender inequity in health: why it exists and how we can change it. Submitted September 2007 on behalf of the Women and Gender equity Knowledge Network to the WHO Commission on Social Determinants of Health.
4. Ellsberg M, Jansen HA, Heise L, Watts CH, Garcia-Moreno C. WHO Multi-country Study on Women's Health and Domestic Violence against Women Study Team. Intimate partner violence and women's physical and mental health in the WHO multi-country study on women's health and domestic violence: an observational study. Lancet. 2008;371:1165–72.
5. Heise LL. Violence against women. An integrated, ecological framework. Violence Against Women. 1998;4(3):262–90.

Preface

Many books about psychopathology have been written, some by psychiatry and psychology professionals with mainly descriptive perspectives and some of them from the psychoanalytic point of view. However, the main aim of this book is to introduce the gender paradigm perspective in a narrative format to understand symptoms in a different way from that in which they are usually presented in psychopathology.

Most doctors, psychiatrists, and psychologists still study descriptive psychopathology by following Jaspers' model and completely fail to display or introduce the gender dimension into the construction of symptoms. Without doubt, this is the core fact that distinguishes human beings at birth. The first thing asked when a baby is born, and even beforehand, is whether it is a boy or a girl. Despite biological diversity and the existence of Turner syndrome (X0), Klinefelter syndrome (XXY), hermaphroditism, and pseudohermaphroditism, a binary model is usually presented and where gender is one of the most difficult taboos to break in our culture. Gender commences at birth; it is learned, it is interpreted, with values in our families, social contexts, and cultures. It is necessary to broaden the area in which psychopathology is built. As in science, it is necessary to include gender in research; not to do so is bad science. In its 2001 report *Exploring the Biological Contributions to Human Health: Does Sex Matter?*, the Institute of Medicine called on biomedical researchers to step up their investigations of sex and gender as critical variables affecting health. Wizeman et al. (2001) proposed that increased understanding of the roles of gender and sex at every level of existence, from the sociological level down to the molecular level in health and disease, could advance preventive, diagnostic, and therapeutic health care practices. Gender (subsuming masculinity and femininity) seems to possess its own significance in the study of health and disease. In fact, several studies suggest that individual differences in the degree of masculine and feminine gender characteristics assessed in early adulthood were significantly related to morbidity, mortality, and health behaviors. For instance, a large longitudinal study demonstrated that greater levels of masculine gender characteristics assessed in early adulthood were significantly related to increased mortality over the next several decades, even after adjusting for unhealthy lifestyle habits (e.g., smoking, obesity, risk-taking). Importantly, this finding held true for both sexes; female and male participants who manifested higher levels of masculine gender characteristics than did their same-sex peers were also more likely to die at any given age. In the Terman study (2000), *Is Masculinity Hazardous to Your Health?*, mortality rates were highest for the most masculine men and lowest for the most feminine women.

An updated history of gender needs to be included in the history of psychiatry for psychiatrists and psychologists. When dynamics change, symptoms change through history. A discourse should be created, not only for scholars, for historians, anthropologists, and sociologists, but for public mental health overall, including gender in psychopathology. The first question to ask ourselves in the construction of our reality is basically how we know what we think we know, to open fissures in the discourse to include what is hidden. Public space should be a space for negotiation for a changing world and changing symptoms.

Very recently, in November 2013, Germany started to allow indeterminate gender to be recorded at birth. Parents are now allowed to leave the gender blank on birth certificates, creating a new category of indeterminate sex. Germany has become Europe's first country to allow babies with characteristics of both sexes to be registered as neither male nor female.

The problem with psychopathology is that it is built using the masculine model as a benchmark. What has shaped us as human beings and what we are nowadays are dependent on the possibility of creating fractures or breaches in the orthodox medical discourse in which scientific vocabulary is masculine. In the words of the Spanish philosopher, Amelia Valcárcel, the problem is power. We do not have the power to solve the problem.

Sex and gender differences as they relate to the causes and expression of medical conditions are established for a number of diseases, including selected mental disorders. Revisions to DSM-5 included reviewing potential differences between men and women in the expression of mental illness. In terms of nomenclature, sex differences are variations attributable to an individual's reproductive organs and XX or XY chromosomal complement. Gender differences are variations that result from biological sex as well as an individual self-representation that includes the psychological, behavioral, and social consequences of one's perceived gender. However, some differences are based on only biological sex, as pointed out in DSM-5.

To return to the definition of gender as the term that subsumes masculinity and femininity (male versus female) would clear the confusion and could also have implications for the study of health and disease. Gender, in this sense, is related to sex, instead of to masculinity and femininity with regard to behavior and psychology, which tends to be associated with men and women respectively. However, it is important to note that both men and women differ widely in the degree to which they manifest gender characteristics that are typically viewed as either masculine (e.g., aggressive, stoic) or feminine (e.g., nurturing, expressive) as Ristvedt explained in *The Evolution of Gender* in *JAMA* in November 2013. Sex and gender are associated, but they are not the same. Each variable is worthy of study in its own right. Gender is a continuous and not a categorical variable in the investigation of various health outcomes. Studies of relationships between gender characteristics and health outcomes could lead to insights into mechanisms that underlie broader categorical differences between the sexes in terms of morbidity, mortality, and health behaviors.

Gender bias in research could be defined as a systematically erroneous gender-dependent approach related to social construct, which incorrectly regards women and men as similar/different. Most gender bias can be found in the context of discovery (development of hypotheses), but it has also been found in the context of justification (methodological process), which must be improved. In fact, one of the main effects of gender bias in research is the partial or incorrect knowledge contained in the results, which are systematically different from the real values. This is a serious mistake in scientific research. The problem is not only with gender and different role gender, but masculine gender is still considered superior than female gender nowadays.

There is inequality in the access to certain jobs; inequality in power, the glass ceiling, unequal access to healthcare; all this is a reality in our society nowadays. Moreover, in the journal *Nature*, published in March 2013 "*Science Remains Institutionally Sexist*." Despite some progress, women scientists are still paid less, promoted less, win fewer grants, and are more likely to leave research than similarly qualified men. The reasons range from overt and covert discrimination to the unavoidable coincidence of the productive and reproductive years. In this special issue, *Nature* takes a hard look at the gender gap and at what is being done to close it. A survey of the data reveals where progress has been made and where inequalities still lie, from salary to tenure. A news feature reveals a particular dearth of women in some commercial spheres, such as on the scientific advisory boards of biotechnology firms, and an article by historian Patricia Fara traces the wearying stereotypes perpetuated by the biographers of women scientists. This special section of *Nature* finds that there is still much to do to achieve gender equality in science. Science remains institutionally sexist. Abundant research has demonstrated gender bias in many demographic groups, but has yet to investigate experimentally whether science faculties exhibit a bias against female students that could contribute to the gender disparity in academic science. In a randomized double-blind study ($n = 127$) published in 2012 by Moss-Racussin, science faculties from research-intensive universities rated the application materials of a student—who was randomly assigned either a male or female name—for a laboratory manager position. Faculty participants rated the male applicant as significantly more competent and hireable than the (identical) female applicant. These participants also selected a higher starting salary and offered more career mentoring to the male applicant. The gender of the faculty participants did not affect responses, such that female and male faculties were equally likely to exhibit bias against the female student. Mediation analyses indicated that the female student was less likely to be hired because she was viewed as less competent. They also assessed faculty participants' pre-existing subtle bias against women using a standard instrument and found that pre-existing subtle bias against women played a moderating role, such that it was associated with less support for the female student, but was unrelated to reactions to the male student. These results suggest that interventions addressing faculty gender bias might advance the goal of increasing the participation of women in science.

Psychiatry concerns meanings as much as physiological facts. Central to psychiatry is the aim of understanding individuals as much as explaining diseases, but understanding meaning is a different kind of intelligibility from framing causal and etiological reasons. It includes psychosocial, cultural, and historical aspects too.

Karl Jaspers in the *Phenomenological Approach in Psychopathology* portrays the meaningful connections between life history and psychosis. The culmination of this approach came when he was commissioned by the publisher, Springer, for a textbook on psychopathology. This resulted in *General Psychopathology* (*Allgemeine Psychopathologie*), which appeared in its first edition in 1913. At a time when psychiatry was dominated by the brain mythologists, Jaspers' major aim was to bring psychiatry back within the domain of the human sciences. Descriptive psychopathology is based on Jasper's view and clinical psychiatry is still based on this text.

Professor Berrios always states that every generation of psychiatrists should participate in the construction of a psychopathology because it influences historical, cultural, and social aspects in every part of the world. In a biopsychosocial model for mental health problems we always forget the social part that would be included. On the other hand, the paradigm of gender has been omitted along with the history of psychiatry. This book is an attempt to include gender in the way in which psychopathology is expressed by the human being.

The term "feminism" defined in the Oxford Dictionary is the advocacy of women's rights on the grounds of the equality of the sexes. Etymologically (http://www.etymonline.com), feminism comes from the French (1893). Alexandre Dumas (son of the famous writer, Alexandre Dumas) used the word to name the men who defended women rights. At the end of the nineteenth century and the early 20th, suffragettes fought for the right to vote and to possess equal rights to men in public life. However, in the origins of feminism, it was first used in 1871 by Ferdinand Valére Faneau de La Cour in *Du Feminisme et de l'Infantilisme chez les Tuberculeux* to put a name to the feminine appearance of men affected by tuberculosis. He stated that some men with tuberculosis have breasts, changes of voice, and their attitudes and movements resemble those of women. So, from the very beginning, the term feminism was used for men. It seems questionable nowadays that in the Pantheon of Paris, which contains the tombs of famous French citizens like Voltaire and Victor Hugo, there are only two women, Sophie Berthelot ("*Cette distinction lui a été attribuée en hommage à sa vertu conjugale, étant morte à quelques heures de son mari*") and Madame Curie, and this is in 2013. Moreover, to speak about human rights in the French language *droits de l'homme* is used.

In the UK, it was not until the emergence of the suffragette movement in the late nineteenth century that there was significant political change. A "second wave" of feminism arose in the 1960s, with an emphasis on unity and sisterhood (http://oxforddictionaries.com/us/definition/english/feminism?q=feminism).

Gender is not a feminist concept. The first person who used this word was Dr. John Money, a sexuality researcher and pediatrics teacher from John Hopkins

University to distinguish that intersexual sex was another way of presenting sexuality in human beings.

Gender anthropology constituted an important part of critical reflection and also contains questions about the universal and particulars of human cultures, and studies of how androcentric prejudices and ethnocentric structure were a way of viewing the world. It implied a revision of theoretical models and its consequences.

The distinction between sex and gender, as sexual identity, and the social and cultural construction of sexual identity, provoked an epistemological change in the conception of female identity. The consequences of these concepts were very significant in addition to the philosophical contribution made by Simone de Beauvoir and the anthropological contribution of Margaret Mead.

However, gender and sex have usually been used as synonymous concepts in the medical literature. In fact, there are no studies in which gender is the main perspective in viewing how psychopathology is differently expressed in relation to it in social studies and the humanities. Gender studies have been included as a growing field by including gender as a main object of study, doctoral thesis, articles, books, university studies, and it is still a controversial area. Medical studies are still in the Paleolithic Age from a gender perspective and this is real.

It is time to demand an equality that sustains biological differences in human beings, especially in women. This book has been divided into five parts. The first part and introduction of this book is written by Professor Berrios, who is a referee in epistemology of psychiatry. The second part includes general aspects with social, neurobiological, and psychological aspects of sex and gender differences. The third part, on general psychopathology, includes an extensive section on the psychopathology of trauma, corporality, somatomorphic, and eating disorders because they are a significant part of psychopathology in women, including anthropological and social perspectives that change the vision we usually have. The fourth part includes psychopathology related to hormonal aspects, including physiological and mood changes in hormonal cycles that are not pathological at all. Reproductive life cycle events, including estrogen variations, also contribute to gender differences in risk and expression of illness. The fifth part is a gender perspective of the main psychiatric disorders and pharmacological aspects of psychiatric treatment. In this last part, as happens in the medical literature, sex and gender are sometimes used in the same way. This is a reality that we cannot change. But we want to highlight it. The present book is a review that we hope will be significant for psychiatrists and psychologists. We cannot change the horizon, but we can change the perspective. This is our purpose.

Vitoria, Spain Margarita Sáenz-Herrero

Contents

Part IV Gender in Psychiatric Disorders

List of Contributors

Estibaliz Sáez de Adana Department of Psychiatry, Alava University Hospital, Vitoria, Spain

Kristina Jausoro Alzola Department of Psychiatry, Alava University Hospital, Vitoria, Spain

Batirtze Artaraz Mental Health Outpatients Services, Osakidetza, Vizcaya, Basque Country, Spain

Leonardo Delarze-Carrillo Servicio de Psiquiatría de Chiloé, University of Chile, Chile

Maria Dolores Avia Psychology Faculty, Complutense University, Madrid, Spain

Belén Sanz-Aránguez Ávila University Hospital Puerta de Hierro Majadahonda, Madrid, Spain

Sonia Ruiz de Azua Department of Psychiatry, Alava University Hospital, Vitoria, Spain

University of the Basque Country UPV/EHU, Leioa, Spain

CIBERSAM, Madrid, Spain

Sara Barbeito Department of Psychiatry, Alava University Hospital, Vitoria, Spain

CIBERSAM, Madrid, Spain

Ana Cano Department of Psychiatry, Alava University Hospital, Vitoria, Spain

Leire Celaya Mental Health Outpatients Services, Osakidetza, Alava, Basque Country, Spain

Paz de Corral University of the Basque Country, Leioa, Bizkaia, Spain

Eva Garnica de Cos Zamudio Hospital, Vizaya, Spain

Marta Crego-Meda Cruces University Hospital, Bilbao, Spain

María del Río Diéguez Autónoma University of Madrid, Madrid, Spain

Cristina Díez-Alegría Clinical Hospital San Carlos, Complutense University of Madrid, Madrid, Spain

Enrique Echeburúa University of the Basque Country, Leioa, Bizkaia, Spain

CIBERSAM, Madrid, Spain

Ane Eizaguirre Department of Psychiatry, Alava University Hospital, Vitoria, Spain

Miryam Fernández Department of Psychiatry, Alava University Hospital, Vitoria, Spain

Isidro Fernández-Pérez Cruces University Hospital, Bilbao, Spain

Aranzazu Fernandez-Rivas Department of Neuroscience, University of the Basque Country UPV/EHU, Leioa, Spain

Psychiatry Service, Basurto University Hospital, Bilbao, Spain

Aitor Francos Department of Psychiatry, Alava University Hospital, Vitoria, Spain

Jon Gaviña Department of Psychiatry, Alava University Hospital, Vitoria, Spain

Julia García-Albea University Clinic Hospital, Madrid, Spain

Pedro García-Parajuá Clinical University Hospital Puerta de Hierro, Madrid, Spain

Itxaso González-Ortega Department of Psychiatry, Alava University Hospital, Vitoria, Spain

CIBERSAM, Madrid, Spain

University of the Basque Country, Leioa, Bizkaia, Spain

Ana González-Pinto University of the Basque Country UPV/EHU, Leioa, Spain

Department of Psychiatry, Alava University Hospital, Vitoria, Spain

CIBERSAM, Madrid, Spain

Miguel Angel González-Torres Department of Neuroscience, University of the Basque Country UPV/EHU, Leioa, Spain

Psychiatry Service, Basurto University Hospital, Bilbao, Spain

Maria Haarmans Clinical Psychology, Institute of Psychology, Health and Society, Liverpool, UK

University of Liverpool, Liverpool, UK

Karim Haidar Department of Psychiatry, Alava University Hospital, Vitoria, Spain

Inmaculada Hurtado CEU Cardenal Herrera University, Alicante, Spain

Izargi Lacunza Department of Psychiatry, Alava University Hospital, Vitoria, Spain

Irantzu Lago Department of Psychiatry, Alava University Hospital, Vitoria, Spain

Purificación López University of the Basque Country UPV/EHU, Leioa, Spain

Department of Psychiatry, Alava University Hospital, Vitoria, Spain

Jose López-Gil Valdecilla University Hospital, Santander, Spain

Saioa López-Zurbano Department of Psychiatry, Alava University Hospital, Vitoria, Spain

Magdalena Marino Roberto Clemente Center, New York, NY, USA

Mónica Martinez-Cengotitabengoa Department of Psychiatry, Alava University Hospital, Vitoria, Spain

Iñaki Markez Basque Institute of Psychotherapy, Bilbao, Spain

Carmen Meneses Comillas Pontifical University, Madrid, Spain

Juan Miguel García Moncho La Fe University Hospital, Valencia, Spain

Olatz Napal Department of Psychiatry, Alava University Hospital, Vitoria, Spain

Paloma Navarro Department of Psychiatry, Marina Baixa Hospital, Alicante, Spain

Marta Navas Department of Psychiatry, Infanta Leonor Hospital, Madrid, Spain

Emma Noval-Aldaco Department of Psychiatry, Valdecilla University Hospital, Santander, Spain

Nuria Nuñez Department of Psychiatry, Alava University Hospital, Vitoria, Spain

Beatriz Payá-González Department of Psychiatry, Valdecilla University Hospital, Santander, Spain

Patricia Pérez Department of Psychiatry, Alava University Hospital, Vitoria, Spain

Rocío Polo-López University of the Basque Country, Leioa, Bizkaia, Spain

Beatriz Rodriguez-Paz Lucus Augusti University Hospital, Lugo, Spain

Agueda Rojo-Pantoja Department of Psychiatry, University Hospital Complex, Vigo, Spain

María Ruiz-Torres Department of Psychiatry, Valdecilla University Hospital, Santander, Spain

Margarita Sáenz-Herrero University of the Basque Country UPV/EHU, Leioa, Spain

Department of Psychiatry, Alava University Hospital, Vitoria, Spain

Mª Luisa Sánchez-Bernardos Complutense University in Madrid, Madrid, Spain

Miriam Santamaria Department of Psychiatry, Alava University Hospital, Vitoria, Spain

Rafael Segarra-Echebarria University of the Basque Country UPV/EHU, Leioa, Spain

Psychiatrist Cruces University Hospital, Bilbao, Spain

Jaime del Corral Serrano Clínica Nuestra Señora de la Paz, Madrid, Spain

Josep Toro-Tralleras University of Barcelona, Barcelona, Spain

Anibal Arrillaga Trueba Cruces University Hospital, Bilbao, Spain

Amaia Ugarte Department of Psychiatry, Alava University Hospital, Vitoria, Spain

Ana Villamor Department of Psychiatry, Alava University Hospital, Vitoria, Spain

Iñaki Zorrilla Department of Psychiatry, Alava University Hospital, Vitoria, Spain

Eider Zuaitz Mental Health Outpatients Services, Osakidetza, Guipuzcoa, Basque Country, Spain

Marta Zubia Department of Psychiatry, Alava University Hospital, Vitoria, Spain

Part I

General Aspects

1 Women's Mental Health Around the World: Education, Poverty, Discrimination and Violence, and Political Aspects

Kristina Jausoro Alzola and Magdalena Marino

Abstract

In this chapter, we will discuss the specific challenges that women face in the healthcare system, including the lack of access that much of the world's female population suffers. We will defend a change of approach to women's health issues whenever they need to use the health system.

To this end, we will describe some of the gender inequalities that arise from family microsystems as well as from the social and political macrostructures of power and world organization that are some of the causes of female pathological conditions. We refer here to some that particularly affect women: gender violence, poverty, migration, human trafficking, and violence used against women during armed conflicts. To conclude, we talk about lack of justice.

After analyzing these aspects, we suggest some recommendations for mental health professionals with regard to possible lines of work in the healthcare system, with the objective of making a change possible, a change based on the empowerment of women, considering health professionals as active agents and enablers of that empowerment.

1.1 Introduction

"All symptom is, in essence, a precipitate of meanings related to different dimensions of human life: childhood history, psychic suffering, intersubjective conflicts (couple or family), social failure, situations of helplessness, conceptual breaks with reality, and are

K. Jausoro Alzola
Department of Psychiatry, Alava University Hospital, Vitoria-Gasteiz, Spain
e-mail: kristina.jausoroalzola@osakidetza.net

M. Marino (✉)
Roberto Clemente Center, New York, NY, USA
e-mail: magdalena.marino-campos@nychcc.org

M. Sáenz-Herrero (ed.), *Psychopathology in Women*,
DOI 10.1007/978-3-319-05870-2_1

presented as manifestations of a malaise that cannot be reduced to an absolute determinism, whether biological, psychic or cultural. Epidemiological studies reveal a female, general and mental, excess morbidity in adulthood, which highlights the need to reflect on this situation" [1].

There is no society or community in the world where women are treated as equals to men, with inevitable consequences for their health. Thus, "women's mental health can only be understood if their life's context is taken into consideration; biological, sociocultural and the person" [2].

The World Federation of Mental Health announced in 1996 that often psychological stress in women has social origins; discrimination against women in employment, education, food distribution, health access, and the resources for economic development render them vulnerable to physical and sexual violence, psychiatric disorders, and psychological stress.

According to the 2009 World Health Organization (WHO) report "Women and Health," women and men face many similar health problems; nevertheless, the differences are so great that women's health requires special attention. Taking into account the same report it is fair to say that some disorders affect men and women to the same extent, but only women face more difficulties obtaining the healthcare assistance that they need. Gender inequalities in education, freedom, or income, for example, limit girls and women when it comes to protecting their own health.

Health problems faced by women share common features worldwide, but many great differences are also observed, determined by various living conditions. Girls and women's health is influenced by social and economic factors, such as access to education, family health, and place of residency. These differences are established not only in developing countries, but also in developed ones.

The differential prevalence of psychological disorders has led to the investigation of more accurate differential diagnoses that take into consideration the importance of culture in the construction of subjectivity. Defending the need to work with a differential diagnosis does not imply establishing differences and defending unequal illnesses, but presupposes taking into consideration living conditions and different risk factors affecting men and women. We need to develop approaches that consider a range of discriminations suffered by women, and these approaches must include the effect of poverty, lack of cultural resources, violence, and social devaluation [3].

To achieve this approach work is needed to shed the gender bias underlying theoretical models and healthcare practice. The gender bias, as pointed out by Carmen Valls-Llobet [4]:

- Extrapolates to the general population (meaning women) research results obtained from the male population. Assuming that risk factors and health protection are the same for everyone leads us to suppressing the gender differential morbidity and mortality.
- The belief that men and women get ill in different ways. The weight of this belief is so great that many "women's problems" are sent from primary care or women's health centers, limiting women's health to reproductive health. Other

symptoms are usually ignored, and after repeated demands for medical attention, analgesics or anxiolytics are prescribed; as a result, the demand is psychologized and medicalized.

- The clinical approach, especially biomedical and pharmacological, is derived from framing the claim as pathology.

In this context, "the increased use of psychotropic drugs for women can be a source of self-regulation of the exogenous elements in order to reduce discomfort" [5].

It is true that during the last few decades the health sciences have evolved, allowing some of the problems of women to be visualized, but much work remains. To contribute to breaking down gender bias, Professor Valls-Llobet [4] puts forward five proposals.

1. Democratization of knowledge production. Health research should consider experimental subjects in both men and women.
2. Research designs, in addition to the biological differences between sexes, must also consider gender, and the positions and social roles that each plays.
3. To achieve a better diagnosis, family life and work conditions should be taken into consideration.
4. Sex is a demographic control variable and gender should be considered a relational analytical variable.
5. Innovative designs should be implemented to detect the attitudes of health workers during their clinical practice in order to detect any inequalities.

With the conviction of the universal right of all people to a public healthcare system that ensures their welfare, this system should work within all scopes incorporating the gender perspective transversely. This involves two main axes of action:

- Enhances the participation and role of women as active agents in the protection of her own health.
- The incorporation of interdisciplinary teams (physicians, psychologists, social workers, social educators) trained in addressing health issues from the perspective of gender. It would have to boost the collective empowerment of healthcare system workers, with the objective of introducing the gender perspective into their daily practice, training them and stripping them of the aforementioned gender bias.

Interdisciplinary work is not only essential in the field of health, but also the answer to many of the problems that arise in the field of women's health. Women's health should be addressed from the social health domain where different institutions (health, justice, social services, education, employment, etc.) are involved.

1.1.1 The Social Health Approach

The traditional structure of health and social services is not well suited to the mixed nature of women's needs. Between the scopes of the health and social services, zones of confluence are particularly confusing and present coordination difficulties because they are dependent on various government agencies. These difficulties may have a negative impact on people's quality of life.

There are elements that are considered fundamental and defining in terms of the social health approach:

- It is a response to complex needs that require mixed interventions, social and health, simultaneously or sequentially, but always complementary.
- It is has the objective of guaranteeing the continuity of care, avoiding mismatches, gaps or waiting times between the different services.
- It is ruled by the interdisciplinary principle.
- It is based on an integral interventional approach focusing on the person and oriented toward guaranteeing the maximum level of quality of life and autonomy.

The principal objective of the social health approach is a response to complex needs. There are certain populations for whom, because of their nature and their healthcare and social characteristics, maximal coordination between the two fields is required. Among these population groups are the elderly dependent and people with chronic disease (major disabilities, mental disorders, etc.). To these groups we can add those whose diagnoses are conditioned to their gender role, highlighting the urgent need for coordination regarding gender violence.

There are many advantages of the social health approach; we emphasize the main ones below:

- It introduces greater facilities in the articulation of services of different kinds in the context of community action, therefore responding better to new social demands.
- Favors permanence in the community, articulating the means of preventing hospitalization or long-term residencies.
- Offers greater possibilities of developing an interdisciplinary approach that enriches professional practice.
- Facilitates access to the most vulnerable population groups that otherwise present significant barriers in access to care owing to social isolation.
- Favors a more rational use of resources and higher levels of efficiency and effectiveness.
- Promotes continuity of care.
- Favors reduction of dysfunction at different levels and in different fields of care.

If we consider that women's health is conditioned from childhood by the gender roles imposed, the treatment approach must come from within the scope of social health and with incorporation of several disciplines into the two work teams of primary and specialized care.

1.2 Gender Violence

1.2.1 Violence Against Women as a Public Health Problem

The declaration of violence against women as a social problem has been accompanied by the recognition by the health sector of violence against women as a public health problem.

In 1996, the World Health Organization (WHO) declared gender-based violence an international priority for health services, owing to its grave consequences on health, its magnitude, and the significant economic impact involved. That same year, the WHO carried out several actions that paved the way for the recognition of this problem, among them resolution WHA 49.2513 of the 49th World Health Assembly.

The WHO's commitment to addressing the problem of violence against women was reinforced in 1998 with the declaration of this matter as a public health priority through the publication of the document "Violence against women. A priority health issue" [6], and with the development of the "World Report about Violence and Health" [7].

In addition, the WHO urged its Member States to assess the problem and take measures to prevent and solve it.

1.2.2 Classification of Gender-Based Violence

In most of the literature on the subject, there is agreement that violence against women takes three main forms: physical, psychological, and sexual violence [8].

However, and although this is the most common differentiation, based on the proposal of the "Expert Report on Combatting Violence Against Women" of the Council of Europe (1997) [9], there are frequently other forms of violence, giving rise to description of the following types:

- Physical violence: all action carried out voluntarily that causes or may cause damage and personal injury to women. It includes the use of physical force or objects to threaten their physical integrity.
- Sexual violence: any threat to the sexual freedom of women in which they are obliged to bear or carry out acts of a sexual nature. It includes any act or sexual expression carried out against their will that violates their physical or emotional integrity, such as jokes, rude expressions, unpleasant comments, obscene phone calls, undesirable sexual proposals, forcing them to watch pornography, any non-consensual act or sexual intercourse (harassment, rape, incest), any

relationship or sexual act deemed by women to be humiliating or painful, or the obligation to prostitute themselves.

- Psychological violence: any action, generally of a verbal or financial nature, that causes or may cause psychological damage in women. It includes the use of mechanisms of control and communication that threaten women's psychological integrity, well-being, self-esteem or consideration, in both public and private, in front of other people, such as: to denigrate them; to despise what they do; to make them feel guilty; to treat them as if they were slaves; to make unpleasant comments about their physique; to humiliate them in public or in private; to give them a bad reputation, to force them to be accountable for their relationships and contact with other people; to force them to break off with friends; to prohibit them from talking to people of the opposite sex; to show jealousy of friendships; to limit them in their living space or show it disrespect; to make jokes: sexist jokes of denigrating nature, to undervalue their contributions or action; insults made in public or in private; threats and intimidation; emotional blackmail; threats of suicide if the couple expressed their desire to separate, etc.
- Economic violence: inequality of access to common resources. It includes denying or controlling women's access to shared sources of money, generating economic dependency, impeding their access to employment, education or health, denying their rights of property, etc.
- Structural violence: intangible and invisible barriers that impede women's access to basic rights. It includes the denial of information on their fundamental rights, the relationships of power in school or at work, or discriminatory legislation in all social spheres.
- Spiritual violence: the destruction of women's cultural or religious beliefs through punishment, ridicule, or the imposition of a system of beliefs that is alien to their own. It includes the submission and invisibility of women's cultural or religious beliefs or analyzing them from an ethnocentric perspective.

1.2.3 International Recommendations for the Prevention of Gender-Based Violence

> "Violence against women is perhaps the most shameful human rights violation. It knows no geographical or cultural limits, or economic position. As long as it continues, we cannot say that we have actually made progress towards equality, development and peace." Kofi Annan, Secretary-General of the United Nations

The Declaration on the Elimination of Violence Against Women, adopted by the General Assembly of the United Nations in 1993, shows international understanding and recognition that violence against women is a violation of human rights and a form of discrimination against women.

The human rights norms that emerge from the Convention on the Elimination of all Forms of Discrimination against Women, subsequently ratified by the World Conference on Human Rights of the United Nations (UN) of 1993 and other international instruments, not only extend the validity of areas that were previously not considered the subjects of rights, but also establish differences between formal equality and substantive equality. It is recognized as well that so-called universal human rights—even though they guarantee in formal terms the legal equality of men and women—were defined according to the lives and experiences of men and do not take into account the needs and everyday existence of women.

Therefore, the following are recommended:

- Expanding democracy based on the effective participation of citizens and the full observance of human rights.
- Developing a National Plan with the State guarantees compliance with the principle of gender equity.
- Creating government initiatives to improve the social status of women.
- Promoting the production of up-to-date statistical information permitting visualization of the gaps and iniquities of gender at all levels.
- To penalize the media and professionals involved in cases that through promotional campaigns use women as objects or marginalize women's social, intellectual, racial or economic status.

The Platform for Action document adopted at the Fourth World Conference on women, held in Beijing in 1995, defines violence against women as one of the 12 critical areas of concern that should be given particular emphasis by Governments, the international community, and civil society.

At its 42nd session, in 1998, the Commission on the Social and Legal Status of Women of the United Nations proposed new measures and initiatives that should be applied by the Member States and by the international community in order to put an end to violence against women, including the incorporation of a gender perspective in all policies and relevant programs. Among the conclusions agreed upon during the session, there are measures to provide support to the work of nongovernmental organizations: to combat all forms of trafficking in women and girls, to promote and protect the rights of migrant workers, in particular women and children, and girls, and promoting the coordinated activities of research on violence against women.

In relation to violence against women in the domestic sphere, the WHO multi-country study results on the health of women and domestic violence against women underscore the need to take urgent measures on a wide variety of instances, ranging from local health authorities and community leaders to national governments and international agencies [10].

As the study graphically shows, violence against women is a widespread and deeply rooted practice that has serious consequences for the health and well-being of women. Its persistence is morally unacceptable; the costs are immeasurable for individuals, for healthcare systems, and for society in general. However, until relatively recently, no other relevant public health problem had been so widely neglected and misunderstood.

The wide differences in the prevalence and patterns of violence found between one country and another, and mostly between one context and another within the various countries examined, suggest that there is nothing "natural" or inevitable about this problem. Attitudes can and must change, the conditions of women can and must be improved, and men and women can and must convince themselves that violence cannot be accepted in human relationships.

The following recommendations have been extracted, primarily from the conclusions of the study, although they are also based on studies and lessons learned from experiences in numerous countries. Specifically, the recommendations corroborate the conclusions and recommendations presented in the WHO's World Report on Violence and Health [11]. Recommendations are grouped into the following categories:

- Strengthening the commitment and actions at the national level.
- Promoting primary prevention responses.
- Involving the education sector.
- Strengthening the health sector response.
- Supporting women living with violence.
- Sensitizing those who are part of the criminal justice systems.
- Supporting research and collaboration.

In order to address and prevent violence against women, it is necessary for many sectors (educative, legal, health, economic, etc.) to take action in many areas. However, it is important that the State takes the final responsibility for the security and well being of its citizens. In this sense, the national governments, in collaboration with nongovernmental organizations and international organizations, must give priority to this issue.

Following international recommendations, State is called upon to implement prevention programs of gender-based violence, to investigate such acts, and prosecute and punish perpetrators, as well as to ensure the female victim's rights to care and assistance.

Various strategies and different models of legislation have been established in different countries; some include educational measures and preventive actions, while others establish specific courts or police offices for the matter. In the best cases, prevention, education, and integrated services for victims (from health to legal assistance in the same agency) conform to a comprehensive approach to the elimination of gender-based violence. Thus, not all approaches define violence against women in the same way, nor do they act against all of its manifestations.

1.2.4 Prevention and Response

Further assessment is required to determine the effectiveness of violence prevention measures [12]. Some of the interventions with more promising results are the promotion of education and work opportunities for women and girls, the improvement of their self-esteem and their negotiating skills, and the reduction of the inequalities of gender in communities.

Other efforts that proved to be effective are: intervening with adolescents to reduce violence in their relationships; supporting programs for children who have witnessed acts of violence between partners; massive public education campaigns; and adopting measures of collaboration with men and boys to challenge attitudes to gender inequities and the acceptability of violence.

The defense of victims, greater awareness among health workers about violence, and a broader knowledge of the resources available for battered women (such as legal assistance and/or accommodation and care of children or other dependants) can mitigate the consequences of violence.

1.3 Women Around the World in Situations of Social and Structural Violence: Poverty, Migration, and War

1.3.1 Defining Poverty and Its Gender Distribution

"Poverty is the worst form of violence" Mahatma Gandhi

"Overcoming poverty is not a task of charity, it is an act of justice" Nelson Mandela

The association between poverty and mental disorders appears to be strong and universal, occurring in all societies, irrespective of the levels of development of the country [13]. Traditionally, poverty has been defined in purely economic terms as the amount of income per day. In terms of income, women make up 70 % of the world's one million poorest people [14]. Women work two-thirds of the world's working hours, produce half of the world's food, but earn only 10 % of the world's income and own less than 1 % of the world's property [14]. On average, around the world, women earn half of what men earn [14]. Informal employment offers more employment for women than for men. While it can offer opportunities to earn money, the low pay and lack of social protection makes women vulnerable and open to exploitation. Added to unemployment, the lack of equal and fair opportunities for women to work has contributed to the feminization of poverty [15]. Thus, if these data are not indicative enough of the economic discrimination and structural violence against women, poverty means much more than income.

Poverty was defined in the UN's Human Development Report 1997 as denial of the opportunities and choices most basic to human life—the opportunity to lead a long, healthy, and creative life, and to enjoy a decent standard of living, freedom, dignity, self-esteem, and respect from others [16]. The lack of opportunities and choices for women and girls around the world because of gender is immeasurable. Of the world's 800 million illiterate people, more than two-thirds are women [16]. Fifty million of the 72 million of children out of school are girls [14]. Women's political presence in parliament around the world is only 19 % [14].

Poverty and its structural causes limit women's ability to be active and productive members of society, to realize their potential, and ultimately to be mentally as well as physically healthy [13]. The negative social and economic factors associated with poverty, furthermore, act as a barrier to health and mental health care services. Similarly, restrictions in women's ability to participate fully and actively in the community, to be part of the decision-making process on issues affecting one's life, or to have the opportunity to improve one's social and economic situation and status also adversely affect the mental health of women. Mental health professionals have the responsibility to acknowledge the challenges and external barriers that poverty—in its broadest definition—brings to women. Also, an approach focusing on strengths and resilience, instead of just psychopathological personality traits stigmatize and limit them even more.

The eradication of global poverty requires a strong change of the deep-seated structural causes of poverty that we cannot discuss here. However, we want to pay special attention to structural violence and discrimination against women, a solid compromise with the promotion of women's human rights, from the basic right of education, and the incorporation of gender equality and mainstreaming into all legislation to decrease gender-related poverty.

1.3.2 The Feminization of Migration

Owing to the globalization of the economy and its effect on the labor market, migration has risen to the point where it has almost doubled during the last 50 years. Traditionally, women migrated with men as dependants or as part of a family reunification process, but recently they are migrating as autonomous breadwinners. Some are highly skilled workers, but most are running away from poverty and other human rights violations. Women now constitute almost half of all international immigrants, i.e., 95 million [17].

Despite migration being a complex, multi-cause phenomenon, there is an agreement on suggesting as principal causes for this change in the gender of migration in the country of origin ("push" factors), such as gender-based violence, gender inequality, feminization of poverty, unemployment, human rights violations, war, and discrimination [18]. Even when economic causes are the main reason for moving, women often migrate to escape from abusive and patriarchal traditions that limit opportunity and freedom [17]. On the other side of the frontiers, the most common "pull" factors (anticipated benefits in the destination country) are the increasing demand for women in domestic positions and service and care-related jobs, the opportunity to receive higher wages, and family reunifications.

For many women, migration means a safer place, a new world of more equality, a relief from oppression and the discrimination that limits freedom, and an opportunity to develop their potential. For the country of origin and the receiving country, the contribution of women migrants can transform the quality of life. In the countries of origin, the economic contribution can palliate poverty, provide education and health care, and generally improve the quality of life of their families and even whole communities. Beyond the economic factors, the social change brought about the belief that the new and renovated ideas, values, knowledge, or the skills of women can contribute to promoting human rights and gender equality. In the receiving countries, they contribute their work and expertise, pay taxes, and support a life-style in developing countries that most take for granted, allowing, for example, other women to delegate childcare and responsibilities regarding the elderly to immigrant women for going out to work. However, migration also has its negative side.

Women migrants experience common and severe stressors that potentially affect the well-being of all migrants. While traveling, they are exposed to severe abuse, including kidnapping, extortion, physical violence, and trafficking. In the destination country, immigrants face language barriers, culture shocks, isolation, and loss of support systems, loss of socioeconomic status, unemployment or working under unsafe or unhealthy conditions, poverty, social exclusion, prejudice and discrimination, lack of knowledge of existing services, and barriers in accessing the healthcare system, and feelings of vulnerability owing to their legal status [19]. In addition to all these stressors that can affect (in different proportions) all migrants, women of undergo the unique experience of sexual and gender-based violence [20]. Because of their status as women and as foreigners (in addition to being of different race, ethnicity, class, or religion), female migrants face a disproportionate risk of abuse and violence at home, in the streets, or in the place of work [17].

The International Organization worldwide recognized a feminization of migration in 2000, and compromised to promote equal access to projects and services for immigrant women, even creating specific programs to address their specific needs [21]. However, despite this acknowledgement of the challenges and risks for immigrant women, both international and national regulations failed to adequately address their problems. The trafficking and exploitation of domestic workers, two kinds of modern enslavement that affect mostly females, testify to the lack of adequate opportunities for women to migrate safely and legally.

Even though migration can be a positive experience for millions, there are serious risks to female migrants that can compromise their physical and mental health, and even their survival. In the following, we will describe two phenomena relating to immigration that require the special attention of mental health professionals and, even more than ever, a culturally and gender-sensitive perspective: transnational motherhood and human trafficking.

1.3.3 Transnational Motherhood

The feminization of migration changes the structure, organization, and hierarchy of the family and has an impact on the life cycle of its members. As women are increasingly migrating alone to find work, this has reconfigured the shape of the immigrant family and transnationalized the meaning of motherhood [22]. Hondagneu-Sotelo and Avila [23] were the first to employ the term "transnational mother" to describe these women who have migrated to another country in order to become the family breadwinner, leaving their country, culture, family, and children behind. In describing the paradox of having to leave their children, they relate the experience as being simultaneously "here and there"; here as breadwinners and there as caregivers and emotional mothers. Transnational mothers are "in the process of actively, if not voluntarily building alternative constructions of motherhood" [23].

As we said, there are some advantages for the family and the community in the migration of one of its members, especially economic ones. However, the existing literature on transnational families finds that the migration of mothers is a traumatic event, with devastating consequences for these women, and inflicts substantial social and psychological negative changes on the family left behind [23].

Several studies find devastating psychological effects, such as anxiety, anger, somatic symptoms, depression, guilt, symptoms of post-traumatic stress disorder related to separation from children, and guilt, experienced by women with family fragmentation [22, 25, 26]. Miranda et al. [27] found that the odds of depression for Latina transnational mothers were 1.52 times greater than those of Latinas whose children were currently living with them. Further, the reunification phase is not as easy and dreamlike as it might seem. It affects the entire functioning of each person of the family in their environment. When reunification occurs in Latino immigrants, families are faced with difficult processes of adjustment that can include acculturation challenges, the addition of new family members, missing caretakers in the homeland, authority conflicts, depression, anxiety, and behavioral problems. In Suarez-Orozco et al. [28], mothers after reunification verbalized their struggle with asserting authority and frustration because their financial and emotional sacrifices were not fully appreciated by their children.

It is important to note that there are not only the frontiers, but also the social inequalities that create the ambiguous loss of separation and provoke emotional consequences for mothers and children. The current migration policies are creating "illegal persons," and there is an emotional consequence of that "illegality" [22]. An undocumented status creates huge vulnerability to oppression, discrimination, violence, and inequality in transnational mothers. Experiences of racism, discrimination, or exploitation affect them physically and mentally, and often negatively form and transform their identities [29]. Like many immigrants, these women have an internalized sense of powerlessness and not deservedness that again makes them an easy target for abuse and exploitation, perpetuating the vicious circle.

Even when they attempt to receive assistance, the limitation of services for undocumented persons aggravates the barriers that transnational mothers already face, and these limitations are extended to their children when they arrive here [26]. These challenges make it more necessary than ever to incorporate into clinical practice with these women a social justice framework that resists oppression by combating the effects of power differences and differential access to resources based on gender, race, class, and legal status [29].

Despite these challenges, transnational households continue to exist across space, and mothers and children may only connect across borders. These families need to develop their own norms for functioning, their own strategies in communicating, and particular emotional connections based on their cultural context [30]. When these experiences are meaningful for the family and all members in both countries participate, a sense of coherence and continuity is created that promotes the healthy development of its members [31]. To create these coherent narratives, it is therapeutically necessary to process the multiple traumas related to immigration, separation, violence, discrimination, or poverty that transnational mothers suffer.

However, the clinical work will not be completed according to any intrapsychic intervention. In clinical work with transnational mothers, the whole family and the psychological and virtual relationships among members need to be addressed and empowered [29]. It is imperative to work with alternative social constructions of normal families. There are two stories in transnational mother–children relationships. Mothers might describe a story of trauma and sacrifice for their family, and as a consequence might expect gratitude, while children might tell a story of abandonment, even neglect, and will present anger. Validating both experiences and promoting the listening and empathy between family members will establish the basis for a new relationship among members where narratives are linked. Assisting transnational mothers and their children to create a meaningful and coherent narrative at a distance that promotes the adaptation and growth as a family will decrease the damage that migration provokes under these conditions.

1.3.4 Human Trafficking

> "Trafficking demonstrates the weaknesses of global capitalism and the disparity caused by the economic rules of the countries most powerful; but mostly reveals normalization of human cruelty and cultural processes that have strengthened"
> Esclavas del poder, Lidia Cacho [32]

Human trafficking is defined as the recruitment and movement of persons by threat, force, coercion, or deception for the purposes of exploitation (sexual exploitation, forced labor or slavery) [33]. Because of its underground nature, statistics on the scale of the problem are unreliable, but the International Labour Organization (ILO) estimates that globally 2.5 million persons are currently in situations of exploitation as a result of trafficking, and that another 1.2 million are trafficked annually [34]. Human trafficking is a particularly abusive form of migration, and one of the most severe human rights violations in the world. Reports from around the world include descriptions of the extreme forms of physical, psychological, and sexual abuse perpetrated toward persons who are trafficked for exploitation in the sex industry and a multitude of labor settings, including construction, agriculture, and domestic servitude [35].

While trafficking affects both men and women, it is not a gender-neutral phenomenon. Up to 80 % of trafficked persons are women and girls [17]. Women are particularly vulnerable to trafficking owing to their social and economic position, as well their position in the migratory process. Poverty, unemployment, a high demand for (and low regulation of) cheap labor and services in female-designated sectors of work, discriminatory immigration laws, and a cultural context in which violence against women is tolerated, are the most important and well-recognized causes of women trafficking [15]. These causes have a common root: gender inequality and the lack of rights afforded to women. By failing to protect and promote women's civil, political, economic, and social rights, governments create situations in which trafficking arises. A real political response and compromise with the respect, protection, and promotion of women's human rights in all the arenas (social, economic, politic, educative, health) is the first step toward ensuring an end to trafficking in women.

While the solution to trafficking is being found, the United Nations requires governments to implement measures to promote the physical, physiological, and social recovery of human trafficking victims, including medical and psychological responses to the health needs of trafficked people [33]. To meet these international agreements, countries will have to provide psychological support services for trafficked persons. Yet, the physical and mental health consequences and potential public health implications of human trafficking have generally received little attention, and the mental health community is just beginning to respond to these persons' needs [35].

Human trafficking victims enter into a vicious circle of terror, violence, and cruelty that denies them their right to safety, dignity, freedom, equality, health care, work, and education, among others. Often, victims have already come from a history of gender-based violence, and are re-victimized. As a result of such exposure—and re-exposure—to trauma, the limited research on the mental health consequences of trafficking consistently reports high levels of symptoms indicative of anxiety (48–97.7 %), depression (54.9–100 %), and post-traumatic stress disorder (PTSD) (19.5–77 %) [35]. Comorbidity among these disorders is also common [36]. The literature describes a broad range of reactions related to trauma: fear, guilt, rage, sense of betrayal, distrust, helplessness, shock, suspicion, feeling lost, sense of apathy and resignation, extreme forms of submissiveness to authority, maladaptation in social situations, and the loss of personal autonomy [37]. The length of time spent being exploited and the level of violence and injuries sustained while being trafficked increase the risk of suffering anxiety, depression, and PTSD symptoms [35, 36, 38]. Also, a higher prevalence of PTSD was found among women who had been trafficked for sexual exploitation compared with women trafficked for labor exploitation [39].

When authorities encounter trafficked women, they are likely to be suffering physical pain and exhaustion, confusion, disorientation, amnesia, strong emotional reactions, and the inability to recall events or to communicate that may affect their ability to obtain assistance [40]. Even after being liberated from a trafficking experience, women and girls face huge stressors, including entering into a complicated legal system for obtaining assistance, possible participation in criminal proceedings, immigration and asylum procedures, the stigma associated with sex work, the return to families who may be unaware of their experience—or who are aware and reject them as a consequence— and not least, the same concerns about poverty and unemployment that caused them to leave their home in the first place [36]. Subsequently, the lack of social support and additional life stress may affect the severity of the symptoms.

The patterns of severe symptoms and the post-trafficking risks and challenges for victims indicate that treatment services should be available immediately [38]. However, some victims are quickly deported back to their country of origin, finding the same context of poverty and discrimination that they had left and where assistance is non-existent, or they are forced to participate in criminal investigations as pre-conditions to assistance. As a consequence of the abuse of power suffered and the intensity of the trauma, the engagement and creation of a therapeutic relationship may be a challenge. In the early period after trafficking, a sensitive approach is required, with the problems of memory, the lack of trust, and the fear of talking about their experience. It is essential to accord trafficking survivors a period of recovery and reflection before making decisions about their future and well-being (such as going back to their family or participating in criminal investigations).

Although multidisciplinary teams are usually important, they are crucial in this field. These interdisciplinary teams should involve law enforcement personnel and social agencies that provide legal, educational, vocational, economic, and other vital life resources. However, this collaboration should not liberate clinicians from a general awareness of immigration policies.

Mental health professionals working with trafficking survivors must have specific training in trauma, especially sexual and interpersonal trauma [37]. Most treatments to date have followed the direction of trauma treatments for victims of domestic violence, sexual assault, torture, and immigrants and refugees. In addition, clinicians need a culture-sensitive approach and the multicultural competence required to work with immigrants in order to provide these women with appropriate care.

We cannot forget that human trafficking is not only a personal experience, but also a communal and global matter that severely attacks social justice and human rights, and we as professionals and as human beings have a responsibility to combat it.

1.3.5 Women in Armed Conflicts

Since 1945, there have been an estimated 150 wars in the world [41]. Despite the new techniques of warfare, the sophistication and precision of weapons, and international conventions that forbid the use of civilians as targets, it is the noncombatants who die in greater number than soldiers. Children and women, being more vulnerable, are the first victims of these wars. Even when conflicts officially end, violence against women continues and often worsens [42].

Violence against women during wartime is recognized by international humanitarian organizations as a fundamental violation of human rights, a primary public concern, and a major impediment to peace making, reconstruction, and development of war-torn countries [42]. In 2000, the United Nations passed Resolution 1325 on women and peace and security. This historic resolution called for the equal participation and full involvement in all steps of conflict resolution and peace building, as well in the promotion and maintenance of peace and security. It also demanded that all parties to the conflict take special measures to protect women and girls from gender-based violence, particularly rape and other forms of sexual abuse, in situations of armed conflict [43]. This resolution sought to give a voice to the silenced women survivors and to include the perspective of women in the construction of peace, but sadly it had (and still has) a very limited impact.

Historically, sexual violence against women during war can be tracked from the eleventh century to the present day. For centuries, sexual violence against women has been barely prosecuted and often even considered "an unfortunate product of war" [44]. In Resolution 1325 it is still considered gender-based violence. In June 2008, the United Nations in Resolution 1820 denounced that "women and girls are particularly targeted by the use of sexual violence, including as a tactic of war to humiliate, dominate, instill fear in, disperse and/or forcibly relocate civilian members of a community or ethnic group" [45]. This means that in the context of a war, sexual violence is a deliberate (and effective) military weapon designed to tear apart individuals, families, and communities.

In 2009, the UN Security Council openly recognized, through the voices of Hillary Clinton and Ban Ki-moon, that violence against women had not diminished, but has even increased in some places, being used as a brutal weapon in armed conflicts with total impunity. Two new resolutions (S/RES/1888 and S/RES/1889) were approved, asking for the immediate cessation of all acts of sexual violence and reiterating the importance of women's participation in peace processes and promoting women's leadership respectively [46, 47]. These resolutions, along with the S/RES/1960 in 2010, repeat and strengthen the same petitions.

Recently, two new resolutions in *women and peace and security* were adopted. On 24 June 2013, the Council adopted Resolution 2106, which defined sexual violence as a crime against humanity and encouraged Member States to adopt national penal legislation to prosecute perpetrators [48]. On 18 October, S/RES/2122 supported the petition of women's leadership and requested from the UN more active involvement in protecting human rights, pursuing gender equality, and empowering women in areas of conflict [49]. The Secretary has reported some advances in this fight, but there is some distance to go before there is at least a gender-egalitarian respect for the human rights of women and girls.

> "If we do not have the capacity to prevent war, we have a collective responsibility to better understand and treat its psychiatry, medical, and social consequences."
> Michael Hollifield ([49], p. 1284)

Hagen [50] describes five characteristics that distinguish war-time sexual violence against women from other kinds of sexual violence during "peace time": (1) massive in scale; (2) approximately 90 % occur in the presence of other women to infuse fear, in the presence of other soldiers to promote solidarity, and in the presence of other community members to show power and total suppression; (3) extreme levels of brutality; (4) often includes slavery; and (5) serves ethnic cleansing purposes.

The consequences of these brutal attacks against women are felt on multiple levels. On the individual level, women who survive war rape suffer multiple and severe forms of physical and psychological trauma. From severe and permanent physical damage and disabilities, through AIDS, to post-traumatic stress disorder, depression, anxiety, a sense of helplessness, and a total destruction of self-identity and sense of belonging, the wounds of war rape in an individual are atrocious [44]. Adding to these wounds, and to the personal shame and humiliation that public, brutal, and mass rapes bring, many women suffer rejection by their own family and the community because of socio-cultural values regarding sexuality [42]. On a macro level, these women face a destroyed society that does not have the economic, political, sociocultural, and health care infrastructure to assist them, and they are forced to migrate into refugee camps where education, work, and recovery opportunities are limited. Displaced and removed from their community, they are condemned to a life of extreme poverty and complete dependence that places them at risk of further victimization [51].

As the consequences are felt in all dimensions of a person's life, interventions should also address the full impact in all areas. Refugees and war survivors in destroyed societies have multiple physical and psychiatric symptoms, cultural individualities, language barriers, and polytraumas that complicate the experience and diagnosis of illness from a traditional western perspective [50]. Biomedical models of trauma are too limited to attend to the reality of these survivors [41]. These complex realities need a holistic model that understands the peculiar experience of women in a society in war, and the women's voices should guide it.

In the continuing absence of that holistic model, some recommendations are appearing in the literature:

- Disempowerment, gender inequality, stigmatization of sexual violence, self-identity, and body objectification are some of the central themes to work on in the therapeutic space [51].
- There is a change from labeling these women victims to labeling them survivors, resilient women who are capable and should participate in their healing process. The resilience of women needs to be recognized and supported by mental health providers as a way of promoting their adequate access to their rights of health care and justice [41].
- There is also a change in the focus from psychopathological manifestations to resilience, protective factors, and methods of coping for the purposes of developing interventions and services [41].
- Physical and mental health services for war survivors need to be culture- and gender-sensitive.
- It is necessary to understand the social reality where the services are being offered, such as political instability, uncertainty about settlement, migration stressors involved, and the effect of collective trauma [51].
- It is important to include the protection and promotion of human rights, the search for social justice, and the empowerment (at a personal and social level) in work with female war survivors [41].
- Coordinated, multi-agency services are suggested [41].

In summary, mental health interventions with war survivors need to take into account the environment and ecological reality of the person and the community. They need to be complemented by individual and collective legal, social, and political actions designed to build or restore the empowerment of women and address all the types of social inequalities and discrimination that exist.

1.4 The Empowerment of Women

There are many definitions of the concept "empowerment," depending on the discipline that uses it: psychology, political science, education, law, etc., although this concept is not widely used in medicine, since it is related to the field of social sciences.

The concept of empowerment has become widely recognized in the last 20 years, women's studies and the development of gender having placed the term at the axis of discussion. However, even in this field there is no total consensus on its meaning, as it is used much like a substitute for integration, participation, identity or development, and loses its proper meaning.

Empowerment as a term was first introduced at the IV World Conference on Women in Beijing to refer to the increase in women's participation in the processes of decision-making and access to power [52]. Currently, however, this expression also takes into consideration another dimension: the awareness of the power that women possess individually and collectively that is concerned with the recovery of women's own dignity as people.

Empowerment is "the process of gaining control over an ideology and the resources which determine power" [53]. These resources may be human, intellectual, financial, physical and belong to each person. Any process of empowerment has as its objective to change and transform, whether for an individual or a collective goal. For Young in 1997, empowerment is "to assume control over their own lives, to set their own agendas, to organize themselves to help each other and raise demands to the State requesting support and societal change" [54].

Empowerment, a strategy especially promoted by and for the women's movement in developing countries, has become the central axis of the gender perspective and represents a strengthening of the social, economic and political positions of women, and we could add that it also involves the strengthening of their health.

Gender relations are basically subordinate power relationships where everything related to the female is of inferior value to the male. Thus, in order to obtain true development for women it is necessary to modify these relationships, their acquisition of power being the only way to redress the imbalance. Popularly, there is the belief that the empowerment of women represents the disempowerment of men. Yet, from a different point of view, Magdalena Leon argues that women's empowerment can also lead to the psychological and emotional empowerment of men, through which they might advance by removing the restrictive breastplate in which gender stereotypes have placed them [55].

Empowerment is a personal process, each woman has to empower herself, but society in all its dimensions should encourage a favorable arena and grant the possibilities for this process to unfold. As women empower themselves, they can actively participate in societal changes that will promote the human rights of women and other possibilities of empowerment for further generations. Numerous authors emphasize the two spheres of empowerment: the individual and the collective. Individual empowerment should be stronger in the cognitive processes, and in the context of personal control. This individual empowerment process must be integrated into collective empowerment in order to change oppressive and discriminatory socio-political structures in the hands of a dominant, inadequate power.

The public health system must become an enabling agent of empowerment. In the context of health services, it is necessary to program health promotion activities, allowing women to learn strategies for the control and care of their own health. To achieve this, it is necessary to create an environment that favors women's confidence in themselves, in their autonomy and self-esteem, and that promotes the ability of collective action for them to achieve personal change with a projection in public life. These health promotion activities must serve as a space for sharing personal and collective experiences and for acquiring personal and social skills to find alternatives in order to change the unfavorable circumstances as a result of the gender roles women hold.

References

1. Tubert S. Deseo y representación. Madrid: Editorial Síntesis; 2001
2. Psicopatología de la mujer. Eduardo Correa D y Enrique Jadresic M, Editores. Ediciones de la Sociedad de Neurología, Psiquiatría y Neurocirugía de Cile. Imprenta Salesianos S.A.; 2000.
3. Isabel Martínez Benlloch. Universidad de Valencia "Actualización de conceptos en perspectiva de género y salud". Cursos de formación de formadores en Perspectiva de Género en Salud.
4. Valls-Llobet C. Desigualdades de género en salud publica En AAVV: género y Salud. Madrid: Instituto de la Mujer; 2000, p. 16–2.
5. Burin M. El Malestar de las mujeres. La tranquilidad recetada. Paidós: Buenos Aires.
6. Salud familiar y reproductiva OPS, División de Salud y Desarrollo, OMS. Violencia contra la mujer. Un tema de salud prioritario. Washington: OMS/CPS; 1998. http://www.paho.org/Spanish/HDP/HDW/violencepriority/themesp.pdf
7. Organización Panamericana de la Salud (OPS). Informe Mundial sobre la Violencia y la Salud: Resumen. Publicado para la Organización Mundial de la Salud. Washington, DC: Author; 2003. http://www.paho.org/Spanish/AM/PUB/Violencia_2003.htm
8. Bosch E, Ferrer VA. La voz de las invisibles. Las víctimas de un mal amor que mata. Valencia: Cátedra. Colección Feminismos; 2002.
9. Council of Europe. Informe del Grupo de Especialistas para Combatir la Violencia contra las Mujeres. Estrasburgo: Mimeografiado; 1997.
10. OMS. Estudio a fondo sobre todas las formas de violencia contra la mujer. p. 119–9. http://www.observatorioviolencia.org/upload_images/File/DOC1164822961_N0641977.pdf

11. Informe mundial sobre la violencia y la salud: resumen. Washington, DC: Organización Panamericana de la Salud, Oficina Regional para las Américas de la Organización Mundial de la Salud; 2002.
12. World Health Organization (WHO) (2009). Violence against women. Descriptive note November.
13. Herrman H, Saxena S, Moodie R. Promoting mental health. Geneva: World Health Organization; 2005.
14. Globalpovertyproject.com. Welcome|United Kingdom|Global Poverty Project. [On line]. Available from: http://www.globalpovertyproject.com/
15. Blokhuis B. Violation of women's rights: a cause and consequence of trafficking in women. Amsterdam: La Strada International; 2008.
16. Fukuda-Parr S. What does feminization of poverty mean? It isn't just lack of income. Feminist economics [serial on the Internet]. (1999, July); 5(2): 99–103. Available from: Business Source Complete.
17. Alcala M. The State of World population 2006: a passage of hope. New York: United Nations Population Fund; 2006.
18. Gouws A. The Feminisation of Migration. Afr Insight [serial on the Internet]. (2010, June);40 (1):169–80. Available from: Social Sciences Full Text (H.W. Wilson).
19. Thurston W, Vissandjée B. An ecological model for understanding culture as a determinant of women's health. Crit Public Health [serial on the Internet]. (2005, Sep);15(3):229–42. Available from: CINAHL.
20. Dimmitt Gnam A. Mexico's missed opportunities to protect irregular women transmigrants: applying a gender lens to migration law reform. Pac Rim Law Policy J [serial on the Internet]. (2013, June);22(3):713–49. Available from: Academic Search Complete.
21. Martin S. World migration report 2000. Geneva, Switzerland: International Organization for Migration; 2000.
22. Horton S. A mother's heart is weighed down with stones: a phenomenological approach to the experience of transnational motherhood. Cult Med Psychiatry [serial on the Internet]. (2009, Mar);33(1):21–40. Available from: CINAHL Complete.
23. Hondagneu-Sotelo P, Avila E. "I'm here, but I'm there": the meanings of Latina transnational motherhood. Gender Soc [serial on the Internet]. (1997, Oct);11548–571. Available from: Social Sciences Full Text (H.W. Wilson).
24. Lahaie C, Hayes J, Piper T, Heymann J. Work and family divided across borders: the impact of parental migration on Mexican children in transnational families. Community Work Fam [serial on the Internet]. 2009;12(3):299–312. Available from: Business Source Complete.
25. Sternberg R, Barry C. Transnational mothers crossing the border and bringing their health care needs. J Nurs Scholarsh [serial on the Internet]. 2011;43(1):64–71. Available from: CINAHL Complete.
26. McGuire S, Martin K. Fractured migrant families: paradoxes of hope and devastation. Fam Community Health [serial on the Internet]. 2007;30(3):178–88. Available from: MEDLINE with Full Text.
27. Miranda J, Siddique J, Der-Martirosian C, Belin T. Depression among Latina immigrant mothers separated from their children. Psychiatr Serv [serial on the Internet]. 2005;56 (6):717–20. Available from: PsycINFO.
28. Suarez-Orozco C, Bang H, Kim H. I felt like my heart was staying behind: psychological implications of family separations and reunifications for immigrant youth. J Adolesc Res [serial on the Internet]. 2011;26(2):222–57. Available from: ERIC.
29. Falicov C. Working with transnational immigrants: expanding meanings of family, community, and culture. Fam Process [serial on the Internet]. 2007;46(2):157–71. Available from: CINAHL Complete.
30. Mazzucato V, Schans D. Transnational families and the well-being of children: conceptual and methodological challenges. J Marriage Fam [serial on the Internet]. 2011;73(4):704–12. Available from: Social Sciences Full Text (H.W. Wilson).

31. Walsh F. Normal family processes: growing diversity and complexity. 3rd ed. New York: Guildford; 2003.
32. Cacho L. Esclavas del poder. Mexico, DF: Grijalbo; 2010.
33. United Nations. Optional protocol to prevent, suppress and punish trafficking in persons, especially women and children, supplementing the United Nations Convention Against Transnational Organized Crime; 2000. Available from: http://www.unodc.org/documents/treaties/UNTOC/Publications/TOC%20Convention/TOCebook-e.pdf
34. International Labour Organization. A global alliance against forced labour. Geneve: International Labour Organization; 2005.
35. Oram S, Stoöckl H, Busza J, Howard L, Zimmerman C. Prevalence and risk of violence and the physical, mental, and sexual health problems associated with human trafficking: systematic review. PLoS Med [serial on the Internet]. 2012;9(5):1–13. Available from: Academic Search Complete.
36. Hossain M, Zimmerman C, Abas M. The relationship of trauma to mental disorders among trafficked and sexually exploited girls and women. Am J Public Health [serial on the Internet]. 2010;100(12):2442–9. Available from: Social Sciences Full Text (H.W. Wilson).
37. Yakushko O. Human trafficking: a review for mental health professionals. Int J Adv Couns [serial on the Internet]. 2009;31(3):158–67. Available from: PsycINFO.
38. Zimmerman C, Hossain M, Yun K, Gajdadziev V, Guzun N, Watts C, et al. The health of trafficked women: a survey of women entering posttrafficking services in Europe. Am J Public Health [serial on the Internet]. 2008;98(1):55–9. Available from: CINAHL Complete.
39. Tsutsumi A, Izutsu T, Poudyal A, Kato S, Marui E. Mental health of female survivors of human trafficking in Nepal. Soc Sci Med [serial on the Internet]. 2008;66(8):1841–7. Available from: CINAHL.
40. Bjelajac Z, Spalevic Z, Banovic B. Psychophysical status of human trafficking victims. Health Med [serial on the Internet]. 2013;7(4):1341–6. Available from: Academic Search Complete.
41. Sherwood K, Liebling-Kalifani H. A grounded theory investigation into the experiences of African women refugees: effects on resilience and identity and implications for service provision. J Int Womens Stud [serial on the Internet]. 2012;13(1):72–94. Available from: LGBT Life with Full Text.
42. Jones A. War is not over when it's over. New York: Metropolitan Books; 2010.
43. Un.org. Landmark resolution on women, peace and security (Security council resolution 1325). Available from: http://www.un.org/womenwatch/osagi/wps
44. Trenholm J, Olsson P, Ahlberg B. Battles on women's bodies: war, rape and traumatization in eastern Democratic Republic of Congo. Glob Public Health [serial on the Internet]. 2011;6 (2):139–52. Available from: CINAHL Complete.
45. Un.org. Women, peace and security. United Nations peacekeeping. [Online] Available from: http://www.un.org/en/peacekeeping/issues/women/wps.shtml
46. United Nations Security Council. Resolution 1888 (2009). Available from: http://www.un.org/womenwatch/daw/vaw/securitycouncil/S-RES-1888-(2009)-English.pdf
47. United Nations Security Council. Resolution 1889 (2009). [Online] Available from: http://www.womenpeacesecurity.org/media/pdf-scr1889.pdf
48. United Nations Security Council. Resolution 2106 (2013). [Online] Available from: http://peacemaker.un.org/sites/peacemaker.un.org/files/SC_ResolutionWomen_SRES2106(2013)(english).pdf
49. United Nations Security Council. Resolution 2122 (2013). [Online] Available from: http://www.peacewomen.org/assets/file/sgres2122.pdf
50. Hollifield M. Taking measure of war trauma. Lancet [serial on the Internet]. 2005;365 (9467):1283–4. Available from: CINAHL Complete.
51. Hagen K, Yohani S. The nature and psychosocial consequences of war rape for individuals and communities. Int J Psychol Stud [serial on the Internet]. 2010;2(2):14–25. Available from: Academic Search Complete.

52. http://www.un.org/womenwatch/daw/beijing/pdf/Beijing%20full%20report%20S.pdf "\o" Report of the Fourth World Conference on women "\t"_blank.
53. Batliwala S. El significado del empoderamiento de las mujeres: nuevos conceptos desde la acción. In: León M (comp) Poder y empoderamiento de las mujeres. Bogotá: Tercer Mundo SA; 1997.
54. Young K. el potencial transformador en las necesidades prácticas: empoderamiento colectivo y el proceso de planificación. In: León M (comp) Poder y empoderamiento de las mujeres. Bogotá: Tercer Mundo SA; 1997.
55. León M. el empoderamiento de las mujeres: encuentros del primer y tercer mundos en estudios de género. In: La ventana, Revista de estudios de género, nº 13. Universidad de Guadalajara; 2001. p. 94–116.

2 Psychosexual Development and Sexual Dysfunctions

Rafael Segarra-Echebarría, Isidro Fernández-Pérez, Juan Miguel García-Moncho, and Leonardo Delarze-Carrillo

Abstract

Within human sexuality three basic pillars are entwined: biological factors; individual personality or psychosexuality, which encompasses the sexual identity of the subject concerned, as well as the interaction and conveyance of the different types of affection for those closest to them (together with the relational aspects derived) and the life circumstances at each moment; and the sociocultural environment in which it is lived.

The sexual development of an individual bears a resemblance to a relay race: genetic and chromosomal influences and hormonal, environmental, and psychosocial factors appear in a chronological sequence. Each of them, regardless of the opinion of different authors and schools, plays the main role at certain moments, although in the end all need the others to achieve the ultimate goal of being a grown, sexually mature, and healthy individual (according to an interactionist model), which in turn leads to the enhancement of the personal identity (including sexual identity and narcissism itself).

Sexuality is therefore a more general phenomenon than plain physical sex. In this regard a curious paradox is worth noting: human sexual behavior is scarcely known, at least from a scientific perspective and through epidemiological and

R. Segarra-Echebarría (✉)
Cruces University Hospital, Bilbao, Spain

University of the Basque Country, UPV/EHU, Cruces, Spain
e-mail: rafaelsegarraechevarria@osakidetza.net

I. Fernández-Pérez
Cruces University Hospital, Bilbao, Spain

J.M. García-Moncho
La Fe University Hospital, Valencia, Spain

L. Delarze-Carrillo
Chiloé Health Service. Castro Hospital, Chile University, Castro, Chiloé, Chile

M. Sáenz-Herrero (ed.), *Psychopathology in Women*,
DOI 10.1007/978-3-319-05870-2_2

gender-relevant studies. Finally, sexual dysfunctions represent a group of heterogeneous disorders and include an array of processes that affect the general population, generating a high impact at the quality of life and interpersonal relationship levels, and they are analyzed here from the perspective of the new DSM-5.

2.1 Introduction: The "Normal" or "Healthy" Sexuality

Sexuality (or sexual behavior) constitutes one of the most complex aspects of human experience. The human being is a social animal who needs a connection to others for his physical and psychological development. In all the different academic fields of study of the human being, a broad consensus seems to exist when it comes to being considered in terms of an ape that couldn't possibly exist if it was outside a close relational network that provides emotional and material support. Biologists who study the central nervous system (CNS) tend to picture the human being as a brain interconnected with other brains, and authors such as Damasio [1] point out that encounters with other human beings constitute the basic element in the construction of the Self and of human conscience. Bonding with an "other" shapes us and changes us, and the constant recording of those changes in our CNS determines the emergence of a nuclear conscience that develops until it evolves into the so-called extended conscience, supporting our biographical identity, which connects our present to the life history that went before us.

That interpersonal bond acquires the highest complexity in the couple relationship, which involves the close and continuous cohabitation of usually two people who consider themselves to be a living pair. A union between two human beings, common in all of the species' groups, is seen as the predominant way of life. This close cohabitation implies an adaptation to the needs, preferences, and fears of the other.

That same complexity is stressed during the sexual encounter, which in the context of an emotionally significant relationship constitutes possibly the most complex bonding experience between human beings. For this reason it is not surprising that this is a complex area of exploration and evaluation in which alterations and problems arise with an enormous frequency. Furthermore, we as mental health professionals tend to consider sexual life as an interpersonal area that works at its best as soon as all the other spheres of personal life are problem free. Nothing could be further from the truth, and from desire.

Desire is the driving force behind sexuality that propels us toward each other and that, from an academic point of view, has received much less attention than it should. Sexual relations generally start with desire, and nowadays it is understood that desire can take place spontaneously (innate desire) as much as it can be stimulated externally or either through cognitive and emotional motivations. External or cognitive incentives include feeling closer to the partner, experiencing sexual pleasure, enhancing the self-image, easing tension, diminishing the feeling of guilt that arises from infrequent sexual intercourse, and that of conceiving a child [2].

We should not forget that sexual life and affective life are two sides of the same bond. In evaluating deep interpersonal relationships attention must be paid to the subject's ability to fall in love and to build a meaningful relationship that includes the sexual sphere. There is "love pathology" beyond sexuality, which deserves deeper attention.

When we talk about "normal" or "healthy" human sexuality we find ourselves facing an extremely complex phenomenon that is difficult to define. Attempting to disentangle what the normal patterns might be is of little use, given the variation between life experiences and the polymorphism of sexual behaviors from different people and across different cultural settings.

In that regard a curious paradox is worth noting: human sexual behavior is scarcely known, at least from a scientific perspective and through epidemiological and relevant studies. In the mass media the attention paid to this sphere is constant, and debates and comments on different aspects of sexual behavior and its problems take up much space in a great quantity of magazines. This could lead us to think that there was ample scientific literature providing a basis for explaining in detail people's normal and pathological sexual behaviors. Nothing is further from the truth. Studies of general populations are scarce, and they are becoming outdated. Even today in the USA, studies are still dependent on data from a big study by Chicago University [3] published 20 years ago (*Sex in America*). Taking into account the influence that cultural and social features bring to bear on sexual behavior, the need to replicate any study on sexuality in different countries, ethnic groups, cultures, religious beliefs, etc., seems clear.

The scarcity of information regarding the general population is even larger when we focus on concrete collectives, for instance, psychiatric patients. There are scant publications on this matter [4], which still offer a partial view of that collective.

Within human sexuality three basic pillars are entwined, as described next:

Biological Factors; Individual personality or psychosexuality, which encompasses the sexual identity of the subject concerned, as well as the interaction and conveyance of the different types of affection to those closest to them (together with the relational aspects derived) and the life circumstances at each moment; and the Socio-Cultural Environment in which it is lived.

The sexual development of an individual bears a resemblance to a relay race, according to Money [5]: genetic and chromosomal influences and hormonal, environmental, and psychosocial factors appear in a chronological sequence. Each of them, regardless of the opinion of different authors and schools, plays the main role in certain moments, although in the end all need the others to achieve the ultimate goal of a grown, sexually mature, and healthy individual (according to an interactionist model).

2.2 Psychosexual Development

The sex of the embryo is determined at the moment of fertilization, depending on the chromosome of the spermatozoid, either X or Y. However, during human embryogenesis some weeks go by without any noticeable differences, even under an electronic microscope, between a female and a male fetus. This is known as the sexually undifferentiated period of sexual development [6].

During the undifferentiated period the gonadal crests, the outlines of the future gonads, are bipotential, and evolve into testicles or ovaries depending on the genetic make-up. In parallel, in the same mesoderm, we find Wolff's mesonephric duct and Müller's paramesonephric duct, both outlines of the internal genitalia as well but unipotentials in this case.

With regard to the external genitalia, they result from the cloaca and the cloacal membrane, the urorectal septum being in charge of the uro-genital division of the rectum. All the genital outlines are bipotential, with a differentiation dependent on the presence or absence of testicular hormones.

Sexual differentiation is established, under normal conditions, around the seventh week of embryonic development, considered to be since the last menstruation date.

Thus, in XY individuals the gonadal crests are differentiated, forming the fetal testicles, the germinal cells of which, differentiated into spermatogonial cells, divide through mitosis, not entering meiosis until puberty. These cells are accompanied, forming the seminiferous tubules, by the Sertoli cells, of somatic origin, and the Leydig cells, at an interstitial level, in charge of the expression of proteins that are key to the consequent sexual differentiation, among which we can find the anti-Müllerian hormone (AMH).

In the case of XX fetuses, the gonads retain an undifferentiated appearance for a longer period of time. Moreover, unlike the XY fetus, the germinal cells, differentiated into oogonial cells, proliferate through mitosis until the 4th month, when they initiate the meiosis stage until the diplotene stage, which stops shortly before birth, restarting at puberty with each ovarian cycle.

The presence of the Y chromosome becomes the determining factor of the sexual development of the fetal gonad. Concretely, in its short arm we find the SRY gene (Sex—determining Region Y—chromosome). Although the cell mechanisms through which it works are not yet precisely known, the gene SRY is deemed to perform the migration function and to differentiate all three main cell structures:

- We find the differentiation of germinal cells into spermatogenic cells.
- The Sertoli cells start to show a specific pattern of expression characterized by an increase in SOX9 (protein of the SRY family) and in AMH, together with a reduction of DAX1 levels, its gene being located in the X chromosome.

There is experimental evidence that SRY and DAX1 interact in early stages of the gonadal crests. Thus, in XY individuals there is only one allele of the SRY gene, and just one allele of the DAX1 gene. Under such conditions SRY seems to be dominant, and allows testicular differentiation with the resulting expression of genes that are typically testicular, such as SOX9 and AMH. Nevertheless, not only the SRY levels but also their chronology of expression are determining, given that a delay in the expression of SRY would allow an anti-testicular action of DAX1.

In XX individuals the absence of SRY results in an increase in DAX1 levels in the gonad that is differentiated in an ovarian sense. In spite of that, DAX1 does not seem to be essential for the development of the ovary, for mice DAX1 Knock-out do present, a fact that has classically led to the conclusion that the mere absence of SRY results in ovary development. However, although the absence of SRY is imperative, it seems logical to imagine that some of kind pro-ovarian genes must exist, but this is unknown to date.

- Finally, from the eighth week of pregnancy, the Leydig cells control the androgen production.

On the basis of such provisions we can sum up the sexual differentiation process as follows (Figs. 2.1 and 2.2):

- Internal genitalia. Under the action of the testicular androgens, the Wolffian mesonephric ducts give rise in the male fetus to the epididymis, vasa deferentia, and seminal vesicles. In the female sex, given the absence of AMH, the Müllerian paramesonephric ducts form the uterine tubes, the uterus, and the upper third of the vagina. Therefore, the Wolffian ducts degenerate in the XX fetus owing to the lack of androgens, whereas the Müllerian ducts return in the XY fetus by the action of the AMH. It should be noted that the action time frame of the AMH is short: the testicular secretion starts by the end of the 7th week, and the Müllerian ducts become refractory to its action from the 10th week.
- External genitalia: the undifferentiated outlines evolve into male structures under the action of the dihydrotestosterone, a powerful androgen derived from the action of the 5-α-reductase enzyme on the testosterone. Thus, the penis originates from the genital tubercle, whereas the labioscrotal folds enlarge and fuse in the ante-posterior sense to form the scrotal sacs. In the female fetus, the lack of androgens allows the clitoris to originate from the genital tubercle, and the urogenital folds to remain separate, forming the labia majora. However, the mere presence of testosterone and AMH is not enough, for the final action depends on the binding of each molecule to its specific receptor, and on the proper functioning of the subsequent molecular cascade.

The same sexual differentiation phenomenon proves to be more complex and determinant, given that under the influence of the sexual hormones circulating in the fetus the dimorphic development of certain brain areas is produced too.

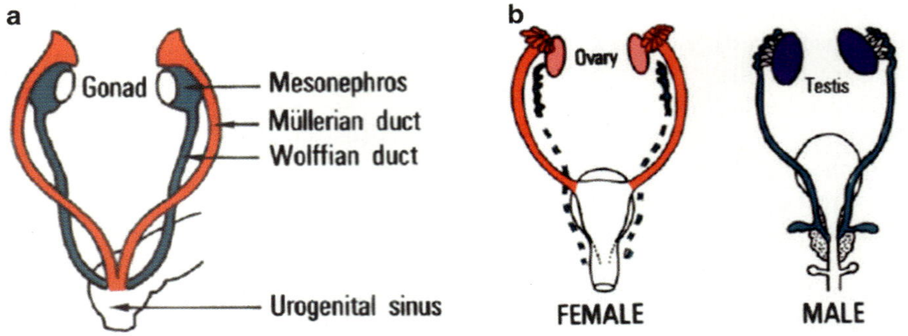

Fig. 2.1 Embryo–fetal sexual differentiation

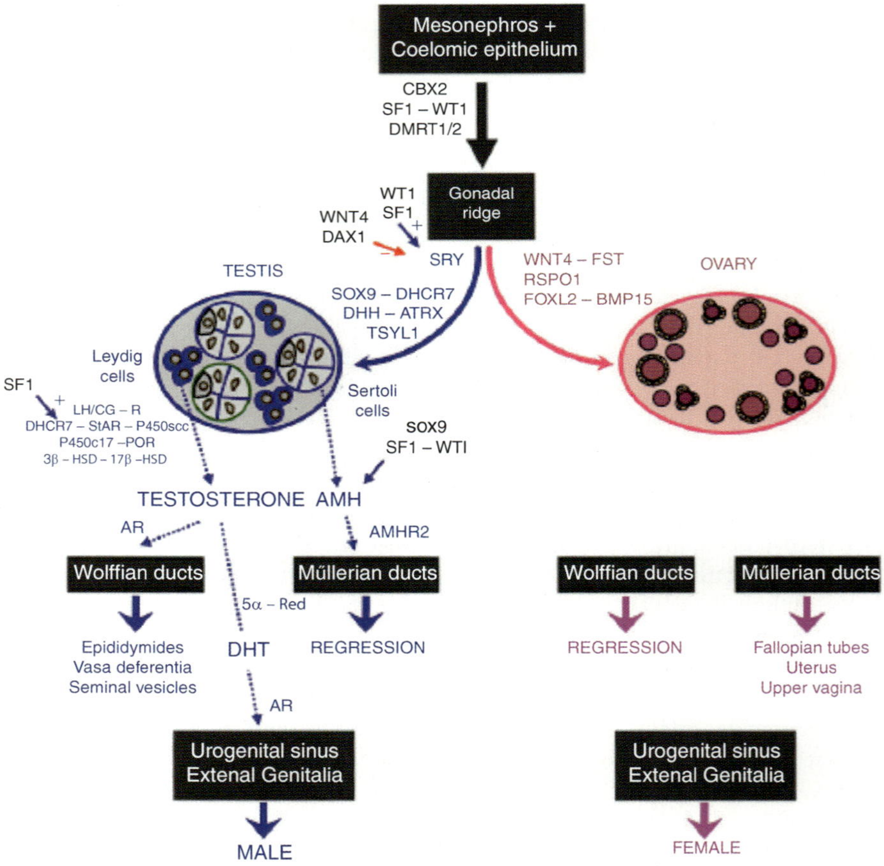

Fig. 2.2 Male and female embryo–fetal sexual differentiation

Furthermore, the brain, like the internal genitalia, is monotypic, and in it the feminization principle also prevails, unless there is an adequate level of circulating androgens [7].

Sexual differentiation of the human brain takes place approximately between weeks 16 and 28 of embryonic development, and the specific hypothalamic and hypophyseal functions (cyclic in women and noncyclic in men) are determined at that moment.

The hypothalamus is considered to be the main regulating center of sexual behavior in humans. In the pre-optic nucleus the hormone that releases gonadotropins (GnRH) is produced, which stimulates the anterior pituitary so that it can in turn produce luteinizing hormone (LH) and follicle-stimulating hormone (FSH). Both control the steroid hormone secretion by the gonads (estradiol, progesterone, and testosterone).

This complex system of hypothalamus–hypophysis–gonads presents secretory self-regulation by means of positive and negative feedback mechanisms. Moreover, the GnRH modulates the catecholaminergic neurotransmission, direct and indirect arbiter of the sexual output of the individual (while dopamine stimulates the sexual function, and serotonin and prolactin inhibit it, the balance dopamine/serotonin becoming crucial in this field). Other substances implicated in the complex world of the neurochemical interactions that modulate human sexuality are: GABA, ACTH, cortisol-releasing peptide, endogenous opioids, and acetylcholine.

The secondary sexual characteristics are induced by the CNS and controlled by a substantial increase in the circulating androgens or estrogens, as well as the female-specific functions regarding menstruation, gestation, and lactation. The precise way in which CNS "rules" the beginning of puberty is still unknown. It has been considered that one of the mechanisms implicated is the reduction of the sensitivity of the hypothalamus to hormonal negative feedback [8].

Since puberty, hormonal imbalances may alter secondary sexual characteristics, generating different physical alterations. Nevertheless, the influence of the hormone levels on desire and sexual behavior is much less clear at this point of development and at subsequent stages.

Once the fundamental biological factors in the formation of human sexuality are determined, it is worth going deeper into the other fundamental pillar, that is to say, that related to the formation of a sexual identity or psychosexuality.

Communication and early social learning are of paramount importance in determining early sexual behavior. Therefore, control over sexual behavior as well as of mating within our species, is to a great extent determined by the earliest social interactions, together with the aforementioned biological determinants.

In both sexes the inadequate availability of sexual hormones in the blood plasma reduces the intensity of sexual desire. But when the levels are adequate, the dependence of sexual desire on their fluctuations is negligible in comparison to the relevancy of the psychosocial kind of stimuli. McConaghy [8] believes that female sexual desire can be more influenced by psychosocial factors than masculine desire. Even so, the paucity of scientific research concerning this issue is surprising.

The development and maturation of the individual's sexuality, as well as the personality, go hand in hand with the establishment of the ability to experience love for certain objects, sexual or not (parental, filial, narcissistic, group). In the case of sexual love we can say that "healthy" sexuality is accompanied by the foundation of a certain degree of intimacy, empathy, and confidence in the beloved object, which in turn leads to the enhancement of the personal identity (including the sexual identity and narcissism itself). These values become the fundamental basis of a relationship in which sexual activity plays the role of positive reinforcement and affective catalyst, aside from its reproductive function.

Sexuality is therefore a more general phenomenon than plain physical sex and a more restricted one than the set of behaviors derived from the libidinal drive and directed according to Freud toward the achievement of pleasure, and according to many post-Freudian authors (such as Fairbairn), toward the establishment of interpersonal relationships.

There is a widespread consensus in the psychoanalytical literature on the key importance of earlier relationships in the construction of gender identity and sexual orientation. Authors such as Kernberg [8, 9], from a conciliatory perspective based upon the theory of object relations, emphasize the relevant role of the relational configurations that populate the internal world of boys and girls. They are the result of the incorporation of the so-called object relations dyads, consisting of one representation of the Self, another of the object, and an affection that bonds them together.

Contemporary authors such as Stoller [10–13], who was especially dedicated to this sphere of knowledge, point out how gender identity seems to be acquired in very early stages.

The utmost significance that used to be attributed to the "Oedipal Complex" is no longer ascribed to it, and it consists now of nothing but a cultural construction of mythical proportions. It must be noted that from certain sectors of psychoanalysis it is also highlighted that the sense of the Self and of the other evolves through the fact that separate minds are able to share feelings and intentions in a process of mutual recognition. This recognition can be established through a dyad mother/son, or father/daughter, or any asymmetrical relationship, as long as the needs of the other are not falsified through constructions or representations that justify and disguise domination.

The androcentrism of psychoanalytical theory concerning sexual differences stems from that point, of the double absence and invisibility of what the father does in the scenario where the girl and the mother end up finding their place and developing their subjectivity [14].

In fact, the dominant factor in humans that determines the intensity of sexual desire, leaving aside the aforementioned hormonal factors, is of a cognitive–affective kind, and is clearly constrained by psychosocial factors. It is worth noting at this point how the affective memory is related to the limbic system, which is the nervous substrate of affection and of the rest of the appetitive functions.

Because sexual activation also includes the implementation of the limbic system under the influence of a particular cognitive–affective state, which stimulates the peripheral and central nervous systems that determine the congestion and lubrication, and increases the focused sensitivity of the genital organs, providing a central feedback "self-realization" of that genital activation and the subsequent psychological excitement.

In that regard, Kernberg [8,9,15,16] adds that sexual arousal is a specific affection that shows all the features of the affective structures, and constitutes the central building block of the so-called sexual or libidinal drive as a general motivational system. Sexual arousal is the basic affection that constrains the appearance of a more complex psychological phenomenon, erotic desire, in which the sexual arousal seems to be bound to the emotional relationship with a specific subject.

The source of desire is not an anatomical body but a body that is built through the array of discourses and intersubjective practices. Both girls and boys organize themselves through their relationship with other subjects (for instance, the mother) who aren't just objects for the child, because both the girl and the boy are able to recognize that subject as different from them and, at the same time, as akin to them. In this way, the intersubjectivity plays a role in the structuring of the psychological world. It may be noted that uneven consequences arise from a double sexual standard, the fact that admiring women or giving them recognition only for their physical attributes poses a difficulty for their mental balance, as well as the extra work to which the female psyche is subject if it intends to reconcile the multiplicity of demands of its motivational systems [17].

To conclude this introduction we attempt to define in a simple and operational way a general consensus as to what constitutes "abnormal or deviant" sexual behavior, that is:

Anything that is destructive or damaging to the subject who displays it and to those who get involved in it.
Anything that is not oriented to the other in the strict sense.
Anything that excludes the stimulation of the subject's own genital organs and those of their partner.
Anything that is inappropriately associated with feelings of guilt and/or anxiety.
Anything that shows a compulsive repetitive nature.

We share with many authors a preoccupation that has arisen from the manifest neglect in clinical practice in documenting the medical/sexual history and its psychopathological manifestations in the individuals who visit the doctor. More frequently than would be desirable, it is the health professional themselves (unlike the patients) who perceive this issue as a complicated area to explore, and thus a subject to be avoided. It is essential to explore the patient's love life, including sexual patterns, as well as their fantasies and the nature of the object relations that are established in the context of their sexual behavior [16].

2.3 Sexual Dysfunctions

Sexual dysfunctions represent a group of heterogeneous disorders and include an array of processes that affect the general population, generating a high impact on quality of life and interpersonal relationships.

They are usually underdiagnosed and undertreated, and in them etiopathological aspects of biological, psychosocial, and interpersonal nature overlap. It is important to determine any underlying disorder or incurring psychosocial factor when evaluating a patient who has sexual problems, to such an extent that it has been stated that the sexual dysfunction may in fact be a symptom or side-effect, and not a primary pathology [2]. Additionally, in all cases carrying out surveillance of the possible organic causes is unavoidable (highly frequent in the case of a man's erectile dysfunction), as well as toxic and pharmacological causes or other psychiatric disorders, pre-dominantly of an affective nature.

Historically, sexual response has been understood as a linear process in various stages, initially defined by Masters and Johnson (excitement-arousal-orgasm-resolution), and later modified by Kaplan into a triphasic model of desire arousal and orgasm [2].

From this model, sexual dysfunction has been historically classified with regard to a disturbance of the sexual act, attributable to various causes. Among them [18]:

Disturbances in the physiological processes specific to each stage of the sexual response cycle (excitement-arousal-orgasm-resolution).

Algesic disorders that hamper either the performing of sexual intercourse (dyspareunia, vaginismus) or its achievement (post-sexual dysphoria).

All share a common trait: the anxiety they cause to sufferers and/or their partners. This anxiety may trigger the dysfunction, or act as a factor that prolongs it once it has set in [18].

However, as we see later, today a new, more complex and nonlinear model of sexual response has been adopted, which includes emotional and relational factors, as well as the interference from outside sexual stimuli, together with those of a cognitive kind.

Another peculiarity to be taken into account, as reflected in the new edition of the DSM, is that sexual excitement includes both a subjective and a physiological or genital arousal [19]. These two are often different from each other, and studies have shown that there is a poor correlation between subjective and physiological arousal. Thus, healthy women with sexual arousal disorder have shown normal genital vessel congestion as a response to erotic stimuli, despite protesting that experience a low level of subjective arousal [20].

The epidemiology shows us how regular medical practice is not in accordance with the facts regarding disorders associated with sexuality, and the underrated perception of this psychopathological characteristic that is so frequently neglected.

*Women

The prevalence of sexual dysfunctions in women has been estimated for years to be about 43 %, on the basis of a National Health and Social Life Survey Study, which examined a cohort of adults in USA in 1992

More recent data from a transversal female population-based case-control study in the United States (Prevalence of Female Sexual Problems Associated with Distress and Determinants of Treatment Seeking) determined a prevalence for any sexual dysfunction of 44.2 % [21].

According to the National Health and Social Life Survey more women (43 %) than men (31 %) gave information about their sexual problems. Among those women who gave information about any kind of sexual difficulty, problems related to sexual desire were the most common (average 64 %), followed by difficulties with orgasm (average 35 %), difficulties with arousal (average 31 %), and sexual pain (average 26 %) [22].

It is worth noting that women vary significantly when it comes to assessing the importance that they attach to the practice of sexual intercourse, as well as their sexual practice of preference, their views on the optimal sexual frequency, and the amount of stimulation necessary to obtain adequate sexual arousal and satisfaction [23]. It is not hard to imagine that the multidimensional gender variable explains such a wide variability.

Another factor to be taken into account is age. Most studies offer evidence that sexual activities, as well as sexual function, decrease with age. This decline has usually been seen to start from the 30–40s age bracket. In addition, many women describe a decline specifically associated with menopause. Only a small percentage of women in longitudinal studies (5–15 %) informed of an increase in sexual function and activities with age. Nevertheless, it must be clarified that a decline in sexual function and activities does not automatically imply the presence of a dysfunction or a sexual disorder [24].

*Men

Different studies show a high prevalence of sexual dysfunction symptoms in men, reaching 64.3 % in those over 40 [25].

A recent study on an Australian male population aged between 20 and 64 years who have been sexually active in the last year, confirms that 34 % of men refer to at least one sexual difficulty: 48 % of men with any sexual difficulty presents with problems maintaining an erection, and 24 % refer to delayed ejaculation; 11 % of the sample related to having experienced a loss of interest in sex in the last year, and 7 % complain about premature ejaculation [26].

Also, the lack of interest in sex or a decrease in the libido is associated with erectile dysfunction, premature ejaculation, and delayed ejaculation in 38 %, 28.3 %, and 50 % of men respectively [27].

As regards nosology, in the first versions of the Diagnostic and Statistical Manual of Mental Disorders (DSM) of the American Psychiatric Association only two sexual dysfunctions are set out: frigidity (with regard to women) and impotence (with regard to men).

The category psychosexual Disorders was included for the first time in the third edition of the Manual (DSM-III) in 1980, where it was defined as "inhibitions in sexual desire or the psycho-physiological changes that characterize the sexual response cycle" [28]. The diagnostic of "inhibited sexual desire" includes inhibitions within any of the sexual stages indicated by Masters and Johnson in 1966 [29]: excitement-arousal-orgasm-resolution. In 1987, in the DSM-III (DSM-III-R) revision, "inhibited sexual desire" was subdivided into two categories "hypoactive sexual desire disorder" (lack of interest in sex) and "sexual aversion disorder" (phobic aversion to sex). Since then, progress has been made with regard to both the diagnostic classifications and the definition of sexual dysfunctions.

The DSM-IV (published in 1994, followed by its revision, or DSM IV TR, in 2000) gathers four categories of sexual dysfunction, following again the linear model of sexual response by Masters and Johnson: "disorders of sexual desire, arousal, and orgasm, and disorder of sexual pain." In addition, in order to perform a diagnostic of the disorder, the sexual performance must cause significant upset or interpersonal difficulties [30]. The DSM-IV also frames the disorder in terms of the nature of its inception ("lifelong vs acquired"), the context in which it takes place ("generalized vs situational"), and etiological factors (due to primarily psychological factors, with the contribution of medical factors, or due to substance use).

While waiting for better adaptation and implementation of the DSM 5, as of today, the DSM-IV TR diagnostics are still the most frequently used by the majority of psychiatrists. Therefore, and because the new DSM edition feeds on them in different ways, a detailed analysis of the different sexual dysfunctions based on the linear model of sexual response is carried out below, later moving forward to revise, in a briefer way, the different nosographic changes as set down in the DSM 5 [19].

2.3.1 Sexual Desire

2.3.1.1 Hypoactive Sexual Desire

By hypoactive sexual desire, sexual frigidity or a decrease in sexual desire we understand a clinical condition characterized by an absence (anaphrodisia) or decrease in sexual fantasies and in the desire to engage in sexual intercourse with the partner concerned. This clinical picture is often (but not necessarily) accompanied by difficulties with other stages of the sexual cycle (arousal, orgasm), or by a previous history of adverse previous sexual experiences (dispareunia, vaginism).

The decrease or absence of sexual desire appears, from an epidemiological point of view, more frequently in women, in their adult life and after a period of normal sexual activity, coinciding with extrinsic stressing factors or with periods of psychological unease, sometimes influenced by various psychiatric disorders (major depressive disorder or anxiety disorder) and/or organic disorders.

Frigidity can in its turn come to be an important source of psychological upset associated with low self-esteem. Another possibility is that this clinical picture represents in itself a defense mechanism against unconscious fears that are unacceptable to the individual, such as fantasies of a homosexual or paraphilic nature. Nor is the situation unusual in which hostile feelings toward the partner, a deterioration in the loving relationship, or the expression of a situation of abuse or gender-based violence lie beneath hypoactive sexual desire.

The actual prevalence of this clinical picture can approach 20 % of the general population, being:

A global illness that extends to all sexual relationships of the individual, and reveals difficulties with emotional bonding and in facing intimate relationships.
Or an affection circumscribed to certain situations, such as with a certain partner or featuring a certain sexual practice.

Aspects such as the kind of couple relationship that has been established, the sociocultural environment to which the individual belongs, as well as his or her intellectual and educational level, should all be checked, running joint interviews if necessary. In fact, it is not uncommon for the decrease in the sexual desire of one of the members of the couple to be a response to an increase in the desire and demands of the other, or that the decrease in desire alternates and is transitory for both members of the couple.

2.3.1.2 Sexual Aversion

In this clinical picture, what was noted in the previous subsection reaches its most extreme manifestation in the shape of a rejection of everything related to sexual practices, with an active and lasting avoidance of sexual intercourse.

The patient who suffers sexual aversion experiences disgust and rejection of some particular aspect of genital or sexual contact, suffering a real terror at the mere possibility of it happening, accompanied by great anxiety. The association of symptoms frequently observed in anxiety disorders with those of mood disorders forces us to effect an exhaustive differential diagnostic for all of them.

2.3.1.3 Erotomania or Hyper Erotism

At the polar opposite of the decrease in or rejection of sexual desire is hyper erotism or excess libidinal desire or sexual impulse. This picture, which is also known as erotomania (or hypererosia if we make reference to the same phenomenon in the animal kingdom) [31], is accompanied by a predominance of cognitions and mental images full of sexual content, generic or specifically crystallized around certain people, absolutely independent and detached from any coital and reproductive function.

This phenomenon is more akin to young individuals who can find in their excess of sexual desire a source of conflict and concerns given its unadaptive nature.

The ICD 10 [31] includes in this section two classical forms, the male form (satyriasis) and the female form (nymphomania). In both cases reference is made to serious disorders dealing with an excess of sexual desire, with significant repercussions in the social and psychic life of the patients, who live under the clear constraints of a disorder that acquires a compulsive nature.

A differential diagnostic with other psychiatric disorders should also be carried out, such as pseudo erotomania or pseudolism [32], and with erotomaniac delusion [33].

2.3.2 Excitement Phase

During the excitement stage we can find different kinds of dysfunction, depending on the type of sex that is the object of analysis.

2.3.2.1 Male Impotence

The male can find it difficult or even impossible to obtain or maintain a penis erection that enables penetration and the achievement of coitus. This phenomenon is known as erectile dysfunction or impotence.

It is a frequent phenomenon, provided that it happens occasionally, as an episode, and does not create difficulties when it comes to establishing future interpersonal relationships. In the elderly a further delay in obtaining the erection and orgasm is also relatively frequent (responding to a physiological cause typical of advanced age), or in those cases in which there is inadequate sexual stimulation in terms of the stimulation object, intensity, and/or length. When the problem is more relevant and lasting, this is known as actual psychogenic impotence.

In an epidemiological study carried out throughout the world by GOSS (the Global Online Sexuality Survey) in a cohort of 1,133 English-speaking men, a prevalence of male impotence of 33.7 % was found [34].

In a recent study, Giuliano and collaborators [35] indicate a prevalence of male impotence less than 10 % of men under 50 and 20 % of those over 60. Risk factors associated with erectile dysfunction are age, cardiovascular diseases, diabetes mellitus, hypercholesterolemia, smoking, depression and other mental illnesses, psychological conflicts, and unfavorable socio-economic constraints.

However, it is worth underlining that there is a medical basis for the disorder of between 20 and 50 % of men who suffer erectile dysfunction, and this is also the case in 72 % of men under 40. The pathologies most associated are vascular, endocrinological, neurological diseases, and Peyronie syndrome, not overlooking the side-effects due to the use of pharmaceuticals [36].

Spanish psychiatrist Castilla del Pino [37] links sexual impotence to various psychogenic causes, such as the response of frustration to a previous failed sexual experience, which provokes in the individual a depreciation of his Self, of his self-esteem, and of his erotic narcissism, and which triggers a inhibition with regard to any other future sexual experience. Or he links it to feelings of guilt regarding a relationship considered morally reprehensible or because of the choice of a particular sexual partner. When the erection disappears at the moment when penetration is attempted, this is known as vestibular impotence. In this case, as long as the erotic foreplay lasts the erection is maintained, disappearing the moment the partner adopts a "passive" role and allows penetration, the moment at which anxiety appears. Impotence can also be interpreted as being the result of latent homosexuality.

Castilla del Pino [37] is interested to see the high frequency in which in a clinical setting impotent subjects maintain a stable relationship with a partner that does not add too much "conflictuality" to the dysfunction concerned. Sometimes they even seem to enjoy and benefit from it. He proposes as possible explanations for this enabling behavior from the partner the adoption on her/his part of a role similar to that of the mother, or the presence in the partner herself/himself of a diminution of sexual desire.

The presence of a satisfactory erection during masturbation or during the REM sleep stage directs us towards the psychogenic origin of the clinical picture. On the other hand, multiple primary psychiatric disorders can be accompanied by difficulties with the male erection, among them major depressive disorder, schizophrenia or obsessive compulsive disorder [18], all of which, however, entail an exclusive chapter in the DSM 5 [19].

2.3.2.2 Sexual Excitement Disorder in Women

In women, the prevalence of a sexual excitement disorder can be as high as 35 % [18], depending on the study. The women have been assigned a role with psychological factors, including anxiety, guilt or fear phenomena, as well as factors linked to the moment during the menstrual cycle at which the patient is found, according to the prolactin, estrogens, testosterone, and even thyroxin levels circulating in her blood.

The absence of sexual excitement in the woman manifests through an absence of the physiological changes that characterize this stage: vaginal lubrication, vascular congestion of the labia minor with flushing, hardening, elevation, and retraction of the clitoris after the pubic symphysis, constriction of the lower third of the vagina (orgasmic plateau), increase in the size of the breasts, as well as elevation of the heart and breathing rhythm, and of the arterial pressure.

Otto Fenichel [38], from a psychoanalytical perspective, interprets female frigidity as the existence of anguish before the damage arising from the complete satisfaction of sexual interests, anguish that culminates in different ways:

Women, who, through the educational constraints of class, status, and personal beliefs suffer a pejorative internalization of the vital aspects related to sexuality (mostly female sexuality), which results in a true horror with regard to the penis, filth, violence, and the aggressiveness of the male, all symbolic representations of the sexual act.

Women who show more or less conscious rejection of their sexual partner.

Women whose frigidity reveals problems inherent to the lack of resolution of the oedipal conflict, or either the pre-oedipal fixation with the mother and rejection of the masculine role.

Women, who, through their frigidity, find masochistic gratification in the shape of passivity, or either use it as a defense against the intense feelings of guilt arising from sexual satisfaction that is considered despicable at an unconscious level and culturally constrained (concept of "habitus" coined by Pierre Bourdieu).

Dispareunia and Vaginism

Among the main causes of a diminution of the sexual desire in women (which can also happen in men, although it is less frequent, a reason for it to have been rejected from the DSM 5) [19] we find psychogenic dispareunia, that is, pain during coitus, and even before or after it.

This type of disorder, according to the psychoanalytic theory, is framed in "conversion hysteria". Painful coitus can be a consequence of the tension and anxiety triggered by the sexual act in the individual, which mostly provoke in women the involuntary contraction of the perineal and vaginal muscles, hindering performance (vaginism), although this is not its only cause.

Vaginism consists in the involuntary, episodic or persisting contraction of the perineal muscles in the lower third of the vagina at the introduction of various objects, such as the penis, specula, fingers, sexual toys, and even tampons.

In some women the mere idea of vaginal penetration can induce a muscular spasm, which can be mild or intense and painful. It is possible that the other areas of sexual response are preserved, even the ability to experience excitement and achieve orgasms, as long as real or imaginary penetration is avoided.

Vaginism is a more frequent disorder in young women, of a high educational level and belonging to high socio-economic groups, with a negative attitude regarding sex because of previous traumatic experiences, because of a history of sexual abuse, or because of social and educational constraints. The systematic search for potential situations of past abuse in this group of patients is mandatory.

These clinical pictures are often accompanied by a decrease in the subjective feeling of excitement in both women and men, as well as a decrease in sexual desire, that can mimic previous experiences of traumatic and painful sexual relationships and be the origin of the active avoidance of them in the future, with subsequent damage to the couple's relationship and the psychological distress that it entails.

As in previous cases this disorder should not be considered pathological, as long as it only happens occasionally and does not generate difficulties when it comes to establishing satisfactory interpersonal relationships. Likewise, the possibility of incorrect sexual stimulation in terms of object, intensity, and duration must be researched. Frequently, there are also underlying difficulties in the couple's relationship, as well as religious, cultural, and social constraints.

At this point we would like to point out how psychoanalysis systematically tends to monopolize the discourse of truth on female sexuality. A discourse that narrates the truth of the logic of that same truth, precisely, that femininity is only prevalent within models and laws that have been enacted by masculine subjects. This implies that there are not two sexes but just one. One only (unique) practise and representation of the sexual, with its own story, its needs, its reversals, its shortcomings, its negative side or sides, whose support is still the female sex.

The thesis of the psychosexual development maintained by Freud since 1908 implies that girls aged 3–5 years discover that they do not have a penis and come to the conclusion that they lack something, that they have been castrated. This is the concept of "penis envy," which, together with boys' "fear of castration", operates not only at an individual level but also in the collective consciousness.

This fact has had negative effects, depriving women of a self-determined sexuality, dispossessing them of their creative ability. By the end of the nineteenth century the terms "vulva" and "labia" do not appear in Webster's Dictionary (derived from An American Dictionary of the English Language, by Noah Webster, 1928) to refer to the female genitalia, staying confined to the term "vagina." The problem is that Freud went even further, stating that the greatest desire of every girl, and later of every woman, would be the desire to possess a phallus ("penis envy"), and that that desire could only be replaced by the desire to conceive a baby.

Irigarary [17] relates it thus: the woman would only complete herself through maternity, in bringing to the world a child who is a "penis substitute" and, if she is completely lucky, a child with a penis of his own. The perfect fulfillment of becoming a woman would consist, according to Freud, in reproducing the male sex, neglecting one's own.

Together with the imaginary non-existence of the female genitalia, other non-existent items are addressed. Jacques Lacan, for example, wrote something like this: "A woman only exists if excluded from the nature of things, which is the nature of words, and it must be said that if there is something that women themselves complain about enough for the time being, it's just that they don't know what they're saying, and that's the whole difference between them and me" [14].

The rivalry between the two sexes in psychoanalysis has been formulated, pre-eminently, in genital terms, confusing form with content, genitalia with the wide scope of human actions that masculinity symbolizes. While it pretends to provide a scientific explanation of the sexual behavior, psychoanalysis is limited to the reinforcement of the myth. Women and men inserted into that cultural and allegedly scientific discourse picture all creativity and empowerment in a woman (in non-traditionally female areas) as some kind of usurpation or transgression: phallic women and men threatened with mutilation. The disguising and reinforcing of the hierarchic order of the sexes through an insisting recurrence of the differences between them continues to be made, reducing the complexity of the conflicts that are inherent to them, and widening alterity and human inequality [14].

2.3.3 Orgasm

Orgasm constitutes the climax or fulfillment of sexual pleasure, lasts an average of between 3 and 25 s (with great interindividual variability), and is accompanied by a rhythmic contraction of the perineal and anal muscles, of the pelvic reproductive organs, and by a massive relief of the sexual tension, followed by a muscular relaxation and by a subjective feeling of psychological and physical well being. It is followed by a certain decrease in the consciousness level and can be accompanied by a drowsiness that is generally superficial.

In the case of the male, the orgasm is announced by the subjective feeling of an immediate and inevitable ejaculation, followed by the rhythmic contraction of the prostate, the seminal vesicles and urethra, culminating in the emission of semen. In the case of the woman, the orgasm is accompanied by an involuntary contraction of the lower third of the vagina as well as of the uterus in its entirety. After the orgasm men experience a refractory period of between some minutes and several hours, during which they are not able to experience a new orgasm. This period is not usually experienced by women.

2.3.3.1 Female Anorgasmia

Anorgasmia or inhibited female orgasm is understood to be the recurring absence or the delayed onset of the orgasm in women for whom the rest of the sexual response stages are normal, either in the context of the sexual relationship of the couple or during the practice of masturbation.

In women the orgasm is usually achieved through the simultaneous stimulation of the clitoris and of the vaginal walls. Female anorgasmia can be primary if the woman has never experienced an orgasm, or secondary if there have been previous orgasmic experiences (including masturbatory practices or the orgasm during sleep). On the other hand anorgasmia can be accompanied by physical discomfort (somatic equivalents), in the form of pelvic pains, itching, vaginal discharge, mammary tension, and dispareunia.

Primary anorgasmia is more frequent in women without a partner, and its prevalence diminishes with age, being more frequent during adolescence and youth, probably because of the decrease in psychological inhibition at an older age, not being forced to adhere to social conventions, greater sexual experience, or a combination of them all [18].

Secondary anorgasmia is a frequent disorder in clinical populations that can generally reach up to 30 % of women and involve a variety of causes [18]. Among them, certain disorders of a psychological kind stand out, such as the disproportionate fear of a pregnancy, the rejection of a sexual partner or of any potential partner, the previous negative conditioning toward sex, accompanied by an excessive fear of sexual intercourse, and the fear of a loss of control of the impulses (represented by the orgasm), that may symbolize a dyscontrol of the aggressive or destructive kind toward the partner. Female anorgasmia is generally accompanied by difficulties at the excitement stage, and on occasion, by anankastic personality traits.

Other causes of anorgasmia in women are found in certain adverse constraints of the sociocultural, educational, and religious kinds.

2.3.3.2 Female Multiple Orgasms

As in the literature there is no record of the clinical presence of a premature female orgasm (the equivalent to premature ejaculation in males), cases of spontaneous multiple orgasms have been described, without sexual stimulation, in women suffering from temporal lobe epilepsy, as well as cases of spontaneous multiple orgasm associated with different physiological functions such as yawning or laughing in women under different pharmacological antidepressive treatments (fluoxetine, mirtazapine, trazodone, clomipramine), among others [18].

On the other hand, and taking into account that the presence in women of a refractory period following an orgasm is exceptional, if during sexual intercourse the stimulation performed by the partner is maintained, it is common for the female to experience several consecutive orgasms in proportion to the time length of the stimulation. The same goes for cases in which the stimulation takes place during masturbatory practices.

2.3.3.3 Male Anorgasmia or Delayed Ejaculation

The orgasmic disorder in males, male anorgasmia or delayed ejaculation, is less frequent than that in women, with a prevalence of around 5 % [18], and as in the previous case, it can be primary or secondary. This picture is much less frequent than impotence or premature ejaculation, and it should be differentiated from orgasmic anhedonia (ejaculation without orgasm).

Primary anorgasmia in males usually reveals serious pathological dysfunctions in those who suffer from it, including obsessive ruminations (for instance: of guilt, or of filth and contamination) associated or not with rituals of atonement, rigid and restrictive familiar and social environments, difficulties with interpersonal relationships, and in some cases the co-occurrence of an attention deficit disorder that may condition the difficulty in achieving sufficient excitement to trigger the sexual climax [11].

There are two antithetic points of view to explain this dysfunction: inhibition and models of desire deficit.

In the inhibition model behaviorists suppose that the male does not receive enough stimulation to reach his orgasmic threshold. The advocates of a psychodynamic model who support the same idea suppose that the symptoms are a conscious (or unconscious) expression of male aggression, someone who deprives or holds away from his partner something they covet.

In the desire deficit model, Apfelbaun [39] postulates that the delayed ejaculation is a desire dysfunction that is mistaken for a performance disorder.

When it comes to secondary anorgasmia it almost always reveals unresolved interpersonal and couple problems, of which the subject is more or less aware, obsessive–compulsive disorder or a clear hostility toward potential sexual partners.

2.3.3.4 Orgasmic Anhedonia

By orgasmic anhedonia we understand those male cases (in women it is simply termed Anorgasmia) in which the patient shows both the sexual excitement and the physiological components of penis contraction and ejaculation but do not experience the physical feeling of well-being provided by the orgasm.

In these infrequent cases possible medullary injuries to the sacral area and to neurological afferent pathways to the frontal lobe must be ruled out, as well as psychological causes, including intense feelings of guilt related to physical pleasure, and which determine the emergence of dissociated states that override the conscious pleasure of the orgasmic experience [18].

2.3.3.5 Premature Ejaculation

Among men the main cause of sexual dysfunction that appears in their questions to the medical practitioner (close to 40 % of cases) is premature ejaculation [18], which consists in repeatedly reaching orgasm and ejaculation before they would wish to, practically at the moment of penetration, with subsequent repercussions for their sexual relationship.

It is estimated that up to 30 % of the world's male population suffer from premature ejaculation. Among its etiological factors, a polymorphism of the dopamine and serotonin transporter genes has been found in patients with permanent premature ejaculation. In contrast, acquired premature ejaculation has been associated with factors of a urological, endocrinological, neurological, and psychological nature [40,41].

This clinical picture is more frequent among young men and is fostered by factors of a psychological kind, such as anticipatory anxiety based on the fear of not being able to sexually satisfy the partner, or adverse conditions of a cultural and educational kind. It has also been observed a certain biological predisposition in the form of a briefer latency in the ejaculation in those people under intense sexual stimuli.

2.3.4 Resolution Stage

During the resolution stage different alterations may arise, among which post-coital dysphoria and post-coital cephalalgia stand out.

It is worth noting that in the case of the interruption of coitus and of the non-achievement of orgasm (interrupted coitus), the resolution phase can be extended for between 2 and 6 h, and it is accompanied by an increase in the muscular tension in the genital area of both men and women, as well as by irritability and dysphoria.

2.3.4.1 Post-Coital Dysphoria

The term post-coital dysphoria refers to a particular psychophysical state subsequent to the performance of the coitus, more frequent in men, that can last from some minutes to several hours and includes a mixture of asthenia or superimposed fatigue and a clinical picture of anxiety, somatic anguish, irritability, and affective lability, which varies in terms of severity, it being possible to reach a state of true psychomotor agitation and the development of phobic symptoms and of avoidance behaviors related to the sexual act. Nevertheless, most frequently the clinical picture is mild and the recovery from it total.

2.3.4.2 Post Coital Headache

The post coital headache is characterized by the appearance of a headache immediately after coitus that can last several hours, and generally responds badly to conventional analgesic treatments.

The classic presentation of this disease is in the form of a pulsating headache, in the frontal and occipital regions, which is apparently more prevalent in women [18]. Its ultimate cause is still unknown, with vascular, muscular (tensional headache), and psychogenic factors having be found to be involved. Coitus can also trigger migraine attacks in those who have a predisposition to them.

2.3.5 Masturbation

Masturbation, or onanism, is a universal sexual practice of genital self-stimulation that usually consists of the more or less intense and rhythmic massage of the clitoris in women, and of the more vigorous kind of the penis in men (in both cases stimulation can reach other erogenous zones), which practically all men incur, as well as 80 % of women, at some point in their lives [18].

This practice has been frequently censored and forbidden by different societies and more or less developed cultures, on the basis of restrictive medical, moral, and religious stances, going so far as to consider it a causal factor of severe physical and psychiatric illnesses. However, none of these assumptions has been substantiated.

Masturbation is common during childhood, within a self-exploratory behavior that starts between the 2nd and 3rd year of age in which pleasure is sought. After the work of Freud, supposed discoverer and demystifier of the relevance of the sexual life of children, it started to be understood to be a normal form of sexuality, as the final step of self-eroticism toward the search for an outside object with erotic connotations [37].

In later times, coinciding with an increase in the socialization of children, masturbatory behaviors play a key role and enable interest and curiosity about one's own genitals and those of another, a basic fact in the maturation of the sexual identity and in the discovery of the opposite sex, with exhibitionist behaviors in both boys and girls being frequent at this age, thus increasing the feeling of pleasure, as long as an unfortunate and disproportionate restrictive and/or punitive attitude on the part of parents and caretakers does not foster a disproportionate sense of guilt in them.

In puberty, and later during adolescence, the onanistic activity increases in conjunction with the hormone "apocalypse" that entails the development of secondary sexual characters, an increase in sexual desire, as well as the conflict typical of the teenager, who on the one hand strives for the strengthening of his sexual identity through the achievement of coitus, and who on the other hand must comply with social and moral demands that impose on him a control of his sexual impulses.

It should be noted that during adolescence, masturbation is accompanied by coital fantasies that do not take place during childhood. These fantasies indicate a crucial step forward in the development of sexual identity, as well as in the positive reinforcement of the egosyntonic adult sexual role. In this sense, non-objectal masturbation can turn out to be a psychopathological manifestation, revealing an underlying psychical disorder.

Castilla del Pino [37] considers the masturbatory activity at these ages to accomplish two fundamental tasks:

On the one hand the concretion of sexual excitation in the genital sphere.

On the other hand, fantasies accompanied by masturbation target almost invariably real sexual objects; thus, we are talking about the first (fantasized) rehearsal of an alloerotic sexuality.

Masturbatory activity is usually maintained until adult life, when it is substituted by coitus, even though this substitution is not absolute and masturbation usually persists in adults, sometimes as another component of the general activity of the couple within the sexual encounter, other times with the adaptive function of substituting in a more or less persisting way an unsatisfying or non-existent couple relationship, or in parallel to the couple relationship, regardless of the satisfaction it grants, providing an experience of intimate enjoyment.

An exception to this view on masturbation occurs when it acquires compulsive or restrictive characteristics, or when it is accompanied by other psychopathological manifestations. In many cases compulsive masturbators hide a fear of impotence and substitute real sexual relationships (non-existent) for others that are fantasized and accompanied by masturbatory activities.

2.4 Changes in the Diagnostic Criteria of the Sexual Dysfunctions in the DSM-5

Once the different epigraphs have been analyzed and described, it is worth going deeper into how they have been adapted or reformulated in the recently published new diagnostic classification. Because the DSM criteria for sexual dysfunctions, like those devised for other disorders, aim to reflect the prevailing psychiatric opinion at the moment of their issue [19].

As we discussed earlier, previous editions of the DSM were based on the sexual response model suggested by Master and Johnson and on its later development by Kaplan. Recent research questions the validity of this model, given that both the strict distinction between the excitement phases and the linear sexual response model were inadequate to explain sexual behavior.

The changes that have been carried out in the chapter on sexual dysfunction widen and clarify the different diagnostics and their respective criteria. Although some of the changes are subtle, others are remarkable: such as the addition of gender-specific sexual dysfunction, of time and frequency patterns, or the merging of some previous diagnostics [42].

Classification of sexual dysfunctions has been simplified in only three sections in the case of women, and in four in the case of men:

***Females** Female Hypoactive Sexual Desire and Sexual Excitement Disorders, which appeared in the DSM IV, are now gathered in one single disorder, called Female Sexual Interest/Arousal Disorder. Research on this topic suggests that making a separation would seem too artificial. The fact is that, according to the increasing rejection of the sexual excitement linear model, a high comorbidity of desire and sexual excitement disorders has been proved [43,44].

Similarly, the previously independent dispareunia and vaginism disorders are gathered now under the chapter Genito-Pelvic Pain/Penetration Disorder.

There are two main reasons: first, the definition of vaginism as a "vaginal muscular spasm" is not supported by scientific evidence; second, fear of pain or penetration is shared by clinical descriptions of dispareunia and vaginism. With regard to the female orgasm disorder, this has not been modified [45].

The sexual aversion disorder has also been eliminated from the DSM-5 owing to its lack of empirical support, sharing a great number of features with phobias or other anxiety disorders; for that reason, it has not been included in the Sexual Dysfunctions chapter [46].

***Male** Male Hypoactive Sexual Desire has now an independent epigraph. In the case of erectile dysfunction character, the term "male" is suppressed. The male orgasm disorder is substituted by delayed ejaculation, the premature ejaculation epigraph not having been modified. Male dyspareunia or male sexual pain, present in the DSM IV TR, was not included in the DSM-5, because of its low prevalence [47].

It has been decided that the classification sexual dysfunctions due to medical reasons has been excluded, and the NOS category ("not otherwise specified") has been substituted with "other specific sexual dysfunctions" and "non-specific sexual dysfunctions". All these changes are included in Chart 2.1.

Another big change consists in the requirement for any given disorder to be present within the 75–100 % range of occurrences to be able to support a specific sexual dysfunction diagnostic, with the notable exception of those disorders induced by substances or medication. In addition, a 6-month minimum duration of the disorder is required. The condition of provoking interpersonal difficulties, as was specified in the DSM IV TR, has been modified into a condition resulting in a significant upset. On the other hand, a new exclusion criterion has been added: the disorder should not be explained by a non-sexual mental disorder and/or must result from serious difficulties in the relationship (for instance, gender-based violence) or other significant stressors.

DSM-IV-TR Diagnoses	Changes in DSM-5
Female dysfunctions	
Female hypoactive desire disorder	*Merged into:* **Female sexual interest/arousal disorder**
Female arousal disorder	
Female orgasmic disorder	*Unchanged*
Dyspareunia	*Merged into:* **Genito-pelvic pain/penetration disorder**
Vaginismus	
Male dysfunctions	
Male erectile disorder	*Changed to* Erectile disorder
Hypoactive sexual desire disorder	*Changed to* **Male** hypoactive sexual desire disorder
Premature (early) ejaculation	*Unchanged*
Male orgasmic disorder	*Changed to* **Delayed ejaculation**
Male dyspareunia	***Not Listed***
Male sexual Pain	
Other dysfunctions	
Sexual aversion disorder	***Deleted***
Sexual dysfunction due to a general medical condition	
Substance/medication-induced sexual dysfunction	*Unchanged*
Sexual dysfunction NOS	*Replaced by* **Other specified sexual dysfunctions** *and* **Unspecified sexual dysfunction**

Note: Individual changes to DSM nomenclature and criteria are in **bold**.

DSM: Diagnostic and Statistical Manual of Mental Disorders; IV-TR: 4th Edition-Text Revision; NOS: Not Otherwise Specified

Chart 2.1 Diagnostic changes proposed by the DSM 5 regarding sexual dysfunction

To the already existing specifications of "for life vs acquired disorder" and "generalized vs situational," a new importance dimension scale has been added, i.e., it is now possible to catalogue as mild, moderate and serious.

In addition, a new group of criteria named "associated characteristics" is included, where we can find:

1. Partner factors, such as sexual or health problems
2. Relationship factors, such as lack of communication or discrepancies regarding sexual stimuli

3. Individual vulnerability factors (such as poor self-image, history of sexual abuse), psychiatric comorbidity (depression, anxiety) or environmental stressors (loss of job)
4. Cultural and religious factors, such as prohibition regarding sexual intercourse and pleasure, and different attitudes toward sexuality
5. Medical factors for the prognosis, course or treatment [42]

The most important innovation, besides time and frequency requirements, is the introduction of a "list of criteria," appearing as an essential specific diagnostic criterion "A," which demands a certain number of sub-criteria for its diagnostic.

***Female** in the Female Sexual Interest/Arousal Disorder: four new criteria are added to the absence or diminution of sexual interest or in erotic thoughts or fantasies, and they take into account the absence or diminution of activity in four additional aspects of sexual life: beginning of the activity or ability to respond to the partner's attempts to make it start; excitement and pleasure; response to sexual signals, and feelings during the sexual activity (genital and nongenital). For the diagnosis, at least 3 of the 5 criteria are necessary.

For the diagnosis of female orgasm disorder it is necessary that one or both of the following criteria are present in 75–100 % of sexual intercourse episodes: absence, low frequency or delay of the orgasm and/or diminished intensity of the orgasm.

For the new genito-pelvic pain/penetration disorder to be diagnosed the following must take place in a persistent or recurring way: difficulty in vaginal penetration, stressed vulvovaginal pain during or at the moment of attempting vaginal penetration, associated fear or anxiety before, during or after penetration, and hardening or tension of the pelvic floor muscles when attempting penetration.

***Male:** Changes in the male sexual dysfunctions are more limited. Requirements for the diagnosis of hypoactive male sexual desire are the same as those in the DSM IV TR.

The criteria for erection disorder are similar to those present in previous editions, with the addition of the rate criteria (75–100 %), as well as diminished erectile rigidity. The epigraph of delayed ejaculation is similar to that of the DSM IV TR, as well as that for premature ejaculation, except for the time limit: ejaculation must occur approximately a minute after vaginal penetration. Although the diagnosis of premature ejaculation applies in the context of intercourse without vaginal penetration, in this case specific duration required is not defined. Finally, the criteria for substances or medication-induced sexual disorder [32] remain unchanged.

Despite its recent publication, the current nosography has not forestalled all criticism, and different authors such as Sarin et al. [48] argue that the new criteria exclude an important number of patients with desire and excitement diminution. Clayton [49] supports the same argument and states that the majority of women who fulfilled DSM IV TR criteria for sexual excitement disorder would not fulfill any of the criteria proposed for the female sexual interest/arousal disorder of the DSM 5 [19].

References

1. Damasio A. The feeling of what happens. New York: Harcourt Brace; 1999.
2. Latif EZ, Diamond MP. Arriving at the diagnosis of female sexual dysfunction. Fertil Steril. 2013;100(4):898–904.
3. Laumann E, Michael RT, Kolata G. Sex in America. A definitive survey. New York: Warner Books; 1995.
4. González-Torres MA, Salazar MA, Inchausti L, et al. Lifetime sexual behavior of psychiatric inpatients. J Sex Med. 2010;7(9):3045–56.
5. Money J. Handbook of sexology. New York: Elsevier/North Holland; 1977.
6. Rey RA. Fetal sex differentiation: from molecules to anatomy. Rev Chil Anat. 2001;19(1):75–82.
7. Rey RA, Grinspon RP. Normal male sexual differentiation and aetiology of disorders of sex development. Best Pract Res Clin Endocrinol Metab. 2011;25(2):221–38.
8. Kernberg O. Love relations. Normality and pathology. New Haven: Yale University Press; 1998.
9. Kernberg O. The sexual couple. A psychoanalytic exploration. Psychoanal Rev. 2011;98:217–45.
10. Stoller RJ. The transsexual experiment. London: Karnac Books; 1975.
11. Stoller RJ. Sex and gender. London: Karnac Books; 1984.
12. Stoller RJ. Presentations of gender. New Haven: Yale University Press; 1985.
13. Stoller RJ. Perversion, the erotic form of hatred. London: Karnac Books; 1986.
14. Bleichmar ED. La sexualidad femenina. Barcelona: Paidós; 1997.
15. Kernberg O. Limitations to the capacity to love. In: Kernberg O, editor. The inseparable nature of love and aggression. Washington, DC: American Psychiatric Publishing; 2012.
16. Kernberg O. Sexual pathology in borderline patients. In: Kernberg O, editor. The inseparable nature of love and aggression. DC: American Psychiatric Publishing. Washington; 2012.
17. Irigaray L. Das Geschlecht das nicht eins ist. Berlin: Merve Verlag; 1979. Spanish translation: Ese sexo que no es uno. Madrid: Akal; 2009.
18. Sadock VA. Normal human sexuality and sexual dysfunctions. In: Sadock BJ, Sadock VA, Ruiz P, editors. Kaplan & Sadock's comprehensive textbook of psychiatry. 9th ed. Baltimore: Lippincott, Williams & Wilkins; 2009.
19. APA. Diagnostic and statistical manual of mental disorders, DSM 5. 5th ed. Arlington, VA: American Psychiatric Association; 2013.
20. Basson R, Wierman ME, van Lankveld J, Brotto L. Summary of the recommendations on sexual dysfunctions in women. J Sex Med. 2010;7:314–26.
21. Shrifen JL, Monz BU, Russo PA, Segreti A, Johannes CB. Sexual problems and distress in United States women: prevalence and correlates. Obstet Gynecol. 2008;112:970–8.
22. Hayes RD, Bennett CM, Fairley CK, Dennerstein L. What can prevalence studies tell us about female sexual difficulty and dysfunction? J Sex Med. 2006;3:589–95.
23. Potter JE. A 60-year-old woman with sexual difficulties. JAMA. 2007;297:620–33.
24. Hayes R, Dennerstein L. The impact of aging on sexual function and sexual dysfunction in women: a review of population-based studies. J Sex Med. 2005;2:317–30.
25. Corrêa LQ, Cozzensa da Silva M, Rombaldi AJ. Sexual dysfunction symptoms in men age 40 or older; prevalence and associated factors. Rev Bras Epidemiol. 2013;16(2):444–53.
26. Smith AM, Lyons A, Ferris JA, et al. Incidence and persistence/recurrence of men's sexual difficulties: findings from the Australian longitudinal study of health and relationships. J Sex Marital Ther. 2013;39(3):201–15.
27. Corona G, Rastrelli G, Ricca V, et al. Risk factors associated with primary and secondary reduced libido in male patients with sexual dysfunction. J Sex Med. 2013;10(4):1074–89.
28. American Psychiatric Association. DSM-III: diagnostic and statistical manual of mental disorders. 3rd ed. Washington DC: American Psychiatric Press; 1980.
29. Masters WH, Johnson VE. Human sexual response. Boston: Little-Brown; 1966.

30. American Psychiatric Association. DSM IV TR: diagnostic and statistical manual of mental disorders. 4, text-revisionth ed. Washington, DC: American Psychiatric Press; 2000.
31. International Statistical Classification of Diseases and Health Related Problems. The ICD-10. Geneva: World Health Organization; 1992. Spanish translation: Trastornos Mentales y del Comportamiento, CIE 10. Madrid: Meditor; 1992.
32. López JM, Higueras A. Psicopatología de las tendencias instintivas y de las necesidades vitales. In: López JM, Higueras A, editors. Compendio de Psicopatología. 4th ed. Granada: Círculo de Estudios Psicopatológicos; 1996.
33. Ey H, Bernar P, Brisset Ch. Manuel de Psychiatrie. Spanish translation: Las psicosis delirantes crónicas. In: Ey H, Bernard P, Brisset Ch, editors. Tratado de Psiquiatría. 8th ed. Masson: Barcelona; 1978.
34. Joe Lee KC, Fahmy N, Brock GB. Sexual dysfunction in 2013: advances in epidemiology, diagnosis and treatment. Arab J Urol. 2013;11(3):194–202.
35. Giuliano F, Droupy S. Erectile dysfunction. Prog Urol. 2013;23(9):629–37.
36. Ludwig W, Phillips M. Organic causes of erectile dysfunction in men under 40. Urol Int. 2014;92(1):1–6. doi:10.1159/000354931.
37. Castilla del Pino C. Conductas paradigmáticas sexuales. In: Castilla del Pino C, editor. Introducción a la Psiquiatría. Tomo I. Problemas generales. Psico(pato)logía. 4th ed. Madrid: Alianza Editorial, S.A.; 1993. p. 215–62.
38. Fenichel O. The psychoanalytic theory of neurosis. New York: Routledge; 1999.
39. Althof SE, Schreiner-Engel P. The sexual dysfunctions. In: Gelder MG, López-Ibor JJ, Andreasen N, editors. New Oxford textbook of psychiatry. New York: Oxford University Press; 2001.
40. Santtila P, Jern P, Westberg L, Walum H, Pedersen CT, Eriksson E, et al. The dopamine transporter gene (DAT1) polymorphism is associated with premature ejaculation. J Sex Med. 2010;7:1538–46.
41. Janssen PK, Bakker SC, Réthelyi J, Zwinderman AH, Touw DJ, Olivier B, et al. Serotonin transporter promoter region (5-HTTLPR) polymorphism is associated with the intravaginal ejaculation latency time in Dutch men with lifelong premature ejaculation. J Sex Med. 2009;6:276–84.
42. IsHak WW, Tobia G. DSM-5 changes in diagnostic criteria of sexual dysfunction. Reprod Sys Sexual Disorders. 2013;2:122.
43. Graham CA, Sanders SA, Milhausen RR, McBride KR. Turning on and turning off: a focus group study of the factors that affect women's sexual arousal. Arch Sex Behav. 2004;33:527–38.
44. Janssen E, McBride KR, Yarber W, Hill BJ, Butler SM. Factors that influence sexual arousal in men: a focus group study. Arch Sex Behav. 2008;37:252–65.
45. Binik YM. The DSM, diagnostic criteria for vaginismus. Arch Sex Behav. 2010;39:278–91.
46. Brotto LA. The DSM, diagnostic criteria for sexual aversion disorder. Arch Sex Behav. 2010;39:271–7.
47. Binik YM. The DSM, diagnostic criteria for dyspareunia. Arch Sex Behav. 2010;39:292–303.
48. Sarin S, Amsel RM, Binik YM. Disentangling desire and arousal: a classificatory conundrum. Arch Sex Behav. 2013;42(6):1079–100.
49. Clayton AH, DeRogatis LR, Rosen RC, Pyke R. Intended or unintended consequences? The likely implications of raising the bar for sexual dysfunction diagnosis in the proposed DSM 5 revisions: 1. For women with incomplete los of desire or sexual receptivity. J Sex Med. 2012;9:2027–39.

Gender and Psychological Differences: Gender and Subjectivity

3

María Dolores Avia and Mª Luisa Sánchez-Bernardos

Abstract

Different units of analysis to study gender differences in psychological domains have been proposed. Basically, the present chapter is focused on the trait domain, characteristic adaptations, the objective biography, self-schemas, and character strengths. The main results point to some differences between men and women at the trait level, but the magnitude of this difference is generally small. Although the basic tendencies that represent traits are strongly dictated by heredity, some cultural and environmental influences have been signaled. Vital pathways, different patterns for managing work and the private life, interpersonal ways of treating others, etc., are among the different adaptations that men and women have to accomplish. At this level more gender differences have been found, although they are not stable because of cultural and historical changes. Research has found male/female differences in the structure of the self-schema, and some data on a few of the many character strengths also have appeared. According to all this, it is argued that differences can also be found in the objective biography of men and women. The conclusion, however, is that we should not emphasize peculiarities, since in the five domains of personality the differences are generally not large.

M.D. Avia (✉)
Psychology Faculty, Complutense University of Madrid, Madrid, Spain
e-mail: mariavia@psi.ucm.es

M.L. Sánchez-Bernardos
Complutense University of Madrid, Madrid, Spain

M. Sáenz-Herrero (ed.), *Psychopathology in Women*,
DOI 10.1007/978-3-319-05870-2_3

3.1 Introduction

Over the past few years, gender studies have become increasingly popular. Feminist orientations, sociological perspectives, and psychological models, among others, offer disparate points of view on the differences between men and women, often impregnated with ideological connotations that do not help researchers to properly understand this topic. Meanwhile, public opinion holds that gender differences are associated with deep psychological differences and with different ways of structuring subjectivity. How much about these approaches in society is true? Are they only social stereotypes about men and women, or do they have a firm basis?

Such types of questions require a complex, interactional answer, which could not possibly be set forth here. Instead, we offer information, some from our own research, that give us a few hints in examining the complex reality of gender.

If we want to study psychological differences, we have to start by choosing the units of analysis, that is, the kind of basic variables we are going to use. The different units may all be appropriate, but they provide various information about our subject. One unit of analysis that has been extensively studied is the concept of *trait*. A trait refers to the typical ways in which we behave, think, and feel, often showing that people are consistent over time and situations. A much respected area in personality deals with the study of personality traits. One researcher, Nettle [1], has made the point that in all lives there is a *leitmotiv* and has referred to traits that provide the leitmotiv in our lives. Whether we are a curious person, often changing from one interest to another, or an ill-tempered individual with frequent uncontrolled bursts of anger, the leitmotiv of our lives would appear once and again: in one case, the tendency to go from initial enthusiasm to boredom; in the other, the proclivity to be easily disturbed.

3.2 Gender Differences in Personality Traits

Psychological studies have shown that personality differences can be reduced to a few general traits. One group of studies (the lexical approach) analyzed the way in which ordinary people talk about personality. Careful analysis of those personality adjectives found five main global traits or dimensions, which were called the Big Five [2]. There is growing evidence that people in diverse cultures, using very different languages, view individual differences in personality traits in ways similar to the Big Five.

Personality researchers have investigated this five-factor personality structure, and most have used the NEO-PI-R developed by Costa and McCrae [3]. In 2005, McCrae and Terracciano [4] conducted a crosscultural study in which researchers from 50 cultures (our research group was one of them) took part, with a total of 11,985 subjects. The personality traits were assessed by the personality questionnaire NEO-PI-R (R form), which measures the factors neuroticism, extraversion, openness to experience, agreeableness, and conscientiousness. Neuroticism is the susceptibility to experience emotional instability and strong negative emotions, such as anxiety, anger, sadness, frustration, or hostility, to be easily worried, and to have unrealistic thoughts and ideas; its opposite is emotional stability. Extraversion is the tendency to show behaviors typical of a sociable, energetic, enthusiastic person, who is active, talkative, optimistic, and fun-loving. The opposite is introversion, a tendency to be aloof and reserved. Openness is the tendency to feel curiosity, to show open and imaginative behaviors, and to be interested in new ideas and unconventional values; conventional, down-to-earth people would be at the other end of the trait spectrum. Agreeableness involves a tendency to behave in a kind and pleasant way to others and to be compassionate, empathetic, soft-hearted, trusting, and attentive, just the opposite of the other pole, which shows cynical, suspicious, and uncooperative attitudes. A person with a high level of conscientiousness is likely to be organized, a hard worker, punctual, an achiever, and persistent, while a low level of conscientiousness involves being aimless, unreliable, lazy, and negligent.

Besides the general score for the trait, the NEO-PI-R also offers scores in specific aspects, which are called facets. Every trait is composed of six facets. In the study by McCrae et al., the five-factor structure emerged not only in the combined sample, but also in the great majority of cultures, showing that the same personality traits appear in very different environments. Regarding gender differences, considering the whole sample, it was found that women scored higher than men in the big five dimensions: they were more neurotic, extravert open, agreeable, and conscientious than men. The differences were more pronounced in the traits of neuroticism and agreeableness. In relation to facets, men were found to score higher than women in assertiveness, sensation-seeking, openness to ideas, and competence, while women exceeded men in anxiety, vulnerability, and openness to feelings and sensitivity to others.

Some female/male differences were modulated by age. This was the case of achievement motivation: in older people, men were higher achievers than women, but in younger subjects female scores in achievement motivation were higher than men's, perhaps revealing a generational effect of an increase in women's professional aspirations all over the world. Other male/female differences were modulated by the gender of the person who made the assessment. Thus, women (scoring higher in agreeableness) offered more positive assessments of others, especially when they assessed other women (i.e., they described them as scoring lower in neuroticism and higher in agreeableness).

The above differences, obtained with the combined sample of 50 countries, were also obtained when the analyses were carried out in the specific countries that participated in the study. Thus, it was found that differences between men and women were systematic and consistent with social stereotypes. They appeared despite variations in culture, age, and methods (self-report/other reported data). Therefore, as far as personality traits are concerned, it can be said that gender differences seem to be universal. However, these differences were quite small (0.5 standard deviation). Recently, Vianello and coworkers [5] found even smaller differences using implicit measures of traits in a large sample of more than 14,000 participants.

Different studies have tried to examine the relation between those five factors and mental health, psychological adjustment, and well-being. In general, the most predictive factor is neuroticism, which shows a systematic positive relation to maladjustment, a low level of well-being, and poor mental health. Neuroticism predisposes individuals to a wide range of psychiatric disorders: generalized anxiety disorder, panic disorder, phobias, major depression, dysthymic disorder, and borderline personality disorder are diagnosed more often in women than in men. Extraversion, on the contrary, emerges as a protective factor, being consistently associated with a higher level of well-being and good mental health. The openness factor is basically unrelated to the above variables, although specific facets may be related to maladjustment, and both agreeableness and conscientiousness show positive connections, although generally quite small, with well-being and adjustment.

Feingold [6] conducted four meta-analyses to examine gender differences in personality in the literature (1958–1992) and in normative data for well-known personality inventories (1940–1992). The results are consistent with those of the Big Five studies: men were found to be more assertive and had slightly higher self-esteem than women. Women scored higher than men in extraversion, anxiety, trust, and, especially, tender-mindedness. Gender differences in personality traits were generally constant across ages, years of data collection, educational levels, and nations.

In a much smaller study, Carrillo et al. [7] asked participants (half male, half female) to fill in the NEO-PI(R) and the Beck Depression Inventory. We were interested in the role that one of the Big Five factors, the trait of openness to experience, played in the development of symptoms of depression. It was found that one specific facet of the trait, openness to actions, was negatively related to experiencing symptoms of depression (it appeared to be adaptive), while the facet of openness to fantasy functioned as a predictor of dysphoric symptoms in the case of women, who scored higher in this facet.

It is well known that across the lifespan women are twice as likely as men to suffer from depression. Carrillo et al. [8] found a cluster of personality aspects that were related to the probability of having symptoms of depression, most of them related to experiencing highly negative emotions. The authors attribute this result to women having learned more negative emotional responses to life stimuli than men.

A very different personality trait that has received attention and shows differences between men and women is Snyder's self-monitoring construct, a less comprehensive trait than the Big Five categories, which belongs to a long tradition in psychology, the dramaturgical model [9, 10]. According to this, we behave the way others expect us to, we are alert to subtle cues in our social environment, and, in general, we engage in self-presentation. Research has examined interpersonal differences in the degree in which persons are able to control their expressive behavior, the emotional, non-verbal cues emitted, and the adequacy of their representations in different contexts. All of this is encompassed in the self-monitoring construct developed by Snyder in 1974. Typically high self-monitors are greatly concerned with the situational and the interpersonal appropriateness of their social behavior, are particularly sensitive to the expression and self-presentation of relevant others in social situations and use this as a guideline for regulating and controlling their own self-presentation [11]. Low self-monitors, on the contrary, are frequently guided by internal aspects, are less concerned with the social environment surrounding them, and value more the congruence among what they feel, think, and do. Low self-monitors, in turn, appear to have a lower repertoire of self-presentation skills and lower expressive control than high self-monitors, who show a rich range of skills with which to present themselves in society and a good ability to control their performance.

Many studies have been conducted to explore the consequences of these two interpersonal orientations. Data show that both the relation attitude–behavior (the congruence between what we believe and what we do) and the consistency across situations are mediated by self-monitoring: congruence is higher for the low self-monitor, and so is behavioral consistency. Executives, business managers, and salesmen, among others, are used to scoring highly in self-monitoring; accountants or researchers tend to score lower. As readers may have guessed, men frequently have higher scores on the self-monitoring scale than women (see Rojo and Carrillo [12]). One problem with high self-monitors is that usually they do not communicate their internal states; the problem with low self-monitors is their dependency on their internal states and the poor control they have over them when negative. Several studies have found a significant relation between self-monitoring and psychological maladjustment, basically social anxiety and negative emotions (see Sanz and Graña [13]). There are reasons to expect that those subjects with high coherence and high situational consistency would be especially vulnerable to developing depressive symptoms in the presence of stressful events. Results consistent with this hypothesis have been found [13].

A very relevant part of research on self-monitoring concerns the social worlds of the two groups. Results suggest two different orientations toward friendship and sexuality: friends of high self-monitors are chosen "to do activities", while low self-monitors have "friends for everything" [14]. In terms of sexuality, the first group shows "unrestricted" attitudes and values toward sexuality, while low self-monitors have relationships that are more monogamous and faithful [15]. In a replication of the latter study, Avia et al. [16] assumed that sexual orientation would be explained in part by gender. We considered that the social/interpersonal words, as well as the sexual orientation of men and women are often different, due in part to the role structure in western culture. Our hypothesis was that a restricted sexual orientation, defined by the need to have close emotional links and commitment within the sexual relation would be related to being a female, being of a lower age, and having a low score in self-monitoring. Results were consistent with our hypotheses, gender being the most discriminative variable.

To conclude this section, in many studies differences between women and men are found at the trait level, but these are generally small. The largest differences that have been found are in the domain of motor performance, some measures of sexuality (masturbation and attitudes toward uncommitted relationships), and physical aggression [17]. The cause of these differences is not easy to explain. Costa and MacCrae have a clearly biological viewpoint, and results in psychological literature are consistent with this. Other researchers, however, are more cautious: "Drawing conclusions about differences between men and women is a very tricky matter. Even if one finds such differences, it is hard to interpret them. Men and women differ biologically, but also socially. They often develop within societies which do or treat men and women unequally. Gender differences may be socially constructed rather than being biologically caused" [18]. In fact, some studies show that personality traits can change according to historical conditions. In one longitudinal study, Twenge [19] analyzed the mean levels of anxiety and neuroticism from 1950 to 1990, and found that anxiety increased significantly throughout this period. The authors conclude that cultural and historical changes produce parallel changes in personality. McCrae and Costa [20] recognized that a number of results suggest an environmental influence on traits: in women, the experience of divorce was related to decreased dominance and increased extraversion, while in Chinese undergraduates, openness and agreeableness increased when they lived in Canada.

3.3 Gender Differences in Characteristic Adaptations

Personality traits, although important, are not the only way to examine human personality. Personality traits are considered *basic tendencies* that determine recurring patterns of acting and feeling, but other concepts have also been used [20]. *Characteristic adaptations* are the particular forms in which people adapt to the environment. They are supposed to result from the interaction between basic tendencies and specific external influences (environment, situation, culture, etc.). While basic tendencies are assumed to be strongly determined by heredity, characteristic adaptations are culturally conditioned phenomena. Many personality psychologists have considered personality to be the particular way in which the person adapts to the environment, and have used concepts such as *personal projects* [21], *personal strivings* [22] or *personal narratives* [23] to capture relevant psychological differences. This level is related to processes, rather than structures. As has been said, the focus here is on "doing," while structural models are based on "having" [24]. In an influential paper, Dan McAdams asked readers a very deep question: "What do you know when you know a person?" [25]. Most of us would think that to say that we know somebody, we would need to know his/her interests, values, preferences, and motives; what would make this person happy or sad, what would be the type of behaviors that, as far as our comprehension goes, he/she would never do, and what others would be expected instead. Clearly, traits do not give us that information. Personality, at this level, is related to goals, plans, and particular ways of talking about ourselves.

Men and women have shown different patterns when handling work and private life. Levinson [26] studied the kind of dreams that encourage men and women, and found that men tend to place all their expectations in work, while the great majority of women give more importance to interpersonal relations. In general, women who have entered the labor market have not generated a change in competitive attitudes, nor they have considered professionalism as a focal aspect in their lives. Eagly and Johnson [27] proved that in the workplace, women often use a more democratic and participative style of decision-making than men, and some authors have found that even when the achievement levels of both were the same, men used to manifest an achievement style that was direct and competitive, while women had a relational style based on cooperation (see Barberá and Lafuente [28]). Since the seminal study by Helson et al. [29] was published, two different pathways in life have been associated with men and women: the pursuit way, or the commitment to work for him and the family/motherhood way for her. In this influential study, Helson et al. found that for women from 22 to 27 years old, motherhood was associated with more responsibility, self-control, and tolerance, and with decreases in self-confidence and sociability.

What are the processes through which the male and female universes emerge? What are the developmental processes that lead to differences in behaviors, attitudes, motivation, and self-concept? According to Gilligan [30] men subordinate their interpersonal relations to work, since society drives them to be dominant and self-confident, to value their goals and success at work, and to control their emotions. Women, in turn, are prepared to assume caregiving tasks, to dispense with aggressive attitudes, and to favor dependency, since they are expected to be loving and obedient, and to take good care of their physical appearance.

In the last 30 years, however, society and the expectations associated with men and women have changed both in the public and in the private domain. Newton and Stewart [31] have analyzed similarities and differences concerning personalities of women at midlife who had taken non-normative life courses. The results showed that women with a high professional status versus those in more traditional female professions were characterized as being more power-oriented, rational, "objective," and proud of themselves – traits conventionally associated with masculinity. Nevertheless, these high-status women did not score lower than women with more traditional professions on characteristics typified as feminine, such as warmth in interpersonal relationships, caring for others, and so on. Women without children scored lower than women with children on traits conventionally associated with femininity, that is, they were less compassionate, less protective of the people close to them, and tended to score higher on conventional masculine traits such as keeping people at a distance, value their own independence, and avoiding close interpersonal relationships. Have their personality traits impelled women to take one or another pathway, or has it been the pathway that has effected changes in these sub-traits? So far, we have not been able to answer this question.

In any case, at the level of characteristic adaptations more gender differences are found than when basic dispositions are studied. These differences are not stable, since they are affected by time, context, and working conditions.

3.4 Objective Biography and External Influences: The Role of Gender

From the above point of view, typical adaptations, in conjunction with the direct influence of the environment, shape our objective biography.

One of the fathers of personality psychology defined personality as simply biography [32], and indeed personality can be inferred from a person's life story. From a sociological point of view it is clear that, in addition to our particular ways of adapting to private and working life, external influences of the environment differ greatly according to our gender. For example, within the same family the social roles of men and women determine different expectations about them that may eventually lead to differences in important life events. There is already ample evidence that certain developmental processes operate differently for men and women.

One experiment illustrates neatly the ways in which girls and boys react according to gender stereotypes. Hoffner [33] interviewed children aged 7–12 about their favorite TV character. Nearly all boys and about half of the girls selected same-sex favorites. Regression analyses used perceived character traits (attractiveness, strength, humor, intelligence, and social behavior) to predict wishful identification and social interaction with characters. For male characters, wishful identification was predicted by intelligence and (for girls only) humor; social interaction was predicted by intelligence, attractiveness, and (for boys only) strength. In marked contrast, for female characters (chosen only by girls), attractiveness was the only significant predictor.

Research into gender differences has expanded to reach technological domains; a great deal of interest is focused on the way in which men and women present themselves on the Internet in relation to personality and social behavior. Dunn and Guadagno [34] have found that teenage girls and adult women are more prone to reveal information about themselves or about their family than boys and men. At the same time, girls and women present themselves more positively on socio-emotional characteristics than men. What is actually interesting is that although both groups used different strategies for self-presentation in the virtual world (creating a more attractive personality, for example), men and women selected "characters" that differed from themselves, but fitted neatly with the social norms (i.e., thinner, warmer, and so on, for women).

3.5 Gender Differences in Self-Schemas

The particular way in which we see ourselves is in part determined by our history. We cannot see ourselves in the same way if we fail or if we succeed. We learn what we are in part by observing what we do. But the self-concept is also determined by our basic tendencies and by the regular way in which we adapt to situations.

Research into self-schemas has found that there are two basic types: an independent construction, separate from others, and an interdependent, structure, connected to others [35]. Self-schemas are important: they determine how we process information, the way in which we make comparisons with others, the information we remember and how we compensate when under threat. According to several results, men are more inclined to have an independent self-schema, while women usually show a connected type of self ("individuality" versus "sociality" [36]). A study by Guimond and his coworkers [37] about the processes by which self-stereotyping is construed found that women score higher in interdependent self-construal, whereas men score higher on independence.

Joseph and others [38] nicely illustrated how gender norms influence the way in which we establish our self-esteem. For men, thinking of themselves as independent and unique was associated with high self-esteem, while for women self-esteem was linked to thinking of the self as connected. Block and Robins [39] found that in the age range 14 to 23, self-esteem (concordance between the real and the ideal self) increases in boys and decreases in girls. Throughout that time, men become more self-confident, but women lose confidence in themselves. Women with high self-esteem valued close relationships with others; men with high self-esteem were more controlled and emotionally distant in relationships with others. The authors conclude that these differences in relationships reflect the very different expectations society holds for what it means to be a man or a woman. People whose personalities fit the cultural expectations are more likely to feel good about themselves and have a self-concept close to their ideal self.

Differences in self-esteem, however, are not stable. One meta-analysis by Kling et al. [40] showed that self-esteem grew for boys, but not for girls from childhood to adolescence and high school, but this difference was smaller in adults and in old age.

The literature on gender differences in autobiographical memory, on the other hand, (the recollection of personal events), is consistent. Women construct autobiographical narratives in a more detailed, longer, more emotional and coherent form than men, a difference that can be traced back to the way parents talk to their children [41]. Very early in development, the parents teach their children which events are reportable and how to relate them, and these lessons are contoured by culture and gender. Particularly, the findings have signaled that talking about emotional events is a gender-typed activity. Mothers talk more about emotions with her daughters than with her sons.

Parents can also encourage their children to play music, to tell or read stories, to play "as if" and other activities related to fantasy that, in the course of development, make fantasy-prone individuals [42]. Several studies showed that women [43] and adolescent girls [44] are greater fantasizers than men and boys.

3.6 Character Strengths of Men and Women

In the few last decades, positive psychology, a school of thought that has become very popular, has advocated that we should devote more time and effort to studying the positive, adaptive parts in our lives [45]. Although not centered properly in personality aspects, the positive psychology movement has offered an alternative way of looking at human behavior and has proposed 24 "character strengths" that make a good life possible and provide a new, healthy way of assessing people. Thus, strengths of creativity, curiosity, temperance, justice, courage, wisdom and knowledge, transcendence, open-mindedness, love of learning and ability to have a perspective in life (related to the virtue of wisdom and knowledge), love, kindness and social intelligence (which belong to the virtue of Humanity), forgiveness, humility, prudence and self-regulation (included in the broader virtue of temperance), bravery, persistence, integrity, and vitality (virtue of courage), citizenship, fairness, and leadership (belonging to the virtue of justice), and appreciation of beauty and excellence, gratitude, hope, humor, and spirituality (considered part of transcendence), have become significant areas in which to examine the psychological universe of people.

Are there gender differences in strengths? From the many studies conducted, only a few show systematic differences between men and women. There is a well-documented advantage of women over men on scales of *emotional intelligence*: they score between one quarter and one half a standard deviation over men, a moderate sized group difference [46]. In citizenship or social responsibility, women are more likely than men to exhibit *altruism and empathy* and to feel guilty when they do not attend to the needs of others, and they are also more likely to engage in voluntary services in their community [47]. A number of studies suggest more *modest self-presentation* in women than in men [48]. Although a small difference, self-esteem tends to be lower in women and narcissism higher in men [49]. As for transcendent strengths, women score higher in connectedness, transportation, and elevation [50]. Regarding the strength of *spirituality*, it is ubiquitous in empirical research that women *are more religious* than men, although that may reflect social and cultural rules. Gender differences in *humor* have been reported, in which men are more likely than women to joke, tease, and kid, but the differences could be ascribed to role differences in accepted standards of behavior and status. With regard to other strengths, the differences are negligible.

Recently, Biswas-Diener [51] evaluated character strengths across cultures. Kenyan Maasai, Inughuit in Northern Greenland and University of Illinois students filled out the Valued in Action Classification (VIA) to assess strengths of character. Results showed strong similarities among cultures, but also gender differences between and within them. Lindley et al. [52] presented data on the character strengths of a large UK sample and found that women typically scored higher on strengths than men. However, four of the top five "signature strengths" of the UK men and women overall were the same (open-mindedness, fairness, curiosity, and love of learning). Shimai and others [53] investigated gender and cultural differences in the distribution of character strengths in Japan and North America and found that women were more likely than men to report strengths of love and kindness, whereas men were more likely to report bravery and creativity.

Conclusion

In the 1970s Maccoby and Jacklin [54], in a frequently cited study, reviewed studies of gender differences using qualitative methods. Their conclusion was that there were many popular beliefs about differences that were unfounded, since gender-related differences were generally small. Political and scientific elements intervene when comparing men and women. When the first approaches to gender differences were made in the 1970s, scholars were skeptical about differences, gender stereotypes were challenged, and sameness was promoted [55]. During the 1980s and 1990s, evidence on differences was gathered, especially concerning personality and social behavior. A more recent study by Hyde [17] again proposes the similarity between genders. Men and women are more alike than they are different.

At the trait level, psychological differences have been found between men and women that are similar in different cultures and times and that have appeared with different measurement methods [56]. These differences, however, are small, smaller than individual variation within genders. Greater contrast is found at the level of characteristic adaptations, where remarkable differences appeared in the way in which men and women manage both their private life and their work. Perhaps because of this, the objective biography would generally include distinct life events for both. As a consequence, the structure of the self also becomes different. Among the many character strengths proposed, only a few show gender differences and those are favorable to women.

The strikingly similar male/female differences in personality traits over cultures have allowed researchers to propose biological explanations. In contrast, trait differences could also be thought of as the sediment of a series of specific culture and society-based differences that have stabilized through time, social impact, and behavior itself. In both cases, stable trait differences are expected, but the explanations would differ. The exact nature of gender differences and the roles of the evolutionary hardwiring versus social structure in bringing them about remain to be defined. In the meantime, however, we should be aware that too much emphasis on differences can be costly for individuals and society. Dorothy Parker wrote:

Man delights in novelty.
Love is woman's moon and sun;
Man has other forms of fun.
Woman lives but in her lord;
Count to ten, and man is bored.
With this the gist and sum of it,
What earthly good can come of it?
Despite (small) real differences, we can communicate with each other.

References

1. Nettle D. Personality. What makes you the way you are. New York: Oxford University Press; 2007.
2. Goldberg LR. Language and individual differences: the search for universals in personality lexicons. In: Wheeler L, editor. Review of personality and social psychology. Beverly Hills, CA: Sage; 1981. p. 141–65.
3. Costa P, McCrae R. NEO-PI- R: professional manual. Odessa, FL: Psychological Assessment Resources; 1992.
4. McCrae RR, Terracciano A, and 78 members of the project "Personality Profiles of Cultures", among them Avia, M.D. and Sánchez Bernardos, M.L. Universal features of personality traits from the observer's perspective. Data from fifty cultures. J Pers Soc Psychol 2005;88:547–61.
5. Vianello M, Schabel K, Sriram N, Noreck B. Gender differences in implicit and explicit personality traits. Pers Individ Dif. 2013;2013(55):994–9.
6. Feingold A. Gender differences in personality: a meta-analysis. Psychol Bull. 1994;116:429–56.
7. Carrillo J, Rojo N, Sánchez-Bernardos ML, Avia MD. Openness to experience and depression. Eur J Psychol Assess. 2001;17:130–6.
8. Carrillo J, Rojo N, Staats W. Women and vulnerability to depression: some personality and clinical factors. Span J Psychol. 2004;7:29–39.
9. Goffman E. The presentation of self in everyday life, Anchor books. Garden City, NY: Doubleday; 1959.
10. Snyder M. Public appearances, private realities. New York: Freeman; 1986.
11. Snyder M. Self-monitoring processes. In: Berkowitz L, editor. Advances in experimental social psychology, vol. 13. New York: Academic; 1980.
12. Rojo N, Carrillo J. La presentación de uno mismo a los demás: ¿habilidad o defensa? (The presentation of self to others: skill or defense?). In: Avia MD, Sánchez-Bernardos ML, editors. Personalidad: aspectos cognitivos y sociales (Personality. Cognitive and social aspects). Madrid: Pirámide; 1995. p. 413–25.
13. Sanz J, Graña JL. Factores psicosociales y síntomas depresivos: el caso de la auto-observación (Psychosocial factors and depressive symptoms: the case of self-monitoring). Psicothema. 1991;3:381–99.
14. Snyder M, Gangestad S, Simpson JA. Choosing friends as activity partners: the role of self-monitoring. J Pers Soc Psychol. 1983;51:181–90.
15. Snyder M, Simpson JA, Gangestad S. Personality and sexual relations. J Pers Soc Psychol. 1986;51:181–90.
16. Avia MD, Carrillo J, Rojo N. Personalidad y diferencias sexuales: el papel del sexo, la edad y la experiencia (Personality and sexual differences: the role of sex, age and experience). Revista de Psicología Social. 1990;5:7–22.
17. Hyde JS. The gender similarities hypothesis. Am Psychol. 2005;66:581–92.
18. Pervin LA, Cervone D, John OP. Personality. Theory and research. New York: Wiley; 2005.
19. Twenge J. Birth cohort, social change and personality: the interplay of dysphoria and individualism in the 20th century. In: Cervone D, Mischel W, editors. Advances in personality science. New York: Guilford; 2002.
20. McCrae R, Costa P. The five-factor theory of personality. In: John OP, Robins RW, Pervin LA, editors. Handbook of personality: theory and research. New York: Guilford; 2010.
21. Little BR, Salmela-Aro R, Phillips S. Personal projects pursuit: goals, acting and human flourishing. New York: Psychology Press; 2006.
22. Emmons RA. Personal strivings, daily life events and psychological and physical well-being. J Pers. 1991;59:453–73.
23. McAdams DP. Personal narratives and the life story. In: Pervin LA, John OP, editors. Handbook of personality. New York: Theory and research. Guilford; 1999. p. 478–500.
24. Cantor N. From thought to behaviour: "having" and "doing" in the study of personality and cognition. Am Psychol. 1990;45:735–50.

25. McAdams DP. What do you know when you know a person? J Pers. 1995;63:365–96.
26. Levinson DJ. A conception of adult development. Am Psychol. 1986;41:3–13.
27. Eagly AH, Johnson BT. Gender and leadership style: a meta-analysis. Psychol Bull. 1990;108: 233–56.
28. Barberá E, Lafuente MJ. Procesos de sexuación e implicaciones de género en la etapa adulta (Sexuation processes and gender implications in adulthood). In: Fernández J, editor. Varones y mujeres. Desarrollo de la doble identidad del sexo y del género (Men and women: development of dual identity of sex and gender). Madrid: Pirámide; 1996.
29. Helson R, Mitchell V, Moane G. Personality and patterns of adherence and nonadherence to the Social Clock. J Pers Soc Psychol. 1984;46:1079–96.
30. Gilligan C. In a different voice: psychological theory and women's development. Cambridge: Harvard University Press; 1982.
31. Newton NJ, Stewart AJ. The road not taken: women's life paths and gender-linked personality traits. J Res Pers. 2013;47:306–16.
32. Murray HA. Explorations in personality. New York: Oxford University Press; 1938.
33. Hoffner C. Children's wishful identification and parasocial interaction with favorite television characters. J Broadcast Electron Media. 1996;40:389–402.
34. Dunn RA, Guadagno RE. My avatar and me: gender and personality predictors of avatar-self-discrepancy. Comput Human Behav. 2012;28:97–106.
35. Markus H, Kitayama S. Culture and the self: implications for cognition, emotion and motivation. Psychol Rev. 1991;98:224–53.
36. Lang-Takac E, Osterweil Z. Separateness and connectedness: Differences between the genders. Sex Roles. 1992;27:277–89.
37. Guimond S, Chatard A, Martinot D, Crisp RJ, Redersdorff S. Social comparison, self-stereotyping and gender differences in self-construals. J Pers Soc Psychol. 2006;90:221–42.
38. Joseph RA, Markus H, Tafarodi RW. Gender and self-esteem. J Pers Soc Psychol. 1992;63: 391–402.
39. Block J, Robins RW. A longitudinal study of consistency and change in self-esteem from early adolescence to early adulthood. Child Dev. 1993;64:909–23.
40. Kling KC, Hyde JS, Showers CJ, Buswell BN. Gender differences in self-esteem: a meta-analysis. Psychol Bull. 1999;125:470–500.
41. Nelson K, Fivush R. The emergence of autobiographical memory. A social cultural development theory. Psychol Rev. 2004;111:486–511.
42. Sánchez-Bernardos ML, Avia MD. Fantasy. In: Levesque JR, editor. Encyclopaedia of adolescence, vol. 2. New York: Springer; 2011. p. 984–89.
43. Merckelbach H, Horselenberg R, Muris P. The Creative Experience Questionnaire (CEQ): a brief self-report measure of fantasy proneness. Pers Individ Dif. 2001;31:987–95.
44. Sánchez-Bernardos ML, Avia MD. Personality correlates of fantasy proneness among adolescents. Pers Individ Dif. 2004;37(5):1069–79.
45. Seligman MP. The president's address. Am Psychol. 1999;54:559–62.
46. Mayer JD, Salovey P, Caruso DR. Models of emotional intelligence. In: Sternberg JR, editor. Handbook of intelligence. Cambridge: Cambridge University Press; 2000. p. 396–420.
47. Flanagan C. Citizenship. In: Peterson C, Seligman MP, editors. Character, strengths, and virtues. Washington, DC: American Psychological Association; 2004. p. 369–89.
48. Exline JJ, Lobel C. The perils of outperformance: sensitivity about being the target of a threatening upward comparison. Psychol Bull. 1999;125:307–37.
49. Kachorek L, Exline J, Campbell W, Baumesiter R, Joiner T, Krueger MJ. Humility and modesty. In: Peterson C, Seligman MP, editors. Character, strengths, and virtues. Washington, DC: American Psychological Association; 2004. p. 461–75.
50. Haidt J, Keltner D. Appreciation of beauty and excellence. In: Peterson C, Seligman MP, editors. Character, strength, and virtues. Washington, DC: American Psychological Association; 2004. p. 537–51.

51. Biswas-Diener R. From the equator to the north pole: a study of character strenghts. J Happiness Stud. 2006;7:293–310.
52. Lindley P, Maltby J, Wood AM, Harrington J, Peterson C, Park N, Seligman MP. Character strengths in the United Kingdom: the VIA inventory of strengths. Pers Individ Dif. 2007;43: 341–51.
53. Shimai S, Otare K, Park N, Peterson C, Seligman MP. Convergence of character strengths in American and Japanese young adults. J Happiness Stud. 2006;7:311–22.
54. Maccoby EE, Jacklin CN. The psychology of sex differences. Stanford, CA: Stanford University Press; 1974.
55. Eagly AH. The science and politics of comparing women and men. Am Psychol. 1995;50:145–58.
56. Costa P, Terracciano A, McCrae R. Gender differences in personality traits across cultures: robust and surprising findings. J Pers Soc Psychol. 2001;81:322–31.

Self-Identity and Gender Differences 4

Miguel Angel González-Torres and Aranzazu Fernandez-Rivas

Abstract

After reviewing the origins of the concepts of identity and Self, departing from historical psychoanalytical proposals, special focus is placed on the complex process of identity construction in both genders, including core gender identity and gender role identity. Different ways of approaching sexual orientation and sexual behavior are examined, introducing the concept of sexual fluidity and studying the importance of individual variations in those dimensions. The role of others in the process of identity building is analyzed, from the impact of others' sexuality to the influence of large group processes. Depositation phenomena and mechanisms of transgenerational transmission are debated. In the social context, special attention is paid to the imbrication of violence and sexuality, showing differences between men and women regarding this combination throughout history. Finally, a point is made on how social considerations of the respective value of men and women may have a very real and deleterious impact, much beyond feelings of worthlessness or superiority.

4.1 Introduction

Identity is a concept that in its own way eludes us. Intuitively, we know what it is, but it is not easy to define and it has nuances that are overwhelming to those who venture into its depths. Its richness covers the fields of psychology, biology, sexuality, history, sociology and—why not?—economics and politics. Without question, if we're talking about identities that are anomalous, psychiatry should be introduced into the scenario in order to provide comprehension and meaning. To

M.A. González-Torres (✉) • A. Fernandez-Rivas
Department of Neuroscience, University of the Basque Country (UPV/EHU), Leioa, Spain

Psychiatry Service, Basurto University Hospital, Bilbao, Spain
e-mail: miguelangel.gonzaleztorres@osakidetza.net; aranzazu.fernandezrivas@osakidetza.net

M. Sáenz-Herrero (ed.), *Psychopathology in Women*,
DOI 10.1007/978-3-319-05870-2_4

attempt to examine all of these fields in-depth would surpass the limits of this text, which is why a choice is necessary. In order to provide the reader with some orientation, we are planning to emphasize particular aspects of self-identity as it relates to gender, from a perspective that gives precedence to a psychological point of view, and specifically one in which psychoanalytical theory serves as a guide that is not unique, but certainly preferential.

There are not many references in Freudian writings relating to the concept of identity. It was Erikson [1] who established the key aspects of the concept, which we still consider relevant. Erik Erikson described identity as a global synthesis of functions of the Self on one hand and on the other hand the consolidation of a sense of solidarity with the ideals of a group and group identity. He thus indicated that identity also implied the rejection of a series of unacceptable roles, in a manner in which this constructive process could have affirmative (this is how I am) and negative aspects (this isn't how I am).

Otto Kernberg [2] developed this vision of identity, broadening it, observing that the definition of the ego identity formulated originally by Erikson included the integration of the concept of self. For Kernberg, an approach from the theory of object relations extends this definition by adding the corresponding integration of the concepts of significant others. Westen [3, 4] had previously revised the empirical and theoretical literature on identity and self, signaling the primary components of identity: a sense of continuity in time, an emotional commitment with a set of representations of the Self that have been self-defined, relationships consisting of nuclear roles and values, and ideal standards of the Self, the development and acceptance of a *weltanschauung* that grants significance to life, and a sort of acknowledgement from the significant others regarding our place in this world.

Identity is found to be continually under construction and in this substantial process, the people with whom we establish relationships (the others) play a key part. In his famous concept of the "mirror stage," Lacan [5] describes the so-called imaginary dimension in the creation of the I. This is a period of child development in which the child sees himself through the eyes of his mother, and upon seeing this image he builds his identity. In this complex process, the desires of the mother and the others are introduced, such as the need to reconcile our identity with those that others assign to us. To that end, we feel obligated to hide aspects about ourselves that may be fundamental, generating an identity and a presence that is always partial and at the same time a continuous longing to recover what we felt obliged to hide. The pressure toward conformity, toward a more-or-less subtle accommodation of the far-removed desire, is grounded in the deepest parts of our nature. For this reason, in a certain way, within each personal identity, we can find traces of the society to which that individual belongs, traces that indicate the pressures taken in so that the subject, in development, should occupy the space for growth available and no more. In this sense, Fromm [6] assures us that the development implies "mystification", a process that provides us with a costume in which we can present ourselves, and with which we can relate to others.

Identity is very topical in psychoanalytical publications, with whole issues dedicated to it (e.g., Ermann [7]). Undoubtedly, this multiplicity of attention, in a world as heterogeneous as that of psychoanalysis, challenges us with definitions that are very different with regard to the concept of identity, which are sometimes difficult or impossible to integrate. The idea of identity that we deal with below, in this text, reflects a mode of thought regarding this term that is characteristic of current psychoanalytical authors belonging to various theoretical schools, from the North American ego psychology, the most contemporary version, to the theory of object relations or relational or intersubjective lines of thought.

In order to clarify our position further, we will say that we consider identity to be an internal representation of our global person, which incorporates a significant temporal aspect: a vision of the past, which explains where we have come from, including a social and familial narrative, a vision of the present that includes our place in the world and a vision of the future that includes our ideals and desires for tomorrow.

4.2 Concept of Self

When reviewing psychoanalytical literature regarding the Self, there is a degree of confusion about the term. Different authors utilize the same terms in order to indicate different realities. The concept of "I" overlaps with that of the Self, or with that of the "ego," or even with that of the person. The peculiar translation by Strachey does not help in this process, taking the German "*Ich*," seemingly under pressure from Ernest Jones, and instead of changing it to the English "I," as in other languages, ended up transforming it into the peculiar "ego," which has had so much success in Anglo-Saxon psychoanalytical literature and even in international popular literature. Even Freud utilizes the term "ego" (*Ich*) in two ways: to refer to a part of the psychic apparatus in his structural theory of the mind, and also in order to indicate the entire person, or Self. This equivalence between the person and the Self continues to this day, from authors such as Meissner [8], a true exegete of the work of Freud, reaching levels of analysis of extreme complexity.

Meissner [8] points out some fundamental characteristics of the Self, especially in its role as generator of structure.

- The Self is equal to the person, therefore is a source of agency
- The Self includes the three components (Id, Ego, Superego) as substructures
- The Self includes experiential and non-experiential dimensions
- The Self-as-agent is the source of all the actions of a person
- The Agency of the Self is shared by the Id, the Ego, and the Superego
- The relation of the Self with the tripartite model is supraordinated
- The intrasystemic and intersystemic conflicts reflect patterns in the diversification and interaction of the functions of the Self
- The concept of the Self as a structure contrasts with that of the Self as representation
- The internationalisations are primarily modifications of the system of the Self and may be ascribed secondarily to substructures or representations

We can see that the concept of Self varies according to various schools of thought and authors. We observe two fundamental ways in which the Self can be conceived. One is as a substructure, considering the Self as being equivalent to the I, or rather, taking the Self as a structure of a greater entity that contains within itself all of the parts of the psychic apparatus. In this sense, the concept of the Self runs parallel to that of the I in the work of Freud, which alternates between the two uses described. On the other hand, there is a different usage, which we consider to be greater today. This would be the use of the Self as representation, equivalent to the global person, especially in the context of object relations. This is the more standard use in contemporary psychoanalytical literature. Applebaum [9] considers the structure to be composed of "stable configurations of the Self and the object," thus developing the classic formulations of Kernberg [10].

In summation, we should say that in this text we consider the Self to be equivalent to the global person, following the extensive use of the concept indicated in the work of Meissner [8], as well as many other authors. To that end, the idea of the identity of the Self (self-identity), in our case, reflects the very conception of our person in the most global sense, including one's generic identity, with all of the subtleties that we describe below.

We should also indicate that the confluence of the concepts of self-identity and gender lead us to different analyses. One is the examination of the process of acquisition of gender identity and of gender role identity. The other is a reflection regarding the different factors that affect the construction of self-identity in men and women. We will touch upon the first topic and concentrate more on the second, which, to our understanding, has not been sufficiently dealt with in the literature, and is of great interest.

4.3 Gender Identity and Gender Role Identity

What are we talking about, in natural terms, when we refer to gender identity?

1. What I am. This is the result of what my biological body affirms and the response that society provides in the face of it. It is important to highlight this aspect: contemporary research indicates that feedback from parents is vital for this initial identity construction relating to gender to take place. The body alone is not sufficient. To paraphrase Freud, we should say that anatomy is, normally, destiny.
2. How I feel. Independently of the body, I can feel like a woman or a man, or perhaps something intermediate between the two. Certainly, 1 and 2 tend to coincide, but that is not obligatory.
3. How I act. I represent a social role in front of the others, which includes a multitude of subtleties relating to attire, language, movement, interaction.
4. Whom I desire. Men and women exclusively, or fluidly, one or the other, according to the moment. . .
5. Whom I select as a life partner. This can be a choice in line with the above, or not.

Within this conceptual variety, two elements occupy a preferential position [11]. They are core gender identity, based on biological and constitutional aspects, and gender role identity, built on a foundation of social and collective provisions. We direct our reflections here toward those points in particular.

The concept of bisexuality in Freud occupies a very central position in his thoughts regarding human sexual development. The social and academic attitude toward this proposal has gone back and forth throughout the years. Often, it has even been vehemently rejected. Nowadays, it has been accepted once again, in line with the increased attention currently paid to the very early relationship with parental figures, especially the mother. The processes of identification and fusion with the mother are today considered key to generic identity formation, which for Stoller [12, 13] is firmly established before the age of 2 years, before any type of Oedipal eventuality. Authors such as Benjamin [14] draw attention to the limitations of the classic Freudian theory on the subject and propose a more integrated vision of the processes that constitute gender. For this author, the boy and girl want what they don't have, in addition to what they have, not instead of what they have. Logically, from this point of reflection, the classic lines of thinking regarding "fault," "injury," "envy," or even "castration," acquire different nuances.

Some people, including some researchers, are uncomfortable with this complex reality and even reject it. It is certain that a good part of the population, possibly the majority of the population, displays a consistency between inner life, social role, desire, and partner choice, but undoubtedly there is another group, perhaps larger than we believe, that does not comply with this generality. For a while now, homosexual men and women have also been becoming a field of study and every day we know more about their lives and their internal world as well as their relationships. However, we still know little about those who do not fall under that narrow definition of homosexuality. Those who show orientation or identities that are more complex tend to be considered outliers in the world of science and academia, set apart from normal studies. The result is a general loss. A loss, perhaps, for these people, who could see themselves being more integrated into the social norms in which they live, and without question a loss for us, since the study of different lives can enormously enrich our comprehension of key phenomena such as identity, sexuality, and gender.

Without question, the study of "different" sexualities and their construction is perceived as a danger within society in general. Sexuality, understood in the broader sense of Stoller [15] as that which has to do with gender identity and desire, is a fundamental pillar of individual and collective identity. To establish other possible sexual identities would provoke a furious reaction in some and a more discreet rejection from almost everyone else. There is something intimate that breaks when we are faced with things that might be different, that we might desire other people or feel differently. It seems like the acquisition of this generic identity, especially the masculine identity, is a laborious and fragile process that we should take care of and protect. The conduct of these extreme minorities that go from rejection to frank aggression to those who are different show a major trace of tendencies and movements that affect society as a whole. Some turn their attention toward the social–political background of the gender roles, and the unequal distribution of power that they entail, considering social forces, expressed through certain individual attitudes, as the ultimate cause of the anxiety that is felt in the face of the possibility of there being differences. In our opinion, the anxiety has a deeper origin. Damasio [16] describes the so-called extended Self, which originates in the autobiographical conscience and thus comes from that identity continuity through time: I am who I was yesterday and who I was before then. We should say that gender identity and the disposition of our desire constitute aspects that are absolutely nuclear within this extended Self. When the final certainties relating to gender are called into question, panic comes to the fore.

The situation regarding sexuality in contemporary psychoanalytical theory deserves reflection, even if it is brief. We should say that the central position that sexuality occupied within the origins of psychoanalysis has changed greatly. Amazingly, in spite of the growing attention that biological matters are awakening in many neighboring disciplines such as cognitive theory, psychoanalysis has moved away from what were its first signs of identity. The relational perspective, already present in the works of Erikson [17], more intensely in the contributions of Klein et al. [18] and followers, and today more so in the relational theories of Mitchell [19], has in a way desexualized the sexual encounter to the point of considering it simply a variation of the way in which humans connect with each other. Nonetheless, as Fonagy indicates in a review [20], the reality around us, which shows us the constant presence of sexual inhibitions and lack of satisfaction, conflicts, and perversions, the tremendous intensity of guilt, jealousy, and rage that are involved in sexuality, still remind us the central role of sexual function. Possibly Kernberg [21], with his more integrated model that assigns a greater role to drives, is one of the few contemporary theorists, together with Laplanche [22], who continue to consider sexuality to be central to the internal world and to human behavior.

Nancy Chodorow [23] warns us of the necessity of valuing sexuality in an individual manner and of avoiding empty generalizations. She criticizes overgeneralization, universalism, and essentialism and advocates consideration of the individual route, which each subject goes through, and of the thousand different ways of creating global and gender identity. She indicates to us, referring to the woman: "It is apparent that gender, like selfhood, must be individually unique. . .There are many psychologies of women. Each woman creates her own psychological gender through emotionally and conflictually charged unconscious fantasies that help construct her inner world, that projectively imbue cultural conceptions, and that interpret her sexual anatomy. By making some unconscious fantasies and interpretations more salient than others, each woman creates her own prevalent animation of gender." It is difficult to synthesize the description of such a complex process any better. It might be possible to extend this reflection to men as well.

We frequently talk about gender identity or about sexual orientation as if we were talking about traces that, once fully formed at the end of adolescence, remained immovable forever. Recent works, such as that of Lisa Diamond [24], put the concept of sexual fluency on the table. They use this term to refer to a characteristic pertaining to an unknown but significant number of women who feel attraction toward different genders at different points in their lives, without identifying completely with one stable gender role. Diamond points to some facts that require explanation: changes in sexual identity over time, the sensation that identity and orientation do not presuppose anything definitive with regard to the future, the fact that for a group of women, non-exclusive attractions are more often the norm than the exception, and the diminished importance of early experiences with regard to predicting future identity and orientation. This sexual fluidity seems to affect women more than men, who may keep themselves more rigidly glued to their identity and choice of sexual object starting in adolescence. Nonetheless, as the author indicates, these groups of the population have not been sufficiently studied, and have been considered anomalies, outliers, that have distorted the vision of the whole. A specific study could lead us to reconsider this matter in the case of men as well.

4.4 Construction of Identity

The construction of a global identity within which gender identity occupies an important place deserves specific attention. Do men and women develop a different constructive process? Boys and girls depart from a psycho-biological structure, which develops later within a familial and social context. The possible differences between men and women within this process have been explored insufficiently, but it seems clear that, given the existing differences relating to genetics, biology, psychology, experience, social relations, etc., there could be differences worth mentioning. The identity structure of an individual is always complex, made up of multiple layers, the product of successive significant interpersonal links over time.

Freud presents a famous dictum: "Anatomy is destiny," signaling the fundamental importance of all things biological in defining the identity of the individual, in general, and especially in the sexual realm. In his opinion, the structure of our body was the frame of identity, the scaffold upon which the perception that the individual has of himself and his place in the world is construed. Over the years, different authors, inside and outside psychoanalysis, have called into question Freud's dictum, ascribing more value to all that is acquired throughout one's experiences, be they within the confines of the family or in society in general.

Possibly, the concept of identity and representation of the Self are accepted as equivalent in the contemporary psychoanalytical world. Authors today often link this representation of the Self with representations of the object, thus forming pairs of representations that are internalized and that would form the basis of that global identity. Along these lines, personal identity includes a vision of the object in relation to the Self, and not just of the Self alone. In other words, the internal presence of the other is a fundamental element in our identity; those whom we know form a part of our own selves. Taking gender into account, we could consider that within the inner structure of each person is a representation of the other sex and thus in some manner the other sex forms part of the basic building blocks of our personality and of our global being. We have come close to the most complex manner that individuals employ to construct their gender identity, their gender role and, finally, their desires. Obviously, each one of these aspects should play a relevant role in the construction of our Self, of our global persona, and with that, of our identity in the broadest sense of the word. The man contains the woman and the woman contains the man.

If we approach this from a vision of the Self as the result of the incorporation into the internal world of internalized representations of object relations, it is clear that the image that we maintain of ourselves and that which others give back to us come to form part of this identity. There is no Self without the object; there is no representation of the Self without representation of the other. How I feel leads to how I act and this second part produces a reaction within the environment that simultaneously conditions the response of the former. There is a fluctuation of experiences and reactions that generate identity. As with the mother, in the period that Lacan calls the "mirror stage," who gives the child the image that he seeks, the others are mirrors in front of which we pose. In them we seek something with which to build the representation of our Self, which is, so to speak, our own identity.

It could be that this "other" of the opposite gender that each one of us has within has to do with the intense effect men and women have on each other with their mere presence. Popular wisdom is aware of this powerful force. When asked if she saw a possible relationship between religious people of different genders, Saint Teresa of Ávila affirmed: "Between a saintly man and saintly woman. . .; a bolted and barred-up wall." Phryne before the Areopagus, the mermaids charming sailors with their songs, or the horrific stare of Medusa, are but examples that demonstrate this influence, well-known from the dawn of time.

Coming back to the psychoanalytical literature, we see that Freud warns Jung in a letter: "The way these women manage to charm us with every conceivable psychic perfection until they have attained their purpose is one of nature's great spectacles" (quoted in Fonagy [20]). In this ambivalent line that Freud was expressing to his favorite disciple, prior to their definitive break, we see that the Viennese genius acknowledges the difficulty that comes with seeing oneself liberated from the influence of the other sex, since only trained and vigilant clinicians could isolate themselves from that influence.

If we consider the construction of identity as construction of the Self, we should pay logical attention to Kohut in particular, founder of the Self Psychology School [25]. Kohut and Wolf indicate how the construction of the identity, parallel to the development of narcissism, implies the relationship with three types of objects that cover different necessities. He would call those objects "self-objects." The self-object of idealization would be that which allows the child in development to cast an admiring stare toward a powerful and capable person. The mirroring self-object would be that which gives the child back a valuable image of himself. Lastly, the twin object would correspond to a peer, an equal with whom the relationship would be built based on symmetry. The connection with objects of these characteristics allows the subject's Self to develop soundly, reaching the necessary intensity with regard to his ambitions, ideals, and goals. It is interesting that Kohut and Wolf do not pay much attention to the differences between men and women on this journey. It is possible that in setting aside Freudian structural theory and in so doing, taking away the importance of the drives, they downplayed the study of sexuality. Consequently, in their opinion, gender and desire do not represent an area of special interest. Characters in Kohut and Wolf's theoretical narrative seem strangely asexual.

Spitz [26] describes a series of stages that are essential in the development of the human infant, which he calls "organizers" and which include steps that are indispensable for understanding the development of the child's identity. The first is the social smile, which presupposes the acknowledgement of oneself as a member of the human species. The child does not smile at objects or at animals, only at humans and thus, to smile is to belong to the human race, to be a part of us It happens by the second or third month. The second organizer described by Spitz is anxiety in the face of strangers, which allows for fundamentally connected figures to be differentiated (those who do not cause anxiety) from the rest (those who do cause anxiety). This occurs at 8 months. Last, the third organizer is the NO, which appears in the second year. This is the simplest way to distinguish oneself: I am not you. In adolescence the NO appears again, with a force that did not exist at 2 years of age. The process of the construction of gender identity is concluded at around 3 years of age. Nonetheless, the process of the construction of the identity in general continues until the end of adolescence. Mahler [27], with his proposal regarding the initial process of separation/individuation, and Blos [28], through his approach to adolescence as the second period of separation/individuation, completes the proposals that are essential in this context.

Volkan [29] describes in detail the process of "intergenerational transmission," which he explains as a set of ideals and fears that pass from one generation to the next, having a powerful effect even within the span of decades and centuries. Standing out in this process is the phenomenon of "depositation," which overlaps with that of projective identification. The mother "deposits" within the child her dreams, hopes, and fears and the way in which the child can escape this destiny that is written out for him. There is also a gender problem present here in the sense that the dreams of the mother relating to the social tribe (large group) to which she belongs especially refer to the values placed on the masculine figure in the society in which they live. The heroes are, in particular, men, and the stories relating to them are transmitted by the mother in particular. Collective identity, the feeling of belonging to the large group that is the nation or homeland has to do with processes of generational transmission and thus with depositation phenomena in which the mother, with her inevitably sexualized and sexualizing vision, plays a primordial role.

The obvious influence of the environment does not impede in any way the valuation of the importance of genetics in the construction of identity. The field of epigenetics [30] shows us how the environment is capable of powerfully influencing the expression of genetic material, thus offering a bridge that helps us to understand how early interpersonal connections are capable of acting over the chains of nucleotides and generating different proteins.

Emilce Dio Bleichmar, in her extraordinary text *The Spontaneous Feminism of Hysteria* [31], reveals how hysteria represents, in our culture, the largest exponent of the profoundly conflictive dimension of feminine sexuality. In the face of the devaluation of her gender, the woman, in our culture, tries out vicarious forms of narcissization, adding certain phallic-like traits to her femininity, or addressing a man who tells her who she is. Thus, the infantile/dependent personality, or rather the hysterical personality and the phallic/narcissistic personality, makes up a psycho-pathological type whose pivot is the acceptance or rejection of stereotypes relating to gender roles. For us, the sexual enjoyment of women who freely desire and obtain sexual satisfaction poses a transgression. This "spontaneous feminism" of the hysteria constitutes a form of reaction in the face of the devaluation of the feminine gender role among us. The hysterical conduct can thus be a manifestation of the distancing of women from the positions of power still in force.

Those who surround us serve a key function in the construction and development of our identity. Others act as a mirror and as a counter-point, signaling what we lack and also what value we hold. Without question, others contribute to the generation within ourselves of a sensation of pertinence to a group, they show us who is the other, and likewise they help us to build the experience of otherness. In a game of projections and introjections, such as the relationship between mother and baby, we build an individual identity that is still collective, mirroring those who are other. However, we must not forget that the image that we are given back by others undoubtedly contains aspects that do not belong to us and therefore there is always something that is ours in the vision that we have of others, and something of ours in that of theirs. Kristeva [32] bluntly affirms that only the acceptance of one's own otherness, of the strangeness that inhabits us, can lead us to more human levels of relationships with others who surround us. Our internal world is certainly a world, conceived of diverse parts that blend together in different harmonies in order to create an interior landscape that mimics the variety and conflict of the external world.

Two events of the last few decades illustrate that strange fluctuation in identity that affects both genders. On the one hand, the development of feminist proposals that seek a different place for women in 20th century society, a place that is not the traditional one for the wife/mother or lover, in order to recover in some way the place of the warrior woman, in the broadest sense of the term; the woman who is capable of thinking and acting freely and at the same time expressing her aggressive drive: to struggle, compete, and, why not, to win over the man who travels at her side. This appearance, for some, accompanies previous and parallel changes that occurred within the role of the man and the view that he had of the woman. The 20th century man becomes more misogynistic, more contemptuous of the woman, searches more for his identity through the rejection of all things feminine that may reside in him, including, of course, any satisfaction derived from submission. At the same time, in an almost parallel fashion to the feminist movement are proposals, especially literary ones, that talk about the attractive side of submission and the surrender on the part of women who freely choose that path among many others. From the *Story of O* to *Fifty Shades of Grey*, there is a whole tradition of narratives that are openly masochistic and that in some way demonstrate a sensitive part of the woman, and the entire social body. At a moment of almost complete liberty of thought and narration in the developed world, some women, and men, observe in fascinated fashion how the duality of sado-masochism seems to offer new modes of thought regarding parts of our desires that were previously unmentionable. Jean Paulhan, the prestigious Parisian man of letters and lover of Anne Desclos, the secret author (even for him) of the *Story of O*, indicates with what we can guess is a certain relief, that masochistic fantasies express a true feminine desire to be submissive and dominated. However, some authors, such as Anita Phillips [33], observe that, as always, there are things that hide beneath the surface. The young woman who chooses to be submissive may be in search of something that goes beyond what her fascinated or proud partner may provide for her. The submission of her Self seems to open unknown doors and allow for the exploration of new inner worlds, and in this journey of discovery the partner who exercises dominance can be merely a useful tool. Stoller [34] warns us that the simple search of pathology in sado-masochism presupposes a view that is too restrictive, and which loses the importance of nuances related to the identity and personality of the protagonists.

4.5 Social Aspects of Self-Identity

Psychosocial identity is composed of social and personal components, the shape of which can vary from context to context [11]. Surroundings beyond one's family, spanning the entire society, exert a continuous influence in the construction and development of identity. Society as a whole is constantly changing; therefore, this influence varies throughout different times and places.

Our Western society has changed its ways and the ways in which it organizes itself in recent decades, bringing about notable changes in the roles expected of individuals according to gender. In general, there has been a massive incorporation of women into the workplace, at a different pace and intensity depending on the specific countries, of course, and this has obviously changed aspects of the family, economics, health, education, and politics in the whole of society. Speaking about our contemporary welfare society, sociologist Javier Elzo [35] says: "The mother has had to leave the house; the father still hasn't returned." The new role that women play has been accompanied by an apparent sense of anxiety in their masculine counterparts, unsure of their role in this new society and going back and forth between indifference and hostile rejection, or even voluntary over-involvement in the new order. The answers to questions such as "who am I?" or "what is my role?" are more complex than ever before, for everyone: for women who are developing a professional career without abandoning the traditional position of taking care of their own, and for men who add to their usual role an attitude of care-giving, which has never before been their role.

Society hopes and fears different things regarding the conduct of boys and girls. Parents and adults in general are attentively watching both, and reacting in different ways. Concern over sissy behavior in a boy far outweighs concern over tomboy activity in a girl [11]. There is a conviction that is implicit within society, in the sense that masculine identity is more fragile and carries with it more risks than the feminine identity, because of which it is considered necessary to understand and provide a continuity with regard to the conduct and attitudes of masculine children, in order to avoid anomalies in future gender identity. It is as if that masculine identity requires constant validation from the environment and particularly from women within that environment. As they have done time and again, poets depict these complex problems with great precision: "...it is said that a man is not a man / unless he hears his name / come from the lips of a woman / this could be true..." It is fascinating to witness how the personal value of the man seems linked to the mere idea of being one. Thus, it is others, especially women, who give or take away value from the individual. In women, gender identity seems to be not so linked to personal value. Feminine gender identity is provided as a given and does not depend as much on confirmation from third parties, such as is the case with men. To summarize, we would say that the woman needs confirmation of her worth, not of who she is. The man, on the other hand, needs to have who he is confirmed, because that is where his value lies.

Sexuality, especially adult sexuality represented by a couple that enjoys that union, always makes the social group uneasy. This group, submitting to primitive forces, observes the couple with mistrust, and promotes the disengagement of men and women in order to return to that primitive and infantile sexuality pertaining to large groups. The couple has to constantly protect itself from that pernicious influence, knowing that the struggle has no end. Large groups in which aggression has taken place and therefore functioning is even more primitive do not tolerate mature sexuality among their ranks and they make moves to articulate rules that regulate the sexuality of couples, looking upon love and happy desire with hostile envy [36]. From this we surmise that two human qualities that any totalitarian system will try to stamp out are doubt and personal intimacy, for both threaten the total control of individuals by the state [37]. In his novel *1984*, Orwell [38] describes how Big Brother watches and regulates love and hunts down the protagonist couple that has escaped its control. In one startling scene, the police savagely torture the male protagonist and in his desperation he tries to provide the information that would stop the pain. But there are no questions and therefore he finds no answer. This goes on until a terrifying conviction overcomes him; he shouts, asking for her to be the one who is tortured so that he might be spared. We can imagine the smile on the torturer in having achieved his objective: there is no bond that resists the State; love and sex are at the service of the group and do not exist without it.

Throughout history the same discovery is repeatedly found: the enormous difficulty in combining aggression and sexuality in woman. However, we find a long tradition of mixing violence and sexuality in men. The rape and capture of the enemy's women is a historical act sustained throughout cultures and time periods, from remote antiquity up to today. Sudan, Rwanda, and Bosnia are recent scenarios in which violence against women and forced sexuality become another aspect of combat. It is a part that serves various ends, as with any other act of war, from the sowing of terror within the enemy, to the punishment of the enemy for his actions or even for the victor to humiliate him, leaving him with offspring that will perpetuate the humiliation. Also, the possibility of an animalistic and irresponsible sexuality that would never be allowed within the group may make up another part of the spoils of war. This is why, for the man, there is no difficulty in combining his roles as lover, father, and warrior. Together with this terrible custom, which is well known, we find a historic footprint of another means of fusing eroticism and militarism. The homosexual link among men who fight together, more or less disguised and/or sublimated, forms a long tradition. The military fraternity shows a discreet path for the comrades to express affection, desexualized at first, that tends to be considered "purer" than the affection between a man and a woman. A classic example that has stayed in the collective memory is that of the so-called Sacred Band [39], the elite unit of the Teban infantry in the 4th century BC, which remained undefeated for 40 years until its complete annihilation by Philip II of Macedon in the Battle of Chaeronea. This combat group was, in accordance with tradition, composed of a 150 couples, of lover and beloved who fought and died together. The history of this undefeated phalanx, which contrasts with the famous 300 Spartans who, guided by Leonidas, contained the Persians in the Battle of Thermopylae, has inspired poets and narrators throughout the centuries, turning the love, sexual or otherwise, between warriors into something that is not only acceptable but sublime. The permanence of this legendary group in historic memory tells us, without question, about the fascination that the combination of violence and sexuality in men has instilled in our culture.

Giuliana Galli-Carminati [40] and other researchers of the feminine identity approach the concept of the "woman warrior," considering it the third pole of the female archetype. This would be a pole that throughout time will be left lacking all sexual and identity-related nuance before finally disappearing to the benefit of the two other mythological female figures: the mother/wife and the lover. To briefly analyze the history, the authors demonstrate that in some of the most ancient civilizations, the figures of warrior goddesses occupied a distinguished place in the religious pantheon. In the majority of the cases, these warrior women could not maintain a complete sense of sexuality: or they were virgins in the current sense of the word (Greece), or they were limited to sexual relations without ending up as mothers or wives (Sumer). In Semitic cultures in particular, those from which our Western culture derives, the view was rather misogynist, placing the woman in positions that are socially valued less and therefore taking her away from violent action. It would be tempting to venture a possible relationship between this strict separation of sexuality and violence in the Greco-Roman culture and the historical difficulty of the Christian civilization in accepting a passionate and happy sexuality that goes beyond the reproductive function. The myths of the Amazons, the Gorgon or the Furies, free and virginal, indicate to us how, starting in antiquity, the absence of sexuality was considered the key to achieving a life free from submission to man. The warrior woman, independent and capable, had to pay a price, her own sexuality, and she renounced being part of a couple as well as maternity. The reappearance among our cultural myths of feminine figures (cinema, comics, TV series, etc.), who are independent and capable of violence continue to demonstrate these ancestral parameters, as if we still lived in classic antiquity: the sexuality of these heroines is partial or absent. It continues to be impossible to integrate loving passion, maternity, and violence within the same feminine figure.

The fact that the overwhelming majority of serial killers have been men could shed some light for us too on identities and genders. It may be said that in the internal world of women there is no possibility of a representation of the Self that is charged with such meanness. The intense anti-social traits that are accompanied by the total lack of compassion that characterizes psychopaths seem to characterize women less, perhaps through pressure and expectations that are social, cultural, genetic, hormonal, etc. Of course, there are some women capable of carrying out very violent and ruthless acts, but they are very rare outliers in a masculine world. In general, their participation in extreme sadistic acts is usually in the role of companion or assistants to the men, who take the initiative in these crimes, either luring the victim into a trap or collaborating in the very torture and related assignments [41]. Remember the young attractive woman who accompanies the magician in her role of distracting the public and helping the master to execute his tricks. Lest we forget, anyway, that is precisely this diverting of the audience's attention that allows the performer to carry out his final surprise.

The impact of the social attitudes and views toward individuals according to their gender is not limited to the internal world of the protagonists and in favor of the development of rather conflicting identities. Sometimes this effect has a vitally transcendent aspect, literally. The winner of the Nobel Prize in Economics, Amartya Sen, has analyzed a worrying phenomenon [42–44]. In 1992, Sen published in the *British Journal of Medicine* a brief paper of great impact: *The Missing Women*. It analyzed how in some Asian countries such as India, China, Korea, and others the small preponderance of women vs men that can be found in the rest of the world simply did not exist. These countries were "lacking" many women, with an estimated number of many millions. In order to counteract the argument of some regarding the determinant importance of poverty in this phenomenon, Sen referred to the comparison of countries that were similarly poor in Africa, confirming that in those the proportion of women compared with men in the general population was similar to France or UK, and much different from the populations of the Asian countries indicated. The reason for this tragedy was, for Sen, the disparity in healthcare for girls compared with boys, which was related to a clear preference within these social groups for men instead of women. In his first analysis, Sen had already indicated the general education of the population and in particular of the women and girls as being one of the fundamental ways of overcoming this scourge. Returning to the problem, years later, Sen found that medical attention to boys and girls has partially balanced out in many of these countries. Nonetheless, the proportions of men and women have continued in the same vein. One new test of the data reveals a reality that has not been perceived before: the advances in medical technology have now allowed many of those Asian countries to find out the gender of babies before birth, and have brought about the selective abortion of female fetuses. In this way, even though health-care had been balanced for both sexes, the number of births of girls decreased and the end result was the reassertion of previous proportions, and thus, a lack of large numbers of women. In a recent review of this reality (2013), Sen shows that in some of these social groups, the level of education of the population has risen clearly and many women have obtained access to levels of training that are much greater than those of their mothers. These women are now more capable of providing the same care to their own daughters and sons, although these are the women who access that technology and opt to selectively abort according to the gender of the baby prior to birth. Undoubtedly, there is a very important social aspect when acquiring an identity, and of course, at when assigning value to that identity. The reality of the "missing women" obliges us to face this absence of value in persons of the female sex in different social groups. The lack of value that is undoubtedly also transferred by women in the group, women who cannot escape those general values in which they are immersed and from which their lives, family, work, ideals, and desires are forged.

We men and women weave the web of oppression. Every knot we tie submits us inexorably to the influence of forces beyond ourselves, which make up our identity, as individuals, as men, and as women.

References

1. Erikson E. On the generational cycle. Int J Psychoanal. 1980;61:213–23.
2. Kernberg OF. Identity: recent findings and clinical implications. Psychoanal Q. 2006;75: 969–1003.
3. Westen D. Self and society: narcissism, collectivism and the development of morals. New York: Cambridge University Press; 1985.
4. Westen D. The cognitive self and psychoanalytic self: can we put ourselves together? Psychoanal Inq. 1992;3(1):1–13.
5. Lacan J. The mirror stage as formative of the/function as revealed in psychoanalytic experience. In: Fink B, Trans. Ecrits: the first complete edition in English (p. 75–81). New York: Norton & Company; 2006.
6. Fromm E. Psicoanálisis de la sociedad contemporánea: hacia una sociedad sana. México: Fondo de Cultura Económica; 1989.
7. Ermann M. Special issue on identity. Int Forum Psychoanal. 2004;13(4):209–83.
8. Meissner WW. The self as structural. Psychoanal Contemp Thought. 2000;23:373–416.
9. Applebaum A. Psychotherapeutic routes to structural change. Bull Mennin Clinic. 1994;58: 37–54.
10. Kernberg OK. Object relations theory and clinical psychoanalysis. New York: Jason Aronson; 1976.
11. Meissner WW. Gender identity and the self: I gender formation in general and in masculinity. Psychoanal Rev. 2005;92:1–27.
12. Stoller RJ. Sex and gender. London: Karnac Books; 1984.
13. Stoller RJ. Presentations of gender. New Haven, CT: Yale University Press; 1985.
14. Benjamin J. Sameness and difference: toward an "overinclusive" model of gender development. Psychoanal Inq. 1995;15:125–42.
15. Stoller RJ. Sweet dreams: erotic plots. London: Karnac Books; 2009.

16. Damasio A. The feeling of what happens: body and emotion in the making of consciousness. New York: Mariner Books; 2000.
17. Erikson E. Childhood and society. New York: Norton; 1950.
18. Klein M, Heinman P, Isaacs RJ, editors. Developments in psychoanalysis. London: Hogarth Press; 1946.
19. Mitchell SA. Relational concepts in psychoanalysis: an integration. Cambridge, MA: Harvard University Press; 1988.
20. Fonagy P. Psychosexuality and psychoanalysis. An Overview. In: Fonagy P, Krause R, Leuzinger-Bohleven M, editors. Identity, gender and sexuality. London: Karnac Books; 2009.
21. Kernberg O. Love relations. Normality and Pathology. New Haven, CT/London: Yale University Press; 1995.
22. Laplanche J. Seduction, persecution, revelation. Int J Psychoanal. 1995;76:663–82.
23. Chodorow NJ. Theoretical gender and clinical gender: epistemological reflections on the psychology of women. J Am Psychoanal Assoc. 1996;44S:215–38.
24. Diamond LM. Sexual fluidity* Understanding human love and desire. Cambridge/London: Harvard University Press; 2008.
25. Kohut H, Wolf ES. The disorders of the self and their treatment: an outline. Int J Psychoanal. 1978;59:413–25.
26. Spitz RA. The first year of life: a psychoanalytic study of normal and deviant development of object relations. Oxford, England: International Universities Press; 1965.
27. Mahler MS. On the first three subphases of the separation-individuation process. Int J Psychoanal. 1972;53(3):333–8.
28. Blos P. On adolescence: a psychoanalytic interpretation. New York: Simon and Schuster; 1966.
29. Volkan V. Psychoanalytic technique expanded: a textbook on psychoanalytic treatment, vol. 2. Charlottesville, VA: Pitchstone Publishing; 2012.
30. Szyf M. Epigenetics, DNA methylation, and chromatin modifying drugs. Annu Rev Pharmacol Toxicol. 2009;49:243–63.
31. Dio BE. El feminismo espontáneo de la histeria. Madrid: Adograf; 1985.
32. Kristeva J. Strangers to ourselves. New York: Columbia University Press; 1991.
33. Phillips A. A defense of masochism. New York: Saint Martin's Press; 1998.
34. Stoller RJ. Pain and passion. New York: Da Capo Press; 1991.
35. Elzo J. Tipología y modelos de relación familiar, vol. 21. Congreso La familia en la sociedad del siglo; 2003. p. 17–8
36. Kernberg OF. The sexual couple: a psychoanalytic exploration. Psychoanal Rev. 2011;98: 217–45.
37. Lemann N. The new deal we didn't know. The New York Review of Books, September 26; 2013. p. 23–5.
38. Orwell G. 1984. London: Signet Classics; 1950.
39. Leitao D. The legend of the sacred band. In: Nussbaum M, Sihvola J, editors. The sleep of reason. Erotic experience and sexual ethics in ancient Greece and Rome. Chicago: The University of Chicago Press; 2002.
40. Perroud N, Galli-Carminati G, Carminati G, Garbino MV. Le troisieme pole de l'archetype feminin. In: Galli-Carminati G, editor. La femme guerriere. Le troisieme pole de l'archetype feminin. Firenze: L'Autore Libri Firenze; 2009.
41. Stone M. The anatomy of evil. New York: Prometheus Books; 2009.
42. Sen A. Missing women. Br Med J. 1992;304:587–8.
43. Sen A. Missing women. Revisited. Br Med J. 2003;327:1297–8.
44. Sen A. India's women: the mixed truth, vol. LX. The New York Review of Books, Number 15, October 10–23; 2013. p. 24–7.

Improving Our Science in Psychosis Research with a Sex- and Gender-Based Analysis

5

Maria Haarmans

"From the moment of birth, if not sooner. . ." writes Kaschak, ". . .the body is gendered" (1992, p. 44). "There is no existence in our culture prior to and separate from gender. Almost invariably, the first question parents ask, even before birth, is: 'Is it a boy or girl?'" (p. 45).

Abstract

The World Health Organization has identified gender as a "critical determinant of mental health and mental illness." In the schizophrenia field, however, while there has been an increased focus on sex differences, little is known about how gender impacts the risk of psychosis, its expression (e.g., content of hallucinations), coping, or recovery. In this chapter, I argue for a sex- and gender-based analysis (SBGA). I outline the literatures on gender and mental health, describe SGBA, related constructs and corresponding scales, and delineate some of the barriers to conducting SGBA, equipping the interested reader with the tools to conduct SGBA in psychosis research.

The term 'psychosis' is increasingly being used in preference to 'schizophrenia' due to the poor scientific validity and reliability of the schizophrenia classification [157–159] and thus is used in this paper to encompass schizophrenia, schizoaffective disorder, and first episode psychosis diagnoses. Generally, the term 'psychosis' refers to the 'symptoms' or anomalous phenomena such as hallucinated voices or unusual beliefs. Increasingly research focuses on these experiences specifically as opposed to diagnoses. In this paper, I will therefore use the terms 'psychosis' or 'psychotic' to refer to the anomalous phenomena as described in psychiatry and am using the term 'schizophrenia' where researchers have referred specifically to this diagnosis or to refer to the field in general.

M. Haarmans (✉)
Clinical Psychology, Institute of Psychology, Health and Society, University of Liverpool, Liverpool, Merseyside L69 3BX, UK
e-mail: maria.haarmans@liverpool.ac.uk

M. Sáenz-Herrero (ed.), *Psychopathology in Women*,
DOI 10.1007/978-3-319-05870-2_5

5.1 Introduction

In the health field, sex and gender are increasingly being recognized both nationally and internationally as important determinants and indispensable aspects of research [1–3]. The Canadian Institutes of Health Research's Institute of Gender and Health promotes "…the integration of gender and sex as routine considerations in all domains of health research" (p. vi) [161]. In the UK, government health policy has incorporated gender as a key determinant of health, service need, and service planning [4]. The World Health Organization [3] has identified gender as a "critical determinant of mental health and mental illness" (undated), and its 2004 report *Gender in Mental Health Research* states: "Integrating gender considerations in health research contributes to better science and more focused research, and, consequently, to more effective and efficient health policies and programmes" (p. 2). However, since Nasser et al. [5] criticized the status of schizophrenia research, more than a decade ago, for "the profound neglect of the role of socio-cultural factors…" (p. 351) and the role of gender in particular, few advances have been made in the field. One notable exception is the surge of research examining the relationship between trauma and psychosis, particularly the association of sexual abuse and hallucinations [6]. However, even with this line of inquiry, when it is known that there are differences in the rates and impact of sex and gender between men and women who have experienced sexual abuse in the general population [7–9], a sex- and gender-based analysis (SGBA) is lacking. It seems that people diagnosed with schizophrenia are still considered "genderless" [5].

One probable reason for the relative lack of attention to gender is that current conceptions of schizophrenia continue to emphasize the role of biogenetic factors. However, sociocultural and psychological factors are also clearly important. For example, studies in several countries have observed that migrants have a fivefold elevated risk of psychosis [10], suggesting that experiences of discrimination, social capital, and social defeat may contribute to the risk of illness [11]. Other studies found associations between early life adversities such as socioeconomic disadvantage [12], urbanicity [13, 14], early parental separation [15, 16], bullying at school [17, 18], and, as mentioned previously, sexual and other types of abuse [6] and the development of psychosis.

Psychological approaches, particularly cognitive behavioral models of psychosis, have implicated the role of core beliefs about the self, others/world, and future in the maintenance of delusional beliefs and hallucinated voices and emphasize links between life experience and/or trauma and psychotic phenomena [19–21]. For example, Morrison [22] suggests that negative beliefs about the self and the world are thought to be developed in response to trauma and are predicted to mediate the distress experienced in relation to psychotic phenomena. Birchwood et al. [23, 24] demonstrated parallels between the experience of subordination by voices and subordination and marginalization in the social world. Hayward et al. [25] recently reviewed 18 studies examining the nature of the voice-hearer's relationship with their hallucinated voices and found, as with the aforementioned studies, that collectively the studies suggest a correspondence between voice hearers' relationship with their voices and their interpersonal relationships in the social world.

While all of the aforementioned studies underline the importance of context, life experience, and sociocultural factors in the etiology, development, and expression of psychotic phenomena, none conducts an SGBA. An SGBA takes into account the role of both biogenetic and sociocultural factors by utilizing an analysis of the biological construct of sex and the sociocultural construct of gender.

Although there has been an increase in the research into sex differences in schizophrenia, it is still relatively neglected in comparison to research on other mental health disorders such as depression. Barker-Collo et al. [26] point out that a Medline analysis estimated that only about half of all articles on schizophrenia up to 2010 even record sex and a scant 2.5 % analyze research findings by sex. When sex differences have been examined, the authors indicate the focus is on the supposed biological base of such differences. To conduct SGBA, we must take into account both sex and gender for, as Nowatzki and Grant [1] argue, "Sex is a poor proxy for gender, as it is not capable of capturing the full range of social, political, and economic forces that affect health" (p. 265). Several researchers have suggested that examining gender could, in addition to increasing our understanding of the heterogeneity in expression and subjective experience of psychotic phenomena, clarify of some of the reported sex differences [5, 27–29], such as why more women than men seem to hear voices—findings that are observed in both clinical [30–32] and nonclinical populations [33, 34]. Much of the sex difference research is purely descriptive and does not identify the mechanisms responsible for producing any such differences [35, 36]. A gender analysis could possibly contribute to understanding the etiology and illuminate mechanisms involved elucidating the variability in some reports of sex differences (e.g., prevalence) [37].

An interesting example of research that demonstrates the importance of using an SGBA is illustrated by Lewine and Daniel et al. [29, 38] who examined sex differences in cerebral blood flow using positron emission tomography (PET) and found a higher rate of blood flow in women than in men (all healthy individuals). When femininity and masculinity was measured, however, it was discovered that high blood flow related far more strongly to femininity than biological sex.

In this chapter, I make a case for the importance of an SBGA, which is long overdue in schizophrenia research, outlining the literature on gender and mental health. First, I review relevant theoretical constructs for conducting an SGBA and describe how to conduct an SGBA.

5.2 Sex and Gender: What's the Difference? Constructs and Corresponding Research Measures for Conducting an SGBA

Several methodological problems plague gender research in the schizophrenia field. One of the most fundamental is the conflation of the terms sex and gender, which are often used inconsistently and/or interchangeably in the literature [5, 29]. As Johnson et al. [2] point out: "This conflation leads to confusion about the contributions of sex and gender to health, and missed opportunities for developing appropriate medical interventions and policy responses" (p. 1).

Sex refers to: "The biological characteristics such as anatomy…and physiology…that distinguish males and females" [39]. Gender refers to "…the array of socially constructed roles and relationships, personality traits, attitudes, behaviours, values, relative power and influence that society ascribes to the two sexes on a differential basis…" [39]. It has been argued that: "The complex interconnections of sex and gender affect who we are, what we do, and how we are treated, and have profound effects on our health" [2].

5.2.1 What Is SGBA?

Sex- and gender-based analysis originated in international development research where, owing to significant evidence that biological, economic, and social differences between women and men contribute to differences in health risks, use of health services, health system interaction, and health outcomes, research began integrating a gender and sex perspective [40, 41].

Health Canada [41] has defined SGBA as:

> … an approach which systemically inquires about biological (sex-based) and socio-cultural (gender-based) differences between women and men, boys and girls, without presuming that any differences exist. The purpose of SGBA is to promote rigorous sex/gender-sensitive health research, which expands understanding of health determinants in both sexes, in order to provide knowledge which can result in improvements in health and health care. Gender-blind science fails to account for disparate life trajectories that are influenced by genetic endowment, environmental exposures and social and political environments.

Sex- and gender-based analysis incorporates multiple levels of analysis from the micro-individual level to the macro-social level, integrating other social determinants of health or diversity indicators:

> SGBA is meant to be applied within the context of a diversity framework, that attends to the ways in which determinants such as ethnicity, socioeconomic status, disability, sexual orientation, migration status, age and geography interact with sex and gender to contribute to exposures to various risk factors, disease courses and outcomes. Using a SGBA lens brings these considerations into focus and can help to formulate research, policies and programs that are relevant to the diversity of the Canadian populace [42].

Nasser [43] has advocated approaches to researching women's (and men's) mental health that:

> …take into account gender differences between men and women in a sociocultural context including differences in pay, social status, political power, burdens of domestic care, and mothering, relationship inequalities and rates of domestic violence as well as gender differences in social pressures and expectations (p. 25) [43].

An SGBA is one such approach.

Conducting SGBA occurs throughout all phases of the research process, starting with clearly differentiating and defining the concepts of sex and gender [41]. First,

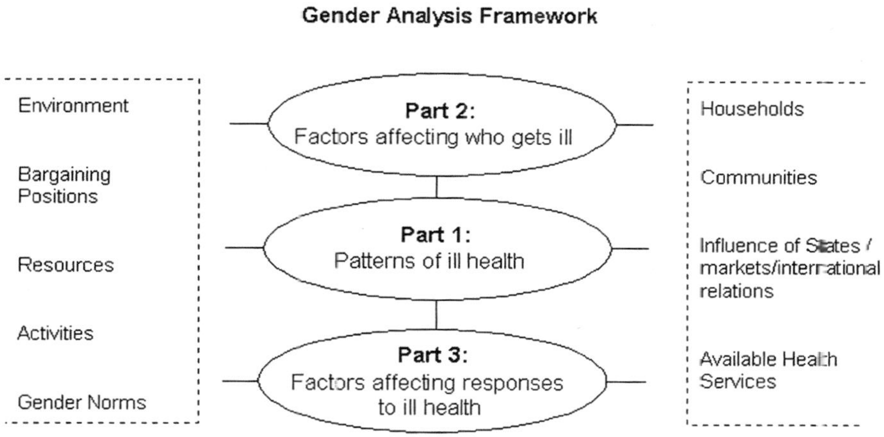

Fig. 5.1 Gender analysis framework (*Source*: Liverpool School of Tropical Medicine, Gender and Health Group, University of Liverpool, Reproduced with permission)

it is essential to include gender and sex in the research question(s) and/or hypotheses. Examining the extent to which past research has taken gender or sex into account is an important part of the literature review. Using representative samples is also very important in order to be able to conduct SGBA, as well as collecting data that are disaggregated by sex, a major methodological barrier in schizophrenia research. Whether conducting quantitative or qualitative methodologies, using an analytical approach that captures gender- and sex-based factors is also a very important part of the process in addition to considering diversity factors as they interact with sex and gender and affect exposure to various risk factors, illness course, and outcomes.

In order to conduct an SGBA, researchers not only examine sex differences but pay attention to the broader theme of gender, gender relations, institutionalized gender, and the larger social context as demonstrated in Fig. 5.1. This diagram, developed by the Gender and Health Group at the Liverpool School of Tropical Medicine, University of Liverpool for researching health problems and services, provides an excellent framework for SGBA that can also be applied to psychosis research. Multiple levels of gender (the interactional, the organizational/institutional, and the cultural) [44] are represented. A gender analysis makes explicit the social, cultural, historical, and political context of the lives of research participants, combining both micro- and macro-levels of analysis as shown in Fig. 5.1. This framework offers a range of approaches to assess the relationship of gender to a particular health problem, issue, or system. It also raises the issue of how gender guides the research methodology to be employed. Parts 1, 2, and 3 involve three stages of gender analysis. In the first stage, Part 1, gender-related differences in patterns of ill-health (or "health outcomes data") are examined: who gets ill (i.e., men and women of different ages, socio-economic and ethnic groups; *what* types of illness women and men get; *when* women and men become ill (e.g., time of year); and *where* women and men become ill. Parts 2 and 3 provide guidelines for investigating the interplay of gender and social, cultural, and economic factors that affect health and responses to ill-health. It is suggested that examination of these factors may require contextualized, descriptive, and analytical sources of information, dictating qualitative, participatory, and/or mixed research methods where perceptions, attitudes, and subjectivity are of interest. Each of the factors listed on the left of the matrices—environment, activities, bargaining position, resources, and gender norms—is an area of enquiry to be examined in the context of each of the levels of society—households, communities, and states/markets/international relations, available health services—or contexts—listed to the right of the matrix. *Environment* refers to women's and men's living and working context including the general social and economic milieu. *Bargaining positions* denotes decision-making power within gender relations. Gender differences in women's and men's access to and control over *resources* such as money, transport, time, information, political power, and influence is also an important consideration in this analytical framework. *Activities* represent activities of daily living, including what women and men do at home and at work. These are based on culturally prescribed roles and include:

- *Productive* roles, i.e., paid work, or production of goods for subsistence or sale
- *Reproductive* roles, i.e., domestic tasks including cooking, cleaning, caring for children and sick people
- *Community* roles, i.e., participating in various tasks associated with managing community organizations, and operating and maintaining community services [45].

Different activities carry different mental and physical health risks. *Gender norms*, often implicit and unspoken, are the beliefs, prescriptions, and proscriptions for women and men's capacities, characteristics, social behaviors, roles, and interests (Liverpool School of Tropical Medicine, undated). This framework incorporates the four core concepts of SBGA: sex, gender, diversity, and equity as outlined by Clow et al. [40]. Examining the intersection of other social hierarchies with gender is a necessary aspect of approaching gender as a multidimensional construct.

Marsh [45] has criticized the mental health services for ignoring the context of individual's lives, in particular, women with severe mental illness who, like women in general, because of gender norms, are affected by the burden of caring for others, often prioritizing their needs above their own, placing more emphasis on their relational environment, which can both undermine health and act as a social buffer to stress [46]. Examining such differences in a life context has also been ignored in schizophrenia research. Using the above framework for SGBA in psychosis research has utility in exposing the possible impact of these variables on well-being by utilizing the various matrices, such as *environment*, *gender norms*, and *activities*, for example, with obvious implications for gender-responsive interventions.

5.2.2 The Constructs

5.2.2.1 Gender: A Multidimensional Construct

Recent conceptualizations of the feminine and masculine have moved beyond a simplistic understanding of global and opposing personality traits based on a unifactorial, bipolar model to a multidimensional and multifactorial construct [47, 48] operating "...on multiple levels including the subjective and intrapsychic, the interactional, the organizational and institutional and the cultural" [44] and encompassing the dimensions of gender-typed personality traits [49, 50], gender-related interests, global gender role behaviors [42], masculinity ideology [51], gender role conflict [52], gender role strain [53, 54], gender role stress [55], gender role conformity [56, 57], gender identity [48], and femininity ideology [42]. In order to represent the complexity of gender, research must, therefore, address gender as multivariable. Knaak [44] suggests delineating three overarching dimensions for the purposes of research: the subjective (e.g., man/woman/transgendered); the cultural (e.g., masculinities/femininities), and the institutional (e.g., social–structural). She argues that this multidimensional interpretation demands that "...gender cannot be adequately understood in isolation from other social hierarchies" (p. 306) and thus it is important to examine how the dimensions of class and race, for example, shape and interact with gender. Another obvious implication of the multiplicity of gender for research design is the need to utilize several measures, as any one gender measure may tap only a small portion of the gender construct [47].

While a robust body of literature examining gender exists in the fields of social psychology, developmental psychology, and women's and men's psychology, clinical psychology has paid scant attention to issues of gender [58]. Several constructs with corresponding measures generated from these fields are defined below. A lack of awareness of their existence may constitute another barrier to conducting SBGA in schizophrenia research.

Gender ideology is defined as: "...an individual's internalization of cultural belief systems regarding gender roles" [42], operationally defined by gender role stereotypes [59]. It is distinct from the identity/trait approach where one is presumed to *possess* particular sex-based personality traits, in that the ideology approach views gender norms as being socially constructed. In this approach one can endorse the ideology that men and women should have these sex-specific characteristics without necessarily possessing them oneself. The process of internalization of cultural messages may often be barely noticed on a conscious level and taken for granted as a common place and natural aspect of daily life. The term *ideology* is used to convey "...the superordinate, organizing nature of these beliefs at both the individual level and the social-structural level," thus constituting a belief system [54]. Masculinity ideology [51] refers to the internalization of cultural beliefs regarding masculinity specifically; similarly, femininity ideology refers to the internalization of cultural beliefs regarding feminine gender role norms [42, 60]. The Male Role Norms Inventory-Revised (MRNI-R) scale was developed to measure masculinity ideology, identifying seven factors: avoidance of femininity, negativity toward sexual minorities, self-reliance, aggression, dominance, non-relational attitudes toward sex, and restrictive emotionality. The following is a sample item: "A man should not react when other people cry." Items are rated on a seven-point Likert-type scale ranging from 1 (strongly disagree) to 7 (strongly agree), with higher scores indicating higher levels of endorsement of traditional masculinity ideology. Levant et al. [42] also developed the Femininity Ideology Scale (FIS), which has five domains: stereotypical image and activities, dependence/deference, purity, care-taking, and emotionality. An example item is: "Women should dress conservatively so they do not appear loose," rated for agreement on a five-point Likert-type scale.

Gender schema refers to a cognitive structure in which information is processed according to sex-linked associations or *sex-typing* defined as: "The process by which a society thus transmutes male and female into masculine and feminine" [50]. Bem [61] argues that these schemata form in response to societal prescriptions, norms or standards constituting appropriate masculine and feminine behavior socialized through such forces as family, school, peers, and the media. These norms shape gender identity and can contribute to gender role strain [50, 62]. The Bem Sex Role Inventory was developed to measure sex-typed traits and gender identity. However, more recent research has criticized the scale with regard to its validity in terms of measuring self-perceived, gender-linked personality traits [59].

Gender roles "...are the behavioural norms applied to males and females in societies, which influence individuals' everyday actions, expectations, and experiences. Gender roles are expressed and enacted in a range of ways, from how we dress or talk, to what we may aspire to do, to what we feel are valuable contributions to make as a woman or a man" (p. 5) [2]. The Gender Role Socialization Scale was developed to assess the degree of internalization of gender-role messages in women (e.g., "I feel embarrassed about my own sexual desires" rated for agreement on a seven-point Likert-type scale), and how these messages may affect health and well-being. The developers suggest that the scale "...can also be used to examine the relationship between internalized gender role messages and the various types of mental health concerns that women experience in order to facilitate the development of prevention and treatment protocols" (p. 190) [63].

Gender identity refers to how we see ourselves as female or male constructed in the context of strong societal messages and prescriptions for the *acceptable* gendered role for one's presenting sex [2]. Gender identity influences our aspirations, social interactions, behaviors, characteristics, and body image [2, 64–66].

Institutionalized gender represents the unequal power distribution between the sexes in the political, educational, religious, media, medical, and social institutions in any society through different expectations and opportunities for women and men and girls and boys, such as social and family roles, job segregation, job limitations, dress codes, health practices, and differential access to resources such as money, food, or political power [2].

Gender role stress denotes the cognitive appraisal of specific situations as stressful when individuals judge themselves to be failing to live up to imperatives of traditional gender roles [67]. Corresponding scales have been developed for each sex: the Masculine Gender Role Stress Scale and the Gillepsie and Eisler FGRSS [67]. Each has five scales comprising particular situations that might cause stress owing to a feeling of not meeting feminine or masculine gender role norms. The following are examples of items on the MGRS: "Admitting that you are afraid of something"; "Staying home during the day with a sick child." Sample items from the FGRS are as follows: "Having others believe you are emotionally cold"; "finding that you have gained 10 pounds."

Gender role strain refers to the negative psychological consequences experienced by individuals when they try to live up to an idealized gender role schema [53]. Within this framework, gender role strain occurs partly because stereotyped gender role norms are often contradictory, unattainable, and inconsistent. This construct is embedded in the overarching theoretical framework of the gender role strain paradigm developed by Pleck [53]. This paradigm "emphasizes the centrality of gender ideology as a cultural script that organizes and informs everything from the socialization of small children to the emotions, cognition, and behaviour of adults" (p. 130) [42]. Conceptions of gender roles in the gender role strain paradigm depart from the older personality trait—orientations of gender role identity in that they are understood to be acquired via a "...variable process strongly influenced by prevailing gender ideologies, which themselves vary according to social location and cultural context" (p. 131) [42]. Pleck identified three subtypes of gender role strain: discrepancy strain, dysfunction strain, and trauma strain.

(1) Discrepancy strain suggests that stereotypical gender role standards are exist and that individuals attempt to conform to them to varying degrees. Pleck hypothesized that "not conforming to these standards has negative consequences for self-esteem and other outcomes reflecting psychological well-being because of negative social feedback as well as internalized negative self-judgments" (p. 13) [54].
(2) Dysfunction strain applies to the negative consequences of those who do conform to normative gender roles such as aggression and emotional constriction as prescriptions for *masculinity*, which are psychologically harmful, promote unhealthy behavior, and as such cause psychological strain. Similarly, the very same qualities that characterize depression and low social rank such as passivity, submission, perceptions of self as inferior or in an unwanted subordinate position, and low self-confidence [68], for example, have been regarded as normal and desirable qualities of *femininity*. These gender role norms are encouraged through socialization, *tradition*, and discrimination [69–72].
(3) Trauma strain refers to the traumatic experience of certain groups of men whose gender role strain has been particularly severe such as war veterans, survivors of child abuse, and marginalized groups such as men of color and gay and bisexual men.

When Pleck developed the gender role strain paradigm, it was within the context of a critical examination of masculinity ideologies. Since then it has been widely used as a framework for understanding and researching gender, primarily in the field of men's psychology [59, 73]. However theoretically, the gender role strain paradigm is also relevant for women, as has been demonstrated by other researchers

[53, 54, 74, 75, 154]. Some researchers have suggested that men experience more social pressure to adhere to gender roles than women [59, 76]. In fact, Levant has described the need to transform traditional notions of masculine ideology, which he has termed "a new psychology of men," as "overdue and urgently needed" (p. 259), pointing to the disproportionate representation of men experiencing public and social health problems resulting from the male role socialization process, such as substance abuse, homelessness, perpetration of family and interpersonal violence, estrangement or detached fathering, sex offenses, fatal automobile accidents, and lifestyle and stress-related fatal illnesses [73].

Gender role conflict (GRC) is defined as "a psychological state in which socialized gender roles have negative consequences for the person or others [that] occurs when rigid, sexist, or restrictive gender roles result in personal restrictions, devaluation, or violation of others or self" (p. 130) [77]. In other words, GRC refers to the interpersonal and intrapersonal conflict that arises from the rigid enactment of traditional gender roles, from the violation of gender roles, or from gender role devaluations (e.g., men who freely express emotions may be devalued by others because emotionality is associated with femininity). An example where both inter- and intrapersonal conflict could potentially occur is when men "...internalize masculine gender role ideals that encourage for example, aggressiveness, overemphasis on achievement, and relational emotional disconnection" (p. 334) [61]. Gender role conflict is related to the concepts of gender role strain and gender ideology. Patterns of gender role conflict have been hypothesized as observable negative outcomes of *gender role strain* [78]. O'Neil and colleagues [52] developed the Gender Role Conflict Scale-I (GRSC-I), an empirically derived measure of male gender role conflict or gender role strain, that has been described as "...readily complementing masculinity ideology measures" (p. 151) [78]. The scale assesses men's gender role attitudes, behaviors and conflicts in four domains: restrictive emotionality, success/power/competition, restrictive affectionate behavior between men, and conflict between work and family relations. The GRSC-II was developed to measure men's degree of comfort or conflict in specific gender role conflict situations.

5.2.3 Methodological Issues: Barriers to SGBA in Psychosis Research

5.2.3.1 Underrepresentation of Women in Research Studies

A significant limitation with schizophrenia research inhibiting a sex- and gender-based analysis is the underrepresentation of women in research studies [79–81]. In fact, Longenecker and colleagues [79], in their analysis of epidemiological incidence and non-epidemiological study participation, found "...a widespread mismatch between the incidence of schizophrenia in females and their participation in research" (p. 242). They cite the incidence rate of 1.4 male schizophrenia patients to every female patient, or 58 % men, taken from a recent meta-analysis by McGrath and colleagues in 2008. Their analysis reveals that this imbalance is exaggerated in non-epidemiological studies, where 66 % of research participants are men. They report that this overrepresentation of males in the literature has been consistent over the last two decades. Focusing on the incidence of first-episode psychosis, Iacono and Beiser [82, 83] describe an excess of men in most studies and report that in many instances the male to female ratio among study participants exceeds 3 to 1, which they attribute to a higher incidence of schizophrenia in men than in women.

5.2.3.2 Aggregated Data/Controlling for Sex

A further factor in schizophrenia research inhibiting an SGBA is that most studies do not provide information on sex or gender separately or where they do in some of the few studies where large numbers of women have been recruited, researchers have "controlled for sex" rather than treating women and gender as important areas to explore [81, 84, 85].

5.2.3.3 Sex Bias in Diagnosis/Sampling Bias

Both sex bias in diagnosis and sampling bias confound the actual rates of incidence and prevalence. For example, women in older age groups are at a higher risk of developing psychosis than men; thus, male–female incidence ratio studies should ideally include participants of all ages [86]. Studies that are limited to inpatients may also promote sampling bias owing to the overrepresentation of men, which Aleman et al. [86] suggest is because of a less favorable course of the disorder for the male sex citing the example of violence and aggression being more common in men. Psychosocial aspects of gender role norms may be partly related to this overrepresentation. For example, Walker and Lewine point out that male patients are more likely than female patients to display antisocial behavior and have police contact and criminal records, leading to the perception by treatment providers and families that men are more aggressive and threatening. Conversely, female patients are viewed as more helpless, withdrawn and depressed. They suggest that these perceptions, in addition to self-perceptions of men and women (women are more likely to view themselves as ill, as needing treatment and to seek and comply with treatment), partially influence whether a person is in treatment, particularly in an inpatient setting. Seeman [87] and Falkenburg and Tracy [88], in their reviews of sex differences, have also pointed to higher expectations of families for sons with regard to education and achievement than daughters, resulting in higher expressed emotion (EE) in families toward sons and perceptions of greater need for treatment for sons.

In addition, some authors have also suggested that because there are more women experiencing co-morbid affective symptomatology, women are predominantly diagnosed with schizoaffective disorder and it may be more difficult to assign categorical diagnoses to women than to men [89, 90].

Epidemiological research adopting SBGA in schizophrenia is an important factor in the reduction of methodological artifacts.

5.2.3.4 Gender in Context

Another major methodological challenge in conducting SGBA involves how to incorporate the multiple social categories and determinants, such as ethnicity, social class, sexual identity, age, and culture, that intersect with gender, and that have an impact on the distribution of health and illness within and across populations [64, 65]. Researchers advocating an SGBA highlight the need to include social and biological determinants, which overlap and work together to produce health, but at the same time acknowledge both the conceptual and analytical challenges this creates. Researchers are increasingly improving ways of doing this. Johnson et al. describe some promising models that facilitate the investigation of both biological and multiple social influences in a single study [64, 65]. For example, they recommend employing intersectional analyses, which acknowledge a person's multiple social identities, and multilevel and systems modeling, as they can simultaneously analyze both individual-level and group-level factors that have an impact on health and disease. An in-depth discussion of these approaches is beyond the scope of this chapter; suffice it to say, awareness of the available analytical models to address some of these challenges is a helpful first step in promoting an SBGA in schizophrenia research.

5.3 Gender: A Critical Determinant of Mental Health

5.3.1 Institutionalized Gender: Social–Structural Level Oppression

> Emerging evidence indicates that the impact of gender in mental health is compounded by its interrelationships with other social, structural determinants of mental health status, including education, income and employment as well as social roles and rank. There are strong, albeit varying, links between gender inequality, human poverty and socioeconomic differentials in all countries [3].

Referring back to the definition in the first section of this paper, we saw that *institutionalized gender* refers to the distribution of power between the sexes at the system level within political, educational, religious, media, medical, and social institutions in any society. These institutions shape the social norms that delineate different expectations and opportunities for women and men, such as social and family roles and practices, job limitations, for example, and differential access to resources such as money, food, or political power. Such differential opportunities and access may lead to differences in health risks, health services use, health system interaction, and health outcomes for men and women [2, 3, 40].

We have known for quite some time that subordinate group status affects mental health [3]. In the *American Journal of Psychiatry* 30 years ago, Carmen et al. [91] pointed out that the:

> . . .link between women's disadvantaged status and their mental health creates an obligation for mental health professionals to understand how the social context contributes to the origin and persistence of the problems of their patients (p. 1319).

With increasing evidence of this link, particularly research emphasizing the role of trauma, social inequality, and migrant status in psychosis, a lack of gender-based analysis is conspicuous. This section underlines the relevance of conducting both micro- and macro-levels of analysis through SGBA in psychosis research.

5.3.1.1 Gender-Specific Determinants

The Gender in Mental Health Research Report [3] outlines several gender-specific determinants of mental health, such as gender-based violence (physical, sexual, psychological), gender-based income disparity, unpaid labor, and lower social rank. In their review of sex differences in schizophrenia, Falkenburg and Tracy [88] cite studies that demonstrate the differential gender-exposure and risk patterns that disproportionately affect men and women with psychosis. For women these include sexual abuse, socioeconomic disadvantage, and duty to assume responsibility for the care of others [3]. Other researchers have also reported that women with serious mental illness are also at a greater risk for revictimization and for post-traumatic stress disorder [92]. Falkenburg and Tracy point out that despite lower fertility rates than community samples, over 50 % of individuals with a schizophrenia diagnosis become parents with the male partners often absent and approximately one-third losing custody of their children [88]. Single parenting has been identified by the World Health Organization [3] as a risk factor for living in poverty, and an especially high risk for poor physical and mental health.

Gender-specific risk factors for men with psychosis include different responses from relatives [37] where differential gender role expectations lead to, for example, more consistent and severe criticism from relatives (or high EE), increasing relapse and having a negative impact on illness course [87, 88]. Several studies examining high EE report differential responses and attitudes of relatives toward men and women with psychosis [30]. For example, in their review, Falkenburg and Tracy identified lower parental tolerance of symptomatic behavior and sense of responsibility for caring for men, higher levels of fear and conflict owing to higher rates of aggression in men, increased guilt and self-blame and lower attendance at therapy in families of men [88]. Even when controlling for symptomatology, gender role expectations of parents influenced the hospital outcomes of their sons or daughters [93].

Al-Issa cites studies where differential gender role expectations for men and women and the lower social status ascribed to women have an impact on access to treatment [94]. For instance, he outlines studies of French–Canadian villages, where communities were helpful to their young men who were suffering from delusions but not their young women, and families were willing to pay for a son's treatment but not for a daughter or wife [95].

In an original 26-year period cohort study in Sweden, Månsdotter et al. [96], grounding their research in gender relational theory, examined the effects of gendered life in childhood and adulthood on mental health, focusing on the spheres of mother's paid/unpaid work, childcare practice, gendered partnership, and gender ideology. The investigators based their research on the well-accepted theory that the improved gender equality of Nordic countries has had an impact on the health patterns of men and women. Women ($n = 421$) and men ($n = 526$) were followed and surveyed at five different time-points, from age 16 to age 42, with a comprehensive questionnaire developed by the investigators. Gendered ideology was measured using a scale indicating support for societal gender equality ranging from 1 (fully supporting a gender-equal society) to 10 (fully rejecting a gender-equal society), and categorized into traditional: "ranking 4–10," and non-traditional "ranking 1–3." Similarly, gendered partnership and gendered childcare also used a five-point Likert-type scale, each asking a question about the perceived overall equality in one's relationship with a partner and division of childcare responsibility, categorized into traditional and non-traditional. The main findings were that for women, reduced anxiety was associated with a more gender-equal ideology at age 30, while for men, reduced depressive symptoms were associated with more gender-equal childcare division at age 42. Månsdotter and colleagues speculate that the reduced depressive symptomatology for men may be related to the health-promoting effects of expanding social roles and childcare per se for mental health and specifically the positive influence of increased intimacy. One of the study limitations identified by the authors includes a lack of statistical power when categorizing individuals into traditional or nontraditional, and when stratifying the analyses by gender. Nevertheless, this type of research demonstrates the utility of employing an SBGA for incorporating both micro- and macro-levels of analysis, as was done here through examining gender relations, institutionalized gender, and gender ideology.

5.3.2 Gender Role Socialization and Mental Health: Internalized Oppression

In addition to the deleterious effects on the mental health of women due to gender inequality, men too suffer adverse effects from limiting gender role norms. A large body of literature spanning decades emphasizes the effects of gender on mental health, with empirical investigations demonstrating harmful psychological impacts (depression, low self-esteem, and substance abuse, for example) of internalized gender role expectations on both men and women [54, 61, 67, 70, 72, 97–101, 154]. More recent research demonstrates an association between higher masculinity ideology and increased PTSD symptomatology in male veterans [102].

5.3.2.1 Gender Role Socialization, Stress, and Coping

Gender role expectations have been shown to correlate closely with differential mental health problems according to sex [67]. For example, rates of depression, agoraphobia, eating disorders, anxiety disorders, and PTSD are much higher for women than for men. Conversely, rates of substance abuse and antisocial behavior are higher for men [3].

> According to gender role stereotypes, women are "expected" to be submissive, dependent, and anxious about appearance, whereas men are "expected" to be indulgent, aggressive, and demonstrate sexual prowess [67].

Empirical investigations provide evidence that cognitive appraisal and coping is influenced by gender role socialization resulting in gender differences in vulnerability to certain stressors [67, 155]. Gillespie and Eisler [156], in 1992, developed models of gender role stress, drawing explicitly on the cognitive stress model [103], in which stress occurs owing to the cognitive appraisal that one has violated gender role imperatives. These models have been tested using the masculine and feminine gender role stress scales described earlier. With the development of these scales, empirical studies have shown an inverse relationship between gender role stress and measures of physical and psychological well-being for both women and men [55].

A review of stress research of the past few decades by Dedovic et al. [104] highlights some recent results from endocrinological, developmental, and neuro-imaging studies that suggest that gender socialization might play an important role in the metabolic effects of stress. Dedovic et al. also suggest that as some differences between men and women in hypothalamic–pituitary–adrenal (HPA) axis responses to psychosocial stressors cannot be explained by biological variables alone, gender is likely to be a critical factor, and propose a model that integrates these specific findings, highlighting gender socialization and stress responsivity [104]. The authors point to research that manipulates the psychosocial stressor context or uses stressors emphasizing achievement versus social integration, which provide strong support for the role of gender in explaining male–female variations in stress responses.

Surprisingly, the impact of gender role socialization on cognitive appraisal and coping with regard to psychosocial stressors has not been explored in individuals experiencing psychotic phenomena, obviously an important area for inquiry considering the role of stressful life events as precipitants for psychotic experiences, in shaping the content of hallucinated voices and delusions [105], and in men's and women's responses to these phenomena. However, Myin-Germeys et al. [106], in a very interesting study examined sex differences in stress reactivity utilizing experience method sampling. They report that the women in their sample of 42 participants meeting the criteria for psychotic disorder (22 men; 20 women) were more likely to display elevated stress reactivity or emotional reactivity (reflected in both an increase in negative effect and a decrease in positive effect) to daily stress than men. The authors suggest that emotional reactivity to daily stress may be an underlying etiological mechanism for psychosis and constitutes part of the liability to psychosis. The authors speculate that as the small stressors and disturbances in daily life are equally distributed among men and women, it may be the case that women develop higher levels of stress sensitivity through a history of increased exposure to life events and possibly also higher levels of exposure to trauma. However, they did not investigate cognitive appraisals regarding why participants found a particular event stressful, which would have extended findings further with regard to possible underlying cognitive mechanisms and gender differences in terms of what constitutes stress for men and women, thus enabling an SGBA. Research employing an SGBA could be useful for examining HPA axis responses in relation to psychotic experiences and other life stressors, for example.

5.3.2.2 Gender and Self-Esteem

Because sex and gender distinctions are central, important, and pervasive in Western culture, it can be argued that gender is the earliest, most central, and most active organizing component of one's self-concept [47].

According to a cognitive psychological framework, individuals learn *shoulds* and *musts* from important persons in their lives and observe how others act and interact and the societal messages conveyed about those people. Mahalik [61] outlines how masculine/feminine gender role socialization contributes to self-schemata or gender role schemata influencing self-esteem. He discusses how gender role socialization contributes to gender-related cognitive distortions for men and women who are experiencing gender role conflict and underlines the implications for cognitive behavioral interventions. Empirical investigations have demonstrated associations between gender role conflict and depression as well as decreased self-esteem in men [100]. The underlying theoretical framework for this work is the gender role strain paradigm. Similarly, a large body of research based on objectification theory [107–109] has examined the impact of gender role socialization, and in particular, its deleterious impact of on female body image and self-esteem.

Mahalingam and Jackson [99] point to ethnographic research that indicates that idealized cultural gender roles shaped by patriarchy, such as chastity and masculinity, play a critical role in controlling women's and men's behavior through cultural gender imperatives, ultimately influencing self-worth. In their research with son preference societies they suggest that such societies resulting in an excessive male population lead to hypermasculine and hyperfeminine ideals, increasing patriarchal power structures, with detrimental impacts on mental health. This research underlines the importance of incorporating the multiple social categories and social determinants, such as ethnicity, social class, and culture, that intersect with gender to have an impact on mental health in research designs.

As it is known that self-esteem is a significant factor in most mental disorders it is not surprising that researchers have suggested that self-esteem might play a role in the origin, maintenance, and consequence of psychotic experiences, similar to that of depression [110–112]. A prospective general population study found that self-esteem was a risk factor for psychosis [112]. Considering that sex and gender are key features of self-esteem and that self-esteem is implicated in psychotic experience it follows that a sex and gender analysis is very important for both enhancing our understanding of psychosis and implementing more meaningful psychological interventions.

An SGBA can increase our understanding of the interplay among gender, self-esteem, and psychotic experiences, particularly in the light of the finding of a recent study that self-esteem is a predictor of hallucinations and persecutory delusions in early psychosis and that women report lower self-esteem than men [113]. In fact the investigators found that sex was a significant predictor of self-esteem in their first episode sample, with women having significantly lower levels of self-esteem than men, even after adjusting for differences in levels of depression. Another study of sex differences from the Danish Opus study of first-episode schizophrenia spectrum disorders, also reported that although women scored higher in global functioning than men, they scored lower on self-esteem and self-confidence [114].

5.3.2.3 Gender and Depression

Much of the research on sex differences in depression (i.e., the consistently reported finding that the prevalence of depressive disorders is greater in women than men at a rate at least twice that of men) [3] has focused on gender roles owing to the lack of empirical research supporting biological theories [115]. Various researchers have emphasized the importance of gender role expectations with regard to marriage, parenting, and employment, for example, in the etiology of psychological disorders [70]. The differing rates of depression for men and women are explained by differing societal expectations, according to several researchers [116]. Interestingly, rates of depression increase dramatically for both boys and girls during the 15- to 18-year age group, but the female rate rises to double the male prevalence rate [117].

In psychosis, the presentation of depression forms a very complex picture [118]. Birchwood distinguishes three core pathways of emotional disorder in psychosis:

(1) As intrinsic to the psychosis diatheses
(2) As a psychological reaction to psychosis and its sequelae referred to as *post-psychotic depression*
(3) As the result of a disturbed developmental pathway

Researchers also point to the difficulty of sometimes disentangling "negative symptoms" and depression, with some researchers suggesting that it is goal-directed behavior and "defeatist beliefs" that might be underlying negative symptom presentation [119–121], features also common in depression. The repeated finding that women with psychosis present with more affective symptomatology than men and men with more negative symptomatology, may be reflecting the differential expression of depression between men and women in the general population [160]. Here, again, an SGBA would be helpful in exploring these complex presentations.

5.3.2.4 Gender and Men's Health

A large body of work from the field of men's psychology has demonstrated the harmful effects of gender role socialization on men's psychological and physical well-being ranging from depression, lower self-esteem, substance abuse, aggression, elevated blood pressure, and high-risk health habits [61, 100]. Some authors have pointed out that men who violate male gender role norms are subject to more social disapproval than women [53].

Good et al. [122], examining male gender role conflict and psychological distress as measured by the Symptom Checklist-90-Revised, found associations of masculine gender role conflict with depression and interpersonal sensitivity as well as paranoia, psychoticism, and obsessive compulsivity in male students from two different US universities who had requested counseling services. The strongest association for psychoticism was with restrictive emotionality. Paranoid ideation was also related to restrictive emotionality in addition to success, power, and competition, components of male gender role conflict. Obsessive compulsivity was associated with men's conflict between work and family relations. The authors emphasize the clinical implications associated with the harmful psychological impacts of male gender role socialization:

> Given the relations between a range of psychological symptoms and masculine gender role conflict, it appears that men in US society might be psychologically healthier if they did not attempt to limit their feelings, cognitions and behaviours to those prescribed by masculine gender roles. In addition, given the relations observed here, counsellors would be wise to examine the extent to which male clients experiencing depression, interpersonal sensitivity, obsessive-compulsivity, and even psychosis have concerns or discomfort related to male gender roles (p. 48).

5.3.2.5 Gender and Impact of Trauma/Sexual Abuse

A number of studies examining gender ideologies and trauma have reported struggles with sexual identity, negative gender schemata, and shame in both men [9] and women who have experienced sexual abuse [8, 123]. They point out how one's core beliefs about themselves, others, and their relationships are often challenged by the experience of childhood sexual abuse. Studies, particularly qualitative research, reveal that the socio-cultural context and gender in particular influence how individuals make meaning of and respond to traumatic experience [8]. As trauma is common in people with psychosis and there is an association of childhood sexual abuse with hallucinations [6, 84, 124, 125], this line of inquiry may be fruitful in terms of increasing our understanding of how gender interacts with trauma. For example, gender shapes illness experience and presentation in terms of the content of hallucinated voices and experience of and relationship with voices and others in one's social world, underlining obvious implications for intervention. Furthermore, in the light of research that suggests that negative beliefs about the self and the world might be developed in response to trauma mediating the distress arising from psychotic phenomena [22], an SBGA has the potential to increase our understanding of how gender role norms have an impact on such negative self-schemata and core beliefs, ultimately influencing self-esteem and distress. Recent studies have revealed that the sexual content of voices and/or delusions predicts a history of childhood sexual abuse [126–129]. These researchers also point out the important clinical implications for assessing childhood trauma and trauma-related symptoms and for offering a range of trauma-focused treatment interventions. Birchwood et al. [24] suggest that earlier experiences of trauma such as abuse and harassment may be related to the sense of powerlessness and subordination the person experiences in relation to their hallucinated voices and others in their social world. In addition, the few studies that examined sex differences in rates of sexual abuse in psychosis samples reported that CSA was almost double for women than men [130–132] (in an epidemiological study, CSA was five times greater for women than men [133]), that it moderated the effect of sexual trauma and psychosis (being stronger for women) [124], that the prevalence of sexual trauma was higher in ultra-high-risk (UHR) women [129], and in a large epidemiological case–control study of first-episode psychosis, an association of sexual and physical abuse with psychosis was found in women but not in men [134]. Mixed samples found an incidence (3:1) of sexual abuse among women and conversely a higher incidence of physical abuse among men (3:2) than among women [135]. Furthermore, the finding that sexual abuse increases the chance of conversion in UHR individuals almost threefold has important implications for SGBA when conducting research, for prevention [136], as well as for psychological treatment interventions, underscoring the importance of both trauma-informed/-specific and gender-specific approaches to treatment.

In an attempt to redress the lack of studies examining gender-specific responses to child abuse in psychosis, Barker-Collo and Read [137] examined the relationships between child physical and sexual abuse with psychoticism and other subscales of the Symptom Checklist-90 Revised, in addition to coping styles [26]. The authors indicate that while men and women reported similar levels of psychoticism in the absence of abuse, when abuse had been experienced, men's reports of psychoticism and depression increased more than those of women, peaking with sexual abuse. Men also reported a sharper increased overall severity of difficulties on the Global Severity Index (GSI) than women when abuse was reported, as well as a significant elevation in paranoid ideation for men in the sexually abused only grouping. Other differential responses to abuse reported by the investigators were that men are less likely to employ the coping style: "seeking guidance and support" and more likely to employ "emotional discharge" (when sexually but not physically abused), which refers to "take it out on other people when you felt angry or depressed." The authors point out that the finding that males employ "emotional discharge" to cope is consistent with other research that demonstrates that men typically respond to abuse with "...externalizing and aggressive behaviour, sometimes reaching criminal levels as adults" (p. 37). For individuals who had been both sexually and physically abused, psychoticism and paranoid ideation were elevated for both sexes. Barker-Collo and Read [26] emphasize that, "...sexual abuse is rarely spontaneously disclosed by either gender. Boys are not only less likely than girls to spontaneously tell anyone at the time of the abuse but also take longer to do so, or to seek help for the effects of the abuse, as adolescents or adults" (p. 37). This factor, in addition to the findings demonstrating differential coping styles between both sexes who have been abused, underlines the importance of an SGBA in psychosis research for understanding the pathways from trauma to psychosis and the underlying mechanisms involved. For this reason, the authors urge researchers to incorporate a gender analysis into future psychosis research.

5.4 SGBA: Aiding Clarification of Sex Differences

Understanding the impact of gender roles has utility for clarifying some of the reported sex differences in schizophrenia (to date, the literature has failed to explain [adequately] how these differences came about [138]). For example, the repeated finding that men experience more *negative symptoms* than women could be possibly clarified if examined from a gender perspective. Difficulty experiencing, fantasizing, thinking about, and expressing one's emotions or *alexithymia* [139], is more common in men than in women in the general population [140], and men with higher levels of gender role conflict tend to have higher levels of alexithymia [59, 141, 142]. This research has emphasized that one normative masculine role requirement is the restriction of emotional expression, with empirical research finding a relationship between the endorsement of traditional masculinity, ideology and alexithymia in men. In the psychosis field, emerging research has demonstrated within the negative symptom construct, two subdomains: diminished expression and a motivation that has been found to be related to goal-directed behavior and defeatist attitudes [119–121], with motivation identified as the key component especially with regard to functional outcome [120]. Could the subdomain of diminished expression be related to an exaggerated form of alexithymia? Van't Wout et al. [143] found that men (but not women) with schizophrenia reported greater difficulty verbalizing and identifying their emotions and heightened levels of emotional arousal. Research utilizing a sex- and gender-based analysis could be helpful in exploring this possibility, employing scales such as the Gender Role Conflict Scale I (GRCS-I) [52], an empirically derived measure of male gender role conflict or gender role strain assessing restrictive emotionality as one of four domains that include success/power/competition, restrictive affectionate behavior between men, and conflict between work and family relations. Furthermore, as male role norms emphasized achievement and competition, the subdomain of amotivation as related to goal-directed behavior and defeatist attitudes may also have particular relevance for young men who are struggling with these societal messages in their developmental trajectory. Foussias and Remington [120] remind us that "...the earliest descriptions of schizophrenia emphasized a disturbance of volition/will as the fundamental underlying process in its pathology" (p. 359). This is an interesting area to pursue because psychosis onset appears in late adolescence, earlier in men than women, typically at the time when developmental stressors and social roles such as sociosexuality, achievement, and vocational issues are particularly pronounced for young men [87, 144, 145]. Several authors point out that childhood and adolescence are critical periods for "navigating influential and culturally variable constructs of masculinity/femininity ...as part of a complex set of negotiations of an individual's gendered self that continues throughout the life course..." [146]. Here, we can see how the gender role strain paradigm could be relevant for understanding the social pressures, particularly for young men who may be at an increased risk for gender role strain, impacting self-esteem and resulting in psychological distress. The findings that 1. there is poorer academic, occupational, and interpersonal functioning in men than in women before the diagnosis [147–149] and 2. that personal goals are reflected in men's delusional themes [150] also suggest a role for gender and thus SGBA in psychosis research, and again highlight the importance of gender-responsive psychological interventions.

5.5 Conclusion: SGBA Equals Better Science

In conclusion, this paper has outlined several important factors, summarized below, that emphasize the usefulness of an SGBA in enhancing schizophrenia research. Several of these factors, have led to recent international developments such as

WHO advocating SBGA, not only to improve health research, policy, and services but also to respond to gender-related health inequities as a matter of human rights [40, 151]:

1. Gender influences exposure to risk factors such as sexual violence, socioeconomic disadvantage, and low social rank, all of which have been linked to psychosis.
2. Research has demonstrated harmful psychological impacts of internalized gender role expectations on both men and women; however, this has not been explored in the psychosis field.
3. Research, qualitative studies in particular, has revealed how gender influences the impact of sexual abuse. Cultural beliefs about masculinity, femininity, and sexuality influence how female and male survivors make sense of their traumatic experience [8, 9, 123]. Obviously, this is a very important area to explore in individuals with a psychosis diagnosis in the light of research linking sexual abuse and psychosis and has implications for the need to develop gender-responsive, trauma-informed, and trauma-specific psychological interventions.
4. In addition to increasing understanding of the cognitive and psychological mechanisms that generate and maintain distressing psychotic experiences, an SBGA both implicates and satisfies the need to address social factors and injustices by extending analysis beyond intrapsychic distress at the individual level to the sociocultural level. As Connell [152], advocating a "relational gender analysis," explains: "The analysis needs to consider simultaneously the shape of the gender order and its historical transformations, the pattern of institutional and interpersonal relations, and the body-reflexive practices in which health consequences are produced" (p. 1679).
5. SGBA promotes a theoretical sophistication inherent in the overlapping constructs of *sex* and *gender*, where there are not always clear divisions for the biological, psychological, and sociocultural influences.

Greater sensitivity needs to be paid to sex and gender issues in all areas of health research. Failure to recognize this leads to bad science and avoidable mortality, morbidity, and disability [153], (p. 162).

This paper has illustrated that the same argument applies to schizophrenia research. SGBA in schizophrenia research is long overdue. Let's hope that it does not take another decade before we see a true integration of SGBA, improving the science of our field.

References

1. Nowatzki N, Grant KR. Sex is not enough: the need for gender-based analysis in health research. Health Care Women Int. 2011;32:263–77.
2. Johnson JL, Greaves L, Repta R. Better science with sex and gender: a primer for health research. Vancouver: Women's Health Research Network; 2007.
3. World Health Organization. Gender in mental health research report. Geneva: Author. http://libdoc.who.int/publications/2004/9241592532.pdf; 2004. Accessed Mar 29, 2011.

4. DoH. Women's mental health: into the mainstream. Strategic development of mental health care for women. London: Department of Health; 2002.
5. Nasser EH, Walders N, Jenkins JH. The experience of schizophrenia: what's gender got to do with it? A critical review of the current status of research on schizophrenia. Schizophr Bull. 2002;28(2):351–62.
6. Varese F, Smeets F, Drukker M, Lieverse R, Lataster T, Viechtbauer W, Read J, van Os J, Bentall RPB. Childhood adversities increase the risk of psychosis: a meta-analysis of patient-control, prospective- and cross-sectional cohort studies. Schizophr Bull. 2012;38(4):661–71.
7. Goodman LA, Rosenberg SD, Mueser KT, Drake RE. Physical and sexual assault history in women with serious mental illness: prevalence, correlates, treatment, and future research directions. Schizophr Bull. 1997;23(4):685–96.
8. Lebowitz L, Roth S. "I felt like a slut": the cultural context and women's response to being raped. J Trauma Stress. 1994;7(3):363–90.
9. Lisak D. The psychological impact of sexual abuse: content analysis of interviews with male survivors. J Trauma Stress. 1994;7(4):525–47.
10. Harrison G, Brewin J, Cantwell R, Dalkin T, Fox R, Jones P, Medley I. Increased incidence of psychotic disorders in migrants from the Caribbean to the United Kingdom. Psychol Med. 1997;27:799–806.
11. Selten JP, Cantor-Graae E. Hypothesis: social defeat is a risk factor for schizophrenia? Br J Psychiatry. 2007;51:S9–12.
12. Harrison G, Gunnell D, Glazebrook C. Association between schizophrenia and social inequality at birth: case-control study. Br J Psychiatry. 2001;179:346–50.
13. Krabbendam L, van Os J. Schizophrenia and urbanicity: a major environmental influence—conditional on genetic risk. Schizophr Bull. 2005;31(4):106–12.
14. Pedersen CB, Mortensen PB. Evidence of a dose-response relationship between urbanicity during upbringing and schizophrenia risk. Arch Gen Psychiatry. 2001;58:1039–46.
15. Bentall RP, Wickham S, Shevlin M, Varese F. Do specific early-life adversities lead to specific symptoms of psychosis? A study from the 2007 adult psychiatric morbidity survey. Schizophr Bull. 2012;38(4):734–40.
16. Morgan C, Kirkbride J, Leff J, et al. Parental separation, loss and psychosis in different ethnic groups: a case-control study. Psychol Med. 2007;37:495–503.
17. Arseneault L, Cannon M, Fisher HL, Polanczyk G, Moffitt TE, Caspi A. Childhood trauma and children's emerging psychotic symptoms: a genetically sensitive longitudinal cohort study. Am J Psychiatry. 2011;168:65–72.
18. Schreier A, Wolke D, Thomas K, et al. Prospective study of peer victimization in childhood and psychotic symptoms in a nonclinical population at age 12 Years. Arch Gen Psychiatry. 2009;66:527–36.
19. Bentall RP, Fernyhough C. Social predictors of psychotic experiences: specificity and psychological mechanisms. Schizophr Bull. 2008;34:1009–11.
20. Read J, van Os J, Morrison A, Ross C. Childhood trauma, psychosis and schizophrenia: a literature review with theoretical and clinical implications? Acta Psychiatr Scand. 2005;112: 330–50.
21. Morrison AP, Read J, Turkington D. Trauma and psychosis: theoretical and clinical implications. Acta Psychiatr Scand. 2005;112:327–9.
22. Morrison AP. The interpretation of intrusions in psychosis: an integrative cognitive approach to hallucinations and delusions. Behav Cogn Psychother. 2001;29:257–76.
23. Birchwood M, Meaden A, Trower P, Gilbert J, Plainstow J. The power and omnipotence of voices and significant others. Psychol Med. 2000;30(2):337–44.
24. Birchwood M, Gilbert P, Gilbert J, Trower P, Meaden A, Hay J, Miles JNV. Interpersonal and role-related schema influence the relationship with the dominant 'voice' in schizophrenia: a comparison of three models. Psychol Med. 2004;34(08):1571–80.

25. Hayward M, Berry K, Ashton A. Applying interpersonal theories to the understanding of and therapy for auditory hallucinations: a review of the literature and directions for further research. Clin Psychol Rev. 2011;31(8):1313–23.
26. Barker-Collo S, Read J. The roles of gender and coping styles in the relationship between child abuse and the SCL-90-R subscales 'psychoticism' and 'paranoid ideation'. NZ J Psychol. 2011;40:28–38.
27. Ivezic SS, John N. Gender and schizophrenia. Psychiatr Danub. 2009;21 Suppl 1:106–10.
28. Lewine R. At issue: sex and gender in schizophrenia. Schizophr Bull. 2004;30(4):755–62.
29. Lewine RR. Sex: an imperfect marker of gender. Schizophr Bull. 1994;20(4):777–9.
30. Leung A, Chue P. Sex differences in schizophrenia, a review of the literature. Acta Psychiatr Scand. 2000;101:3–38.
31. Read J. Poverty, ethnicity, and gender. In: Read J, Mosher L, Bentall R, editors. Models of madness: psychological, social and biological approaches to schizophrenia. London: Routledge; 2004. p. 161–94.
32. Sharma RP, Dowd SM, Janicak PG. Hallucinations in the acute schizophrenic-type psychosis: effects of gender and age of illness onset. Schizophr Res. 1999;37(1):91–5.
33. Murphy JA, Shevlin M, Adamson G, Houston J. A population based analysis of sub-clinical psychosis and help-seeking behaviour. Schizophr Bull. 2010;38:360–7. doi:10.1093/schbul/sbq092.
34. Tien AY. Distributions of hallucinations in the population. Soc Psychiatry Psychiatr Epidemiol. 1991;26:287–92.
35. Unger RK. Imperfect reflections of reality: psychology constructs gender. In: Hare Mustin RT, Maracek J, editors. Making a difference: psychology and the construction of gender. New Haven: Yale University Press; 1999.
36. Hare-Mustin RT, Marecek J. Asking the right questions: feminist psychology and sex differences. Fem Psychol. 1994;4(4):531–7.
37. Riecher-Rössler A, Pflüger M, Borgwardt S. Schizophrenia in women. In: Kohen D, editor. Oxford textbook of women and mental health. Oxford: Oxford University Press; 2010. p. 102–14.
38. Daniel D, Mathew R, Wilson W. Sex roles and regional cerebral blood flow. Psychiatry Res. 1988;27:55–64.
39. Health Canada. Health Canada's gender-based analysis policy. Ottawa, ON: Minister of Public Works and Government Services Canada; 2000.
40. Clow B, Pederson A, Haworth-Brockman M, Bernier J. Rising to the challenge: sex- and gender-based analysis for health planning, policy, and research in Canada. Halifax, NS: Atlantic Centre of Excellence for Women's Health; 2009.
41. Health Canada. Health portfolio sex and gender-based analysis policy, vol. 10. http://www.hc-sc.gc.ca/hl-vs/pubs/women-femmes/sgba-policy-politique-ags-eng.php. Accessed Feb, 2010; 2014.
42. Levant RF, Richmond K, Cook S, Tanner House A, Aupont M. The femininity ideology scale: factor structure, reliability, convergent and discriminant validity, and social contextual variation. Sex Roles. 2007;57:373–83.
43. Nasser M. Women, ethnicity, and mental health. In: Kohen D, editor. Oxford textbook of women and mental health. Oxford: Oxford University Press; 2010. p. 23–9.
44. Knaak S. On the reconceptualising of gender: implications for research design. Sociol Inq. 2004;74(3):302–17.
45. Liverpool School of Tropical Medicine, Gender and Health Group (Undated). http://www.lstmliverpool.ac.uk/research/academic-groups/international-health/gender-and-health-group/gaf. Accessed May 15, 2012.
46. Marsh DT. Serious emotional disturbance and serious mental illness. In: Worrell J, Goodheart CD, editors. Handbook of girl's and women's psychological health. New York: Oxford University Press; 2006.

47. Koestner R, Aube J. A multifactorial approach to the study of gender characteristics. J Pers. 1995;63(3):681–710.
48. Spence JT. Gender-related traits and gender ideology: evidence for a multifactorial theory. J Pers Soc Psychol. 1993;64(4):624–35.
49. Bem SL. The measurement of psychological androgyny. J Consult Clin Psychol. 1974;42: 155–62.
50. Bem SL. Gender schema theory: a cognitive account of sex typing source. Psychol Rev. 1981;88:354.
51. Levant RF, Fischer J. The male role norms inventory. In: Davis C, Yarber W, Bauserman R, Schreer G, Davis S, editors. Sexuality-related measures: a compendium. 2nd ed. Newbury Park, CA: Sage; 1998. p. 469–72.
52. O'Neil JM, Helms B, Gable R, David L, Wrightsman L. Gender role conflict scale: college men's fear of femininity. Sex Roles. 1986;14:335–50.
53. Pleck JH. The myth of masculinity. Cambridge: MIT Press; 1981.
54. Pleck JH. The gender role strain paradigm: an update. In: Levant RF, Pollack WS, editors. A new psychology of men. New York: Basic Books; 1995.
55. Eisler RM. The relationship between masculine gender role stress and men's health risk: the validation of a construct. In: Levant RF, Pollock WS, editors. A new psychology of men. New York: Basic Books; 1995. p. 207–25.
56. Mahalik JR, Locke BD, Ludlow LH, Diemer M, Scott RPJ, Gottfried M, et al. Development of the conformity to masculine norms inventory. Psychol Men Masc. 2003;4:3–25.
57. Mahalik JR, Morray EB, Coonerty-Femiano A, Ludlow LH, Slattery SM, Smiler A. Development of the conformity to feminine norms inventory. Sex Roles. 2005;52(7/8):417–35.
58. Boyle M. Making gender visible in clinical psychology. Fem Psychol. 1997;7(2):231–8.
59. Levant RF. Research in the psychology of men and masculinity using the gender role strain paradigm as a framework. Am Psychol. 2011;66(8):765–76.
60. Levant RF, Rankin TJ, Williams CM, Hasan NT, Smalley KB. Evaluation of the factor structure and construct validity of scores on the Male Role Norms Inventory—Revised (MRNI–R). Psychol Men Masc. 2010;11(1):25–37.
61. Mahalik JR. Incorporating a gender role strain perspective in assessing and treating men's cognitive distortions. Prof Psychol Res Pr. 1999;30(4):333–40.
62. Mahalik JK, Talmadge WT, Locke BD, Scott RPJ. Using the conformity to masculine norms inventory to work with men in a clinical setting. J Clin Psychol. 2005;61:661–74.
63. Toner B, Tang T, Ali A, Akman D, Stuckless N, Esplen MJ, et al. Developing a gender-role socialization scale. In: Oliffe JL, Greaves L, editors. Designing and conducting gender, sex, and health research. Los Angeles: Sage; 2012. p. 189–200.
64. Johnson JL, Repta R. Sex and gender: beyond the binaries. In: Oliffe JL, Greaves L, editors. Designing and conducting gender, sex, and health research. Los Angeles: Sage; 2012. p. 39–64.
65. Johnson JL, Repta R, Kaylan S. Implications of sex and gender for health research. In: Oliffe JL, Greaves L, editors. Designing and conducting gender, sex, and health research. Los Angeles: Sage; 2012. p. 39–64.
66. Johnson JL, Greaves L, Repta R. Better science with sex and gender: facilitating the use of a sex and gender-based analysis in health research. Int J Equity Health. 2009;8(14):1–11.
67. Eisler RM, Skidmore JR. Masculine gender role stress. Behav Modif. 1987;11(2):123–36.
68. Gilbert P, Allen S. The role of defeat and entrapment (arrested flight) in depression: an exploration of an evolutionary view. Psychol Med. 1998;28:585–98.
69. World Health Organization. Women's Mental Health: an evidence-based review. Geneva: Author. http://www.who.int/mental_health/media/en/67.pdf; 2000. Accessed Mar 29, 2011.
70. Ballou M, Brown LS, editors. Rethinking mental health and disorder: feminist perspectives. New York: Guilford; 2002.
71. Worell J, Remer P. Feminist perspectives in therapy: empowering diverse women. Hoboken, NJ: Wiley; 2003.

72. Brown LS. Feminist therapy. Washington, DC: American Psychological Association; 2009.
73. Levant RF. The crisis of connection between men and women. J Mens Stud. 1996;5:1–12.
74. Tang TN, Tang CS. Gender role internalization, multiple roles, and Chinese women's mental health. Psychol Women Q. 2001;25:181–96.
75. Tolman DL, Impett EA, Tracy AJ, Michael A. Looking good, sounding good: femininity ideology and adolescent girls' mental health. Psychol Women Q. 2006;30(1):85–95.
76. Sirin SR, McCreary DR, Mahalik JR. Differential reactions to men and women's gender role transgressions: perceptions of social status, sexual orientation, and value dissimilarity. J Mens Stud. 2004;12:119–32.
77. O'Neil JM, Good GE, Holmes SE. Fifteen years of theory and research on men's gender role conflict: new paradigms for empirical research. In: Levant R, Pollack W, editors. A new psychology of men. New York: Basic Books; 1995.
78. Thompson EH, Pleck JH. Masculinity ideologies: a review of research instrumentation on men and masculinities. In: Levant RF, Pollack WS, editors. A new psychology of men. New York, NY: Basic Books; 1995. p. 129–63.
79. Longenecker J, Genderson J, Dickinson D, Malley J, Elvevåg B, Weinberger DR, Gold J. Where have all the women gone?: participant gender in epidemiological and non-epidemiological research of schizophrenia. Schizophr Res. 2010;119(1–3):240–5.
80. Hambrecht M, Maurer K, Häfner H. Evidence for a gender bias in epidemiological studies of schizophrenia. Schizophr Res. 1993;8(3):223–31.
81. Wahl OF, Hunter J. Are gender effects being neglected in schizophrenia research? Schizophr Bull. 1992;18(2):313–7.
82. Iacono WG, Beiser M. Are males more likely than females to develop schizophrenia. Am J Psychiatr. 1992;I49:1070–4.
83. Iacono WG, Beiser M. Where are the women in first-episode studies of schizophrenia? Schizophr Bull. 1992;18:471–80.
84. Read J, Fink PJ, Rudeqeair T, Felitti V, Whitefield CL. Child maltreatment and psychosis: time to return to the genuinely integrated bio-psycho-social model. Clin Schizophr Relat Psychoses. 2008;2:235–54.
85. Taylor PJ, Braqado-Jimenez MD. Women, psychosis, and violence. Int J Law Psychiatry. 2009;32(1):56–64.
86. Aleman A, Kahn RS, Selten JP. Sex differences in the risk of schizophrenia: evidence from meta-analysis. Arch Gen Psychiatry. 2003;60:565–71.
87. Seeman MV. Schizophrenic men and women require different treatment programs. J Psychiatr Treat Eval. 1983;5:143–8.
88. Falkenburg J, Tracy DK. Sex and schizophrenia: a review of gender differences. Psychos Psychol Soc Integr Approaches. 2012;6(1):1–9.
89. Rudden M, Sweeney J, Frances A, Gilmore M. A comparison of delusional disorders in women and men. Am J Psychiatry. 1983;140(12):1575–8.
90. Stone M. The borderline syndromes. New York: McGraw-Hill; 1980.
91. Carmen EM, Russo NF, Miller JB. Inequality and mental health. Am J Psychiatr. 1981;138(10):1319–39.
92. Mowbray CT, Nicholson J, Bellamy CD. Psychosocial rehabilitation service needs of women. Psychiatr Rehabil J. 2003;27:104–33.
93. Goldstein JM, Kreisman D. Gender, family environment and schizophrenia. Psychol Med. 1988;18:861–72.
94. Al-Issa I. Gender and schizophrenia. In: Al-Issa I, editor. Gender and psychopathology. New York: Academic; 1982. p. 153–77.
95. Murphy HMB. Cultural aspects of delusion. Stud Gen. 1967;20:684–92.
96. Månsdotter A, Nordenmark M, Hammarström A. The importance of childhood and adulthood aspects of gendered life for adult mental ill-health symptoms—a 27-year follow-up of the Northern Swedish Cohort. BMC Public Health. 2012;12:493–504.

97. Good GE, Mintz LB. Gender role conflict and depression in college men: evidence for compound risk. J Couns Devel. 1990;69:17–21.
98. Levant RF, Pollock WS. A new psychology of men. New York: Basic; 1995.
99. Mahalingam R, Jackson B. Idealized cultural beliefs about gender: implications for mental health. Soc Epidemiol Soc Psychiatry. 2007;42:1012–23.
100. O'Neil JM. Summarizing, 25 years of research on men's gender role conflict using the gender role conflict scale - New research paradigms and clinical implications. [Review]. Couns Psychol. 2008;36(3):358–445.
101. Sharpe MJ, Heppner PP. Gender role, gender-role conflict, and psychological well-being in men. J Couns Psychol. 1991;38(3):323–30.
102. Morrison J. Masculinity moderates the relationship between symptoms of PTSD and cardiac-related health behaviors in male veterans. Psychol Men Masc. 2012;13(2):158–65.
103. Lazarus RS, Folkman S. Stress, appraisal, and coping. New York: Springer; 1984.
104. Dedovic K, Wadiwalla M, Engert V, Pruessner JC. The role of sex and gender socialization in stress reactivity. Dev Psychol. 2009;45(1):45–55.
105. Raune D, Bebbington P, Dunn G, Kuipers E. Event attributes and the content of psychotic experiences in first-episode psychosis. Psychol Med. 2006;36:221–30.
106. Myin-Germeys I, Krabbendam L, Delespaul PA, van Os J. Sex differences in emotional reactivity to daily life stress in psychosis. J Clin Psychiatry. 2004;65:805–9.
107. Fredrickson BL, Roberts TA. Objectification theory: toward understanding women's lived experiences and mental health risks. Psychol Women Q. 1997;21:173–206.
108. Moradi B. Objectification theory: areas of promise and refinement. Couns Psychol. 2011; 39(1):153–63.
109. Szymanski DM, Moffitt LB, Carr ER. Sexual objectification of women: advances to theory and research 1ψ7. Couns Psychol. 2011;39(1):6–38.
110. Smith B, Fowler DG, Freeman D, Bebbington P, Bashforth H, Garety P, et al. Emotion and psychosis: links between depression, self-esteem, negative schematic beliefs and delusions and hallucinations. Schizophr Res. 2006;86:181–8.
111. Fowler D, Freeman D, Smith B, Kuipers E, Bebbington P, et al. The Brief Core Schema Scales (BCSS): psychometric properties and associations with paranoia and grandiosity in non-clinical and psychosis samples. Psychol Med. 2006;36:749–59.
112. Krabbendam L, Janssen I, Bak M, Bijl RV, de Graaf R, van Os J. Neuroticism and low self-esteem as risk factors for psychosis. Soc Psychiatry Psychiatr Epidemiol. 2002;37(1):1–6.
113. Romm KL, Rossberg JI, Hansen CF, Haug E, Andreassen OA, Melle I. Self-esteem is associated with premorbid adjustment and positive psychotic symptoms in early psychosis. BMC Psychiatry. 2011;11:136.
114. Thorup A, Petersen L, Jeppesen P, Ohlenschlæger J, Christensen T, Krarup G, Jorgensen P, Nordentoft M. Gender differences in young adults with first-episode schizophrenia spectrum disorders at baseline in the Danish OPUS study. J Nerv Ment Dis. 2007;195:396–405.
115. Nolen Hoeksema S. Epidemiology and theories of gender differences in unipolar depression. In: Seeman MV, editor. Gender and psychopathology. Washington, DC: American Psychiatric Press; 1995. p. 63–87.
116. Sparks E. Depression and schizophrenia in women: the intersection of gender, race/ethnicity, and class. In: Ballou M, Brown LS, editors. Rethinking mental health and disorder: Feminist perspective. New York: Guilford; 2002. p. 279–305.
117. Hankin BL, Abramson LY, Moffitt TE, Silva PA, McGee R, Angell KE. Development of depression from preadolescence to young adulthood: emerging gender differences in a 10-year longitudinal study. J Abnorm Psychol. 1998;107:128–40.
118. Birchwood M. Pathways to emotional dysfunction in first episode psychosis. 2003.
119. Beck AT, Grant PM, Huh GA, Perivoliotis D, Chang NA. Dysfunctional attitudes and expectancies in deficit syndrome schizophrenia. Schizophr Bull. 2011 Epub.
120. Foussias G, Remington G. Negative symptoms in schizophrenia: avolition and Occam's razor. Schizophr Bull. 2010;36(2):359–69.

121. Grant PM, Beck AT. Defeatist beliefs as a mediator of cognitive impairment, negative symptoms, and functioning in schizophrenia. Schizophr Bull. 2009;35(4):798–806.
122. Good GE, Robertson JM, Fitzgerald LF, Stevens M, Bartels KM. The relation between masculine role conflict and psychological distress in male university counselling centre clients. J Couns Devel. 1996;75:44–9.
123. Krause E, Roth S. Child sexual abuse history and feminine gender-role identity. Sex Roles. 2011;64(1):32–42.
124. Bebbington PE, Jonas S, Kuipers E, King M, Cooper C, Brugha T, Meltzer H, McManus S, Jenkins R. Sexual abuse and psychosis: data from an English National survey. Br J Psychiatry. 2011;199:29–37.
125. Elklit A, Shevlin M. Female sexual victimization predicts psychosis: a case-control study based on the Danish Registry System. Schizophr Bull. 2011;37:1305–10.
126. Hardy A, Fowler D, Freeman D, Smith B, Steel C, Evans J, Garety P, Kuipers E, Bebbington PE, Dunn G. Trauma and hallucinatory experience in psychosis. J Nerv Ment Dis. 2005;193: 501–7.
127. Read J, Argyle N. Hallucinations, delusions, and thought disorder among adult psychiatric in patients with a history of child abuse. Psychiatr Serv. 1999;50:1467–72.
128. Reiff M, Castille DM, Muenzenmaier K, Link B. Childhood Abuse and the content of adult psychotic symptoms. Psychol Trauma. 2011;4:356–99.
129. Thompson A, Nelson B, McNab C, Simmons M, Leicester S, McGorry PD, Yung AR. Psychotic symptoms with sexual content in the "ultra high risk" for psychosis population: frequency and association with sexual trauma. Psychiatr Res. 2010;177(1–2):84–91.
130. Conus P, Cotton S, Schimmelmann BG, et al. Pretreatment and outcome correlates of past sexual and physical trauma in 118 bipolar I disorder patients with a first episode of psychotic mania. Bipolar Disord. 2010;12:244–52.
131. Lysaker PH, Beattie BA, Strasburger MA, Davis LW. Reported history of child sexual abuse in schizophrenia—association with heightened symptom levels and poorer participation over four months in vocational rehabilitation. J Nerv Ment Dis. 2005;193:790–5.
132. Morgan C, Fisher H. Environmental factors in schizophrenia: childhood trauma–a critical review. Schizophr Bull. 2007;33:3–10.
133. Cotton S, Lambert M, Schimmelmann BG, Foley DL, Morley KI, McGorry PD, Conus P. Gender differences in premorbid, entry, treatment, and outcome characteristics in a treated epidemiological sample of 661 patients with first episode psychosis. Schizophr Res. 2009;114:17–24.
134. Fisher H, Morgan C, Dazzan P, Craig T, Morgan K, Hutchinson G, Jones PB, Doody GA, Pariente C, McGuffin P, Murray RM, Leff J, Fearon P. Gender differences in the association between childhood abuse and psychosis. Br J Psychiatry. 2009;194:319–25.
135. MacMillan HL, Fleming JE, Streiner DL, Lin E, Boyle MH, Jamieson E, et al. Childhood abuse and lifetime psychopathology in a community sample. Am J Psychiatry. 2001;158(11): 1878–83.
136. Bechdolf A, Thompson A, Nelson B, Cotton S, Simmons MB, Amminger GP, Yung AR. Experience of trauma and conversion to psychosis in an ultra-high-risk (prodromal) group. Acta Psychiatr Scand. 2010;121(5):377–84.
137. Derogatis LR, Lazarus L. SCL-90-R, Brief Symptom Inventory and matching clinical rating scales. In: Maruish ME, editor. The use of psychological testing for treatment planning and outcome assessment. Hillsdale, NJ: Lawrence Erlbaum Associates; 1994. p. 217–48.
138. Aschebrock Y. Different realities: challenging conventional ways of conceptualising delusions and hallucinations. Unpublished Ph.D. thesis, University of Auckland, New Zealand; 2005.
139. Taylor GJ, Ryan DP, Bagby RM. Toward the development of a new self-report alexithymia scale. Psychother Psychosom. 1985;44:191–9.
140. Vorst HCM, Bermond B. Validity and reliability of the Bermond Vorst Alexithymia Questionnaire. Personal Individ Differ. 2001;30:413–34.

141. Berger JM, Levant RF, McMillan KK, Kelleher W, Sellers A. Impact of gender role conflict, traditional masculinity ideology, alexithymia, and age on men's attitudes toward psychological help seeking. Psychol Men Masc. 2005;6:73–8.
142. Fischer AR, Good GE. Men and psychotherapy: an investigation of alexithymia, intimacy, and masculine gender roles. Psychotherapy. 1997;34(2):160–70.
143. Van't Wout M, Aleman A, Bermond B, Kahn RS. No words for feelings: alexithymia in schizophrenia patients and first-degree relatives. Compr Psychiatry. 2007;48:27–33.
144. Harrop C, Trower P. Why does schizophrenia develop at late adolescence? Clin Psychol Rev. 2001;21:241–66.
145. Seeman MV. Gender differences in schizophrenia. Can J Psychiatr. 1982;27:107–12.
146. Abrams LS. Contextual variations in young women's gender identity negotiations. Psychol Women Q. 2003;27:64–74.
147. Mendrek A. Sex and gender differences in mental health research. In: Cohen S, Banister E, editors. What a difference sex and gender make: a gender, sex and health research casebook. Ottawa: Institute of Gender and Health of the Canadian Institutes of Health Research; 2012.
148. Morgan VA, Castle DJ, Jablensky AV. Do women express and experience psychosis differently from men? Epidemiological evidence from the Australian National Study of Low Prevalence (Psychotic) Disorders. Aust NZ J Psychiatry. 2008;42(1):74–82.
149. Salem JE, Kring AM. The role of gender differences in the reduction of etiologic heterogeneity in schizophrenia. Clin Psychol Rev. 1998;18(7):795–819.
150. Rhodes JE, Jakes S. Correspondence between delusions and personal goals: a qualitative analysis. Br J Med Psychol. 2000;73:211–25.
151. Commission on the Status of Women. Guidelines for a gender analysis: human rights with a gender perspective implementing the convention on the elimination of all forms of discrimination against women (CEDAW). San Francisco: Commission on the Status of Women; 2000.
152. Connell R. Gender, health, and theory: conceptualizing the issue, in local and world perspective. Soc Sci Med. 2012;74:1674–83.
153. Doyal L. Gender and the 10/90 gap in health research. Bull World Health Organ. 2004;82(3): 162.
154. Zamarripa MX, Wampold BE, Gregory E. Male gender role conflict, depression, and anxiety: clarification and generalizability to women. J Couns Psychol. 2003;50(3):333–8.
155. Sigmon ST, Stanton AL, Snyder CR. Gender differences in coping: a further test of socialization and role constraint theories. Sex Roles. 1995; 33(9/10): 565–587, Nos. 9/10.
156. Gillespie BL, Eisler RM. Development of the feminine gender role stress scale: a cognitive-behavioral measure of stress, appraisal, and coping for women. Behav Modif. 1992;16 (3):426–38.
157. Bentall R. Madness explained: psychosis and human nature. London: Penguin Books; 2004.
158. Bentall RP. Doctoring the mind: why psychiatric treatments fail. London: Penguin Books; 2009.
159. French P, Morrison AP. Early detection and cognitive therapy for people at high risk of developing psychosis: a treatment approach. London: Wiley; 2004.
160. Martin LA, Neighbors HW, Griffith DM. The experience of symptoms of depression in men vs women: analysis of the national comorbidity survey replication. JAMA Psychiatry. 2013;70(10):1100–6.
161. Institute of Gender and Health of the Canadian Institutes Health Research. (2012). What a difference sex and gender make: A gender, sex and health research casebook. Ottawa: Author.

Part II

Gender and Psychopathology

Gender and Corporality, Corporeality, and Body Image

6

Margarita Sáenz-Herrero and Cristina Díez-Alegría

As a woman, I have no country, as a woman I want no country.
As a woman, my country is the world.

Virginia Woolf

Abstract

The body and corporality constitute the nuclear axis of our identity. In Foucault's words, "we are embodied." In this respect, the paradigm of gender is what differentiates human beings at birth in the most nuclear way. The social dimension enters the individual and shapes her/him corporally (embodiment).

This chapter includes the anthropology of gender and the body, together with the cult of the body in Western society, underlining its repercussions for women, the body, and language, with the latter understood in Heideggerian terms as the medium that lives within us and shapes us; the body and gender as a nuclear element in constructing an individual's identity and, more specifically, in constructing female identity; the female body over the course of history and its medicalization and removal from public life; the body and corporality according to psychopathology, postmodern bodies; and body image, providing the global, complex vision that is the construction of human identity and, in particular, female identity.

M. Sáenz-Herrero (✉)
University of the Basque Country UPV/EHU, Vitoria, Spain

Department of Psychiatry, Alava University Hospital, Vitoria, Spain
e-mail: margarita.saenzherrero@osakidetza.net

C. Díez-Alegría
Clinical Hospital San Carlos, Madrid, Spain

Complutense, University of Madrid, Madrid, Spain

M. Sáenz-Herrero (ed.), *Psychopathology in Women*,
DOI 10.1007/978-3-319-05870-2_6

6.1 Introduction

The body, corporality, and its psychopathology are analyzed symptomatologically by descriptive psychopathology. However, many manuals do not even possess a section on the psychopathology of the corporality representing the body, the nuclear axis of our identity. The paradigm of gender is what differentiates human beings at birth in the most nuclear way. The first thing one asks about a baby is its sex. Despite biological diversity and the existence of syndromes such as Turner (X0), Klinefelter (XXY), hermaphroditism, and pseudohermaphroditism, we present ourselves in a binary manner, and gender is one of the taboos that is most difficult to break in our culture. Gender begins from birth; it has been learned, interpreted, as a value in our families and social and cultural environments over the course of history.

Hence, the duality of gender may initially seem inevitable as, in general, sex and the role of gender attributed at birth are interpreted as a permanent element over one's lifetime [1].

Last November, Germany became the first country in Europe (Australia too) to waive the obligation to record the sex of a newly born child on its birth certificate, a modest but important legal revolution enabling intersexual people to select the male or female sex at the hour of their choosing. It is the first European country to legislate on this issue (http://www.bbc.co.uk/news/world-europe-24767225).

Moreover, a transgender couple in Argentina who married in November 2013 are expecting their first child. In terms of their chromosomes and their biological sex, they remain the same. However, in this case these two people are identified (this being the complex process created by beliefs, feelings, attitudes, and models of identification in which each person is identified and by both partners) as possessing the gender opposite to their biological sex. This does not relate to sexual practice, as they are expecting their first child (in this case, the individual identified as the "man" according to gender identity continues to be a woman biologically). Hence, the social construction of gender identity is independent of sexual orientation. The notion of gender challenges the personal and emotional levels of the perception of our culture. What is natural? What is moral? What is normal? What is cultural?

From the sociological viewpoint, the body is individual (our being as a person), social (the use of the body as a metaphor and an organizer of the world around it), and political (the body's disciplines, rules, uses, and ideals, which differ in each culture and are modified over the course of history).

We need to broaden our scope by including gender when psychopathological aspects are involved. When dynamics change, symptoms change over the course of history. There is a need for a discourse that includes these aspects. This should not be limited to academicians, historians, anthropologists, or sociologists but directed at mental health in general. The first question in the construction of our reality must simply be how we know what we think we know: Is gender identity really limited to a binary form? Identity may be more or less masculine, more or less feminine, more or less androgynous (models who are also more socially successful: feminine men—i.e., gentle, sensitive, good communicators—and masculine women, i.e., courageous and determined). The duality is so descriptive that it transfers to sexual orientation, establishing the homo/hetero opposition, with scant consideration of asexual people, such as the celibate like nuns and priests in the Catholic religion or Buddhism.

Therefore, it seems necessary to force open the discourse and incorporate all that is hidden. For many years, men have been regarded as the neutral model and women the sexed one. Masculine education has been preferred for constructing the citizen and a female education for constructing the partner and/or mother of the citizen. Inequalities between men and women reflect the social hierarchization and male domination that is a reality in most societies in our world.

The social dimension is part of the body, if corporality is a process of social interaction, and this demonstrates its potential to us. There are various forms of regulating and disciplining the body in men and in women. With regard to the socialization of women, what is strengthened is the importance of ties and affectiveness. In numerous cultures, public space, decision-making capacity, and the means of production and economic and political power lie in the hands of men.

Femininity provides us with an identity that makes us someone to be perceived, viewed, someone who is in a permanent state of bodily insecurity and symbolic alienation. Appearance plays a key role in this identity. The adolescent girl discovers sexuality for the first time, not through an encounter with her body, but through someone else's gaze that undresses her [2].

From the corporeal experience, women's bodies are markedly represented by instrumentalization, dissociation, and tension. The body is an instrument, the object for performing a variety of functions of a social, reproductive, and productive nature. Maternity and corporal reality would be constitutive elements of an identity that on many occasions is dissociated with a sexuality and sensuality in tense coexistence. Bance [3] mentions the tension that is produced in the experience of sexuality as an area of exploration, pleasure, and action, although at the same time this may lead to distress, repression, and the danger of sexual aggression.

The impact of the feminist movement and gender theories has been crucial in social anthropology. However, psychopathology does not understand this type of paradigm as nuclear in the construction of individual subjectivity and therefore in how it is reflected in mental distress, especially in women, the principal users of community mental health services.

Nevertheless, feminist collectives are not responsible for the appearance of the concept of gender. Rather, it is a researcher into human sexuality, Dr. John Money, who used gender for the first time in its cultural acceptation, based on intersexual states in the human species being a scientific reality [1].

The Spanish philosopher, Amelia Valcárcel [4], sees the problem as power. We lack the power to address the problem. What determines what we are at present depends on the possibility of opening up orthodox medical discourse, given that the vocabulary of science is masculine in the main.

6.2 Body and Anthropological Aspects

A review of anthropological concepts reveals that the hunt was considered the motor of culture in human life. New interpretative models in the study of primates [5] have shown that some *Australopithecus* in Africa ate vegetables, indicating that both genders participated in group production and reproduction.

Anthropologists Marilyn Strathern and Carol McCormack [6] reported that nature is represented as feminine but is subordinate to a culture that is masculine. Reason and mind are related to masculinity but body and nature are related to femininity.

The revolution does not lie in conquering male privilege but in eliminating the distinction, says Marilyn Strathern [7].

Gender anthropology questions the accepted aspects of sexual dimorphism. This includes the difference in height between men and women, which applies neither to the population as a whole nor to all ethnic groups. Not all men are taller than all women, but cultural imperatives exist that give this impression. In numerous societies, couples are formed in accordance with scales of height, creating the impression that women are shorter. This is not true from a biological point of view. Women possess less muscular strength, a smaller breathing capacity, a finer skeleton, and a different weight and fat distribution. However, this does not explain the differences that are currently objectivized in Western societies when we see images of prehistoric women. They are more robust and have much more body hair than seems to exist in a "natural" form in Western women. The latter are increasingly thinner, with less body hair and more infantilized in terms of their genitals, except for their breasts which are increasingly larger.

The impact of Margaret Mead [8] on gender anthropology, the work of Simone de Beauvoir, and the arrival of the contraceptive pill are the three landmarks that marked a change in the twentieth century for women:

> I shared the general belief in our culture that there was a natural temperament which corresponds to each sex, which could, in extreme cases, become distorted or distanced from its normal expression. I failed to suspect that the temperaments we consider innate in a sex, could be rather a change, mere variations of the human temperament, which can be approximated by their education, with a greater or lesser success according to the individual, the members of one or both sexes. [8]

In different cultures throughout the world, body care occupies a main space in female identity along with the history of art. The woman's body and its ornaments are the way to attract the gaze of the opposite sex.

Neck rings are worn in a few African and Asian cultures, usually to create the appearance of a longer neck. Padaung women of the Kayan people begin to wear neck coils as young as 2 years old. The custom of wearing neck rings is related to an ideal of beauty: an elongated neck, giving rise to their name as "giraffe tribes." This can deform the shoulder blades and have medical consequences; if they are removed, the neck muscles are not strong enough to support the head. Nowadays in Western countries, we have height-increasing surgery, using a head implant to increase attractiveness and acquire the height to become a model, for example.

Foot binding is a custom of applying tight binding to the feet of young girls in order to prevent further growth. Called "lotus foot ancestry," it became very popular in China because men considered it highly attractive. It still takes place even today in Guangzhou in China. Tiny, narrow feet in women were considered attractive and made their movements more feminine. Nowadays, Western fashion involves women wearing footwear with high heels that deform their feet. In the nineteenth century, most women possessed a permanently deformed rib cage caused by the habitual wearing of corsets that conformed to the fashion for narrow waists.

Mursi women in Ethiopia wear lip plates that deform their lips, while in some parts of Africa and in Asian countries the lower lip of girls is cut by their mothers or by another woman from their settlement. Western women inject silicone into their lips in an attempt to gain attractiveness.

Ablation of the clitoris, feminine genital mutilation, affects 135 million women and children throughout the world, and the increase in immigration has brought the practice to Europe. Ablation is widespread in a large part of Africa for religious reasons. In recent years, the practice has spread to the indigenous tribes of Colombia's Embera-Chami ethnic group. In Western countries, female genital cosmetic surgery, which includes vaginoplasty, labiaplasty, and hymenoplasty (reconstruction of the hymen to a pre-sexual state) are now more common than years ago. The practice of plastic and cosmetic surgery grows year by year in Western countries.

Muslim women hide their face behind a veil, *hijab* or a burka, which reveals no more than her eyes and sometimes not even those. The member of a religious order, in order to keep her body hidden from others, must remain in cloister, just as Muslim women must accept similar restriction in daily life. The body experience is the place in which psychic disturbances are expressed. In the words of Sartre [9]: "There are no psychic phenomena that must be linked to a body; there is nothing behind a body, but the body is wholly psychic."

Motherhood is the principal aspect of female identity in Western culture and this defines women. In Greek mythology, Zeus brought a baby to Hera to suckle on her milk while she was asleep, but she suddenly woke up and pushed the child away. Hera's spurting milk created the Milky Way, which contains the Solar System.

Upper-class women often did not breastfeed their babies in eighteenth century France, preferring to employ wet-nurses from the poorer classes and reclaim their social lives. Elizabeth Badinter [10] said that this proved that there was no such thing as a maternal instinct. She contends that the politics of the last 40 years have produced three trends affecting the concept of motherhood, and, consequently, women's independence. The first is what she calls "ecology" and the desire to return to simpler times; second, a behavioral science based on ethology, the study of animal behavior; and lastly, an "essentialist" feminism, which glorifies breastfeeding and the experience of natural childbirth, while disparaging drugs and artificial hormones, such as epidurals and birth control pills.

The reasons for this change are various: a series of economic crisis have left women disenchanted with the workplace, while daughters have reacted against the feminism of their mothers. Most of all, we have seen the return of a naturalist ideology not far removed from that of Rousseau, which kept women at home for almost two centuries. Under the pretext of a return to nature, women in our time are being enlisted under the flag of natural child-raising. We decry the materialism and consumerism that made us throw out the timeless wisdom of nature, and we dismiss their offerings as tools of maternal egotism. Today's ideal of motherhood requires that we give birth in pain, without the benefit of an epidural, since this robs us of our first act as a mother. We are enjoined to nurse for 6 months, a year, or longer, day and night, whenever our child wishes, regardless of the mother's situation. The good mother who wants the best for her child is urged to forswear processed baby food, which is seen as a health hazard, and to avoid day-care as injurious to her child's healthy development. With all of its demands, the naturalist ideal of the twenty-first century means that it takes a woman as much time and energy to raise two children as our grandmothers spent raising four. This ideal of the modern mother represents a big change in the condition of women. For some, this new way of life may deliver a kind of joy, allowing women to immerse themselves fully in the act of being a mother, but for others it is a burden, a source of anxiety and isolation. Stuck at home for a year or more, if she decides to quit her job, or equips herself with a breast pump, if she goes back to work, the new mother is forced to choose between renouncing her full adult identity and adopting an expanded and exhausting set of obligations, along with a strong dose of guilt and psychic disturbances.

Nature knows only one way to be a mother. This is not the case for women, who are endowed with consciousness, personal histories, desires, and differing ambitions. What some do well and with pleasure, others do badly or out of duty. By failing to take account of women's diversity, by imposing a single ideal of motherhood, and by pursuing the notion of a perfect mother, they fall into a trap.

The single-minded focus on the ideal of modern motherhood has even more disastrous consequences, which we are just beginning to observe. Women who choose to reject its excessive constraints now have a nuclear option. They can curb their reproduction. They can refuse to have children, as some are doing in many industrialized countries. From Japan to Germany, wherever the duties of the good mother weigh too heavily on women's freedom, the birth rate has sunk too low for the species to continue.

Mithu Sanyal [11] reviews the invisibility of the female sex throughout the history of the Western world. In the first texts, the vulva was seen as principally a wound and then a crack by a world that rejected its existence through denial. Female genitals are the point where the interior meets the exterior. Psychoanalyst Harriet Lerner wrote in the 1970s about the difficulties experienced by many women in naming their own genitals and their inability to explore their own body. What they touched lacked a name. Only boys possessed something external; thus, girls could not touch their clitoris and remain a girl. The absence of an explicit recognition and nomenclature for the girl's genitals had to have pathogenic consequences.

Freud deprives women of a sexuality determined by them and strips them of their creative capacity. To challenge this is to battle a monster, a myth that has taken on a life of its own through two words: penis envy. Sanyal asserts that psychoanalysis has committed matricide by killing the mother and placing the father at the heart of culture. It is odd that Lacan, who created the concept of the "Law of the Father," displayed a reluctance to exhibit *The Origin of the World* in his home. Gustav Courbet's famous painting, which featured a close-up of female genitalia, was kept hidden behind a sliding door created by Surrealist painter, André Masson. *The Origin of the World* was a woman and may be seen today at the Orsay Museum in Paris.

At the end of the nineteenth century, the terms *vulva*, *clitoris*, and *labia* did not appear in the dictionary; just as the only word for female genitals in the dictionary today is *vagina*.

With Freud, there is only one libido, the masculine one, from the moment it is identified with the forms of domination. Simone de Beauvoir in *The Second Sex* [12] criticizes psychoanalysis by stating that the concept of penis envy is symbolic of envy of power. This is a symbol of the privileges that are afforded to boys, the place the father holds in the family, and the universal predominance of boys, with all this reinforcement of masculine superiority. There is poverty in the descriptions of the female libido, the study of which stems from the male libido and not from itself.

There is a permanent relationship between the biological, the cultural, and the construction of what is provided by nature and what is constructed by human beings. It has been variously stated that culture can modify biology by changing meanings and bodies (new technologies enable us to change an individual's sex).

Sexuality, violence, appropriated bodies, and medicated bodies are often related to women, as Michel Foucault [13] expressed in *Histoire de la Folie à l'Âge Classique*, in which he questioned the medical view from the classical hysteria diagnosed by Charcot.

The twentieth century is considered to have been revolutionary for women in Western culture. Society was deeply transformed in the manner in which male and female conception was perceived. Women could join the workforce and take up further education. In the 1950s, the arrival of the contraceptive pill brought a revolution in reproductive control, significantly changing the life of many Western women.

Nowadays, we all know that the revolution has not meant that women have entered the workforce and into social life in the same way as men. The shift from private to public life has not guaranteed a real transformation in real life for women throughout the world. Modern conceptions remain traditional.

In today's world, communication and the market, including the pharmaceutical one, are at the core of women's bodies. The same relates to the female sexual organs, for which a large market has grown, such as the selling of creams to protect women from their own malodorousness. This does not happen in the case of men.

As the philosopher, Pierre Bourdieu [14], affirmed: "There is a symbolic violence against women that leaves them moving from one space to another." The body's increasing power as the identity of the human being turns women into objects. Objects are more easily manipulated economically and symbolically. Anthropology has demonstrated the importance of psychosomatic factors in the construction of diseases [15].

Medical knowledge is very important in producing a reality of the body and the power of social speech in the construction of illness. Nature is understood to be a social construction. The symbolic violence suggested by Bourdieu implies that the androcentric world is presented as neutral. Because of this, most women are trapped inside, trying to do what should be done, while receiving a message that inequality does not exist and that they are to blame for not reaching a certain position. To a certain extent, this resembles the learned helplessness described by Seligman.

6.3 Body and Language

Heidegger [16] recognized that the entire evolution of Western philosophy and science, from the Greek philosophers onward, was based on descriptions of the world as a human observer would see it from God's position. But every human being lives in the world as a part of it, not apart from it. If we fail to take the initial step of creating a state of separation between subject and object, between the human being who does the describing and the world that is described, what different view will we provide of our experience of life? Who am I as an individual? Do I take charge of my life or do others take charge for me?

Heidegger [16] sensed that the evidence was based on the sea of language in which we are immersed from birth. This knowledge is transmitted by two difference mediums: isolated words, as they are pronounced, and the diverse forms of language, teaching, bias, traditions, rituals, and customers that shape culture. People do not create language, but are created by it. "Language is the house of being. In its home, Man dwells," Heidegger said [17].

This vision of language underlines, among other things, that it is impossible to understand language if it is separated from the bodily act of speech. It presents language as the most important way in which a person can indicate to others his/her real world. It demonstrates that language exists in the social space between people within which our sense of being is created in all its aspects: corporal, mental, and spiritual. As Heidegger said in 1971 [16]:

> If we take language directly in the sense of something that is present, we find it in the act of speech, the activation of the organs of speech, the mouth, lips, tongue. Language is reflected in speech as a phenomenon that occurs in Man. It is demonstrated by the names that Western languages have given to it themselves: *glossa*, *lingua*, *langue*, language, *lenguaje*. Language is the tongue. (p. 96)

We can contrast this vision of language with the concept grounded in the twentieth century in which language is a form of communication [18].

Maturana and Varela [19] have called this perspective "the metaphor of the tube" for communication in that language resembles a tube by which a person sends an idea to another person who receives it. However, contained in Heidegger's analysis is the fundamental way in which human beings are physically present, some with others. Language is a form of being. Heidegger's work underlines the critical importance of the ways in which language governs the experience that people have of their bodies and the actions of those who surround them.

Merleau-Ponty, a disciple of Heidegger, believed that our experience of the body comes from the sensations of feeling and being felt. Heidegger and Merleau-Ponty believed that an understanding of language was inseparable from the bodily act of speaking. Language does not exist within individuals but in the social intermediate space. This matrix of language (languages, traditions, custom, and other social uses) creates the identity of each individual. His work on philosophical hermeneutics showed that the division between the mind and the body, upon which modern medicine is based, is an interpretation generated socially and imposed on life as human beings experience it, rather than a reflection of an objective reality situated beyond human experience [20]. From this perspective, biomedical science has continued largely unaware of its own condition; it is neither the only valid tradition nor the mirror of reality but a tradition among others [18].

The perspective of language seen from the cognitive sciences throws new light on the relationship among ideas, language, and the body. The perspectives of philosophical hermeneutics and cognitive science locate language in the interactions between people and not within the mind of each individual. More than a vehicle that transports abstract communications between individual minds, it is coordination of bodily states between members of a social group that preserves the integrity of the group and of each individual [18].

People do not select the history that makes up their personality; nor can they relinquish it easily when its consequences are undesirable. This personal narrative chooses us as much as we choose it; it forms part of the sea of language within which all of us as human beings are born.

Hence, Robin Lakoff argues that language uses us as much as we use it. This means that, just as the thoughts we wish to express guide our choice of forms of expression, the way in which we perceive the real world dominates our form of expressing ourselves on the same things. The relationships among the language, mentality, and social behavior of each human group raise anthropological concerns.

Language, as a symbolic system, is not neutral with regard to gender, just as it is not neutral with regard to ethnicity or social class. Therefore, these categories have a clear impact on individuals. Girls and boys learn to symbolize when they are still young, when they are barely aware of the meaning of their words. Linguistic transformations can influence the form of understanding and interpreting the world. One of the key criticisms by feminists of Foucault's work is precisely the lack of gender perspective in his analysis of language [21].

One of the expressions of sexism in most European languages, especially those of Latin origin, consists of the use of the generic male form to talk of both women and men, giving rise to phrases in which it is impossible to tell whether the speaker is referring exclusively to men in particular or to human beings in general. For example, there are *derechos humanos* in Spain, *human rights* in the UK, and *droits de l'homme* in France.

Women are traditionally labeled as talkers, when ethnographic evidence shows that men speak more than women in conversations between men and women. This contradiction connects to the fact that women are not compared with men in terms of their capacity of communication. Rather, the parallelism established is that of silence, so that any expression is interpreted as "talking too much." Not only do men talk more, they also interrupt more frequently, providing another example of male domination. The stereotype of silence as a quality that is highly valued in women was forged today by reinforcing the negative image of the woman who dares to speak in public, an image that continues to form part of the collective imagination in the contemporary world [1].

For the anthropology of gender, of great interest are Foucault's ideas on the role of language in constructing the body and sexual identities with regard to the distribution of power between men and women. In his view [22], there are normative discourses that transmit the "truth." This implies that certain forms of knowledge are considered truthful and group thinking may be controlled through the discourses that carry the norm. Such discourses would create categories of identity that are closely linked to what is considered to be normal or abnormal in societies, maintaining relationships of domination and power. This exerts a powerful influence on the idea that people possess their identity. The problem is that when Foucault speaks of the sexed body he is speaking of the male body as normative. He does not analyze the attitudes and behavior of women with regard to the social expectations of how their bodies should be.

If de Beauvoir's assertion [12] that "one is not born a woman but rather becomes one" is correct, it follows that woman is in itself a term in process, a becoming, a constructing that cannot rightfully be said to begin or to end. As an ongoing discursive practice, it is open to intervention and resignification. This is the notion of body not as an available surface that awaits signification but as a set of individual and social limits that remain and acquire meaning politically. Referring to an original or authentic femininity is in opposition to the present need to analyze gender as a complex cultural construct [23].

De Beauvoir's theory had radical consequences that she did not initially consider. If sex and gender are radically different, then there is no evidence that a specific sex is the same as a specific gender; in other words, *woman* is not necessarily the cultural construct of the female body and the same is true of *man*. This assertion about the sex/gender division reveals that sexed bodies may be of many different genders. If sex is not limited to gender, it follows perhaps that there are genders, forms of culturally interpreting the sexed body that are not limited to the apparent duality of sex. Another consequence is that gender is a type of transformation or activity.

Monica Wittig is aware of the power of language to subordinate and exclude women. She believes that language is another order of materiality, an institution that can be modified. Clearly influenced by Simone de Beauvoir through the criticism she makes of the female myth in *The Second Sex*, Wittig says: "there is no female writing".

As Wittig asserts, language throws bundles of reality onto the social body. This involves redescribing the options that already exist within the cultural fields that are deemed unintelligible and impossible. The human being, from what it is, accesses reality through language, in a medium "obstructed by words." To describe a man as a *Don Juan* we resort to literature, but in the case of a woman we use psychiatric vocabulary: nymphomaniac. Why has male sexuality been constructed culturally as promiscuous but not its female equivalent? Up to what point is the construction of sexuality related to the survival of the species?

The development of a language that represents women fully and adequately has been necessary to promote their political visibility. This has been of great importance when taking into account the underlying cultural situation, in which the life of women is inadequately represented or not at all.

The new term *transgender* refers to individuals, behaviors, and groups that diverge from the most traditional dual gender roles and cross accepted limits. It includes a varied group of androgynous or transsexual people, in which the desire for surgical reassignment of genitals is not determinant. The term is employed as a synonym to express the third and fourth gender and encompasses the *hijras* of India and Pakistan [24] and eunuchs of eastern harems [25]. It is used to mean *other* in the sense that generic duality is broken [1].

In practice, the expression *queer*, which originally meant strange or unusual, is employed to define a wide group of people: lesbians, gays, bisexuals, transgender, transsexuals, homosexuals, and intersexuals. Basically, these are people, behaviors or groups that transgress normativity. As indicated by the philosopher, Beatriz Preciado [26], in her *Contrasexual Manifesto*, if a woman wants she can become of neither female nor male gender: neither woman nor man.

6.4 Body and Gender

Gender is the cultural construct created by society as a whole with regard to anatomical sex. According to the era and culture involved, it will determine the destiny of the person. Gender is one of the taboos that is most difficult to break in our culture. It is impossible to separate gender from the political and cultural intersections in which it is constantly produced and maintained. One of the problems faced is that the term "women" indicates a common identity [23].

John Waters' film *Female Troubles*, which stars Divine, proposes implicitly that gender is a type of persistent characterization that passes as reality. This is precisely because *female* does not now seem to be a stable notion; its meaning is as vague as *woman*.

As the title by Denise Riley suggests, *Am I That Name?*; this is a question raised by the possible multiple meanings of a name. If one *is* a woman, it is evident that what one is needs not to be everything. This is not because a person with a set gender goes beyond the specific attributes of his/her gender, but because gender is not always constituted coherently or consistently in different historical contexts, and because it intertwines with racial, class, ethnic, sexual, and regional types. Hence, it is impossible to separate gender from the political and cultural intersections in which it is produced and maintained.

Is there a gender that people possess or is this an essential attribute that a person is? This is reflected in the question, what gender are you? If gender is constructed, can it be constructed differently or does its construction entail some form of social determinism that denies the possibility of the agent acting and changing? How and when is gender constructed? The assertion that gender is constructed suggests a certain determinism. In that case, it is culture and not biology that becomes destiny.

As stated above, Simone de Beauvoir [12] asserts in *The Second Sex* that one is not born a woman: one becomes one. For de Beauvoir, gender is constructed, but in its approach it is implicit that gender is something variable and volitional. Can then the construction be circumscribed to a form of choice? De Beauvoir holds that one becomes a woman but always under the cultural obligation to do so. And that obligation is not created by sex. In her study, there is nothing to guarantee that the person who becomes a woman is forced to be of the female sex. If the body is a situation, a body always interpreted by cultural meanings, sex by definition has always been gender [27].

This gives rise to two positions: on the one hand, those who assert that gender is a secondary characteristic in people, and on the other, those who hold that the very notion of person placed in language as a "subject" is a construction, granting the male an original (natural) value and underlining in the female a mask-like nature.

In the philosophical tradition that began with Plato and continued with Descartes, Husserl, and Sartre, the ontological differentiation between soul (conscience, mind) and body always acts in defense of relationships of subordination and political and psychic hierarchy. Not only does the mind subject the body, perhaps it plays with the fantasy of escaping totally from its corporeality. The cultural associations of the mind with masculinity and the body with femininity are well-documented in the field of philosophy [28].

Foucault, in the first volume of *The History of Sexuality* [22], said that the categorization of sexual difference takes place through a form of historically specific sexuality. In his interpretation of the diary of a hermaphrodite, Herculine Barbin, Foucault held that Herculine is not an identity but the sexual impossibility of an identity. The demand for identity is a culturally limited principle of order and hierarchy, a regulatory fiction. Hence, gender is performative, shaping the identity it is supposed to be. Accordingly, gender is always a doing. Nietzsche asserts in *The Genealogy of Morals* that there is no being behind doing, acting, and becoming; doing is everything.

Brigitte Baptiste, the Colombian biologist, university professor, and director of the Humboldt Institute said in *Inventing the Body* [29]: "For as long as I can remember, my body wanted to grow in a different way so I could participate in the world with other attributes, with another vision, without needing to say that I was in the wrong body. I grew and I had to avoid what I imagined my body wanted to be. I learnt to draw my own body, the way I wanted. The pain of not becoming whom I wanted pushed me to become as if I was a woman in the movie world of the sixties, in this case Brigitte Bardot."

There is a cultural construction of gender, a discipline of the body, about what may be done and what may not. That discipline is rigid. However, there is a great biodiversity in nature, which allows different forms of interacting with and perpetuating life. There are different responses in which lives may unfold on our planet. The biodiversity of life is immense. However, gender diversity is one of the most difficult to break in our culture. So, why is there so much biodiversity in nature? This is related to the exploration of diverse possibilities of existing with the presence of ecological relationships and symbiosis. Life is made for difference, to be different. In nature, not all monkeys behave in the same way as gorillas. In the marmoset's world, everyone raises their offspring in the community. Promiscuity is a reality. There is every type of combination of gender and sexuality. We human beings live in cities, upon the asphalt that plays host to millions of persons. These relationships with which the body interacts allows us great creativity. This explains the existence of urban tribes. The city and the world of space change. This enables us to be more than one person. We pretend when we put clothes on. Social media allows us to have different identities. This is a complex ecosystem. We are going to be different people. It allows us to have different bodies. In the world of Greek mythology, male figures mixed with animals such as the Minotaur began to appear. *Trans* people feel this, according to Baptiste: "We feel comfortable in discordance. We don't have identity problems. The body can be imagined. Writing the body is to confirm it. We have no identity problems". This is to give meaning to the bodily territories that have been sealed. Imagining, representing figures, decoding the body. Julia Kristeva sees this as the new humanism, providing the means for this suffering to be recognized as vulnerability.

Some theories are based on Lévi-Strauss's structuralist anthropology. This presents the problematic differentiation between nature and culture in an attempt to support the differentiation between sex and gender: the idea that there is a natural or biological woman who subsequently becomes a socially subordinate woman, with the result that sex is to nature what gender is to culture. If this were the case, we could follow the trail of the transformation of sex into gender as a stable mechanism in all cultures, but this is not so.

In marriage, the woman is not considered to have an identity but a term of relation that differentiates and at the same time establishes links between the various clans of the patriarchal society. The bride, the gift, the object of exchange is a sign and a value that initiates a channel of exchange that not only achieves the functional aim of simplifying the trade but also achieves the aim of reinforcing the internal links and the collective identity of each clan. The bride is a term of relation between groups and does not possess an identity. Nonetheless, the relation of reciprocity between men is the condition of radical nonreciprocity between men and women, and another, as it were, of nonrelation between women [30]. Simone de Beauvoir [12] takes up the ideas of Lévi-Strauss on marriage, stating that this is a link that is not established between men and women but between men through the use of women. Lévi-Strauss's assertion that "the appearance of the symbolic thought must have required women, just like words, to be things which are exchanged" is well known.

Rubin [31] asserts that before the transformation of a biological man and woman into a man or woman with gender, each boy or each girl possesses all the sexual possibilities available for human expression.

Gender stereotypes are social constructions that constitute deeply rooted ideas in the conscience that escape the control of reason. The aim is for it to seem perfectly natural for men to be better equipped for specific roles and women for others. However, gender stereotypes are not stable and change from one culture to another. For example, to be socially masculine and wear a kilt in Scotland is unthinkable for a German boy who wants to wear a skirt to school instead of trousers. The intimacy of girls is exposed differently. People who do not adapt are considered aberrant. Personal adaptation to stereotypes responds largely to people's need to feel socially integrated [1].

However, the problem is not reduced to the existence of culturally constructed characteristics associated with the gender stereotype but those associated with the male gender valued as being superior. There is greater acceptance of women wearing trousers than men wearing skirts. Gender emphasizes that the social differences between men and women are not immutable nor are they universal or objective.

People are educated from infancy in accordance with social paradigms about the interpretations of being a man or a woman. Generally, we accept this without question because we find it *normal*. The precept of being of a specific gender in the case of women generates failures: a variety of inherent configurations that in their multiplicity exceed and challenge the precept through which they were generated [23]. Being of a specific gender is generated through discursive routes, being a good mother, being a sexually desirable object, being a skilled worker. This represents a large amount of guarantees that satisfy a variety of distinct demands. Over history, this has been idealized or manipulated from the perspective of making maternity women's *raison d'être*. Nietzsche asserts that all the values of femininity, all the values of weakness, need to end in order to allow the new world to emerge.

From our viewpoint, this, per se, seems to generate psychic distress and show associated psychopathology. It explains the need to include this paradigm in corporality and body image.

6.5 Body and Historical Aspects

In the history of psychiatry, the pathological condition of the female body is a constant. For Greeks, hysteria is a word that means uterus. Plato [32] in his text *Timaeus* (which has been integrated into Western medical tradition through Galen and the Hippocratic writers) asserted that:

> The matrix or womb in women, which is a living creature within them, longs to bear children. If it is left unfertilized long beyond the normal time, it causes extreme unrest,

strays about the body, blocks the channels of the breath and causes in consequence acute distress and disorders of all kinds. If it is not 'appeased by passion and love' the womb moved from its natural position within the body and, attaching itself to soft internal tissues, gave rise to a wide variety of symptomatic disturbances. (Plato [32])

Through the history of psychiatry, the woman's body has been cataloged as being more prone to illness. Women suffer from nervous disease, neurasthenia, sickness, and gloom more frequently, while chlorotic women are often described in nineteenth century Gothic literature.

Galen thought women to be more likely to suffer mental illnesses and to be weaker and crippled, in reproducing the model of Greek medicine. Galen also believed that they were predisposed to be compliant and servile.

The conception that female organs were inverted and under-developed within the body was held by Galen and subsequently by medieval philosophers. Albertus Magnus believed that women were not in their nature human beings but a failed birth. This conception of the female sex equivalent to the man only within the body was maintained until the sixteenth century. Over history, one sex, the male one, has been constructed and the female has been constructed in opposition to him [33].

From the historical viewpoint, male domination was highlighted from the end of the Middle Ages, with the change in laws on inheritance, the expulsion of women from universities, debates on the duties of women in the Church. Accordingly, the Church had a negative view, with the Dominicans and the Inquisition removing women from other professions. In the Roman era, there were women doctors and translators. Because of the weight of the Church, which confined women within the domestic environment, indissoluble matrimony made women disappear from public life.

The art historian, Julia Varela [34], explains that in the world of art (masculine in the main) it is possible to objectify the inequality in power between men and women, given that every painting is a depositary of the social relationship and encloses an interpretation of the world. This may be objectified in the painting of the Annunciation from the pictorial images of the late fourteenth to the seventeenth century, where the Virgin shifts from being the "mother of God" (occupying the right-hand side, the important one in Western art) to "the Lord's slave" when the weight of religiousness is greater. This is seen in Robert de Campin's painting of the Annunciation in which the Virgin Mary is situated in a house in the Netherlands. The work is housed in New York's Metropolitan Museum. The imbalance of power between men and women becomes an increasingly accentuated process.

In the era of Descartes, rationality was masculine and women moved to the private environment. There were new urban strata in which the arrival of the bourgeoisie meant that the woman was spouse, mother, and housekeeper.

The French Revolution did not bring about a change for women. It was respectful with institutions and bourgeois values. In the fifteenth century the contributions of Olympe de Gouges, who wrote the famous *Declaration of the Rights of Women* (1791), which began with the following words: "Man, are you capable of being just? It is a woman who poses the question," were important. She was subsequently executed by guillotine. Mary Wollstonecraft, the author of the famous *Vindication of the Rights of Woman* (1792) and the feminist John Stuart Mill, who issued the first call in the British Parliament in favor of female suffrage (1867), were also key figures. This was granted in the UK and Germany in 1918, in Spain in 1931, and in France in 1944 (de Beauvoir's book was published in 1949). In Switzerland, women were not allowed to vote until 1971.

Berta Pappenheim was a Jewish feminist in the twentieth century who found fame as the first woman to found an orphanage in Germany. She fought for women's rights and translated Wollstonecraft's *Vindication of the Rights of Woman*. Wollstonecraft was the mother of Mary Shelley (who wrote the novel *Frankenstein*) but died in childbirth, leaving the baby to be cared for by her father, a political anarchist. Mary was cast out by her father when she began a relationship with the poet Shelley, with whom she had to flee the country in order to marry. Some articles show that perhaps the Frankenstein monster, who was able to think and feel emotions but was not human, recalls the situation of women (in the late nineteenth century: they were unable to study, had no access to family inheritance, lacked the vote, and were judged on whether they would form a good marriage).

Berta Pappenheim was known in the history of psychiatry for being the subject of Breuer and Freud's famous case "Anna O." She suffered a "hysterical collapse" when she had to care for her infirm father. Twenty-one at the time, Berta displayed multiple physical symptoms including mood swings and absences, and stopped eating. She also had attacks of rage, during which she broke objects, and suffered from headaches and morphine dependency. According to today's classifications, she might have been diagnosed with emotional instability disorder or borderline personality disorder. However, as mentioned above, her life took a different course. Such was her role in the social reintegration of women that her image was used for West Germany's first set of stamps, which were devoted to the benefactors of humanity. Many people are unaware of how Breuer and Freud's famous clinical case developed.

Another emblematic case was that of Blanche Wittman, a Parisian known as "the Queen of Hysterics." She was admitted very young to the Salpêtriére Hospital where she was known for her famous hysterical crises recorded in paintings of the time.

This took place in the context of what was called "moral therapy" imported by Pinel and implemented in asylums such as the Salpêtriére. The aim was to temper passions and destroy deliria through kindness, persuasion and respect for the doctor's authority.

This theatricality took the form of almost authentic performances, as seen in the famous painting *A Lesson at the Salpêtriére*. We see one of Charcot's famous classes where Blanche, a Salpêtriére resident for many years, is held in Babinski's arms in a show to which members of Parisian high society including painters, writers, and doctors were invited.

The manner of administering the body reached its zenith at the Salpêtriére when Charcot gave his masterclasses on Tuesdays and Fridays. The large number of photographs from this time are well known. At the start of the century, very long exposure times and proper lighting were required for a clear photograph. It was as if the hysterical women were capable of warning of a possible "crisis" to allow the time to create the right conditions for the photographs [35].

The hysterical women of the Salpêtriére led Foucault [13] to question the role of the doctor, who was none other than the great Charcot. However, few people know that following Charcot's death, Blanche left the Salpêtriére to return some years later as an employee, initially in the photographic laboratory and from 1900 in the Radiology Service. She proved herself to be commanding, hardworking, and a good organizer in her work.

The Aimée case, known for "curing" delirium, is perhaps the one that has been least followed. Aimée, who was famed for her "self-punitive paranoia" as Lacan termed it, was destined to be known in the asylums as "the delirium pensioner." With the real name of Marguerite, she ended up working as a cook and governess, without displaying any further signs of madness. She even worked in the house of Lacan's father. That was not all. Marguerite's son, who subsequently became a psychoanalyst, learned on the couch of his teacher, Lacan, that his mother was the subject of the famous case of Aimée ("the loved one").

The study of the body experience, from the perspective of phenomenology and anthropological psychiatry, has provided greater knowledge of the alterations of the experience of one's own body in different mental diseases. This is especially true in those in which there is a confrontation between the body and personal identity, and it is necessary to consider the process of individual identification and a category of personal identity disorders [36].

The gender perspective is essential to explaining body experience and identity and needs to be included in order to understand in depth how certain disorders are more frequent in women in our culture. Husserl believed that subjectivity is the core problem of knowledge and it only exists in embodied form. The integration of the individual in actions is performed through the body, it is expressed in it, and it also reveals the deep sense of fullness of the woman as a person. The question of subjectivity is deeply transformed by gender. Matthew Ratcliffe, in his book, *Feelings of Being*, describes existential feelings such as isolation in Sylvia Plath's novel, *The Bell Jar* [37],

> I knew I should be grateful to Mrs. Guinea, only I couldn't feel a thing. If Mrs. Guinea had given me a ticket to Europe, or a round-the-world cruise, it wouldn't have made one scrap of difference to me, because wherever I sat—on the deck of a ship or a street café in Paris or Bangkok—I would be sitting under the same glass bell jar, stewing in my own sour air. (1966, p. 178)

It is essential to understand what a woman was supposed to be at that time, 1966, in order to understand Sylvia Plath's novels in depth. It seems that something is omitted from history. This is part of the testimony of her friend and writer, Jillian Becker, on the final days of Sylvia Plath (http://www.bbc.co.uk/news/magazine-21336933):

> ... I had met her in September 1962, shortly after her marriage to Ted Hughes had broken up. I felt sorry for her. I admired and envied her talent... Nick was about the same age as Madeleine, a little over one year old. Frieda was nearly three... She told me she would

> 'rather not go home.' It was easy for me to let them stay. . .She seemed to be rambling, and I thought it was because she was growing sleepy. Then her tone changed, and she talked emotionally and energetically about Ted and Assia Wevill, the woman he had left her for. She was bitter, she was jealous, she was angry. Ted had taken Assia to Spain. She wished she could take the children to Spain, to somewhere in the sun, away from this freezing weather. . .Sylvia must look after her children, she must feel that they needed her. So I asked her to come with me, when I took them to the bathroom, when I prepared their meals, when Nick needed feeding and changing. But she didn't pick up soap or a towel, or a spoon, or a safety pin. I'd leave the room, but she'd wait for me to return. My choice was to let them go unwashed, unfed, unchanged, or do the job myself. Mostly I did it. . .Sylvia suddenly said: "I must get back. I have to sort the laundry. . .He parked the car and went to sit on a jump seat opposite Sylvia. As she went on crying, the children began crying too. He took them on his knees. He implored her to let him bring them back to our house. She refused. . .For which thoughts I was to endure long remorse. On the Monday morning at about eight o'clock the phone rang. I answered, and Dr Horder told me Sylvia had put her head in the gas oven and was dead.

Sylvia Plath's work is inseparable from her existence and the feminist view as her contemporary, Anne Sexton, expressed in her poems. (Both were women, poets, and committed suicide). They were diagnosed with depression and were in psychiatric treatment. However, to understand them in depth it is necessary to look at what a woman was supposed to be at that time. As a confessional poet, Anne Sexton exploited the intimate details of her life for her poetry. "Poetry milks the unconscious," she said. Sexton lamented and celebrated female identity, sexuality, and power by revealing painful and shocking personal details about her life. Although she always insisted that her poetry was not autobiographical, her exploration of difficult and taboo female subjects, such as abortion, menstruation, menopause, masturbation, and desires, was made with such frankness that most readers and critics felt that the line between Anne the woman and Sexton the poet was often blurred.

Female subjectivity is constructed in relation to the body, taking care of others, and love as nuclear. Responsibility for others (children, husband, parents) occupies an important part of female identity.

Values such as sacrifice, effort, caregiving responsibilities, and the ability to withstand hardship are part of most religions and culture and are a breeding ground for expressing psychic disturbances in women much more frequently than in men. Elfriede Jelinek (2004 Nobel Prize winner) [38] said that love is working in female lives in her novel *Die Liebhaberinnen* (*Women as Lovers*). Art, literature, and history provide us with many examples of it.

Virginia Woolf, in her essay *A Room of One's Own*, published in 1929, expressed the real position of women at that time and this is still valid now: "For most of history, Anonymous was a woman."

"Suppose for instance, that men were only represented in literature as the lovers of women, and were never the friends of men, soldiers, thinkers, dreams; how few parts in the plays of Shakespeare could be allotted to them; how literature would suffer." If this were the case, literature would be impoverished, and so she argues, this has occurred by closing the doors on women's writing.

Satirically, she describes her perplexity about why are there so many books written by men about women but none by women about men

"A woman must have money and a room of her own if she is to write fiction."

"It is fatal to be a man or woman pure and simple: one must be a manly woman, or a womanly man." [39]

6.6 Body and Corporality

Corporality and *body awareness* have possessed a descriptive basis since the work of Jaspers [40]:

> The body itself is aware for me like my existence and at the same time I see it with my eyes and I touch it with my hands. The body is the only part of the world that is simultaneously felt from within and its surface perceived. It is an object for me and I am that very body. I feel physically and I perceive myself as an object in two ways, but both are indissolubly united.

The body that I am and the body that I have are linked by Jaspers in the form of a simultaneous experience of bodily sensations and of the feelings which arise between them. The body schema articulates all corporeal experiences, providing a clear reference point of what we really are (bodily).

Awareness and corporality are key concepts in Jaspers' psychopathology (1913), and the awareness of self is lived through them. That is, through the feeling of their unity, the feeling of their identity, and finally the feeling of their opposition to the external, the self becomes aware of itself.

Contact with the outside world is made through our body. The latter, on the one hand, belongs to the world of things and, on the other, to the world of ourselves. We are a body and we have a body. When we feel sad and weary, the experience of the spirit and the body itself merge in an overall manner at the same time. Alternatively, as Fernando Colina states in his book *Escritos Psicóticos* [41]:

> What we know and do not know about melancholy comes from the body: it is the source of melancholy as much as its chamber, it is the library, the lesson, the tongue itself. The body refers us to two extremes: the somatic, which is the mute, the organic and the pulsional; and it also sends us to flesh, yearning, language, the writing of desire between the signs of the body. Sadness, as if we were dealing with a blanket, is always that of the body, that is, of what is dying, of the most constant, visible loss.

The German language distinguishes between *Körper* as an object, or objective reality, and *Leib*, as a lived or experienced reality. These two forms of knowing the body are expressed very well in German, although not so well in Spanish. Ortega y Gasset [42] called the former "extra-body" and the latter "intra-body." The intra-body has no color, nor defined form, unlike the extra-body. It comprises fundamentally the feelings of movement or tactile feelings of the viscera and the muscles, the impression of the contraction and dilation of the blood vessels, the small perceptions of the flow of blood in the veins and arteries and the feelings of pleasure and pain. The intra-body is therefore not so much the body seen from within as the body lived from within. The terms are distinguished: the body is something that is anatomical and physiological, and corporality is a lived experience, specifically, that of the body as a phenomenological reality.

Marcel [43] published in 1927 his conception of "*corps vécu*," which includes the notions of "my body in that it is mine, my body as being in the world and the body as a sign of existence".

Sartre [9] distinguishes between the body as a being for itself and the body as a being for another. The body represents a form of being in the world, of occupying it, projecting it, recalling it, sharing it. This is why it occupies a space, projecting and recalling within a time and shared by others. Living corporally is precisely what provides a meaning of reality, or what is the same, a reality with meaning. Being a man and being a woman is to give meaning to the world. The world into which we have been cast, according to Heidegger's expression, is constituted from corporal intentionality. It is the body that, by creating space, time and in meeting with others, makes the world real.

Existential analysts distinguish three types of world, i.e., three simultaneous aspects of the world that characterize the existence of each being-in-the-world [44]:

- First is the *Umwelt*, which is the world that surrounds us: the biological world.
- The second is the *Mitwelt*, literally the co-world, the world shared with our fellow people.
- The third is called *Eigenwelt*, or self-world, and comprises the personal relations of the individual with him/herself.

Health is expressed by corporal silence, by the absence of symptoms. However, at specific moments this intentionality hides itself, concentrates on itself and the body leaves the *Mitwelt* to concentrate on the *Eigenwelt*: i.e., it is ill, or, which is the same, "deprived of all spontaneous coexistence with its body, the patient talks of it as a foreign object" [45].

The experience of the body is therefore ambivalent. Living in one's own body is not only to ensure its ownership or to state its potency, but it is also to discover its servitude and recognize its weakness. It represents the periodic memory of progressive decay and finitude. In depressive states, as asserted by López Ibor and López-Ibor Aliño [46], in the presence of illness, the corporal reality of the subject becomes problematic and his/her attention is concentrated on it. In health, the body is silent or a peripheral awareness, in the words of Lhermitte [47].

The paradigm of this non-availability of the body is its illness. Illness reminds me that I have not got a body (*Körper*; *corps objectif*) alone, as Merleau-Ponty says, but that I am also a lived body (*Leib*; *corps phénoménal* or *corps propre*); it makes me painfully aware that this instrument, body, is escaping from control and availability.

"In situations where it is really important to appear totally serene, I am ashamed when it goes red, it makes me tremble because its voice is quivering, it fails in its accompaniment; it presents itself as an unavailable lived body." [46]

Bodily space is thought to be the place of the self and subject to the experience of "what is one's own." It is simultaneously object and subject; it is in the world and perceives most bodies. The body represents the place of existence of the human being [48]. In fact, for Janet [49], agreeing with Ribot [50], personality is not found in the soul, it is found in the body. Consequently, it is impossible to progress in the study of personality without having previously understood that nature of possessing a body, a body that is distinct from others. This is especially significant in women, in whom the body is much more present in the construction of their subjectivity.

"Being aware of one's body at all times, of always being exposed to humiliation or ridicule and of finding consolation in domestic tasks or in chats with friends. It is not that the needs of biological reproduction determine the symbolic organization of the sexual division of work, but rather a social construction, arbitrary of what is biological and particularly of the male and female body, of its customs and functions which provide a natural basis to the androcentric view of the division of the sexual activity of work and therefore of all the cosmos. It legitimises a relationship of domination by registering it in a biological nature which is in itself a naturalised social construction." [14] Female morality imposes itself above all through a constant discipline that concerns the body, a pressure on clothes, beauty, forms of behavior, and looking after the body. This is the naturalization of an ethic. It includes female subservience, bowing, lowering the head, bending the body, smiling, averting the gaze, accepting interruptions, and in the way women are taught to fill space, walk, and adopt appropriate body positions (keeping their legs open is vulgar). It is as if femininity could be summarized in the act of lessening oneself, limiting territory and restricting movement, and shifting one's body, especially in public places. Equality and respect result from learning. Men and women have to learn and interiorize these aspects that allow them to live in equality.

There is a violence that comes from equality. Women do not know how to behave in the system of equality. They participate in the system when they go down the street and in the face of a provocative gaze that looks into their eyes and says "you are a thing," they avert their gaze. This is part of the program for which they are trained [4]. Women are confused, nobody has taught them how to set limits; they only avail themselves of the recipe of patience and gratitude. Humankind still does not know what it is because it does not know how to behave as a non-natural species. The violence of equality comes from men who experience the situation of equality as a continuous attack on their virility, as exemplified by "putting women in their place." This is related to the maintaining of the brotherhood system. Equality taken in the wrong way can give rise to new violence from a feminist perspective.

The body is the experience of doing, feeling, thinking, and wanting and cannot be separated [51]. From birth, we are designed to seek the relationship that includes the emotional component. Hence, emotions are bodily provisions. Our medium is other human beings. Everything is interconnected. Everything arises in co-dependency. There is no you and them, only us. The mind and the world are one. The body is the medium for the experience of the world and consequently of all learning processes. In this way, the body is the medium with which I have my own world. We perceive the world from and with the body. We are embodied [52].

Some neuroscientists [53, 54] have reached the same conclusions by different routes to phenomenology and psychiatric anthropology. In this, they coincide with contemporary philosophers such as Clark and Noë. Mind, body, and world interact in the adaptation of the individual.

6.7 Body and Postmodernism

The body is a metaphor, container, mirror or barrier. It is the absolute place, the small fragment of space where I am, literally embodied, as Foucault said. The body has become a main topic of contemporary debate and tensions. "I can't move without it. I can't leave it where it is. I can go to the end of world, I can hide under the sheets, I can make myself as small as possible. . .it will always be there" [55]. Contemporary culture is dominated by the omnipresence of the body and the subjecting of it to models whose reproduction is almost impossible for the vast majority of the population, especially for women. A trend has been encouraged toward the continuous modification of the body where it becomes its own show before the mirror. Like Narcissus, who, stunned by the sight of himself, fell madly in love with his own image reflected in water, and caused his own death by throwing himself in.

Many bodies feel increasingly greater dissatisfaction with their image in the mirror and this leads them to begin the path, often with no return, to the continuous and dangerous modification of their bodies. The body is the space in which living with each individual's personal identity is embodied. As Foucault states [48]:

> *Est docile un corps qui peut être soumis qui peut être utilisé, qui peut être transformé et perfectionné.* (Docile is the body which may be subjected, which may be utilized, which may be transformed and perfected.)

According to Laín Entralgo, the body is "the being of man." The problem faced by modern man was already described by Nietzsche: "The most characteristic feature of modern man is the singular contrast between an interior to which no exterior corresponds and an exterior to which no interior corresponds."

In 1976, Foucault wrote at the end of *La Volenté de Savoir* that sex has become "the imaginary point that each individual has to pass in order to have access to their own intelligibility, to the fullness of their body, to their identity. Intelligibility, fullness, identity. The confrontation with oneself has become a confrontation with a body from which we cannot distance ourselves." Foucault said that "sex has become more important than our soul, it has become almost more important than our life." To describe the contemporary situation, it is only necessary to replace "sex" with the word "body" and omit "almost." In our culture, the body has become more important than our soul, it has become more important than our life [41]. Knowledge of oneself is the first step to wisdom. This was engraved as an inscription on the temple of Apollo in Delphi, i.e. in "the navel of the world."

"Know yourself" is at the same time, the cornerstone of philosophy, i.e., of a love for wisdom. It is the first rule of a life for which teaching was proposed. "Knowing yourself has been imposed on all men," in the words of Heraclitus. Practical knowledge appears as a female figure who holds in her hand an instrument, a very valuable one at the time, which enables contemplation and knowledge of oneself: the mirror. He alludes to the importance of the mirror to act correctly; the wise individual must know him/herself. The reason for the mirror also reflects the reverse of knowledge in itself, as self-contemplation may have ill effects. This was Narcissus's big mistake in Schopenhauer's words [56].

In *The Disciple* [57], Oscar Wilde said that when Narcissus died, the nymphs roamed tearful as they missed his presence. Then they went to the lake telling it: "You must certainly be missing Narcissus because he came every day to view himself in your mirror, in your waters." And the response from the lake to the tearful nymphs was: "yes, it's true; I miss Narcissus very much because every day when he came to look at me and to be reflected in my waters, I saw in his pupils, in his eyes, how beautiful I am." This image reveals a narcissistic relationship where one does not see the other, but one sees oneself in the gaze of the other.

There is, on the other hand, a disdain that is born from the body itself as a vulnerable, corruptible, and finite biological space. The disdained body as flesh, weight, a burden, makes it the spirit that vivifies, while the flesh is worthless. The world of art has used bodily distortion as a formula of expression of the modern man, as reflected in the work of painter Francis Bacon: the creation of grotesque bodies. He uses the encroachment of the human figure within the limits of space.

By not limiting itself to its physical dimensions and spreading out, the human body reaches much further from its skin covering, just like the dress and adornments that form part of the body have been incorporated and hence are a manifestation of the individual itself. Even the Neanderthals used pigments for make-up [58]. This is much more important in women where the body image and the body are much more present in female identity. Care of the body and its different ornaments form a way of seducing and therefore achieving the gaze of others.

Through body art, the human body perceives the world through its senses and there is no feeling without contact. It is through the body that the world touches us. As the poet Paul Valery said: "There is nothing deeper than skin." There are artists such as Marina Abramovic who say that what is corporal and suffering may be reconverted through art and the performances in which they use her body as a canvas. This also occurs with the wounded bodies painted by Frida Kahlo, in which the wounds that take time to heal reinforce the artist's creativity. Kahlo was able to transform the terrible chronic pain of the wounded body into pictorial reality.

In body modification culture, bodies used as the location for the oddest modifications and freak and grotesque culture form an expression of postmodernism, e.g., the carnal art of Orlan, who gives her body to artistic creation. She undergoes repeated plastic surgery with the aim of presenting herself as a work of art through a chin like that of Botticelli's Venus or a forehead like the Mona Lisa's. However, this is where the relationship of medical and patient power is inverted. She takes control in progressive body transformation [58]. Artists such as the photographer Cindy Sherman have used their own bodies to portray roles that are culturally defined as female, roles that are earmarked for women in the media using images from B movies: film star, housewife, naïve girl. Films in which women are presented as vulnerable, weak, and even mad. Unlike the photographers who seek locations, Sherman seeks spaces that are interior, private, domestic, and categorized as female. She shows photos of the female body that are increasingly dark, grotesque, and fragmented. In the 1980s, she reduced the female body to its sub-products, vomit, menstrual blood, viscera, and in her photos of the following decade she equipped her body with real and invented prosthetics [58].

De Beauvoir [12] asserts that the female body must be the situation and the instrument of women's freedom and not a defining and limiting essence. This conversion process, which cannot be said to have a beginning or an end, is open to resignification. Hence, the body seems to be a set of individual and social limits. We women are fragments, pieces, and incompleteness; thus, with this lack we find the origin of distress and associated psychopathology. Alluding to an original or authentic femininity is a nostalgic ideal, the philosopher Judith Butler asserts. She proposes that the current need to analyze gender is a complex cultural construction, following de Beauvoir's theory of "one is not born a woman but one becomes one." Hegelian tradition entwines desire with recognition. It asserts that desire is always a desire for recognition and that any one of us constitutes a viable social being only through the experience of recognition. Insofar as desire is involved in social standards, this is linked to the issue of power and the person who meets the requisites of what is recognized as human versus the person who does not [23]. Female human bodies are very often disdained by other bodies and, as a consequence of this disdain, they are subject to abuse, ill-treatment, abasement, and murder. Female desire represents a dangerous energy for the established order. The female body finds itself between disdain and exaltation. We possess many examples of this in literature, cinema, and history: the femme fatale, vamps with come-to-bed eyes, with a dark gaze, provocative clothing, the cult of romantic love and fatal destiny. The diva of this era is Marlene Dietrich in *The Blue Angel*. The dream of the First World War was the devil as a woman, the woman as desire, exotic and sophisticated. The Second World War saw the appearance of pin-ups, girls with big cheeks. In the 1940s and 1950s the most representative pin-up was Rita Hayworth, who was famously slapped in a scene showing the abuse of power [58]. By dint of this type of social determinism, servitude became voluntary and ended up finding pleasure in the renunciation of itself, as in the famous case of the triumphantly beautiful but ill-starred Marilyn Monroe, whose femininity was caricaturized until she took her own life, her sensuality lay in being tragic [58]. To censure the body is to censure, in passing, the breath, the word. The subject is subordinated through language. An individual prefers to exist in subordination than not to exist at all [23]. The pathologization of the female body has been a reality in the history of psychology, just as women do not appear in history until the nineteenth century. For practically the whole of history "anonymous was a woman," as the writer Virginia Woolf [39] reminds us. In *The Portrait of a Lady*, Henry James explains:

"There is no such thing as an isolated man or woman; we are each of us made up of a cluster of appurtenances. What do you call one's self? Where does it begin? Where does it end? It overflows into everything that belongs to us and then flows back again." A kind of collage, with the hope that things endure, however divided and fragmented they may be, like any mind. The body seems to offer, in these conditions, the final anchorage point to cling onto. It is the anchorage point to be grasped as a being, to be organized, manipulated, transformed, exceeded as a person or individual in the eyes of others. This post-human perspective raises questions about certainty over identity and reassurance about oneself, which are also altered by the discovery of other experiences and other constructions of the body through the work of feminist artists (Nancy Spero, Judy Chicago, Cindy Sherman, Barbara Kruger), homosexual artists, and queer culture. Queer culture, according to Beatriz Preciado [26], goes much further by suggesting that this dichotomy does not exist, without even a difference between a true femininity/masculinity and another, impostured one. All gender identity is a performance, a masquerade.

6.8 Body Image

After introducing into the study of the body schema various concepts from psychoanalysis, Schilder [59] in 1935 used a new basic expression in the field of corporality: body image. The author also pointed out that this body image represents an emotional experience, as feelings are states of the self, and the self is above all a corporal self.

Schilder's basic idea is that "there is no perception without action." The postural model of the body is insufficient because it reflects a passive receiving subject. We can only be sure that that perception is correct when the manipulation of the object perceived is correct.

Henri Wallon [60] seeks new responses by studying the childhood origins of body awareness. For him, the genesis of the awareness of the body is a function of the mirror, given that initially children identify the organs of others better than their own. They quickly learn their mother's breast or hands. Postural sensitivity develops from the movements the mother makes with them. Children need to be moved and changed positionally because their bodies cannot be understood to be anything but a "body of relation." The abstract and global idea of their body will not appear, until they are at least 6–7 years old, when it can develop a symbolic function.

Wallon attributes a leading role to the function of the baby as a tonic. When the mother takes the child in her arms, the latter becomes tense or flaccid, resistant or adaptable. Ajuriaguerra [61] goes further and develops a complete child psychopathology based on corporality, classifying children according to body tone. The body is the language between mother and baby, and when there are problems both must search the tonic relationship and work through caresses and relaxation techniques. This first mother–child communication gives meaning to the body as a vehicle of expression of human language for the rest of adult life.

The French philosopher Merleau-Ponty disregards the psychoanalytic components of Schilder's ideas and asserts that they are insufficient because the body schema is defined not through action but through the meaning given to it, which is its function. This connects to the ideas of Wallon and Ajuriaguerra. Merleau-Ponty [45] stresses the classic Heideggerian distinction in the field of corporality and speaks of a "body in itself, a body for self and a body for others." The body's function in each sphere is, for Merleau-Ponty, the unifying element. Hence, for example, to suffer a phantom arm means to miss all the actions that only that arm could perform. The body's practical field is conserved even when the anatomical one no longer exists. This is because the body is the vehicle of "being in the world."

Phenomenology has considerably enriched our knowledge of the experience of the body by enabling Cartesian dualism to be overcome. Setting out from the subject's relationship with its world through the immediate contents of conscience that are phenomena, the body acquires a very special nature. This is the medium in relation to the world, but even more, it is the very condition of the experience lived. The body schema is the form of expressing that my body is in the world. There is no possibility of distinguishing the body as an object that I have from the body as the subject that I am. Marcel [41] expresses this in terms of "I am and I have body" and Marías [62] as "I am installed in my body," that is, I am corporeality.

Until that moment, Cartesian dualism proposed that human nature was the union of the body (*Res extensa*) with the soul (*Res cogitans*). For phenomenology, such a distinction is an abstraction, an intellectual construction, as the phenomenon we experience is of a unitary nature. Corporal experience is accompanied by the experience of a here and now, of oneself in the world, i.e., it is closely linked to the experience of time, of space, of the self, and of the world.

Body and world form an entirety: I am me and my circumstance [63]. I am someone corporal, linked for this reason, through corporeality, to worldliness. For this reason, I am in my body and I am in my world [64]. Corporality is worldly, directed toward the world, related to it from its origin. The eye without light is an organ without a *raison d'être* (actually, it would atrophy). This is why Goethe said that it participates in the sun's nature: "*Wär nicht das Auge sonnehaft/Die Sonne könnt es nie erblicken*"; "were not the eye of the nature of the sun/how could it behold the sun." Therefore, motor functions are seen in their meaning, performance, and expression, which are removed because they refer to the world.

The process by which the brain constructs a body schema requires the integration of exteroceptive, proprioceptive, and interoceptive information, between each other and with the executive activities of the movement associated with it. This achieves a symbolic content that enables a harmonious and effective corporal experience and functioning [65].

The process of overall and harmonious integration of our body requires the participation of what are called mirror neurons, which are both motor and sensory cells, and gives them the capacity to receive and anticipate the movements of other living beings. With this, the individual learns adaptive behaviors and lays the foundations for a social relationship.

The cognitive–emotional genesis of the body image is learned and acquired through life. With the passage of time, the neurobiological mechanisms involved in body image are strengthened by experience, principally in childhood and adolescence, a time when the neuronal networks making this possible are established. For this reason, every individual has a different concept of self body image, which forms part of his/her personal experience [66]. The body remembers everything that it has experienced at any time and all of this is stored.

Somatic markers are emotional and of a different nature, aware or unaware, associated with the brain's representation of the body state to modulate the organism's response beyond mere cognitive aspects. This involves emotional processes that anticipate the rational process and these are established according to past emotional experiences, a concept introduced by Damasio [65].

The representation of oneself gradually develops from the age of approximately a year and a half [66], when a notion of "I" [67] and "I that I know" is acquired [68]. The visual recognition of oneself is the most frequently studied, but there are other important aspects such as emotions, especially embarrassment [69], empathy [70], and altruism [71]. The recognition of oneself is connected with autobiographical memories and with the ability to imitate [72]. Pretense and the denial of oneself are early signs of the ability to understand mental states [73]. Two important aspects are the use of personal pronouns like "me" and "mine" [74], and play [75].

For Schilder [76], body image transcends the knowledge of one's own physical space in which corporal activity takes place to locate itself in a different temporal and mental space that enables one to be able to detach, imagine, symbolize, and even distort the schema itself.

Slade [77] describes body image as the picture we have in our minds on the size, the shape, and the structure of our body, and our feelings toward each of its constituent parts.

The ideal of the male body image has remained unaltered since the Greeks, with Michelangelo's David of the Renaissance continuing to construct the ideal of the male image in the present-day collective imagination.

However, in the case of women, a great transformation in the ideal of beauty has occurred. This began with the prehistoric Venus of large proportions, through Titian's fleshy Renaissance Venus. A progressive slimming of the body image started in the nineteenth century with chlorotic women who suffered from dizziness and "hysterical collapses." This continued to proportions that are impossible to reproduce nowadays without attaining a state of excessive or even extreme thinness while retaining a large bust, leading many women to opt for plastic surgery. Most plastic surgery is carried out in young women aged 20 to 40, with mammoplasty the most frequent operation.

Recent research has expanded the focus of eating disorders to include body image, body dissatisfaction, and channels like the thoughts and cognitions on one's own body affecting body image and the image that one possesses of oneself. Once cognitive schemas on the body are formed, they are maintained firmly and may give rise to distortions in the body image.

Conclusion

We are embodied. The body forms a nuclear part of our being. This review includes anthropological and sociological aspects and those of gender anthropology that demonstrate this influence on the ways in which the body is presented under the influence of history and culture. From the corporeal experience, individuals, and especially women, possess a representation of their body in which it is an instrument, the object for performing various functions of a social, reproductive, and productive nature. Maternity and corporal realities are constituent elements of an identity marked by instrumentalization, on many occasions the dissociation and the tension generated by this. Although much more research is needed and we are aware that many of these theories are speculative, we feel it necessary to include the gender paradigm in the psychopathology of the corporality that represents one of the pillars of the construction of our being in the world. The body seems to offer, under these conditions, the final anchorage point to cling onto. It is the anchorage point to be grasped as a being, to be organized, manipulated, transformed, exceeded as a person or individual in the eyes of others. In the face of binary models of sexuality, other models exist that merit review and which up to now have been denied and ignored (intersexual states).

References

1. Martin Casares A. Antropología del género. 3rd ed. Valencia: Catedra; 2012.
2. Dio BE. La sexualidad femenina. De la niña a la mujer. Barcelona: Paidós; 1997.
3. Bance C. Anthropology rediscovers sexuality: a theoretical comment. Soc Sci Med. 1997; 33(8):875–84.
4. Valcárcel A. Feminismo en el mundo global. Valencia: Catedra UPV; 2010.
5. Sanahuja YU. Modelos explicativos sobre los orígenes y evolución de la Humanidad. Mujeres y sociedad. Nuevos enfoques teóricos y metodológicos La Luna (comp) Universidad de Barcelona; 1991.
6. MacCormack C, Strathern M. Nature, culture and gender. New York: Routledge; 1990.
7. Marylin Strathern M. An anthropological perspective. In: Harris O, Young K, editors. Feminist anthropology. Barcelona: Anagrama; 1979.
8. Mead M (1949) Male and female. A study of the sexes in a changing world. New York: Morow eds; 1952
9. Sartre JP. Being and nothingness. New York: Washington Square Press; 1943.
10. Badinter E. The conflict. How motherhood undermines the status of women. France: Flammarion; 2010.
11. Sanyal MM. Vulva. Barcelona: Anagrama; 2012.
12. Beauvoir S. The second sex. New York: Vintage Books; 1952.
13. Foucault M. Histoire de la folie á lâge classique. Paris: Gallimard; 1972.
14. Bordieu P. Masculine Domination. Stanford, CA: Stanford University Press; 2001.
15. Lévi Strauss C. Las estructuras elementales del parentesco. Barcelona: Paidos; 1998 [1949].
16. Heidegger M. On the way of being. New York: Harper and Row; 1971.
17. Heidegger M. Existence and being. Washington, DC: Henry Regnery; 1949.
18. Griffith JL, Elliot Griffith M. The body speaks: therapeutic dialogues for mind-body problems. New York: Basic Books; 1994.

19. Maturana HR, Varela FJ. The tree of knowledge: the biological roots of human understanding. Boston: Shanmbala; 1987.
20. Gadamer HG. Philosophical hermeneutics. Berkley: University of California Press; 1976.
21. Devaux M. Feminism and empowerment: a critical Reading of Foucault. Fem Stud. 1994;20: 223–42.
22. Foucault M. History of sexuality. London: Penguin Books; 1992.
23. Butler J. Gender trouble. Feminism and the subversion of identity. New York: Routledge; 1999.
24. Nanda S. Neither man nor woman: the Hijras of India. Belmont, ON: Wadsworth Publishing; 1998.
25. Hester D. Eunuchs and postgender Jesus: Matthew 19:12 and transgressive sexualities. J Study New Testam. 2005;28(1):13–40.
26. Preciado B. Manifiesto contrasexual. Barcelona: Opera Prima; 2002.
27. Butler J. Subjects of desire: Hegelian reflections in twentieth century France. New York: Columbia University Press; 1999.
28. Newton E, Walton S. The misunderstanding. Toward a more precise sexual vocabulary. In: Vance C, editor. Pleasure and danger. Boston: Routledge; 1984.
29. Baptiste B. Inventing the body. http://tedxtalks.ted.com/video/Inventando-el-cuerpo-Brigitte-B
30. Butler J. Undoing gender. London: Routledge; 2004.
31. Rubin G. The traffic of women: the political economy of sex. Ann Arbor, MI: University of Michigan; 1975.
32. Plato. Timaeus Dialogue. Stanford Encyclopedia of Philosophy; 2005.
33. Mithu M Sanyal. Vulva La revelación del sexo invisible. Anagrama; 2009
34. Varela J, Alvárez-Uria F. Madrid: Siglo XXI; 2008.
35. Didi Huberman G. Invention of hysteria: Charcot and the photographic iconography of the Salpêtriére. Cambridge, MA: MIT Press; 2003.
36. López-Ibor J, et al. Percepción, vivencia e identidad corporales. Actas Esp Psiquiatr. 2011; 39 Suppl 3:3–118.
37. Plath S. The Bell Jar. London: Faber and faber Eds; 1966
38. Jelinek E. Die Liebhaberinnen (women as lovers) Rowohlt, Reinbek bei Hamburg 1975 ISBN 3-499-25064-0.
39. Woolf V. A room of one's own; 1929.
40. Jaspers K. Psicopatología general. Buenos Aires: Editorial Beta; 1977.
41. Colina F. Escritos psicóticos. Madrid: Dor; 1996.
42. Ortega y Gasset J. Vitalidad, alma y espíritu. Obras completas. Madrid: Revista de Occidente; 1946.
43. Marcel G. Étre et avoir. Paris: Editorial Montaigne; 1955.
44. May R. Existencia. Nueva dimensión en psiquiatría y psicología. Madrid: Editorial Gredos; 1977.
45. Merleau-Ponty M. Fenomenología de la percepción. Barcelona: Editorial Península; 1975.
46. López Ibor JJ, López Ibor Aliño JJ. Cuerpo y corporalidad. Madrid: Editorial Gredos; 1974.
47. Lhermitte J. L'image de notre corps. Paris: Nouvelle Revue Critique; 1939.
48. Pera C. Pensar desde el Cuerpo. Un ensayo sobre la Corporeidad humana. Madrid: Triascatela; 2006.
49. Janet P. L'evolution psychologique de la personnalité. 1st ed. París: Edition Chahine 1929.
50. Ribot T. Les maladies de la personnalité. París: Felix Alcan; 1884.
51. Zubiri X. Sobre el hombre. Madrid: Alianza; 1986.
52. Leder D. The absent body. Chicago: The University of Chicago Press; 1990.
53. Varela FJ, Thomson E, Rosch E. The embodied mind. Cognitive science and human experience. Cambridge: MIT Press; 2004.
54. Damasio AR. Descartes error: emotion, reason and the human brain. New York: G.P. Putnam; 1994.
55. Foucault M. Utopian body. Cambridge, MA: Sensorium, MIT Press; 1966.
56. Schopenhauer A. El arte de conocerse a sí mismo. Madrid: Alianza; 2007.

57. Wilde O. Poemas en prosa. Madrid: Aguilar; 1962. Poems in Prose. The Fortnightly Review 1894.
58. Baecque A. El cuerpo en el cine en Historia del cuerpo vol III. Madrid: Taurus; 2006.
59. Schilder P. Imagen y apariencia del cuerpo humano. Buenos Aires: Editorial Paidos; 1977.
60. Wallon H. Les origins du caractére chez l'enfant. París: Presses Universitaires de France; 1930.
61. Ajuriaguerra J. Evolución y trastornos del conocimiento corporal y de la conciencia de sí mismo. Manual de Psiquiatría Infantil. Barcelona: Toray-Masson; 1976.
62. Marías J. Persona. Madrid: Alianza; 1996.
63. Ortega y Gasset J. Meditaciones del quijote o experimentos de nueva España (1914) en: Obras Completas. 41 ed. Madrid: Revista de occidente; 1957. Tomo II. p. 322.
64. Marías J. Antropología metafísica. Madrid: Revista de Occidente; 1970.
65. Damasio AR. The Somatic marker hypothesis and the possible functions of the prefrontal cortex. Philos Trans R Soc Lond Boil Sci. 1996;351(1346):1413–20.
66. Lewis M, Brooks-Gunn J. Social cognition and the acquisition of self. New York: Plenum; 1979.
67. Lewis M. Aspects of the self: from systems to ideas. In: Rochat P, editor. The self in early infancy: theory and research. Amsterdam: North Holland; 1995.
68. Rochat P, editor. The self in early infancy: theory and research. Amsterdam: North Holland; 1995.
69. Lewis M, Sullivan MW, Stanger C, Weiss M. Self development and self-conscious emotions. Child Dev. 1989;60(1):146–56.
70. Bischof-Köhler D. Self object and interpersonal emotions. Identification of own mirror image, empathy and prosocial behavior in the 2nd year of life. Psychol Z Angew Psychol. 1994; 202(4):349.
71. Zahn-Waxler C, Radke-Yarrow M, Wagner E, Chapman M. Development of concern for others. Dev Psychol. 1992;28(1):126–36.
72. Asendorpf JB. Self awareness, other awareness and secondary representation. In: Meltzoff AN, Prinz W, editors. The imitative mine: development, evolution and brain bases. Cambridge studies in cognitive perceptual development. New York: Cambridge University Press; 2002.
73. Leslie A. Pretense and the representation revisited. In: Stein N, Bauer P, Rabinowitz M, editors. Representation, memory and development. Lawrence Album: Mahwah, NJ; 2002. p. 103–4.
74. Stipek D, Gralinski H, Kopp CB. Self-concept development in the toddler years. Dev Psychol. 1990;26:972–7.
75. Lewis M, Ramsay D. Development of Self-recognition personal pronoun use and pretend play during the 2nd year. Child Dev. 2004;75(6):1821–31.
76. Schilder P. The image and the appearance of the human body. Studies in constructive energies of the psyche. New York: International University Press; 1950.
77. Slade PD. Body image in anorexia nervosa. Br J Psychiatry. 1988;153(2):20–2.

Body and Hysteria: Dissociated Body

7

Agueda Rojo-Pantoja

Abstract

There is a recurring confusion about the terms and names used to describe dissociation and dissociative disorders. By this we mean somatic disorders, conversion disorders, dissociative disorders, Briquet syndrome, depersonalization disorder or split personality disorder, to mention just a few, without clear-cut boundaries among these diagnostic entities. To describe the psychopathology of dissociative symptoms, it is useful to know the genesis of the disorder, the cultural–historical context that saw its birth, and how it has evolved to the present day.

It is common to relate dissociation to hysteria, and hysteria to women. Today, it is a well-known fact that these associations are not always clear. The idea of dissociation was coined by Pierre Janet in France in the late nineteenth century and was used to diagnose female patients who for the most part presented with hysteria, in a historical period and in a city in which hysteria was related solely to women. Prior to Janet, Charcot had already put forward a psychological explanation for hysteria, with traumas as triggers and somatic symptoms as the most significant manifestations. Freud later challenged the conversive mechanism with the dissociative one as an explanation for hysteria, and both terms have found their way into modern-day psychopathological descriptions, bringing about a chaos in terminology. Here we shed light on the confusion created by the different terms and also try to prove that there is insufficient evidence to support the idea that dissociative disorders are predominantly found in women.

A. Rojo-Pantoja (✉)
Department of Psychiatry, University Hospital Complex, Vigo, Spain
e-mail: rojopsastre@yahoo.es

M. Sáenz-Herrero (ed.), *Psychopathology in Women*,
DOI 10.1007/978-3-319-05870-2_7

7.1 Introduction

Modern day psychopathology retains dissociation and dissociative symptoms within the bounds of the psychopathology of consciousness. It defines dissociation as a restriction of the field of consciousness, which denotes a disruption in the normal and continuous flow of ideas, thoughts, perceptions, etc., bringing about a split between cognitive and perceptive elements and behavioral ones, the behavior adopting automatic modes [1]. All of the processes involving a restriction of consciousness have the following psychopathological elements: decrease in the levels of alertness and attention, spatial and temporal disorientation, automatic behavior, post-critical amnesia, absent delirium, and partially preserved sensory reactivity. Other symptoms that are considered dissociative are the dissolution of the self or split personality, dissociative amnesia, depersonalization, derealization, auditory hallucinations [2], trance states [3], and somatoform symptoms.

We owe the term *dissociation* to Pierre Janet, since its genesis can be found in his *désagrégation psychologique* [4], and also to the reformers of eighteenth century associationism, such as Maine de Biran or Herbart, because they provided Janet with a conceptual framework, which was later elaborated upon by Sigmund Freud, another key figure in the emergence of the new concept.

Moving on, we find the *fin-de-siècle* spirit, which reached its zenith in cities such as Paris and Vienna at the turn of the century. The artists in Paris were familiar with Charcot's theories about nervous diseases. Neurasthenia, whose root cause was considered to be the hectic pace of life in the city, became a fashionable affliction. Psychiatry had a strong influence on the spirit of the day, and there is a considerable overlap between the patients described by psychiatrists and the characters portrayed by novelists and playwrights.

Ellenberger [5] cites similarities between Janet's Irene (1907) and Zola's Pauline, from his work *La Joie de Vivre*, between Hofmannsthal's *Electra* and de Breuer's *Anna O*; between Freud's *Dora* and the characters in the short stories by Schnitzler. In this cultural–historical context a predilection for hysteria can be found to be the diagnosis for the women of the day. Consciousness and its alterations become increasingly important and inform the different conceptions that illuminate psychology, psychopathology, and clinical psychiatry [6] throughout the twentieth century.

In 1875, Eugène Azam spoke for the first time of the "French split personality," embodied by Félida. He first described the case as "temporal amnesia," later calling it "double awareness," and finally "split personality." So many cases of split personality were published during the nineteenth century that Ellenberger [5] saw the need for a classification. It is important to point out that all of the cases involved women—Hélène Smith, Estelle, Mary Reynolds, or Miss Beauchamp—and that only one man is mentioned, Ansel Bourne, treated by William James. An interesting point to debate is whether the proliferation of split personalities among members of the female sex was an epidemiological reality or simply the result of the cultural trend in vogue at the time. Two centuries later we can see how this mental disorder has evolved over time. Today its prevalence seems to be greater in the USA than in Europe, and according to the latest studies cited in the bibliography, contradictory information about its prevalence in one sex or the other exists, undermining the notion that women are more prone to suffering from the condition.

However, dissociation not only manifests itself in a split personality, today called multiple personality disorder, but also underlies different mental disorders with different psychological and physical manifestations. Dissociation not only includes dissociative amnesia, depersonalization, derealization, and fragmented identity but also, according to Pierre Janet and other psychiatrists working during World War I, a poor integration of somatomorphic components [7]. Different authors [7] have proposed the name psychological dissociation, instead of somatomorphic dissociation, to illustrate that many somatic symptoms have a dissociative mechanism at their core.

The extremely high number of women among those affected by these types of disorders in the nineteenth century must be understood to be a cultural bias pertaining to the age. In this century the role of the female body was limited to maternity. Women were considered weak and prone to suffering from mental disorders [8]. Many women during this century were labeled chronically sick [9]. In all likelihood, girls and women became sick in no small measure because of the horrible conditions imposed upon them, but few doctors at that time would have seen social factors as being possible etiological causes. With the arrival of psychoanalysis and a new interest in female sexuality, the famous cases of Anna O and Dora appeared, treated by Freud, and these women were considered "hysterical, delirious or depressive" [9]. Once again discrimination was an important factor in the treatment of certain diseases, which were considered to be almost exclusive to women. The stress of modern life was cited to be an aggravating factor that made nervous diseases in women even worse, since women were generally perceived as more delicate and sensitive.

However, whether there is a preponderance of dissociative disorders among women over men is something that has to be ascertained. We will try to use all the facts and figures known at present to see whether the disorder occurs more predominantly in one sex or the other. We think it is important to find an explanation for the statistical data that can be found for different disorders, and to elucidate if these depend on factors specific to women or factors determined by culture.

7.2 Janet and Systematic Anesthesia

There is little doubt that the term dissociation had its origin in Pierre Janet, or more precisely, in his idea of *désagrégation*, at a very specific time and place in history, the French *fin-de-siècle*. Sigmund Freud also deserves a mention, because it is around this time when references to the concept of dissociation start appearing in his work. He will soon drop the idea in favor of repression, and his theories will move in a new direction, leaving hypnosis behind and embracing the new ideas of psychoanalysis. Both authors had conflicting views regarding the origin of dissociation, but their studies overlapped at different points, often leading to the same conclusions [6].

Different concepts start appearing in the works of Pierre Janet (suggestion, subconscious, narrowing of the field of consciousness, psychological misery, fixed ideas) that will lay the foundations and blaze the trail for his *désagrégation psychologique*. His greatest work is *L'Automatisme Psychologique* (1889), the result of the research he carried out in the lab of El Havre hospital, in which he expounds his theory of disaggregation [4].

It was thanks to his clinical observations of patients, and partial catalepsies, that Janet came up with the idea of partial consciousness, the dissociation of the content of consciousness in different compartments. He described women who performed actions subconsciously, that is to say "actions that had all the features of a psychological fact except one, which is that the subject is unaware of what he is doing in the moment he is doing it" [4]. Psychological automatism does not direct all conscious thinking but only a small group of phenomena partially separated from the overall consciousness of the individual that continue to act of their own accord and in a different manner. These partial automatisms have as their simplest form of expression partial catalepsies and suggestions by means of distraction.

For Janet ideas develop into acts. It is no coincidence that his psychological automatism should have carried the subtitle "Experimental-psychological essay on the inferior forms of human activity" [4]. Distraction, according to this author, seems to split the field of consciousness into two parts: one that remains conscious, and another that the subject seems to be unaware of. The distraction would be equivalent to an anesthesia, by means of which we can suggest acts, but also hallucinations. While the distracted consciousness is occupied with other ideas, the suggested act is performed without the subject knowing about it.

By means of suggestion Janet discovers that he can suppress certain sensations, producing in the subject partial blindness or deafness. A suggestion of a negative hallucination or systematic anesthesia was used. The first term came from Bernheim (1886) and the second from and Binet and Fére, the latter seeming more accurate to Janet, since he viewed the phenomenon as being analogous to the systematic paralysis of movement [10].

Janet's understanding is that during conscious perception of sensations, there is an operation in two stages. First, there is a confluence of all of the sensations coming from the different senses and then there is an active synthesis of these sensations as they cluster together, and aggregate themselves to a given perception. It so happens that in the "distracted hysterical" [4] subject there are a set of sensations that during the second operation escape from consciousness. They cannot be linked to the personality of the subject, and therefore, the self is not aware of them. Synthesis is weak and restricted.

Janet considers "systematic or even general anesthesia an injury, a weakening, not of sensation, but of the ability to synthesize sensations, rendering a personal perception, all of which implies a true disaggregation of psychological phenomena" [4].

We can see that this initial concept of dissociation, Pierre Janet's psychological disaggregation, is a concept that stems from the analysis of somatic phenomena, partial catalepsis, and systematic anesthesia, and that it describes "the dissociated body" [4] of sick people, generally hysterical women. Even in the prologue to his philosophy thesis, *Psychological Automatism*, he cites the names of four women, Léonie, Lucie, Rose, and Marie, who were the women that Janet considered as having "the conditions of a good psychological experience" [4]. Later, in 1898, Janet [11] published *Néuroses et Idées Fixes*, in which he gathered all of the articles he published between 1891 and 1897 on the subject of different psychopathological disorders and their therapy, and which were the result of his work in the ward of Charcot in La Salpêtrière, treating hysterical patients, among them were Madame D., Isabelle, Marcelle, Justine, Madame A., etc. One of the few references to male patients is the case of Achilles, who suffered from manifestations of demonic possession.

"It is undeniable that what gave hysteria coherence over a long period of time was its exclusively female nature" [12].

Up until the twentieth century three possible origins for hysteria were considered, the uterus, the brain, and the nerves. The first option justified that only women should suffer from the condition, but later on its origin was generally thought to be located in the brain, and, owing to the analogy between crises of hysteria and epileptic convulsions, it was determined that there had to be only one organ involved in the pathology. This is how the concept of hystero-epilepsy came into existence, consecrated by the Charcot school.

In this *fin-de-siècle* Paris, hysteria continued to be a condition exclusively related to women. Records detailing manifestations of hysteria were always connected with female patients. It was Charcot himself, however, who demonstrated that hysteria was also a male affliction. One of his students, Professor Pierre Maire said to his teacher: "The most salient feature of Charcot's work on the subject of hysteria, the main formulation that will not be lost and that will serve as a guideline to future generations of doctors, is his demonstration that male hysteria exists" [13].

We cannot forget the historical context in which this shift to male hysteria took place. The most important phenomenon in the industrial world of the nineteenth century was the railway, which can be considered, in the words of Hacking "the epic symbol of the psychologizing of trauma" [14]. The railway gave the very idea of accident its modern meaning, that is, among other things, that something can happen randomly or without apparent cause. The term railway spine appears, coined by Johen Eric Erichsen, to refer to those symptoms that did not match any recognizable physical injury. Three years later Russel Reynolds [14] tries to demonstrate that certain disorders such as paralysis, spasms or other alterations of the sensations may depend on the morbid state of a sole idea, or an idea together with an emotion, and such a formulation cannot elude being compared to hysteria. This syndrome was a chance for Charcot to render hysteria potentially male. Gynecologists and obstetricians claimed this territory as their domain; thus, the best way to take the disease away from the gynecologists was to declare that it belonged to both sexes. Up to then male hysteria was recognized, but within the context of an "effeminate" [14] personality. Charcot [15] in his lessons on the disease of the nervous system (1887) discussed the symptoms that Russel Reynolds had described, provoking, by means of hypnosis, the symptoms in a male subject whose masculinity was beyond question. Thus, "memory, hysteria, hypnosis and physical trauma were closely linked together in the lectures by Charcot" [14].

After having worked for 6 or 7 years in El Havre, Janet [16] arrived at La Salpêtrière and followed the teachings of his master Charcot, which ended with his thesis in medicine *L'État Mental des Hystériques*, in which he outlined and completed his studies on the subject of hysteria. According to López Piñero and Morales Meseguer [17], the historical foundations of Janet's initial thinking could be traced back to his being a student first of Ribot and then of Charcot. And it is precisely Charcot's contributions on fixed ideas that were core to certain neuroses and that formed the starting point of Janet's theory of dissociation. In his work *L'État Mental des Hystériques* the author explains the existence of purely somatic phenomenology whose etiology is psychological and Charcot is the first one to link these physical symptoms with traumatic phenomena. According to Janet, hysteria is a mental illness in which there is cerebral stress and also very vague physical symptoms. There is a weakening of the field of consciousness that prevents certain sensations and images from being perceived, and they remain beyond the scope of personal perception. This lack of synthesis enables parasite ideas to form, and since these are completely isolated from the control of personal consciousness, they manifest themselves as disorders in physical appearance. These parasite ideas are the germ of Janet's fixed ideas, which are the cause of mental accidents in hysterics and were how Charcot explained traumatic hysteria.

> Well, gentlemen: thanks to recent findings in the science of hypnotic neurosis, we have been able to intervene to a certain extent, and advance experimentation in the study of cases of this nature. We know that, in individuals in a state of deep hypnosis, it is possible to give birth to, by means of suggestion and intimidation, an idea, a coherent group of associated ideas, which settles in the mind in a similar way to a parasite, becoming isolated from everything else, and which can translate externally in corresponding motor skill phenomena [15].

Charcot devotes himself to the study of hysteria, which affects not only women, but also men and children. It is a disease with multiple symptoms such as contractions, paralysis, anesthesia, convulsions, hallucinations or delirium. From 1878 onwards he becomes interested in hypnosis, a method by which he can provoke in his patients the symptoms of hysteria, and he defends hypnosis and hysteria only being possible in people with weak and degenerate nervous systems.

Charcot is criticized by Liébeault and Bernheim, who deny that there is a link between hypnosis and hysteria and defend that the prerequisite that is necessary for hypnosis to be performed is suggestibility and not the mental disease. After this attack, Charcot begins his work on the psychologizing of hysteria, and, without forgetting its neurological grounding, he proposes a psychological explanation, admitting that personality disorders caused by traumas are a triggering factor in hysteria. This approach permits a therapy to be developed, and such a therapy would be devised by two of his disciples, Freud and Janet [18].

At the end of the nineteenth century and beginning of the twentieth century, the role played by emotion in the triggering of hysteria became controversial. According to Janet past traumatic events that "were forgotten" remained active at the subconscious level, forming fixed ideas, endowed with a life of their own in a dissociated consciousness. From Janet's point of view emotion produced a state of dissociation, narrowed the field of consciousness, and enabled the fixed idea to settle. From Freud's point of view, however, emotion, because of its charge of excitation, submits the body to an overcharge that it is not able to get rid of through the normal channels of abreaction (release of emotional tension).

7.3 Freud and Conversion

In the preliminary Communication of 1893, Freud and Breuer extend to all hysteria the pathogenic formula proposed by Charcot for hystero-traumatic paralysis.

Freud describes in this work two psychological operations in the process of traumatic neuroses [19]. One is a mechanism of dissociation, by which there is a rupture in the association between a function of the body and the rest of its psychological activity. The second is a *clivage* (*Spaltung*), which would keep this separation or diversion completely apart, to the point when it becomes unbridgeable, leaving all these dissociated phenomena inaccessible to any form of association. In order for these mechanisms to kick in, there must be a charge of intense affective value. The difference between Janet's and Freud's understanding regarding this dissociation is that the former explains it as a result of a deficit in the synthesis function or a narrowing of the field of consciousness, while the latter links it to the affective charge.

For Freud the cases of male hysteria described by Charcot could be paradigmatic for female hysteria, because it is in women and in a decidedly female world in which he creates his theories. In these cases, the subjects suffered a trauma, a railway accident, which made them feel terrified, while in hysterical women experiences that could be considered traumatic could be found to be content in their attacks, but it was not the memory that was in itself traumatic, rather, it had happened in a moment of predisposition, and that is the reason why it became a traumatic memory. Freud's understanding is that this memory is unconscious, meaning that it can be found in a second state of consciousness [20].

Freud assumes that the symptomatic complex of hysteria justifies the hypothesis of a dissociation of consciousness, with separate psychic groups being formed, but he does not share the views that were current at the time about the origin of such dissociation. For Janet, dissociation was a primary feature of hysteria and was dependent on a genetic weakness in the capacity for psychical synthesis, which meant that degeneration in hysterical individuals was unavoidable, a hypothesis that is not shared by Freud. At the beginning, this author was in agreement with Breuer's "hypnoid states."

> The split of consciousness, as remarkable as double consciousness, in well-known classic cases, exists in a rudimentary way in all hysteria: therefore, the inclination to dissociate, and along with it, the emergence of altered states of consciousness, which we will summarize under the name of hypnoids, would be the fundamental phenomenon underlying neurosis. [21]

The hypnoid states are singular states of consciousness, of dreamlike qualities, with a diminution in the associative faculty. Any representation emerging from one these hypnoid states is excluded from normal associative connections, broken off from the remaining contents of consciousness, and as a consequence dissociation appears, which is acquired and not primary [6].

In the aforementioned preliminary Communication, the authors defend the idea that traumatic memories retain all of their emotional charge, and the same as a "foreign body" exert an influence on personality, a hypothesis that was backed up by the famous case of Anna O [21].

It will take Freud a long time to leave Breuer's theories behind and formulate his concept of "conversion" in the so-called "defence hysterias." Unlike Janet, who considered the dissociation of consciousness one of the defining features of hysteria, Freud [22] (1894) considered the capacity for conversion one of the defining features.

> In hysteria, the unbearable representation is rendered harmless by transforming the magnitude of stimulus into somatic excitations, a process for which we propose the name of conversion. Conversion can be total or partial, and it happens to the motor or sensory innervation more closely linked in one degree or another to the traumatic event. The mnemic footstep does not disappear because of it, but forms here onward the node of a second psychical group. [22]

His theory explaining hysteria and its evolution can be traced in the medical histories of four of his patients, all of them women, from Breuer's hypnoid state up to his concept of repression [6]. One can see the transition from the hypnoid hysterias of Anna O and Katherina to the defense hysterias of Elisabeth and Lucy, in which the terms dissociation and repression converge, although this is always seen as a defense mechanism.

The concept of repression appears in Freud's work for the first time in the neuropsychosis of defense [22] (1894) and on numerous occasions later on in his *Studies on Hysteria* [21] (1895). Freud explains that the "dissociation of the contents of consciousness (the result of the act of repression) is a consequence of the volition of the patient, being set into motion by an effort of will power, whose motive can be determined" [22]. "I viewed the psychical split as a result of the process of repulsion, that I then called defence, and later on, repression." [22]

The growing importance of psychoanalysis, subsequent to the *Studies on Hysteria* by Breuer and Freud, discredited the concept of dissociation, and it was ultimately replaced by the model of repression. Both Freud and Janet believed that psychological trauma played an important role in the forming of symptoms, but with the advent of Freud's concept of defense, the psychoanalytical theory broke away from the theories about dissociation current at the time, and the popularity of what had been one the most characteristic theories of the late nineteenth century and early twentieth century decreased, until all interest in it all but disappeared [23].

7.4 Dissociation and Conversion in Modern Day Classifications

The concept of dissociation found in the work of Pierre Janet does not refer to the same idea as that found in the work of Sigmund Freud, as we have already seen in this brief analysis of its conceptual and historical evolution. After the French *fin-de-siècle* the term was used to describe psychopathology in a very different nosological field, that of psychosis, bringing about a dramatic change in the understanding of the term. The main goal of this study of dissociation and the dissociated body is, however, concerned with the fact that the notions of Pierre Janet have provided a framework for modern day diagnostic manuals, both the DSM in the USA and the ICD in Europe [24]. In the changes that were proposed for the DSM IV we can already find the term "dissociative identity disorder" (300.14) instead of "dissociative personality", "dissociative amnesia" (300.12) instead of "psychogenic amnesia," or "dissociative fugue" (300.13) instead of psychogenic fugue. All of these terms correspond with manifestations that can be explained by means of Pierre Janet's dissociation.

Pierre Janet defined hysteria as a "form of mental depression characterized by the narrowing of the field of personal consciousness and a leaning towards the dissociation and emancipation of the systems of ideas and functions that make up personality" [25], these systems of ideas and functions belonging either to the psyche or the body.

Classically, there have been different diagnostic visions between American and European psychiatry. The former has avoided the somatic manifestations of the dissociative disorders, in such a way that the DSM-III-R defined the fundamental feature of dissociative disorders as "a disorder or alteration in the integration of functions connected with identity, memory or consciousness" [25] and in the DSM-IV [26] it was added that there could also be a disorder in the perception of the environment. We can see that in these diagnostic systems the somatoform symptoms are not considered to be of a dissociative nature but are labeled a somatization disorder, pain disorder, conversion disorder, sexual disorder, or dysmorphic body disorder. In stark contrast, the International Classification of Diseases, the ICD-10 does contemplate that dissociation can affect somatoform functions. "Dissociative disorders have in common a partial or complete loss of the normal integration of memories from the past, self-awareness and immediate sensations, and control of body movements." [27] This diagnostic manual only deals with dissociative disorders presenting as a loss of sensations or loss of, or interference with, movements. Disorders that may include further sensations such as pain are categorized as somatoform disorders, which are the same as somatization disorder. "Multiple and ill-defined complaints of somatic symptoms must be classified as somatoform disorders (F45.-) or neurasthenia (F48.0)" [27].

We would like to point out once again how confusing such terminology is. In the ICD "Dissociative disorders (conversion disorders)" are discussed as if they are equivalent concepts, although, as we have already seen, they refer to different concepts, according to the two different authors who described them.

To complicate things further, a pseudo-dissociative crisis is classified in the ICD 10 [27] as a dissociative disorder, but as a somatoform disorder in the DSM [26]. As already mentioned, in the American classification the conversion disorder can be found among somatoform disorders and is defined as "the presence of symptoms or deficit that affects motor or sensorial skills, and that suggest a neurological disorder or some other medical condition" [26]. The current DSM-5 renames conversion disorders "functional neurological symptomatic disorder" [28], stressing the need for neurological tests ("consistency in the test is a way of proving incompatibility between the symptom and well-known medical or neurological conditions" [28]) and also implying that the presence of relevant psychological factors cannot always be proven at diagnosis, which seems to give currency to the idea that they should not always be linked to psychological disorders.

The opposite occurs in the case of the somatization disorder, which is now called "somatic symptoms disorder" [28], clarifying that in order to reach this diagnosis there must be somatic symptoms and maladaptive thoughts, feelings, and behaviors. Previously, this disorder was defined as having somatic symptoms that could not be explained medically, but in the current diagnostic this criterion is consigned to conversion disorders and pseudocyesis because these are the only cases in which it is thought that the symptoms can be demonstrated to be inconsistent with medical pathophysiology. There is a substantial difference between these diagnostic criteria and the previous ones, since there is a break away from the classic understanding of the somatization disorder (or Briquet syndrome) belonging to hysteria and therefore of psychological causation. Thus, the possibility of a new medical disorder that has not as yet been identified is opened up.

The depersonalization disorder appears in the DSM IV among the dissociative disorders, but in the ICD 10 it is classified in a category of its own, in the section "Other neurotic disorders" together with derealization, as if they were one and the same. According to the DSM, depersonalization is defined as a "feeling of estrangement or detachment from oneself" [26], and "there can be several different types of sensory anesthesia, lack of affective response and feeling of loss of control of one's own acts" [26], while the ICD 10 speaks of the depersonalization–derealization disorder, which "generally appear[s] in the context of depressive illness, phobic disorders and obsessive-compulsive disorders" [27], with no reference to dissociative disorders, although its definition is similar to that of the DSM.

There are few references in these classifications to the number of manifestations of these disorders in one sex or another. According to Gaviria [29], this approach has been minimal in the DSM I (1952) and II (1968) and was probably due to the lack of research concerning the relation between gender and psychopathology. In the DSM III (1980) there was a slight increase in the interest in sex/gender and in the section on conversion disorder, it is said that "there is no conclusive information" [29], but that globus hystericus is apparently more frequent in women.

The DSM III-R (1987) and DSM IV continued to make some headway in this area, and this time there was information about variations in the expression and length of the disorders according to gender that was included in the section called "specific characteristics including culture, age and gender" [26].

In the DSM IV there are details about the somatization disorder "formerly known as hysteria or Briquet syndrome," [26] indicating that it rarely affects men in the United States, but the high incidence among Greeks and Puerto Ricans suggests that cultural factors can affect prevalence according to gender. Prevalence was in any case variable, between 0.2 and 2 % in women and less than 0.2 % in men, but this could be related to the fact that most doctors were male and a bias may lead him to diagnose more frequently in women. The ICD 10 also concludes that there is a greater prevalence among women, at least in some countries, without taking into account cultural factors. It does mention on the other hand, a link with attention-seeking behaviors (histrionics) [27].

There is only one reference to gender in the description of the depersonalization disorder in the DSM IV-TR, where it specifies symptoms dependent on culture, and that in groups of patients it is twice more frequent in women than in men [30].

Conversion disorders appear more frequently in women than in men, in a ratio ranging between 2:1 and 10:1, and many of these women later present with somatization disorder. In the case of men they find an association with the antisocial personality disorder, in military contexts and in accidents in the workplace [26], which could be interpreted as being based on a sociocultural bias.

Dissociative amnesia is referred to equally in both classifications as affecting men less frequently, and only in extreme cases, such as men subjected to combat stress [26, 27], which definitely is, in our opinion, another cultural bias.

With regard to the rest of the dissociative disorders, the ICD 10 makes no further mention of gender, except in passing when it mentions that young teenage girls suffer more frequently from "moderate and transient variations of dissociative disorders of voluntary motility and sensitivity" [27].

In the case of the DSM IV, there are no distinctions between gender in the rest of the dissociative disorders, with the exception of the dissociative identity disorder, which is diagnosed "three to nine times more in women than in men. . .Women tend to present more identities than men (15:8 by average)" [26].

In the DSM IV-TR (2000) a great effort was made to broaden and deepen the scope of information related to gender [29], but in our opinion, at least in terms of disorders related to dissociation, there is no additional information except that related to the depersonalization disorder.

In the recently published DSM-5 (May 2013), many new additions have been controversial [28]. In terms of the subject we are dealing with here, we have to point out that there is a different structure. The multi-axial evaluation has been dropped and there is a framework of information about age, gender, and characteristics of development of the patient throughout the text. Prior to its publication, we find in the literature critical analysis of the shortcomings to be found in these manuals in terms of the knowledge gathered about variables of age and gender in psychiatric diagnostics [31, 32].

The dissociative identity disorder appeared in a completely different light in the DSM-5 with more information being given about differences in gender, although no specific etiological explanation related to gender is provided, or any other kind. First, it is stated that the condition is more predominant among adult women, but there are no data on children. Denial of the symptoms and traumatic memories among men is postulated as commonplace, and this would account for a high number of false-negatives. Among women, acute presentations are more common (flashback, amnesias, fugues, conversion symptoms, hallucinations, or self-mutilation). Men present more violent or criminal behavior, and the triggers for acute dissociative episodes are combat, being an inmate in prison, or physical or sexual aggression [28].

With regard to dissociative amnesia, in the DSM-5 we find a brief mention of a greater predominance among women. This reference is contextualized within the USA and derived from only one "small" study [28] on the prevalence of the disorder over 12 months: 1.8 % (1 % men, 2.6 % women). Moreover, it includes dissociative fugue within this disorder as just another feature and not as a separate diagnostic entity.

This manual follows the same criterion as the ICD and labels derealization and depersonalization as one and the same disorder, but it remains in the category of dissociative disorders. It adds a prevalence of the disorder of 2 % and a ratio related to gender of 1:1, unlike previous manuals, which claimed that they did not have any information related to this.

As for somatic symptoms disorder, the DSM-5 estimates a greater prevalence than that put forward for the old somatization disorder owing to greater flexibility in the diagnostic criteria, the fact that symptoms that cannot be explained medically should not be required, and the smaller number of symptoms present. It is estimated to be between 5 and 7 %. Also, it does not specify, but it does mention a greater prevalence among women [28].

With regard to conversion disorder, the DSM-5 points to, but once again offers no explanation for, the claim that "the disorder is two to three times more common among women than in men" [28].

7.5 Female Gender in Dissociative Disorders

We start from the assumption that there seem to be differences in how psychical symptoms are perceived in men and women, although this premise could be questionable according to other variables such as social class, ethnic group or cultural environment. In our sociocultural context, women frequently present a subjective perception of lower psychical well-being, worse quality of life, and worse state of health than men and tend to use health services more often [33].

Assuming traumatic events to be factors of vulnerability and triggers of mental disorders, it is known that if these traumatic events take place during infancy, they are more serious. Thus, suffering from sexual abuse in infancy increases the risk of suffering from anxiety disorders. There is, moreover, a different response to a psychical trauma according to gender. In general, women suffer a lower number of traumatic experiences, but they are more vulnerable to them [34].

A subtype of post-traumatic stress disorder is described, which is called "dissociative," and is characterized by dissociative symptoms. Evidence comes from studies on adults and children, which include functional neuroimaging, as well as different types of trauma, including sexual and physical abuse in childhood and traumas associated with military combat. Studies estimate a prevalence of sexual abuse in childhood in this disorder as being 20 % for women and 8 % for men [35]. In a study with veteran soldiers it was found that 15 % of men and 8 % of women suffered from post-traumatic stress disorder 15 years after serving in Vietnam [36].

These international studies demonstrate that boys have a greater probability compared with girls of suffering or being threatened with physical aggression or having a friend or relative who has been assaulted [37]. They also have a greater chance of being hit by a car, getting hurt in a playground, and being witness to violent confrontations. In contrast, girls are at greater risk of sexual assault [37].

We continue to link hysteria with the female gender today. There is a widely-held belief that dissociative symptoms and disorders are predominantly found in women. Empirical studies in the general population and in different clinical trials indicate that there are no differences between genders [38]. One explanation that has been postulated to account for this apparent prevalence of dissociative disorders among women is that women resort more often to health service providers while the condition is usually identified among men in law-related environments such as prisons or forensic institutions [39]. A study in New York [40] did not find any gender differences in the distribution of dissociative disorders. There is a general belief, based on clinical observations and pointed out in the DSM-5 [28], that among clinical populations, male patients easily hide their symptoms and histories of trauma. On the other hand, Sar et al. [41] found in a Turkish study, among high performance university students, that the male students reported more traumas during childhood than the female students.

There are other explanations, determined culturally, that would explain a greater prevalence of dissociative disorders among women, as demonstrated by Wolfrad [42], in his study seeking the relation among dissociative experiences, anxiety features, and paranormal beliefs among a sample of students, in which these were more frequent among women along with higher scores in dissociative experiences. Along the same lines, Pires [43] demonstrated that there was a greater psychological impact on women than on men who have suffered a car accident, but they did not find any significant differences between gender when looking at the peritraumatic dissociation.

Other studies, the vast majority, demonstrate that there is a greater prevalence of dissociative and somatoform disorders among women. Nicolai [44] offers different explanations for these differences in the prevalence according to gender, and one is the occurrence of attachment disorder and abuse in the childhood of these women.

Zona [45] has studied longitudinally the impact of exposure to violence among city teenagers. For both sexes an increase in the number of symptoms was predicted prospectively (externalization, internalization, post-traumatic stress disorder and dissociation). The boys referred on average to greater exposure to violent situations, while the girls were more prone to suffering dissociative experiences, suggesting different specific paths dependent on gender, in terms of the specific psychopathology of the trauma.

Some of the results of the study are of special interest to clinicians who treat somatizations or other somatoform disorders without a clear medical etiology.

The Adverse Childhood Experiences (ACE) [46] in which a direct relation is found between the probability of sexual abuse in childhood and the number of medically inexplicable symptoms in adult age. Women have a 50 % greater probability of having suffered five or more categories of adverse experiences in childhood. Felitti et al. [46] consider that this is key to understanding the greater propensity women have to suffering health problems such as fibromyalgia, chronic fatigue syndrome, obesity, irritable bowel syndrome, and nonmalignant pain syndromes.

Many studies find a higher prevalence of conversion disorders among women [47], although this difference can vary according to the type of disorder. Stone et al. [48] found that the proportion of women was lower in cases of psychogenic weakness syndromes than in cases of epileptic pseudocrises.

Non-epileptic psychogenic crises are recognized in all studies as being more prevalent in women than in men [49, 50], which seems to be consistent with a greater prevalence in conversion disorders as well, and both are included among somatoform disorders in the DSM.

Against a hypothesis explaining this prevalence of conversion disorders in women that would focus on cultural differences, we refer to the comparative study by Cubo et al. [51], who finds a higher prevalence of psychogenic movement disorders among women in different healthcare settings in the USA and in Spain.

Conclusions

Dissociative symptoms are present in different psychiatric disorders, if current diagnostic classifications such as the recent DSM or ICD-10 are used as a yardstick. In order to understand the psychopathology of dissociative symptoms, it is important to know in what cultural–historical context the concept of dissociation was born, and what paths its evolution has followed throughout the history of psychiatry. Down through the years, other related concepts have appeared to have been coined by different authors, among them Jean Charcot or Sigmund Freud.

Different psychological theories have tried to explain somatic and psychogenic symptoms, those whose medical etiology is unknown, and links to hysteria and its phenomenology have been discussed. All of this has culminated in a considerable amount of confusion when it comes to concepts and terminology that we have tried to clarify, insofar as that is possible. From Pierre Janet and his *desagrégation psychologique*, to Sigmund Freud and his conversion, or the somatization disorder described in the DSM IV, there is a descriptive psychopathology that is constantly changing. This conceptual foundation has been addressed in the latest diagnostic manuals, but unfortunately they only add a new dimension to the confusion.

Dissociation has always been related to hysteria and hysteria with women. We have tried to find the cultural and historical basis accounting for this prevalence in the nineteenth century, which is when the concept was born, and remind our readers of the medical references to male hysteria described at the time, now for the most part forgotten, but that were an important part of Charcot's casuistry and his description of traumatic hysteria. Split personality or demonic possession was a condition in no way exclusive to women, and these are clearly considered to be dissociative disorders in modern day psychopathology.

Epidemiological studies indicate that there is a prevalence of conversion disorders among women, but dissociative disorders do not seem to be appearing in the same numbers, and findings are more controversial. There is no explanation as yet for this statistical difference, and it is possible that there may be a reason, dependent on gender psychopathology, accounting for the greater prevalence of somatoform disorders among women. This leads us to the conclusion that further studies are required and that more interest in the field of mental health care for women is desirable. We need to incorporate gender perspective if we want to achieve quality science.

References

1. Gastó C. Psicopatología de la conciencia. In: Ruiloba JV, editors. Introducción a la psicopatología y la psiquiatría. 6ª Edición. Barcelona: Masson; 2006. p. 129–43.
2. Spiegel D, Loewenstein RJ, Lewis-Fernández R, Sar V, Simeon D, Vermetten E, et al. Dissociative disorders in DSM-5. Depress Anxiety. 2011;28(9):824–52.
3. American Psychiatric Association. Manual diagnóstico y estadístico de los trastornos mentales, texto revisado. Primera edición. Barcelona: Masson; 2002.
4. Janet P. L'Automatisme psychologique. 1ª Reimpresión. París: Odile Jacob; 1989.
5. Ellenberger H. El descubrimiento del inconsciente. 1ª Reimoresión. Madrid: Gredos; 1976.
6. Rojo A. El concepto dissociation en el fin-de-siècle: P. Janet y S. Freud [Tesis doctoral]. Madrid: Universidad Complutense; 2005.
7. Ellert R, Nijenhuis S. Somatoform dissociation: major symptoms of dissociative disorders. Journal of trauma and dissociation. 2000;1(4):7–32.
8. Ortega C. Las mujeres y la enfermedad mental. Una perspectiva de género a través de la historia contemporánea. Revista de historia y pensamiento de género. 2011;1(4):208–23.
9. Plumed J. La etiología de la locura en el siglo XIX a través de la psiquiatría española. Frenia. 2004;4(2):69–91.
10. Rojo A. El cuerpo disociado. In: Fuentenebro F, Rojo A, Valiente C, editors. Psicopatología y fenomenología de la corporalidad. Vigo: Feito SL; 2005. p. 119–37.
11. Janet P. Névroses et idées fixes, vol. 1. 4th ed. París: Société Pierre Janet; 1990.
12. Postel J, Quétel C (comps). Historia de la psiquiatría. 1ªReimp. México: Fondo de cultura económica; 1993.
13. Bolzinger A. Freud et les parisiens. París: Campagne première; 2002.
14. Hacking I. L'âme réécrite. Étude sur la personnalité multiple et les sciences de la mémoire. Le Plessis Robinson: Institut Synthélabo pour le progrès de la connaissance; 1998.

15. Charcot JM. Lecciones sobre la histeria traumática. Pereña F, Desviat M (comps). Madrid: Nieva; 1989.
16. Janet P. L'état mental des hystériques. 1ª Reimpresión. Marseille: Laffitte Reprints; 1983.
17. López JMª, Morales JMª. Neurosis y psicoterapia. Madrid: Espasa-Calpe; 1970.
18. Cagigas A. Charcot y las lecciones del martes. In: Charcot JM, editor. Histeria. Jaén: Del lunar; 2003. p. 7–12.
19. Thoret Y, Giraud AC, Ducerf B. La dissociation hystérique dans les texts de Janet et Freud avant 1911. Evol Psychiatr. 1999;64(4):749–64.
20. Freud S. Sobre la teoría del ataque histérico. In: Freud S, editor. Obras completas, vol. 1. Buenos Aires: Amorrortu; 1982. p. 187–90.
21. Freud S. Sobre el mecanismo psíquico de fenómenos histéricos: comunicación preliminar. In: Freud S, editor. Obras completas, vol. 2. Buenos Aires: Amorrortu; 1999. p. 27–44.
22. Freud S. Las neuropsicosis de defensa. In: Freud S, editor. Obras completas. 2nd ed., vol. 1. Madrid: Biblioteca Nueva; 2001. p. 169–77.
23. Pérez S, Galdón J. Los fenómenos disociativos: una revisión conceptual. Rev Psicop Psicol Clin. 2003;8(2):85–108.
24. Garrabé J. La taxonomie actuelle des troubles dissociatifs. Évol Psychiatr. 1999;64(4):717–26.
25. Nijenhuis ERS. Somatoform dissociation: phenomena, measurement, and theoretical issues. New York: Norton & Company; 2004.
26. López Ibor JJ, editor. DSM-IV. Manual diagnóstico y estadístico de los trastornos mentales. Barcelona: Masson; 1995.
27. López Ibor JJ, editor. CIE 10. Décima revisión de la clasificación internacional de las enfermedades. Trastornos mentales y del comportamiento. Descripciones clínicas y pautas para el diagnóstico. Madrid: Meditor; 1992.
28. American Psychiatric Association. Diagnostic and statistical manual of mental, DSM V. 5th ed. Arlington, VA: American Psychiatric Association; 2013.
29. Gaviria SL, Alarcón RD. Psicopatología y género: visión longitudinal e histórica a través del DSM. Rev Colomb Psiquiat. 2010;39(2):389–404.
30. López Ibor JJ. DSM-IV-TR. Manual diagnóstico y estadístico de los trastornos mentales. Barcelona: Masson; 2002.
31. Narrow WE. DSM-V: consideraciones sobre la edad y el género en el diagnóstico psiquiátrico. Barcelona: Masson; 2009.
32. Johnson J, Steward DE. DSM-V: toward a sensitive approach to psychiatric diagnosis. Arch Womens Ment Health. 2010;13(1):17–9.
33. Ezquiaga E. Aspectos diferenciales en los trastornos de ansiedad. In: Saiz J, director. Salud mental y género en la práctica clínica. Madrid: Ars Medica; 2007. p. 59–78.
34. Punamaki RL, Komproe IH, Qouta S, Elmasri M, De Jong JTVM. The role of peritraumatic dissociation and gender in the association between trauma and mental health in a Palestinian community sample. Am J Psychiatry. 2005;162:545–51.
35. Pereda N, Guilera G, Forns M, Gómez BJ. The prevalence of child sexual abuse in community and student samples: a meta-analysis. J Clin Psychol Rev. 2009;29(4):328–38.
36. Schelemger WE, Kulka RA, Fairbank JA, Hough RL, Jordan BK, Marmar CR, et al. The prevalence of post-traumatic stress disorder in the Vietnam generation: a multimethod, multisource assessment of psychiatric disorder. J Trauma Stress. 1992;5(3):333–63.
37. Karestan CK, Roberts AL, Stone DM, Dunn EC. The epidemiology of early childhood trauma. In: Lanius RA, Vermetten E, Pain C, editors. The impact of early life trauma on health and disease. The hidden epidemic. 5th ed. Cambridge: Cambridge University Press; 2013. p. 13–24.
38. Spitzer C. Gender differences in dissociation. A dimensional approach. Psychopathology. 2003;36(2):65–70.
39. Spitzer C, Freyberger HJ. Gender differences in dissociative disorders. Bundesgesundheitsbla. 2008;51(1):46–52.

40. Johnson JG, Cohen P, Kasen S, Brook JS. Dissociative disorders among adults in the community, impaired functioning, and axis I and II comorbidity. J Psychiatr Res. 2006;40 (2):131–40.
41. Sar V, Gamze A, Kugu N, Ozturk E, Ertem-Vehid H, Axis I. Dissociative disorder comorbidity in borderline personality disorder and reports of childhood trauma. J Clin Psychiatr. 2006;67:1583–90.
42. Wolfrad U. Dissociative experiences, trait anxiety and paranormal beliefs. Pers Individ Dif. 1997;23(1):15–9.
43. Pires TSF. Are men more resilient than women after a road traffic accident? Psychol Health. 2012;27(1):104–5.
44. Nicolai NJ. Chronic stress, sex and gender. Tijdschr Psychiatr. 2009;51(8):569–77.
45. Zona K. Gender differences in the longitudinal impact of exposure to violence on mental health in urban youth. J Youth Adolesc. 2011;40(12):1674–90.
46. Felitti VJ, Anda RF. The relationship of adverse childhood experiences to adult medical disease, psychiatric disorders and sexual behavior: implications for healthcare. In: Lanius RA, Vermetten E, Pain C, editors. The impact of early life trauma on health and disease. The hidden epidemic. 5th ed. Cambridge: Cambridge University Press; 2013. p. 77–87.
47. Carson A, Stone J, Hibberd C, Murray G, Duncan R, Coleman R, et al. Disability, distress and unemployment in neurology outpatients with symptoms "unexplained by organic disease". J Neurol Neurosurg Psychiatry. 2011;82(7):810–3.
48. Stone J, Sharpe M, Binzer M. Motor conversion symptoms and pseudoseizures: a comparison of clinical characteristics. Psychosomatics. 2004;45(6):492–9.
49. Reuber M, Elger CE. Psychogenic nonepileptic seizures: review and update. Epilepsy Behav. 2003;4(3):205–16.
50. Reuber M, Pukrop R, Bauer J, Helmstaedter C, Tessendorf N, Elger CE. Outcome in psychogenic nonepileptic seizures: 1 to 10-year follow-up in 164 patients. Ann Neurol. 2003;53 (3):305–11.
51. Cubo E, Hinson VK, Goetz CG, García Ruiz P, García de Yebenes J, Marti MJ, et al. Transcultural comparison of psychogenic movement disorders. Mov Disord. 2005;20 (10):1343–5.

Corporality and Trauma

8

Paloma Navarro and Inmaculada Hurtado

The hands want to see, the eyes want to caress.
[Sehe mit fühlendem Aug', fühle mit sehender Hand.]
Goethe

Abstract
In trauma, silence is broken in giving way to the lived body, but aspects related to corporality as the most frequently lived experience of the traumatic event are not always included. In this chapter we review the different dimensions of the suffering and emergence of trauma in holistic, gender-sensitive, and integrated ways. The body is the epicenter of trauma in its individual experience, impact on identity, and excruciating remembrance of the event. Yet sociopolitical contexts and their ruptures also inhabit the human body: violence, poverty, abuse, and oppression. Thus, understanding trauma requires giving specific attention to the sociocultural fabric in which the wound is inscribed and suffered. It means reviewing integrating models in which the diverse dimensions of suffering are considered, gathering the much-heralded but less frequently performed psychosocial approach to health. In the first part of this article we approach the sociocultural elements surrounding the experience of trauma, without detaching corporeality and its gendered embodied reality. In the second part of this article we approach the concept of trauma from a humanist perspective around the extensive disruption that occurs in identity and in corporeality. The psychopathological conditions that may emerge after a traumatic event are many and varied; even though we do not attempt to cover them all, we provide an approach to two of the expressions more frequently affected by gender: somatization and self-harm.

P. Navarro (✉)
Department of Psychiatry, Marina Baixa Hospital, Alicante, Spain
e-mail: palomacnavarro@medicos.com

I. Hurtado
CEU, Cardenal Herrera University, Alicante, Spain

M. Sáenz-Herrero (ed.), *Psychopathology in Women*,
DOI 10.1007/978-3-319-05870-2_8

8.1 Introduction

The concept of trauma has been ubiquitously defined throughout human history. Body images have been deconstructed and reconstructed over the course of centuries. In our social and political moment, the ongoing debate on the concept of psychic trauma is still in force, and the notion has been changing with the international classifications in the *Diagnostic and Statistical Manual of Mental Disorders* (DSM) and the International Classification of Diseases (ICD) throughout its editions and revisions. To date, there is no universally accepted definition of trauma.

The body is often referred to as a *thing* intersected by society, biology, subjectivity, history, etc. Etymologically, the notion of intersection takes us to cut, to node, to section, to sword. The act of intersection as a concept about the body pierces its image of inscrutability. The body penetrated by trauma is no longer a mere bearer of signs and symptoms; instead, it is be able to capture sense and create meanings to be integrated into its identity. In phenomenology, the corporeality is the lived and living body: "The world is not what I think but what I live through" [1].

Nevertheless, in Western societies, the body has been and is undervalued against pureness and overvalued reason but still does not give way to "*Je sens, je pense en dedans de moi*." Excessive expressiveness and body movements are left in the powerful hands of oblivion and symptoms become central. The body is extremely hierarchized in our culture as an image, a flat image that ceased to be volume to become a glowing silhouette highlighted on the screen, but with no subjective lived events. In trauma, silence is broken in giving way to the lived body. In the diverse contributions to the concept of trauma, aspects related to corporality as the most frequently lived experience of the traumatic event are not always included.

Following the biopsychosocial model, we know that diverse environmental and sociocultural aspects are risk factors in psychopathology and that they manifest complex interactions with neurobiological elements, which are directly connected to gender. In trauma, this panorama is maximized and sociocultural factors such as the absence of social support and the family's exposure to violence are, in this context, determining. Thus, women are more likely to be exposed to some harmful environmental aspects causing the development of the disorder (sexual abuse), whereas men are more likely to be exposed to other factors (physical abuse).

In this article we review the different dimensions of the suffering and emergence of trauma in holistic, gender-sensitive, and integrated ways. The body is the epicenter of trauma in its individual experience, impact on identity, and excruciating remembrance of the event. Yet sociopolitical contexts and their ruptures also inhabit human body: violence, poverty, abuse, and oppression. Thus, understanding trauma requires giving specific attention to the sociocultural fabric in which the wound is inscribed and suffered. It means reviewing integrating models in which the diverse dimensions of suffering are considered, gathering the much heralded but less frequently performed psychosocial approach to health [2]. In the first part of this article we approach the sociocultural elements surrounding the experience of trauma without detaching corporality and its gendered embodied reality.

In the second part we approach the concept of trauma from a humanist perspective around the extensive disruption that occurs in identity and in corporeality. The psychopathological conditions that may emerge after a traumatic event are many and varied; even though we do not attempt to cover them all, we provide an approach to two forms of expression most affected by gender: somatization and self-harm. In parallel, these two expressions are closely related to early sexual abuse, a particular form of psychic trauma. Patients with borderline personality disorder are likely to embody most of those frustrated and blurred identities, those bodies acting as abnormal or altered. The emergence of these clinic cases at this particular time clearly shows a close link between social and cultural factors, which hinge on gender.

8.2 Trauma in Contexts

Following what Bryan Turner [3] calls the context of "emergence of the body," different schools of thought in the social sciences have shifted toward a new model of understanding, the starting point thereof being the bodily experience. In this same light, bodily processes are construed as the core where the complexity of personal, sociocultural, and political reality is articulated. This paradigm shift seeks the disruption of the main western dualisms: nature/culture, mind/body, objective/subjective, passive/active, rational/emotional, etc. [4], since they are now obsolete and consequently inefficient at explaining human experience. Thus, this task requires new languages and narratives to rearticulate what has been split off.

The concept of embodiment allows us to illuminate a more complex understanding of the body. This concept is aimed at transcending the idea that the social is inscribed in the body to talk about corporality as a substantial process underlying its potential, intentional, intersubjective, active, and relational interaction [5]. Nancy Scheper-Hughes and Margaret Lock [6], for their part, respond to the dichotomies mind/body, individual/society, and their effects on the method of configuring health and care, with three perspectives from which the body may be observed: first, the individual body, in a phenomenological sense, as a lived experience of the self; second, the social body as cognitive mapping to represent relations with the natural, the supernatural, the social, and the spatial; and, finally, the political body as an apparatus for social and political control. Body politics constitute the different ways of controlling and disciplining the body—with torture or with more sophisticated maneuvers—which are masked in different socio-political systems and from which we can explain the structural violence with regard to gender.

The term *psychosomatic* has been criticized for setting both a semantic and a methodological dualism in the explanation of pain. In psychosomatic explanations there is a causal link between a psychic and a physical event, with a great correspondence between the royal and the vicarious, and may lead to victim blaming by lumping the failure of therapy together with their alleged mental health problems [7]. Scheper-Hughes and Lock [6] propose the category *mindful body*, understanding the body as a conscious agent, a more holistic approach in which emotions articulate the body, the mind, the individual, society, and the political body:

> Sickness is not just an isolated event, nor an unfortunate brush with nature. It is a form of communication—the language of the organs—through which nature, society, and culture speak simultaneously. The individual body should be seen as the most immediate, the proximate terrain where social truths and social contradictions are played out, as well as a locus of personal and social resistance, creativity, and struggle (p 31).

These authors suggest that many of the subordinated corporal practices related to social suffering or illness carry a *message in a bottle*, a message of resistance and protest that needs to be decoded [8]. The experience of trauma frequently means, in Janzen's terms: "the recurrence of the signs of symptoms of trauma" [9]. It is the body language that emerges in memory (visions, sounds, tactile sensations) recalling the traumatic event. It is also a metaphor of pain as a burden, an inner chaos, an out-of-order engine, an explosion or weariness as energy resource consumption. Or the metaphors: with a heavy heart, with a lump in the throat, with a feeling in the pit of the stomach. The bodily conscience is intersected by the suffering memory; yet, deciphering the materiality of the intangible involves developing our capacity to listen to the bodily expression in which the physical and emotional are indissoluble.

8.3 Identity Intersections

Addressing corporality in the common experience of trauma presupposes a consideration of the gendered dimension of our experience. The sudden shock in a traumatic event and the resultant narrative disruption do not cause a shifting, nor do they override gender; they rather structure common experience. These identity coordinates are analytical tools that enable us to better understand subjectivity and suffering, particularly in women. It is not that women need footnotes or chapters that are different from the *human*, but rather "both from an epistemological perspective as well as in biomedical practice, the 'normality' pattern has been and continues to be the hegemonic masculinity" ([10], p. 42).

Gender inequality is not determined by biological facts. This is the reason why gender perspective neither concludes nor is limited to a gender breakdown in the statistics for psychic distress prevalence and incidence. It is not about searching, describing, and confirming differences between sexes, but rather explaining such differences. Gender is relational and dynamic, a structure of relations that are continually interacting. Thus, gender perspective implies considerations that go beyond the *mystic of numbers* and the essentialist constructions on sexual characteristics of each sex, in order to contextualize data within a well-defined social framework [11].

In fact, feminist authors denounce the fact that the complexity of traumatic experiences of women has not been considered by the prominent model for trauma in a society divided by gender [12, 13]. Other contributions from this same perspective include: the incorporation of some groups neglected by the first diagnosis of PTSD, such as women and children who are survivors of sexual abuse [14], the reformulation of key concepts such as *coping strategies* instead of *symptoms* [15], and the warning that gender violence is a disproportionate everyday occurrence, not only in the context of war but also in peace [11, 16].

Suffering intersects with gender, age, ethnicity, disability, beliefs, economic status, and other global processes affecting local environments. In other words, there is not a single way to suffer and the expression and perception of pain are different, even within members of the same community [17]. Nevertheless, the due consideration to particular contexts with their own cultural and identity settings, their own sources of domination and inequality, enables us to broaden our perspective and in doing so, to better understand the traumatic event, the consequent grief and process of recovery where they unfold. As Janzen reminds us: "[. . .] although war trauma certainly has physical consequences and imprints, it is culturally mediated and that is where its character, causes, consequences and avenues of resolutions may be best understood" ([9], p. 44).

8.4 Violence, Experience, and Care

There are numerous works and studies on trauma, but not so many mainstream ones that have a gender perspective in their design, not so many try to explain the psychological distress and its care in relation to the position women and men have in each society. In particular, I believe that an approach to trauma from this perspective needs to look into these factors, among others: sexual triggers for trauma, diversity in experience, dealing with suffering and expressing suffering, and analytical and health intervention models. Following this approach, in this section, I try to cover research and contributions showing the relevance of gender in violence, experience, and trauma care.

8.4.1 Violence

Certain groups are more likely to be exposed to violence, and consequently, exposed to painful and traumatic experiences [18]. The fact that the main threats to individuals and communities are inscribed in some specific areas and territories proves that violence is not fortuitously distributed. Marginalized populations living in poverty, violence against women, racism, homophobia, and other forms of oppression underline this. As a matter of fact, the proposition maintained in the model of PTSD, which claims that the world is a safe place until exposed to a traumatic event, has been questioned. According to Burstow [15], this could be true for a white, middle-class, straight man, given that trauma is not a neutral but a political experience.

Following the Galtung conflict triangle [19], there are three subtypes of violence. First, direct violence is visible and clear, given that this type of violence is behavioral. Second, structural violence results from an unequal access to resources, material or otherwise, such as education, health, peace, and consequently, power and opportunities. Lastly, cultural violence refers to those aspects of violence that may be used to justify or legitimize direct or structural violence. Gender violence has its roots in culture—in fact, one of the senses of the word *violence* in Spanish, *violencia,* is "the act of raping a woman" (DRAE)—and in terms of its consequences it emerges both direct and structurally. To illustrate this, there are supporting data: 1,161 violations of women are reported every year (Ministerio del Interior, Spain 2011), which means three a day; one every 8 h. Thus, structural violence, as Bourdieu [20] reminds us, is always perpetrated in countless small and great acts of everyday violence, which in most cases continue with impunity.

In the case of internal armed conflict, although they affect the whole population, there is evidence of gender dimension regarding grades of violence and suffering. While men are exposed to the risk of torture and mass killing, women are more likely to be victims of sexual violence and other types of violence, a violence that does not cease when conflicts officially end. Amnesty International (2001) denounced that violence against women is not incidental in war; yet, a weapon deliberately used for different purposes, such as the spread of terror, the destabilization of society, or as a means of rewarding soldiers and extracting information. Such violence includes different assaults of a sexual nature: rape and gang rape, sexual abuse, slavery, mutilation, forced impregnation, and prostitution. In the gruesomeness of war the way the logics of terror operate is made invisible. In fact, the broadcasting of numerous cases of rape and forced pregnancy in Rwanda and the former Yugoslavia drew international attention to the magnitude of this form of cruelty against women in armed conflict.

In her work on the Haitian repression during and after the *coup d'état* in 1991, Erica Caple James [21] examines the influence of gender and its psychosocial aftereffects. In this conflict, women were targeted on account of their active role in politics as well as their small-scale business role. They were also punished on behalf of their husbands, fathers, and brothers, deemed surrogate wives, and taken as "sacrificial substitutes." Their vulnerability to the attacks of different military groups flowed from the responsibilities toward their children and their business activities in local markets, which kept them visible and reachable. The different forms of torture were not only aimed at the delegitimization and bodily disempowerment through pain, but also at destroying the production and reproduction of the victim, breaking social ties with the family and community through the violation of social norms.

Broadly, the after effects of the traumatic event were: embarrassment, humiliation, social isolation from the family and community. Raped women were frequently abandoned—labeled "the rapist's wives"—by their partners and families. Alienated from their social group, they moved to other areas to rebuild and restore their lives, and in most cases their only resource for their survival was the reappropriation of their sexuality as a means of making a living. In male victims of violence, the feelings of shame and humiliation were rooted in their incapacity to protect their families and in the degrading treatment and torture. When working in therapy groups, men's narratives on trauma touched on the loss of property, livestock, and social status. The lack of economic power and the failure to meet societal expectancies forced them to abandon their partners and families, leaving women and children in even more vulnerable conditions.

8.4.2 Experiences

Conception, construction, manifestation, symbolization, and management of suffering are also intersected by gender. As stated by Ana Távora [22], in some determined conflicts, the existing relations between perception and resolution and the mental distress or mental wellbeing of women is determined by the position the dominant system grants them—subordination. In other words, women's distress is framed in a social psychopathology issue.

Inequality between men and women is intertwined by coercive elements, which are eminently corporal, and result in internalized relational models integrated into our subjectivity. According to the author, femininity provides us with such an identity that is centered in a being to be perceived, observed in a continuous state of bodily insecurity and symbolic alienation. In this identity, appearance has a fundamental value. Adolescent women, when bodily changes begin and secondary sexual characteristics appear, face their sexuality not through an encounter with their bodies, but by being mentally undressed by the other [23]. This is what Basaglia [24] calls "being-for" and "being in the being-of-others," which defines a socialization environment for women reinforcing the importance of attachment and the emotional. Following Rosaldo [25] (p. 44), to this we can add: "It now appears to me that woman's place in human social life is not in any direct sense a product of the things she does, but of the meaning her activities acquire through concrete social interaction."

From a bodily experience, women tend to represent their bodies through instrumentality, dissociation, and tension. The body is an instrument, an object with which to perform social, reproductive, and productive functions. In addition, motherhood is the core around which most women build their identities. Motherhood and bodily reality are the constitutive elements of a dissociated reality where sexuality and sensuality coexist in tension [26]. In the same way, Carole Vance [27] narrates the tension produced in the experience of sexuality as a sphere of exploration, pleasure, and performance, yet also how this experience can lead in turn, to helplessness, repression, and risk of sexual violence.

Narratives with their own emphases, (in)consistencies, silence and oblivion are connected to the possibilities of the enunciation of women and the social impact of their experiences. Silences are pervaded by fear, embarrassment, and in the social sense, women stop talking. María Jesús Soriano [28] states that the proportion of sexually assaulted girls is 10 % higher compared with boys. It follows that, in the case of girls, most of the time, the assailant is someone in their immediate environment, and in 70 % of the cases the assailant is a close relative, while in boys it is usually a stranger. This fact allows boys to defend themselves, run, hate or despise the assailant as a means of protection akin to war situations where the enemy is perfectly defined. When there is an attachment, kinship or friendship relation between the assailant and the victim, as happens with girls, if is almost impossible for her to defend herself. Silence reflects how gender-based stereotypes work. Kurvet-Käosaar [29] illustrates this fact in his work on autobiographies by Baltic women during the Stalinist regime. He addresses the difficulties in reporting, giving testimony, considering their limits of self-representation, particularly with socially taboo issues, such as sexual violence.

With regard to words, as stated by Bertaux-Wiame [30], there are differences both in the way in which women and men narrate and in the signification of the narration. Women recall the events in a different way and in more detail, they bind the act of narration to their social experience (family and community networks); thus, they tend to narrate about others [31]. They express feelings and conceive fear from everydayness, thereby granting the testimony a special meaning. This is justified by the fact that *time* in most women is organized according to reproductive events and a different learning process for the emotional [31].

When women speak, they not only do so through words. The work of Kimberly Theidon [32] shows the great variety in response to traumatic experiences and stressful events. In her research on women who had been sexually assaulted and raped by the government forces in Ayacucho (Peru) during the internal war that shook the country, several women asked her: "Why should we remember everything that happened? To martyr our bodies—nothing more?" In these communities, the language of memory is corporal and women carry the burden of pain and suffering in their communities. This research describes the belief that sorrow can be transferred to the child through breast milk. With the term *la teta asustada* (the frightened teat), the researcher sought a way of capturing how the powerful negative emotions alter the body itself and how through blood in utero and breast milk (*the milk of sorrow and worry*) they could transmit this sorrow to their babies. In this division of emotional labor, women embody history [33].

According to Cyrulnik [34], two shocks are required to cause trauma: "a shock in reality (damage, humiliation, loss) and a shock in the representation of reality, that is, in what others say about the person after the assault." Sabine Dardenne, kidnapped in 1996 by a pedophile, stated that she later wrote her story as a means of retrieving her story from under the media spotlight, to express her pain, to put it out there, and to prevent judges from granting shorter sentences for good conduct to pedophiles [34]. Other women, such as the Grandmothers of the Plaza de Mayo continue with demonstrations as a reminder, for social recognition, and for state reparation.

8.4.3 Trauma and Care

The acknowledgement of sociocultural factors is determining the way in which the problem may be seen and nested, and consequently determines the subsequent approach [35]. Thus, these studies provide sex-disaggregated reference data, but the aim in this data collection should be to further elucidate what elements determine such outcomes. Eliana Suárez [36] compiles and questions some of these statements. For instance, several studies suggest that women might be more likely to suffer PSTD than men. One may wonder to what extent these data can be related to differences between women and men in an emotional and biological response to interpersonal traumatic events, or rather consider that such data is mapping the high incidence of gender-based violence. Some other issues must still be addressed, such as the possible overrepresentation of women in the diagnosis of PSTD owing to the gender differences in care seeking behavior after exposure to a traumatic event. At the same time, one may consider that gender intersection with factors such as disability, poverty, discrimination, and ethnicity could be the triggering cause for the greater vulnerability of women to PSTD.

Being sick or suffering is not enough to be cared for or assisted. It has to be socially accepted that the person needs to be cared for. The decision whether to give care or not is based on the societal expectancies in the group and the case given. The decision to care for and assist depends on global criteria through which communities construct the situation based on their past experience, their collective appropriation thereof, and the resources available to them [37].

The hegemonic masculinity model [38] constitutes a hindrance in men's health given that, because of their different way of configuring, dealing with, and solving their health issues, it blocks access to care services. Men have been socialized to be active, be in control, be defensive, be strong, look after themselves, endure pain, use their body as a tool, never ask for help, and cope. This is a model that encourages self-sufficiency, recklessness, competitiveness or omnipotence. It also requires undergoing certain testing to prove that they are on their way to manhood. The predominance of mainstream male education reinforces the idea that care and self-care are feminine; while values such as strength, courage, and boldness are considered masculine. The accident rate and the disproportionate prevalence of men in the suicide rate illustrate this hypothesis [39].

Furthermore, the predominance of a cultural ideology based on "the feminine as the vulnerable" has contributed to reinforcement of such a way of looking at and deeming women's body and health [11]. Sometimes this social construction implies that men's complaints are taken more seriously, while in the case of women there is a tendency to look for psychosomatic explanations for their complaints [10]. Moreover, as stated by Sau [40], in most cases traditional psychotherapies had not only failed to provide suitable answers to women affected by gender violence, but they had also reinforced misogynist myths, and therefore, condemned women to solitude and despair, when these women paradoxically turned to psychotherapy to obtain relief [40].

Complex phenomena need to be observed and constructed in a transdisciplinary, integrated way, taking into account the dialectical relationship underlying in the diverse constitutive dimensions of humanity (biological, psychological, social, cultural, etc.). The intended outcome of such a framework is an approach to the social context in the traumatic event, providing a more comprehensive vision of individual and social pain. A historical overview shows us how the trauma paradigm has been directly linked to social movements such us pacifism and women's rights movement. Therefore, one of the current challenges is to consider the elements that have been sidelined and engage in social justice underlying the traumatic events.

8.5 Concept of Trauma

The concept of trauma relies upon the consideration of trauma as an experience that is seen as unbearable within a given cognitive system. The unbearableness challenges the subject's relational world as it challenges the identity of the self-in-relation [41]. There are different itineraries for approaching traumatic pathology, but not all of them consider the corporal dimension.

The Euro-American psychiatry paradigm on post-traumatic stress disorder (PTSD) needs to be reviewed. Not all the traumatic events cause a similar impact nor are they associated with the same symbolic significance. Thus, trauma responding to extreme experiences is hardly classified in the PTSD diagnosis in that the trauma will have devastating consequences on the psyche, on the corporal experience, and as a result, on the being-in-the-world.

Judith Herman defines these disorders in 1992 as DESNOS (disorders of extreme stress not otherwise specified) or complex PTSD. In this way, the PTSD in its definition of consequence of a traumatic event is distinguished from the chronic trauma associated with extreme horror, such as prolonged domestic violence.

The introduction of this framework expanded the diagnostic criteria with the intention of demonstrating the profound transformation of the personality experienced by persons exposed to this extreme trauma. Although not conceptualized in the DSM, there is a similar category in the ICD-10: *enduring personality change after catastrophic experience*.

Thus, among the symptoms included, there is a broad range of bodily symptomatology (not present in PSTD), such as diverse forms of somatization (chronic pain, digestive, conversive, sexual, and cardiopulmonary symptoms), and an alteration of the affects and impulses, which implies, inter alia, self-destructive behaviors. In many cases the patients experience continued headache, heartburn, and urinary infections [42].

The PTSD is defined as exposure to a traumatic event leading to re-experiencing symptoms (corresponding to the reliving of the traumatic event: images, thoughts, dreams, etc.), avoidance behaviors, increased arousal in the forms of irritability, hypervigilance, concentration problems, etc. However, the DSM-IV lacks a broader definition of the types of trauma; thus, any event resulting in "death or threats to life and limb" was included. The DSM-5 [43] clarifies that a traumatic event may entail threats or death, serious injury or sexual violence. This is the first time that sexual violence seems to be specifically acknowledged as a traumatic event.

A lot has been written about the definition of trauma in its two essential components: as an extreme striking event and as the human response to that event. The DSM-IV required a response accompanied by intense fear, helplessness or horror, not accepting the exposure to a traumatic event as a cause of the disorder.

This has indeed been considered an advance among supporters of the consideration of the subjective response to trauma as equally important in the diagnosis, setting aside the merely situational.

Nevertheless, regarding the diagnostic criteria in the DSM-5, the criterion A2 involving "intense fear, helplessness or horror" has proved to have little utility in the diagnosis and it has been eliminated. The authors point out that the response to trauma, apart from terror or fear, may include dysphoric mood, anhedonia, negative thinking, dissociative symptoms, etc. The variability of human behaviors and expressions of distress were reasons for dropping the A2 criterion from trauma definition.

There remains strong controversy on this subject, given that it has been demonstrated that in traumatic events involving physical integrity such as armed or unarmed rape, the self-perception of menace is the best predictor of PTSD symptoms [44]. Although the incidence of traumatic events is higher in men, studies have demonstrated that women are at double the risk of developing PTSD [45].

From a purely phenomenologist perspective, some reflection might be had as to the consideration in PTSD diagnosis of the multiplicity of the human response to trauma and its heart-rending experience, and the bodily experience in the traumatic event [46]. In the following excerpt by the Auschwitz survivor Jean Améry (1912–1978), we approach the most humane regard of a violence and torture victim. The body, as an intimate territory, is penetrated by the monstrous, the vile, and the evil. The lived body is the fuel for the visibility of a soul tormented to suicide.

Améry, despite having declared: "if being Jewish involves cultural heritage and religious bonds, I have never been one and will never be" was arrested and deported by the Germans:

> The real horror began, however, when the SS took over the administration of the camps. The old spontaneous bestiality gave way to an absolutely cold and systematic destruction of human bodies, calculated to destroy human dignity; health was avoided or postponed indefinitely. (. . .) I must confess that I don't know exactly what that is: human dignity (. . .). Yet I am certain that with the very first blow that descends on him he loses something we will perhaps temporarily call 'trust in the world.' (. . .) But more important as an element of trust in the world, and in our context what is solely relevant, is the certainty that by reason of written or unwritten social contracts the other person will spare me—more precisely stated, that he will respect my physical, and with it my metaphysical, being. (. . .) It is like a rape, a sexual act without the consent of one of the two partners. Certainly, if there is even a minimal prospect of successful resistance, a mechanism is set in motion (. . .) the border violation of my self by the other, which can be neither neutralized by the expectation of help nor rectified through resistance.

This extract underlines some nuclear criteria in the traumatic event being an experience penetrating the body in full: completed rape, frequently linked to extreme emotions, experience of chaos, confusion during the event, memory breakup, absurdity, horror, ambivalence, disconcert, humiliation, despair, loss of control, and helplessness. This delineates the bodily experience through alienation and limit invasion. In fact, the force inflicting physical pain tends to chain victims to their bodies. This tight spatial and temporal control of the body tends to destroy the bodily self-experience in relation to the world in freedom: "Nowhere in the world does reality have such a massive force as in the camp, in any other place is so powerfully real" [47].

8.6 Identity and Corporality: Providing a Framework for Situations of Violence and Trauma

Identity is the sense of self and oneself in the world. Namely, it is the self-image in each context, as there is not only one self defining the person, but multiple selves in coexistence [46]. Thus, we understand that human bodies are recognized in diverse identities/selves in the world in which they live and coexist [48].

However, human beings develop the sense of being one—the sense of self—through the construction of a unique narrative identity. An identity that, while experienced as unique, encapsulates the idea of permanence and change: projection into the future and recognition in the past [41].

Throughout history we are reminded that the sense of self is first and foremost a bodily/corporal sense, experienced not through language, but rather through body motion and sensation [49–51]. This experience of the somatosensory initial corporality eventually forms a narrative self, a sense of conscious versus the emptiness of inconsistency, a self-representation of the being in a dialectical relational process from birth, joint and reciprocal with the attachment relations, which construct and regulate identity.

The theory of attachment has many links with psychoanalytic theory, as it also delves into children's response to trauma in its origin, the body being the first vehicle of identity.

As Humphrey stated "the most interesting thing always happens at the boundaries." The body itself constitutes a limit, a boundary, and a frontier. From the early years of life we come into contact with the world through our skin, which becomes fragmented and altered almost continuously, but also enables us to start to create bonds. The skin, as a porous substrate, in fusion with others, paradoxically generates discontinuity, and gradually configures us in a unique but relational egoic universe.

Our body is our limit, our boundary. This is how Rodríguez relates to this subject "boundaries are the areas of separation or differentiation, but also of connection of the self and the others and the world." Boundaries are configured around the relational experience. In these areas the interchange, the biological and emotional nutrition take place that are necessary to form the mind and self-experience [41].

Along these lines, Bowlby notes that "human beings need the attachment relationship as a regulator of their emotional system for the harmonious development of the self" [52–58]. The body seems to be the first provider of identity and the first vehicle for interpersonal communication between the child and the world. Thus, through primary feelings and physiological sensations, and later with auditory and visual stimuli, children play an increasingly important role. Bowlby accentuates that the groundwork in the first year of life consists of building an attachment relationship and Shore notes that this is the "the affective bond of emotional communication between the child and the primary caregiver." Caregivers, under optimal conditions, help the child to identify and verbalize the affects that are initially experienced, mainly in somatic terms. Thus, the child learns to distinguish somatic experience from psychological experience [41].

This theory is based on the assumption that attachment to affective referents in childhood (mainly parents) configures a *damaged* neurobiological structure that would determine the adult abnormal response to trauma. From a moderate perspective, one would understand that the attachment style marks a tendency toward response patterns that can be activated or not in stressful situations [46].

In this rising corporality, affection, historical condition, values, and beliefs become interwoven and social and subjective features, such as the primary identity and the generic condition, re-engage.

This self is not only fluids, bones, finiteness, and forcefulness, it is rather what sets us apart from others. Dio Bleichmar maintains that the sense of femaleness is constructed in relation to the body, the attachment to others, and to love as the core of identity [59]. In line with this, Husserl claims that the self only exists if embodied. Thus, following Merleau-Ponty, we see ourselves not as *having* bodies, but as *being* bodies.

Human bodies, apart from expiring and being *deteriorable*, following Cristóbal Pera, they are vulnerable, suffer trauma, and become "injured bodies." We are finite bodies exposed to a host of misery, trauma, and pathology. Thus, the abused, raped or beaten body is deeply harmed in its bodily identity, leaving the self helpless, defenseless like a 3 year-old boy. Freud addresses the body and comes to the conclusion that the *ego* is a differentiation from the *id*, owing to the contact of the body with the outside world. In Freud's words, the *ego* comes first and is mainly a corporal self [60].

Identities are relatively stable. There is a tendency toward defending the coherence of the oneness, a tendency that preserves it from the normality and everydayness. There are only some experiences, such as traumatic events, that may cause dramatic changes [46].

The traumatic event (or the recurring of the multiplicity of configurations of violence and trauma) as extreme questioning events resolve key aspects of this identity. In this way, trauma not only acts as a questioning event of the self and the world, but it can also be inscribed as a defining event, a provider of meaning. In fact, the traumatic and painful event unleashes an experience of discontinuity that implies a denarrativization of the body. Thus, it provokes a disruption in the narrative conscience, through which everydayness is configured.

The process of integration of the traumatic experience involves the global readjustment of the person's self-perception in the attempt to relocate the memories of the event. Paul Steinberg, Auschwitz survivor, describes the difficulties in reconciling identities: before Auschwitz, in the camp, and afterward as a parent. Sometimes the force and intensity of these elements of life are so powerful that it becomes nuclear to the identity of the person.

The resultant trauma identity does not necessarily have a negative foundation. Betty Makoni is an African woman, a child abuse survivor, activist, and founder of the Girl Child Network in Zimbabwe, Africa. Betty talks about how girls cope with trauma and the symbol of a tree that is born on the head of a woman whose roots are nurtured by their coping potential [61]. Once again, there are no intrinsically good or bad things, but useful, adaptive and non-adaptive.

Along the lines of managing their own resources and the attribution of new meanings to the events as factors for the protection of the resultant identity, Kimberly Theidon reaffirms the important role of women raped in war as heroines in the defense and protection of their children, leaving the images of humiliation and stigma behind. Anngwyn St. Just notes that the victim's conscience, if we do not strengthen resilience resources and capacity, may have a negative effect on physical and mental health [62].

Pau Pérez [46] notes that a trauma-centric identity only is troublesome if linked to images of vulnerability and powerlessness, dependent relationships, help seeking, and grumbling, hindering the full development of the person. On this basis, Jean Améry asserted that psychiatry, labeling the survivors as "damaged" or "sick," questions their moral legitimacy as privileged witnesses and makes them mere objects of cure and compassion. Thus, their voices are discredited, which is useful for the political class and to society at large.

Importantly, in working with people affected by psychological trauma we must be especially sensitive and consider the risk of possible invalidation of the subjective experience and the subsequent revictimization [63]. In terms of gender violence, but also applicable to other victims, Valiente [64] insists that blaming them for their vulnerability furthers revictimization, even when victims need to understand the elements operating in their vulnerability, be it rooted in unveiled conflicts, fantasies, desires or unadaptive expectations. Chu [65] recommends working in a therapeutic alliance with the patient to prevent self-destructive actions and contribute to the understanding of the mechanism that makes them more vulnerable to revictimization.

Thus, it would be easy to think that *trauma* is embodied as an experience that alters identity. However, it is in that immediacy of life where boundaries and pain awaken the body from its comfortable lethargy that we should broaden choice toward the power of starting afresh and where the infinite possibilities of experiencing living lie.

8.7 Child Sexual Abuse: Perforated Corporality

Bruises healed. Reputation did not.
—*Khaled Hosseini*

Intimacy presupposes the prior concealment of the surface of the body. The relation of intimacy between two bodies is determined by what is hidden and what is revealed. It is social and cultural, but an individual construct as the body itself is. The approximation to bodily intimacy is culturally organized around family rituals and sexual activity. When the *rapprochement*—regardless of the intensity—is not consented to this constitutes an invasion of bodily intimacy and intrusion into the privacy domain.

Many of the disorders that have been linked to adversity in childhood, for instance, depression and anxiety disorders, including PTSD, show in general a higher prevalence among adult women compared with men of the same age [66].

Abuse and PTSD share some symptoms: intrusive and unpleasant memories, dissociations, and flashback sequences. However, a common feature in abuse is the presence of patterns revealing a direct attack on corporality, expressed in different forms: in its pleasure receptor functions, in its capacity of intimacy, conception, and nurture, in fully complying with their own and others' biological destiny, and in the creation of meaningful relationships based on body privacy [67].

When abuse occurs in adulthood, the victim sees himself or herself as having a dubious bodily identity. Adult victims of sexual abuse see their bodies as alienated, as a place owned by another, a settlement for the other, as if the other person articulated their limbs. In this way, physical contact, far from being part of body knowledge and self-perception, deepens the sense of strangeness and distance [67].

More often than not, they express discomfort toward their bodies–dispossession: "I know that somehow this body is mine, but I don't feel it as such" [64]. In Freud's words, *unheimlich*, which literally means *not-at-home* has been translated as unfamiliar, uncomfortable, and eerie. James Chu [65] notes that abuse survivors tend to be ambivalent about self-care and they tend to neglect basic aspects of their physical health.

There is continuing controversy on trauma and memory. Judith Herman wrote in her groundbreaking book *Trauma and Recovery*:

> The study of psychological trauma has a curious history—one of episodic amnesia.
> The study of psychological trauma does not languish for lack of interest. Rather, the subject provokes such intense controversy that it periodically becomes anathema.

Following Herman, Freyd points out that "among the traumatic events that result in *an intense controversy that periodically becomes anathema*, sexual abuse of children seems to be the most revolutionary" [68]. Very often, societies protect themselves from pain and suffering through oblivion, but as it happens, in some cases the best way to forget is through memory and the conscious and emotional recognition of the event. While preserving the memory in the past we displace the painful engravement of the event.

Judith Herman states that the study of psychological trauma always calls into question facts like wars, and intimate family and partner relationships. Thus, we must not forget that the direction in this research field may be influenced by political, ideological, historical, and structural aspects [64].

Psychiatrist Roland Summit explained in 1988 that every society, not only the directly affected, protects the secrecy of sexual abuse of children. In the same way as the victim is silenced, forced into self-punishment, dissociation, and identification with the aggressor, as a society, we are inclined to unthinkingly deny the facts. Jennifer Freyd insists that there are many social interests in child abuse not being revealed and consequently, a great difficulty in discovering the real figures [68].

Neuroimaging studies have shown a decreased function of the medial prefrontal cortex in traumatized persons, clinically resulting in serious attention problems in detecting internal perceptions and sensations. When they finally connect with their inner world they usually find a field mined with perceptions, sensations, and emotions related to trauma. Regarding their corporality, there is often no sense of self-possession over their bodies [64] and they often feel revulsion toward themselves, as well as having a strong negative self-body image; thus, they keep a low profile in order to not to draw attention to their bodies.

Yet, as Pat Odgen [69] comments, we cannot learn to take care of ourselves if we are not in contact with the needs and requirements of our physical self: our physical identity, our bodily identity, what we physically are. This invasion of corporality at an early age is associated with multiple mental disorders in adulthood in the form of depression, anxiety, substance abuse, self-harm, multiple somatization, borderline personality, and PTSD, among others. It is not surprising that these children use their bodies to release tension and manifest their impulses through self-harm [64]. There are findings that suggest that trauma and sexual abuse, more than being linked to a specific disorder, constitute a nonspecific risk factor for psychiatric morbidity [41].

8.8 Psychopathological Manifestations Through the Female Body: Homo Dolorosus (Somatization) and Self-Harm

> Nature has placed mankind under the governance of two sovereign masters, pain and pleasure.
>
> —*Jeremy Bentham*

The suffering body ejects the human being from the island of *sanity* into the world of *sickness*. Through sickness we can re-experience our bodies, we take care of our bodies; we are cared for and looked after. The suffering body is disturbing and creates tension and alarm. Insecurity, weakness, and the intimate connection to the lived body are made visible through pain.

Women frequently express dissatisfaction, and in some cases submission and subjection, through physical pain. The biography of these women is inscribed in the body and its pains, wherein lies a possible identity conflict. Only through this overabundance of the body is it possible to move beyond the severe and disciplining domain of reason in order to acquire “consciousness through pain” [70]. Pain and weakness always set limits and the limit is the intense experience of life. Pain breaks the identity narrative based on ordinariness; the balance of a domesticated lethargy is upset, challenging any established order.

Structural violence directly or indirectly against female identity has led to an individual (identity) subjectivity shaped in a corporal mask, like an eggshell, filled with obstacles, interruptions, tricks, and pain. There is a high occurrence of women with painful multi-symptom disorders without a clear organic cause, in which the body symptoms become the emerging of the unperceived: a body complaining to seek affect, support, and attention. A body that becomes sick in order to say "no" to imperatives, to channel dissatisfaction, and also a body complaining as a possible means of discovering other pathways [22].

Female identity is assimilated into the being-for-others, where the nuclear is the relational and the assigned in androcentric culture, putting aside an intimate story of desire, choices, transcendence, and creation. This requires the self to exist, the possibilities of being to be renewed, and the possible alterations to be produced.

Along the same lines, Hornstein says that the *alteration* is the living substance in identity, to be someone else being oneself (sense of oneness/uniqueness) despite the loss and acquisition of different qualities [71]. To paraphrase García Márquez, one could say that the end of the patriarchal society is "an end foretold," and thus, women and their corporal identity may cease to be so conditioned and pained.

Somatization, fairly common among women, refers to the tendency of experiencing stress through physical symptoms, bodily concerns, and/or experiencing oneself mainly in physical terms. Psychological and physical issues are not integrated. The belief that somatization can be related to trauma as the defensive action of dissociation is not new [41].

Ana Távora runs groups in the mental health center of Santa Fe (Granada) for women with multiple somatoform disorders, where women shift from a discourse focused on the body area to one centered around the detection of conflicts, mostly gender issues.

Janet [59] hypothesized that memories of the traumatic event that are stored outside the person's awareness may contribute to dissociation and somatization in the form of hysteria. Along these lines, Van der Kolk [72] advocates the consideration of dissociation, somatization, and other affect regulation disorders as late-emerging manifestations of trauma. The link among trauma, dissociation, and somatization is empirically supported. In fact, Pribor, Yutzy, Dean, and colleagues [73] found that 90 % of women with somatization disorder had a history of physical, emotional or sexual abuse, and 80 % of them had a history of some form of sexual abuse.

8.8.1 Behavior in Borderline Patients: Self-Injury

> The wound is the memory of the body; it memorizes its fragility, its pain, thus its "real" existence. It is a defense against the object and against the mental prosthesis. —*Gina Pane*

Women in sorrow, with an unbearable feeling of loneliness, in a body in favor of a split identity. Pain often defines their feelings: intense, recurring and dramatic pain, to the extent of giving it the expression: "*the pain of being borderline*" [74]. This deep pain and discomfort rooted in the body turns their lives into a carousel of traumatized corporality. These bodies are cut, attacked, stuffed with food, filled with drugs, in a never-ending emotional swing. The borderline body is the place of respite for their diffused identity, where tension drags out a history of personal pain.

Broadly, all BPD patients are self-destructive and some of them even resort to self-mutilation, but not all of them follow the same pattern. Theodore Millon [75] presents a subtype of BPD in which self-destruction is due to comorbidity in the masochistic pattern: the self-defeating personality. Their bodies filled with scars, like Ulysses, show us their identity, a multi-perforated body. Olivares refers to scars with the following: "a story being told to anyone who will listen, anyone who can understand."

Self-harming behavior is more prevalent in women and is present in 75 % of borderline patients, which for the majority of people has an onset in adulthood and is highest between the ages of 18 and 24 [75].

According to patients with BPD, the reason for self-harm is in some cases related to numbness: "when we don't feel anything special, we don't feel our bodies." Human beings are in constant need of self-perception even if they fall back again, yielding to a quiet lethargy. This intimate experience of physical pain brings them the certainty of the existence of their bodies, the certainty that there is more than emptiness. The way in which they experience life is outside the traditional forms of managing the body in our culture [59]. The wounds, the blood, and the powerlessness denote that they are alive; yet, through all this we can clearly see the expressive function of the body, a pain seeking to be seen and responded to. Even though these behaviors alarm relatives and specialists and may be seen as evidence of suicidal intentionality, self-destructive conduct does not necessarily represent a connecting factor to suicide.

Many self-destructive behaviors have self-punishment motivations [76] and at times are closely related to an experience of relief in painful and unbearable emotional states [77]. Once again, we must not radically condemn homeostasis mechanisms. In many cases, in the interest of preserving what is incorruptible about the human body, we block potential ways of escape. However, the connection between self-harm actions and suicidal intent is complex. It is highly uncertain to assume that self-mutilation is a way of drawing attention. As it happens, borderline patients commit suicide in circumstances that began with a gesture, with no suicidal intention.

The rate of self-harm conduct is in general 75 %, but adding behaviors such as having unsafe sex with strangers or combining alcohol with Antabuse, may bring the self-harm conduct rate up to 90 %. In all this we can see aggression toward the body, a direct act against life, yet it is true that borderline patients put their bodies at risk so that they can experience life. Thus, against social boundaries, there is the individual's chosen limit [70]. The term self-harm describes an act whereby a person intentionally injures or harms themselves. Among the self-injury behaviors we found were cutting or severely scratching the skin (80 %), hitting (24 %), burning or scalding (20 %), banging the head (15 %), and biting (7 %) [78]. If the skin is the damp-proof wrapper, the cut provides an outlet orifice, an exit for pain.

A patient wrote about the self-injury impulse: "I want to cut myself. I want to see pain, because it's the most physical way to show emotional pain. I want to cut myself, cut myself and show it, show it. Taking it out, but taking what? Just pain."

The intentionality of self-harming behavior has been broadly studied. Self-harm has different motivations: to release the pain and tension inside (59 %), to punish (49 %), to control feelings (39 %), to have control over the body (22 %), to express feelings of hate and rage (22 %), to feel *alive instead of feeling numb* (20 %) [78].

Although the conceptualization of the borderline personality and its causes are still unaccounted for, most of the studies suggest a significant relationship between infantile trauma and borderline symptoms, and between childhood sexual abuse and the development of borderline personality disorder [74]. The risk factors that determine borderline patients often include: loss, history of sexual and physical abuse, deep negligence or emotional abuse, witnessing gender violence, drug abuse or criminality in progenitors.

Without further analysis of the factors influencing the resultant gravity of abuse, a piece of research conducted by Silk et al. [79] shows that continued sexual abuse in childhood was the best predictor of serious borderline symptoms, such as parasuicide, chronic helplessness and chronic handicap, transitory paranoia, regression, and intolerance to solitude [75]. Furthermore, sexual abuse by parents and emotional negligence in childhood, both involved in the genesis of borderline personality disorder, are closely related to self-harm behavior [80].

8.9 Conclusions

Sexual abuse and related disorders—such as eating disorder, PTSD, somatization, and others—are categories in which the body is directly attacked, transformed, and frequently negated. Clinical research on these subjects manifests the limitations of the verbal scene, either to understand the phenomena the clinician is facing or to construct a strong therapeutic hypothesis. The narrated body, present in psychoanalysis and other psychotherapeutic disciplines, differs widely from the new forms of trauma management that seem to be moving toward an enhanced approach to corporality. This suggests a comprehensive perspective of the emergence of trauma.

Indeed, it is hard to imagine what cognitive therapies and formats of psychoeducation can better succeed in managing pervasive and existential dilemmas resulting from a traumatic event. In addition to this, therapies with a traumatized person must not leave the body in isolation, as this would mean deficiency and incompleteness. In individuals exposed to trauma, the political, social, and relational context in which the traumatic event occurred is also crucial. Similarly, gender perspective is fundamental in addressing these issues with patients. If we disregard this, we disparage the patient's subjectivity.

For the first time in its history, the DSM includes in its last edition a specific section on gender, giving this construct a profound importance when it comes to instilling a new psychopathology. A need in this matter would be to conduct research that furthers understanding of the way in which trauma affects the subjective reality of gender, experienced, naturally, through embodiment.

Trauma occurs in the body and is revealed through the body. But only through tolerance and respect for every human body, which embodies the dignity of human life, we can hope for better times.

References

1. Merleau-Ponty M. Phénomènologie de la perception. Paris: Gallimard; 1945.
2. Fritz G. The evolution of psychosomatic medicine. Brown Univ Child Adolesc Behav Lett. 2000;16:4–8.
3. Turner BS. Avances recientes en la teoría del cuerpo. Rev Esp Invest Social. 1994;68:11–40.
4. Esteban ML. Antropología del cuerpo: género, itinerarios corporales, identidad y cambio. Bellaterra: Barcelona; 2004.
5. Csordas T, editor. Embodiment and experience, Cambridge studies in medical anthropology, vol. 2. Cambridge: Cambridge University Press; 1994.
6. Scheper-Hughes N, Lock M. The mindful body: a prolegomenon to future work in medical anthropology. Med Anthropol Q. 1987;1:6–41.
7. Helman CG. Culture, health and illness. London: Hodder Arnold; 2000.
8. Scheper-Hughes N, Lock M. The message in the bottle: illness and the micropolitics of resistance. J Psychohist. 1991;18(4):409–32.
9. Janzen JM. Text and context in the anthropology of war trauma: The African Great Lakes Region 1993-95. Suom Antropol. 1999;24(4):37–57.
10. Rohlfs I. El género como herramienta de trabajo en la investigación en epidemiología y salud pública. In: Esteban ML, Comelles JM, Díez M, editors. Antropología, género, salud y atención. Barcelona: Bellaterra; 2010.
11. Esteban ML. Introducción a la Antropología de la Salud: aplicaciones teóricas y prácticas. Bilbao: OSALDE: Asociación por el derecho a la salud; 2007.
12. Wasco SM. Conceptualizing the harm done by rape: applications of trauma theory to experiences of sexual assault. Trauma Violence Abuse. 2003;4(4):309–22.
13. Burstow B. Toward a radical understanding of trauma and trauma work. Violence Against Women. 2003;9(11):1293–317.
14. Herman J. Trauma and recovery. New York: Harper Collins; 1992.
15. Burstow B. A critique of posttraumatic stress disorder and the DSM. J Humanist Psychol. 2005;45(4):429–45.
16. Logan S. Remembering the women in Rwanda: when humans rely on the old concepts of war to resolve conflict. Affilia. 2006;21(2):234–9. doi:10.1177/0886109905285772.
17. Kleinman A, Desjarlais R. Violence, culture and the politics of trauma. In: Kleinman A, editor. Writing at the margins: discourse between anthropology and medicine. Berkeley: University of California Press; 1995. p. 712–189.
18. Farmer P. Pathologies of power: health, human rights, and the new war on the poor. Berkeley: University of California Press; 2003.
19. Galtung J. Cultural violence. J Peace Res. 1990;27(3):291–305.
20. Bourdieu P. La dominación masculina. Anagrama: Barcelona; 2000.
21. James EC. The political economy of 'trauma' in Haiti in the democratic era of insecurity. Cult Med Psychiatry. 2004;28(2):127–49.

22. Távora A. El cuerpo como lugar de expresión de los conflictos. In (coord.): Muñoz Muñoz AM, Gregorio Gil C, Sánchez Espinosa A. Cuerpos de mujeres: miradas, representaciones e identidades. Granada: Universidad de Granada; 2007. p. 143–62.
23. Távora A. Pensando sobre los conflictos y la salud mental de las mujeres. Área 3. Suppl. Género y Salud Mental; 2003.
24. Basaglia F. Mujer, Locura y sociedad. Mexico: Universidad Autónoma de Puebla; 1983.
25. Rosaldo MZ. The uses and abuses of anthropology: reflections on feminism and cross-cultural understanding. Sings. 1980;5(3):400.
26. Hourcade C. Cuerpos fragmentados: Las mujeres y el conflicto con sus cuerpos. Mujeres y salud. Tu cuerpo: Personal e intransferible. CAPS; 2008. p. 24.
27. Vance C. Placer y peligro: explorando la sexualidad femenina. Madrid: Talasa; 1989.
28. Soriano MJ. El abuso sexual en la infancia y su repercusión en la edad adulta. Mujeres y salud. Monográfico Salud Mental. El trasfondo del malestar. CAPS; 2010. p. 29.
29. Kurvet-Käosaar L. Vulnerable scriptings: approaching hurtfulness of the repressions of the Stalinist regime in the life-writings of Baltic women. In: Festić F, editor. Gender and trauma: interdisciplinary dialogues. Newcastle Upon Tyne: Cambdridge Scholars Publishing; 2012.
30. Bertaux-Wiame I. La perspectiva de la historia de vida en el estudio de las migraciones interiores. In: Marinas JM, Santamarina C, editors. La Historia Oral: Métodos y experiencias. Madrid: Debate; 1993.
31. Delgado C. Análisis del testimonio como fuente oral: género y memoria. In: Viejas y nuevas alianzas entre América latina y España. XII Encuentro de Latino Americanistas españoles. Santander, 21 al 23 de septiembre 2006.
32. Theidon K. Entre Prójimos: El conflicto armado interno y la política de la reconciliación en el Perú. Lima: Instituto de Estudios Peruanos; 2004.
33. Theidon K. La teta asustada: una teoría sobre la violencia de la memoria. Ideele. 2009;191.
34. Allué M. La piel curtida. Bellaterra: Barcelona; 2008.
35. Sáenz M. Psicopatología y género: crónica del resentimiento. Norte de Salud Mental. 2012;42: 7–8.
36. Suárez EB. Surviving the "*Sasachacuy Tiempu*" (difficult times): The resilience of Quechua women in the aftermath of the Peruvian armed conflict. Thesis. Factor-Inwentash Faculty of Social Work. Toronto: University of Toronto; 2011.
37. Comelles JM. De la ayuda mutua y de la asistencia como categorías antropológicas: una revisión conceptual. Trabajo social y salud. 2000;35:151–72.
38. Bonino L. Masculinidad, salud y sistema sanitario: el caso de la violencia masculina. In: Ruiz Jarabo C, Blanco P, editors. La violencia contra las mujeres. Prevención y detección. Madrid: Díaz de Santos; 2004.
39. Bergara A, Riviere J, Bacete R. Los hombres, la igualdad y las nuevas masculinidades. Vitoria-Gasteiz: EMAKUNDE-Instituto Vasco de la Mujer; 2008.
40. Bosch Fiol E, Ferrer Pérez VA, Alzamora MA. Algunas claves para una psicoterapia de orientación feminista en mujeres que han padecido violencia de género. Feminismo/s. 2005; 6:121–36.
41. Rodríguez B, Fernández Liria A, Bayón C. Trauma, disociación y somatización. Anuario de Psicología Clínica y de la salud. 2005;1:27–38.
42. Hidalgo R. Daño psíquico en las víctimas de violencia de género. Jornada "Actuar frente a la violencia de género". Pamplona. 2011.
43. American Psychiatric Association. Diagnostic and statistical manual of Mental Disorders. 5th ed. Washington, DC: APA; 2013.
44. Kilpatrick DG, Saunders BE, Amick-Mc MA. Victim and crime factors associated with the development of posttraumatic stress disorder. Behav Ther. 1989;20:199–214.
45. Breslau N. Gender differences in trauma and posttraumatic stress disorder. J Gend Specif Med. 2002;5:34–40.
46. Pérez P. Trauma, culpa y duelo. Bilbao: Desclée de Brouwer SA; 2006.

47. Sáenz M, Díez-Alegría C. Los Alienistas suicidas. In: Fernandez JL, Fuentenebro F, Rojo A, editors. Suicidio. Madrid: Sociedad de Historia y Filosofía de la Psiquiatría; 2008. p. 159–95.
48. Pera C. Pensar desde el cuerpo. Ensayo sobre la corporeidad humana. Madrid: Triacastela; 2006.
49. Damasio A. Descartes' error: emotion, reason and the human brain. London: Vintage; 1994.
50. Damasio A. The feeling of what happens: body and emotion in the making of consciousness. London: Heinemann; 1999.
51. Janet P. L'évolution psychologique de la personalité. Paris: Éditions Chanine; 1929.
52. Bowlby J. The makind and breaking of affectional bonds. I. Aetiology and psychopathology in the light of attachment theory. Br J Psychiatry. 1977;130:201–10.
53. La BJ. Separación Afectiva. Paidós: Barcelona; 1985.
54. Bowlby J. Vínculos Afectivos: Formación, Desarrollo y Pérdida. Madrid: Morata; 1986. p. 90–105.
55. Bowlby J. Developmental psychiatry comes of age. Am J Psychiatry. 1988;145:1–10.
56. Bowlby J. El Vínculo afectivo. Paidós: Barcelona; 1990. 2nd reprint.
57. Bowlby J. La pérdida afectiva. Paidós: Barcelona; 1990.
58. Bowlby J. Postcript. In: J. Stevenson-Hinde, Marris P, editors. Attachment across the life cycle. London and New York: Parkes CM, Tavistock/Routledge; 1991. p. 293–298.
59. Sáenz M. Cuerpo y Género. In: Martínez O, Sagasti N, Villasante O, editors. Del pleistoceno a nuestros días: Contribuciones a la Historia de la Psiquiatría. VIII Jornadas de la Sección de Historia de la Psiquiatría de la AEN; 2011. p. 101–16.
60. López-Ibor JJ. Perception, experience and body identity. Actas Esp Psiquiatr. 2011;39(3):3–118.
61. Shinoda J. Sabia como un árbol. Kairós: Barcelona; 2012.
62. St JA. Trauma: una cuestión de equilibrio. Un abordaje sistémico para la comprensión y resolución. Buenos Aires: Alma Lepik; 2010.
63. Valiente C, Cantero D, Villavicencio P. Reflexiones del suicidio en el contexto de violencia de género. In: Fernandez JL, Fuentenebro F, Rojo A, editors. Suicidio. Madrid: Sociedad de Historia y Filosofía de la Psiquiatría; 2008. p. 299–320.
64. Cantero MD, Villavicencio P. Corporalidad y trauma. In: Fuentenebro F, Rojo A, Valiente C, editors. Psicopatología y fenomenología de la corporalidad. Madrid: Sociedad de Historia y Filosofía de la Psiquiatría; 2005. p. 141–57.
65. Chu JA. Rebuilding shattered lives. The responsible treatment of complex post-traumatic and dissociative disorders. New York: Wiley; 1998.
66. Angold MB, Marcelle C. Una perspectiva evolutiva con consideración especial del trauma psicológico infantil. In: Narrow WE, First MB, Sirovatka PJ, Regier DA, editors. Consideraciones sobre la edad y el género en el diagnóstico psiquiátrico. Barcelona: Elsevier Masson; 2009.
67. Stupiggia M. El cuerpo violado. Aproximación psicocorporal al Trauma del Abuso. Santiago de Chile: Cuatro Vientos; 2010.
68. Freyd JJ. Abusos sexuales en la infancia: La lógica del olvido. Madrid: Morata; 1996.
69. Ogden P, Minton K, Pain C. Trauma y cuerpo. Bilbao: Desclée de Brouwer SA; 2011.
70. Fernández JL. Las vivencias de la corporalidad en el siglo XXI: una aproximación desde el mundo del arte y las nuevas tecnologías. In: Fuentenebro F, Rojo A, Valiente C, editors. Psicopatología y fenomenología de la corporalidad. Madrid: Sociedad de Historia y Filosofía de la Psiquiatría; 2008. p. 69–86.
71. Hornstein L. Autoestima e Identidad. Narcisismo y valores sociales. Buenos Aires: Fondo de Cultura Económica; 2011.
72. Van der Kolk BA, Ducey C. The psychological processing of traumatic experience: Rorschach patterns in PTSD. J Trauma Stress. 1989;2:259–74.
73. Pribor EF, Yutzy SH, Dean JT, et al. Briquet's syndrome, dissociation and abuse. Am J Psychiatry. 1993;150:1507–11.
74. Zanarini MC, Frankenburg FR, DeLuca CJ, et al. The pain of being borderline: dysphoric states specific to borderline personality disorder. Harv Rev Psychiatry. 1998;6:201–7.

75. Millon T. Trastornos de la personalidad en la vida moderna. Barcelona: Masson; 2006.
76. Shearer SL, Peters CP, Quaytman MS, et al. Intent and lethality of suicide attempts among female borderline inpatients. Am J Psychiatry. 1988;145:1424–7.
77. Soloff PH, Lis JA, Kelly T, et al. Self-mutilation and suicidal behavior in borderline personality disorder. J Pers Disord. 1994;8:257–67.
78. Shearer SL. Phenomenology of self-injury among inpatient women with borderline personality disorder. J Nerv Ment Dis. 1994;182(9):524–6.
79. Silk K, Lee S, Hill E, Lohr N. Borderline personality disorder symptoms and severity of sexual abuse. Am J Psychiatry. 1995;152(7):1059–64.
80. Dubo E, Zanarini M, Lewis R, Williams A. Childhood antecedents of self-destructiveness in borderline personality disorder. Can J Psychiatry. 1997;42:63–9.

9 Dysmorphophobia: From Neuroticism to Psychoticism

Batirtze Artaraz, Leire Celaya, and Eider Zuaitz

I am writing as an ugly one for the ugly ones: the old hags, the dykes, the frigid, the unfucked, the unfuckables, the neurotics, the psychos, for all those girls that do not get a look-in in the universal market of the consumable chick.
Virginia Despentes

Abstract

Dysmorphophobia is a concept that challenges psychiatric epistemology. Throughout history it has varied from psychosis to neurosis, from symptoms to syndrome. In the present work we broach the pathoplasty disorder according to sexes and describe its symptoms from a gender-based perspective. This point of view demonstrates that psychopathological symptoms are useless attempts to thoroughly identify oneself with gender stereotypes and beauty ideals.

Anthropological investigations and history have brought to light the esthetic and symbolic importance that a human being has given to his body since ancient times. Since men/women have become self-conscious, they have suffered baseless fears about deformity or ugliness, especially when specular surfaces began to abound.

Body dysmorphic disorder (BDD) or dysmorphophobia is characteristically defined as an excessive preoccupation with a perceived physical defect or with an overestimation of a trivial existing defect. An interference caused by the symptom is produced; the anxiety is very time-consuming and finally damages

B. Artaraz (✉)
Mental Health Outpatients Services, Osakidetza, Basque Country, Spain
e-mail: batirtze.artarazocerinjauregui@osakidetza.net

L. Celaya (✉)
Mental Health Outpatients Services, Osakidetza, Alava, Basque Country, Spain
e-mail: leire.celayaviguera@osakidetza.net

E. Zuaitz
Mental Health Outpatients Services, Osakidetza, Guipuzcoa, Basque Country, Spain
e-mail: eider.zuaitzziztueta@osakidetza.net

M. Sáenz-Herrero (ed.), *Psychopathology in Women*,
DOI 10.1007/978-3-319-05870-2_9

the psychosocial functioning of the individual, which is what distinguishes BDD from normal or "physiological" preoccupations with physical appearance.

9.1 Introduction

Historical and cross-cultural literature suggests that since classical times, people have considered the human body and its appearance the object of a special esthetic and symbolic investigation. These factors can provoke in psychobiologically vulnerable people the development of diverted or pathological ideas about their own body.

Body dysmorphic disorder (BDD), classified by some people as an independent nosological entity of difficult ubication, occurs as dysmorphia or dysmorphophobia. From the psychopathological point of view there are still doubts as to whether its main manifestation consists of an obsessive idea, an overestimated idea, or a delirious idea.

BDD was described at the end of the nineteenth century by Morselli (in an article entitled *Sulla dismorfofobia e sulla talefobia*), who named the preoccupations and complaints about deformity *dysmorphophobia*. This author described dysmorphophobia as an "obsessive and devastating idea" about body deformity and classified it as a "rudimentary paranoia" or "abortive monomania" that affected the integrity of the individual. According to whether it deals with a defense from direct damage or with a manifestation of a more profound disorder, the idea was correspondingly considered principal or secondary [1].

The term comes from *dysmorphia*, which was used by Herodotus when referring to the ugliest woman of Sparta. Etymologically, the word originates from the Greek *dysmorphia*, which means ugliness related to facial appearance. Philippopoulos made an interesting comment: the most appropriate transliteration of this term in English would be *dysmorphophobia*. Since then both limits—one of the concepts and one of the behavior—associated with "dysmorphophobia" have passed through repeated changes. The resultant confusion is attributed to the fact that the term itself is ambiguous as it contains the suffix "phobia." This argument is false because the terms always used to be arbitrary: it is the concept that is important; this has changed since the nineteenth century and it is possible that it will change again.

In his historical analysis, Morselli distinguished one subtype related mostly to body deformity on the basis of a combination of ancient negative attitudes toward the self. This was explained in terms of descriptive and nosological categories of that period. Saying now that he "was mistaken" because "dysmorphophobia" also includes overestimated, delirious ideas, obsessions, and phobias does not make any sense. The term remained, referring to the "symptoms," so there is little empirical evidence that the modern classification is definitive or that it is superior to the classification from the second half of the nineteenth century. In fact, Morselli was aware that the meaning of phobia was changing [2].

During the last years of the nineteenth century and the first years of the twentieth century, different authors approached the clinical phenomenon associated with the term. In 1982, H. Kaan, in his book about neurasthenia and obsession, studies fears of ugliness. In 1901, Hartemberg refers to similar fears in his book about shyness. Contemporaneously, Janet encompasses it into his psychasthenic syndrome and mentions it as "the obsessions and of the shame of the body," also of a nosological phobic–obsessive nature. In 1907, Dupré explains fears of ugliness as a result of proprioceptive alteration. Korkina and Morozov realized a revision at the beginning of the century, when they registered that Korsakov, Betcherev, and Suchanov had already documented similar clinical phenomena in a Russian bibliography. It is Osipov who introduced in 1912 the term *dysmorphophobia* by studying the case of a 27-year-old woman who believed that she was "too tall" and had a deformity of "the lower part of the face" [3].

The term "dysmorphophobia" took time to settle with German and English people. It probably was in the translation of the *Textbook of Mental Diseases* by Tanzi, where it appeared in English for the first time, being mentioned in the section on obsessive ideas under the name Morselli [4]. It was in 1915 when Kraepelin classified it as a compulsive neurosis in his chapter about *Die Zwangsneurose (Dysmorphophobie)*. It was based mostly on the persistent and the repetitive nature of the symptoms and its ego-dystonic nature. He also described the same clinical phenomenon with a different name: *ereuthophobie*. Since then, many other terms appear to have approached the same theme: the shame of the body, the psychosis of ugliness, the hypochondria of beauty, the madness of introspection, etc.

One of the most attention-grabbing names for the disorder was attributed to Stutte, "*The Complex of Thersites*." In the Iliad Thersites is described as the "the ugliest and shameless speaker of Troy." He was cross-eyed and limped, but there is no evidence that he once demonstrated preoccupation about his obvious ugliness [5]. The "Wolf Man" is one of Freud's most famous cases, and he describes the case as a compulsive neurosis, which Brunswick terms hypochondriac paranoia. He detaches how observation of the facial ugliness in a pocket mirror turns into the focus of the patient's whole life.

In the 1930s, Janhureiss makes a reference to the "hypochondria of beauty," mentioning as areas of great interest the nose, skin, and hair. Some years later the term was commented on by Ladee (1966), who pointed out the principal characteristics of the BDD. In 1962, Dietrich defines the term "phobia" on the basis of the fear that patients with a deformed appearance show to other people, and defines the symptom as an "identity crisis." However, Zadiens (1950) describing "dermatological hypochondria," considers dysmorphophobia a form of schizophrenia; Anderson (1964)—a light version of the same disease, and Conollu and Gipson (1978)—a dangerous symptom that frequently leads to schizophrenia. In more recent times, 1971, Schachter defined the "complex of dysmorphia" in contraposition with the "delirium of dysmorphia," distinguishing on the one hand dysmorphical neuroses and, on the other hand, delirium or delirious convictions of dysmorphia. Munro in 1980, distinguishes dysmorphophobia, an excessive preoccupation with minor body defects, from monosymptomatic hypochondriacal psychosis, including in the latter dysmorphic delirium together with delirium of body odor and infestation (already described by Guislan in 1851, but systemized by Ekbom in 193 with the name of presenile dermatozoic delusion) [6].

To turn to the "neurotic" part of the term, in the classification systems used normally, the DSM III (1980) classified dysmorphophobia within the section on somatoform disorder, without specifying its diagnostic criteria, also mentioning the delirious variant in the group of persistent deliriums. In 1987, the DSM III R for the first time introduced the term "BDD" to describe a somatoform disorder of nondelirious nature, characterized by a preoccupation with an imagined or trivial defect in appearance. Those of a delirious nature are included in this classification in the section on delusional disorders of the somatic type.

The DSM-IV and DSM IV TR classifications retain the concept. They add to it the criteria of a "clinically significant defect or deterioration in the psychosocial functioning" [7]. ICD 10 includes both BDD and nondelirious dysmorphophobia in the hypochondriac categories (F45.2) and the above-mentioned delirious dysmorphophobia under delusional disorders. In spite of giving a new name to the combination of the diverted attitudes termed "BDD," they did not dissipate the conceptual ambiguities caused by "dysmorphophobia."

Finally, owing to the evolution of the concept associated with BDD, and with the recent launch of DSM-5, the importance of repetitive behaviors and acts associated with the anxiety about physical defects have been pointed out. They are classified under obsessive–compulsive disorder and other related upsets. The delirious types are no longer included under delusional disorders of a somatic nature. This presentation belongs to the BDD itself, specifying the absence of "insight" or delirious belief [8].

9.2 Symptom or Syndrome

Over the years, one of the main questions was whether BDD could be considered an isolated nosological entity. Some authors believe that dysmorphophobia could be a nonspecific symptom that can result in a variety of psychiatric syndromes, while others consider it to be a separate entity [9]. Thomas is in favor of an average term, pointing out the possible existence of primary and secondary forms, to distinguish cases of principal disorder from those with dysmorphic symptoms, secondary to other psychiatric disorders [10]. As a primary disorder BDD almost always demonstrates other symptoms of comorbidity. According to the relevant data, BDD shows a high comorbidity of major depression, social phobia, obsessive–compulsive disorder (OCD) and substance abuse. In the evaluation of the presence of axis II disorders among patients with BDD, they were singled out as the most common disorders associated with cluster C, including avoidant personality disorder and obsessive–compulsive disorder. The dysmorphic alteration as a symptom has been associated with depression, obsessive mood, personality disorders, and anorexia nervosa [11].

9.3 Dysmorphophobia: From Psychosis to Neurosis

As was referred to in the historical antecedents, the qualifying tradition in different editions of the diagnostic and statistical manual of the American Psychiatric Association included BDD as a somatoform disorder. However, as we have already seen from historical evolution, the relation between obsessive–compulsive disorder and BDD is far from clear [12, 13].

The constant preoccupation about one part of the body can be contemplated, from the descriptive point of view, as an obsession; while repetitive checking, camouflage behavior, and searching for reaffirmation is seen to be compulsive behavior [14]. Many authors consider dysmorphophobia an obsession, suggesting that it might be a part of the obsessive–compulsive spectrum or a type of OCD (Janet, Dietrich, Corbella and Rossi, Noto Campanella, Tomkiewich and Finder, Schachter, Hay, Alby, et al.). More than a century ago, Morselli noticed that BDD patients behave in an obsessive–compulsive manner similar to OCD. As was already mentioned, Janet also classified BDD within a group of syndromes similar to OCD, in his description as an "obsession with shame of the body." Later, Solyom et al. suggested that BDD could be considered an "obsessive psychosis," an atypical and malignant form of OCD. In fact, during the development of DSM-IV, the possibility of classifying BDD in the same section as OCD was evaluated. Nevertheless, according to other authors who demonstrated their disagreement with the theory and believed that taking into consideration only the repetitiveness of the conduct (without other phenomenological variables) was insufficient for a rigorous investigation, it was rejected [15, 16].

On the other hand, the dysmorphic idea is far from being absurd for the patients. They are not aware of the senselessness of their worries. In this aspect we deal with two types mentioned by Schachter: one that is close to obsession (dysmorphobic complex) and another that is more delirium-related (dysmorphic delusion). They are based on the corresponding attitude of acceptance or rejection. Schachter thinks that the difference between an obsessive idea and a delirious idea cannot consist only of different attitudes, as it is not a specific feature of any of them [17].

The difference is found in the disturbance of self-consciousness, which is produced in the delirious idea and not in the obsessive idea. The first is experienced as a duty, a siege outside of the self. However, the obsessive idea does not lose the sense of one's own experience and self-activity [18].

The reality is that a dysmorphic idea can be considered to be closer to the overvalued idea. However, the lack of attention of psychopathology to overvalued ideas and the fact that their origin is not very clear, have an influence on the difficulties in finding the nosological position. The self referential condition that dysmorphophobia sometimes has is because what preoccupies the patients is their appearance. This is why they feel they are being observed, but all this without the phenomenon losing its anankastic character and without the diagnostic criteria of schizophrenia being met [19].

Therefore, it is objectified that the separation of BDD from somatic delirious disorder tends to be difficult on many occasions, as the boundary between overvaluation of the esthetic defect and delirious certainty is sometimes very vague [20]. Some authors consider that both disorders are different, that overvalued ideas and delirious ideas cannot exist at the same time in relation to one aspect [21]. They make the allusion that dysmorphobic ideas can be presented as a simple, unimportant transitory preoccupation, forming an obsessive neurotic syndrome of a very disabling nature, and, in other cases, as a hypochondriac, delirious psychosis.

This difficulty in classifying beliefs and thoughts that people who have BDD show can make us consider that there is no one-of-a-kind way of thinking and that the latter can vary from a light convection of overvalued ideas to the truly delirious ideas [22, 23]. Philips et al. demonstrated patients with no difference between delirious and nondelirious subtypes in the majority of the examined variables, including the response to treatment. Therefore, these authors and their contributors conclude that "a dimensional approach characterized by different degrees of conviction seems to be more precise than a dichotomous approach" [24, 25]. As was shown in the evolutional development of the concept of BDD, this dimensional continuity makes it clear that the difficulty in indicating the limits of BDD is still an aspect of great controversy.

9.4 Gender-Based Epidemiology

Body dysmorphic disorder has been insufficiently studied and according to research, underdiagnosed. We found only three studies that deal with analysis of gender differences [26–28].

According to the data we found, the prevalence of the disorder taking into account the gender aspect does not vary significantly. In an investigation made in Italy in 1997, reference is made to about 1.4 % of women suffering from the disorder, while in the other study carried out the same year in the USA it is reported that about 1 % of women and 1.2 % of men are affected. Because of the lack of information we should carry out more exhaustive epidemiological studies in order to know the prevalence according to gender and the reasons for these differences. The studies mentioned point out the necessity of studying the social cultural influence present in the disorder, although the studies analyzed do not expand on this aspect.

Taking into consideration this request, it is decided to carry out research that would go beyond the clinical medical diagnosis and appeal to other scientific branches such as anthropology and sociology. In this manner, it is very interesting to be able to talk about the body and social theory, which, being a relatively new theoretical methodological model, conveys the body into the center of social and anthropological reflection. From this perspective, it is possible to realize a new reflection on the presence or absence of differences in prevalence according to gender in BDD.

Social theory of the body is taken from the intellectual work of the previous two centuries, as Bryan Turner shows in his article *Recent Developments in the Theory of the Body* [29]. Marcell Mauss in his article *Techniques of the Body* proposes that there is no natural behavior in relation to the body and becoming a social individual implies determined body learning [30]. Douglas in his book *Natural Symbols* refers to Mauss as being the first investigator to try the social anthropological body theory and analyzes the human response to the confusion, the risk, the uncertainty, and the contradiction. This has always been the case since the idea has come about that a human body is the main system of classification and metaphor for the social world in very different cultural realities [31].

In this brief review of the pioneering body theories, Foucault is one of those most responsible for the development that has been taking place in social study of the body in the last few decades. He provided a brilliant explanation of how everything related to the body has been socially and politically processed in different contexts, and how it allowed to the patients to resist their own bodies. Different perspectives included in modern social theory of the body are supported by re-reading and surpassing all these and other previous contributions.

In addition, this is a specialty that is directly connected to the appearance of the new dilemmas and controversies at the epistemological and methodical levels, especially related to the post-structuralist and feminist criticism. Some authors would respond better to this body analysis than to another, to the necessary reformulation of different theories about identity, experience, and culture [32].

Staying on this plan, according to philosopher Celia Amorós, the ethical and political feminist fight has changed into an esthetic fight, in a form in which young girls are regulated by the esthetic aspect while receiving messages of independence that contradict the situation of domination in which they live. During the last 30 years we have faced modifications in the regulations and controls over a woman's body that had consequences for the definitions of the feminine, of being a woman, for configurations of gender, and also for the construction of women's subjectivity.

At the end of the twentieth century, feminism, like other social movements, put the body in the center of the fight and recognition, but it was a reproductive body. Gradually, this body has been converted into an object of exhibition, visibility, within the process that we are all involved in, men and women. The social and political situations have changed and nowadays a woman's body is largely an esthetic body, a visible body, and a political body, which is related to social and cultural dynamics rather than to the gender system. Thus, if the social body is esthetic, the political body should also build on these facts. This has different consequences for young people and adults, because adults are protected by the age, which means that gender standardization affects them in other ways. If we come back to the above-mentioned studies on BDD and nonsignificant differences in prevalence between men and women, we would like to present a theory called *feminist practice theory*, which belonged to authors such as Bourdieu, Giddens or Turner.

This theory influences the appearance of what can be termed study of the "body as agent." One of the most significant authors in this aspect is Connell, who is very critical about body studies generated by both biological and social sciences, and who builds on the premise that both biology and society produce gender differences regarding behavior [33]. From this perspective, the body is seen as a place of resistance, opposition, in different economic, political, sexual, esthetical, and intellectual disputes.

For all these reasons, if an analysis is made from the feminist and social perspective, it is expected that a differentiated prevalence would be found where women would lose. However, this difference has not been observed, according to the data. From the perspective of Connell's theory as a possible explanation of these results, it can be established that a standardized body works as a place of resistance and power. Assuming social requests that are in agreement with diagnostic criteria, these women remain classified as healthy and do not lose their position as healthy social subjects. We may think that the difference between genders is not observed because women would not reveal the symptoms that could have appeared in a subclinical manner. They would consider them socially "normal" and would include them as part of their bodies, accepting or not accepting them, but making them part of society.

We point out one of the main conclusions about the evolution of gender inequalities: a woman's body is regulated, controlled, standardized, and determined by a system of the distinguishing and discriminatory type, by some large-scale institutions (fashion advertising, mass media, sports, medicine). However, as we have already mentioned, this nature of a woman's body, predisposed for confrontation, opposition, and resistance, has given to women all the tools to stay invisible in the face of psychiatric diagnosis and to remain classified as healthy and normal. This is the place of power.

9.5 Clinical Differential Presentation

Pathoplasty is a medical term that refers to the clinical method of disease expression. In the case of BDD, gender is the key aspect of its presentation, clearly distinguishing symptomatology.

According to the results of the studies focused on the clinical diagnosis:

- Men demonstrated an excessive preoccupation with the aspect of genitals and muscle mass, while women showed obsessive thoughts about excess body hair or facial hair and used cosmetics to cover up their imperfections.
- Women tended to look at themselves in the mirror more often and to change clothes, while men dedicated themselves to doing exercises in order to gain muscle mass.
- Women showed a major preoccupation with how other people would perceive them and used to hide their bodies so that other people would not stare at them.

However, in these studies we do not find any reason for these differences, which could be largely explained from a sociocultural and gender perspective. In Western society, men and women are influenced in different and specific ways with regard to their body and appearance. This is related to the definition of the masculine and the feminine, whereby beauty is more commonly associated with the feminine and strength with the masculine, with men and women treating sexuality and desire differently. Women, more than men, take part in jobs in which presence and social interaction are determinants [34].

Naomi Wolf [35], in her book *The Beauty Myth* analyzes how in the eighteenth and nineteenth centuries the beauty myth:

> …in its modern form gained ground after the upheavals of industrialization, as the work unit of the family was destroyed, and urbanization and the emerging factory system demanded what social engineers of the time termed the 'separate sphere' of domesticity, which supported the new labor category of the 'breadwinner' who left home for the workplace during the day. The middle class expanded, the standards of living and of literacy rose, the size of families shrank; a new class of literate, idle women developed, on whose submission to enforced domesticity the evolving system of industrial capitalism depended.

According to the idea of the myth gaining ground, Martínez Benlloch et al. point out that "in the twentieth century, especially since the thirties, fashion has been the mirror into which women look, prevailing in industrialized countries, termed the fetishism of the fit." This changes the beauty stereotype, from the imaginary feminine of pompous forms, represented by the binomial femininity = maternity, to the more androgynous stereotype, of pre-pubescent, slim feminine bodies [36].

However, in this culture, it is not only a certain beauty ideal that is important, but the cult of youth as well, which means to make up not only your face, but also your age [37].

The majority of authors who deal with body image and gender have made an approach to the differentiated reality of men and women. In general, men are shown through the exhibition and the instrumentalization of their body for strength and work, giving priority in male beauty standards to the "masculine vigor" hidden in body strength and fundamentally focused on a muscular and athletic core. This "masculine vigor" also makes allusion to the importance of the genital aspect (for men), which tends to be one of the key areas for the disorder. Nevertheless, the main goals of female body learning are reproduction and seduction. Regarding reproduction, female genital organs are not mentioned, they remain unmentionable in the social sphere, and therefore they are not part of a dysmorphobic female area.

This differentiated instrumentalization leads to constant examination by society of female bodies. On the contrary, male bodies do not suffer that much from the effects of beauty norms, fashion, the constant need to make up, weight loss and gain diets, the effects of esthetic surgery, etc., as there is no need for them to be expressive, just active. As a consequence, women become damaged. In addition, other authors highlight the notion that while men have a holistic idea about bodies, more oriented toward functional aspects such as "keeping fit," women generally function with body images predominantly focusing on form rather than on function. At the same time, women have fragmented views of themselves and try to adjust these fragments to cultural standards [38].

In this way, returning to the headline of this section, the clinical differences of BDD cannot be separated from the existing inequality between men and women taking into consideration image and corporal identity being key elements in the maintenance of this inequality.

9.6 Psychopathology and Gender

> "The critique of gender norms must be situated within the context of lives as they are lived and must be guided by the question of what maximizes the possibilities for a livable life, what minimizes the possibility of an unbearable life, or, indeed, the social or literal death."
> Butler [39]

Although it is important to place on record the fact that body dissatisfaction is not always a disorder; when preoccupation and dissatisfaction with the body do not adjust to reality, occupying one's mind with intensity and frequency, and generating discomfort, interfering in everyday life, we are dealing with body image disorders. Body image is a representation of the human body that every one of us builds in his or her mind [40] and an experience that he or she has with his or her body [41].

Nowadays, there are investigations that demonstrate the relation between body image alterations, dissatisfaction with one's body and how ideas and cognitions about one's body affect the body image and self-image. The acceptance of one's body scheme is the basis of identity. In other words, the body we are born with is unique and unrepeatable; and this uniqueness is exactly what a person needs to recognize himself/herself and to be what he/she is.

The question that in this case a person could ask himself/herself would be why there are some individuals who become obsessed with their look and corporal image and build their lives around changing it, rendering this a characteristic feature of BDD, whereas other individuals experience the corporal image in an unsatisfactory way and believe that by undertaking some changes a normal life can be lived. The primary preoccupation of dysmorphophobic patients is appearance, the image that the body offers to themselves and to other people. They believe that this defect determines or identifies their psychic, intimate, and personal life of a human being, which could be considered a secondary aspect of an identity problem. The patient feels marginalized, rejected, eventually stigmatized by the deformity. This is a stigma that can reveal intimacy; thus, having got rid of it, he/she can be accepted [42].

It is this feeling of wrongness, unfairness, and misconception that strengthens the feeling of desperation and the eagerness to change, alter, and/or hide. Being focused on the defects, the scrutiny, and the constant checking of grooming or hygiene, there is a tendency to avoid comparison with other people and to constantly look for acceptance, either to have the defect minimized or accepted. All this merely creates a vicious circle that increases discomfort.

As previously described, the disorder is structured by two main axes: on the one hand, the distorted self-perception that does not reach the desired beauty or perfection, and on the other the shame of exposing to another individual and not being accepted because of the defect. An explanatory deconstruction of both dimensions and their relationship to gender factors follows below.

9.6.1 Beauty and Defect: To Occupy an Ideal Place Is Actually Not Having a Place.

> "Yes, I know. You haven't the slightest idea what I'm talking about. Beauty has long since disappeared. It has slipped beneath the surface of the noise, the noise of words, sunk deep as Atlantis. The only thing left of it is the word, whose meaning loses clarity from year to year." Milán Kundera

The author Silvia Tulbert develops in her work [43] an explanation regarding the esthetic surgery boom in our society. Such an explanation provides orientation with regard to the actual causes of the increase in defect perception in our society. According to the author's statements, we are facing a complex phenomenon that requires us to take an array of factors into consideration:

1. Subjective factors related to the need to adjust to an ideal model to maintain the level of self-esteem.
2. Relational factors referring to the body image needed to achieve recognition in a business or erotic market.
3. Historic social and cultural factors that place a woman as an object, obstructing the assumption and expression of their subjectivity.
4. Characteristics of our society associated with the rise of the body cult.
5. Supply generates the demand, suitable for the society of the market.

9.6.1.1 Body Image and Self-Esteem

Preoccupation with adjusting the actual body to the ideal image does not only respond to the norm, but it functions like a powerful normalization strategy. It produces bodies able to self-control and self-discipline, ready to transform and improve at the disposal of social mandates and domination and submission relationships. Nevertheless, women experience such practices as power, freedom, and control of sources, and they perceive them as means of achieving beauty, acceptance, and success in the social, work, and sexual arenas, and of having an influence on others. These experiences explain the lack of an increase in the pathological manifestations under consideration, because they are located within the normal standard framework.

This is further complicated by the intersectional position of the body, where there are different aspects that overlap: the body as a material means through which we are included in a social space; the body as a place of embodiment of a subjective position with opportunities and the supposed associated limitations. Finally, a necessity is the support of pleasure and pain, as a reflection of other people's viewpoints and interpretations.

The cultural ideals are originally transferred by families with nuances for the different race, social, educational, labor, national, and regional classes that are modulated by the subjectivity of the transmitters. The corporally ideal self refers to the models that the self tries to emulate to retain his/her self-esteem. The central place for this ideal corresponds to the representations of femininity and masculinity, in the body image and in behavior.

The demand to adjust to a cultural stereotype is more intense in the case of women than in men. The patriarchal culture expects women to be available to satisfy other people's desires. The willingness to be recognized as desirable contributes to the fact that they find themselves more likely to be in a position of an object destined to please others than in a position of being the subject of their wishes. This willingness appears from the identification of women by masculine evaluation, with the corresponding subjective division. Men watch women and women observe how they are watched, and it determines not only how male–female relationships work, but the woman's relationship with herself as well [44]. This position as an object makes a woman more vulnerable in the face of the demands of those who are considered subjects, and the environment.

The gender construction and the attribution to the sexual body start before the birth, and they remain through the life cycle of the individual, taking into consideration the continuous requirement of the necessary correspondence between them. Scientific, philosophical, esthetic or religious discourses are not just abstractions without effect, taking part as a gender technology and working as practical regulations that build the body [45]. Foucault affirms self-discipline, that power does not need to manifest as physical violence to impose rules. It is enough to be under a watchful eye, thus creating self-control. Because women are more attached to this watching, because of their social family subordination, the normalizing mechanism reproduces a cultural code of the differences and power relations between sexes [46].

9.6.1.2 Medical Discourse

It is easy to assess the junction between the body ideal, particularly the female body, and some of the medical proposals that also create body models related to health. The medicine and the aesthetic surgery associate sexual, labor or social success, the ability to seduce, and the essence of identity with the stereotypes imposed on sexual bodies. They define masculinity and femininity, and subordinate the value of the individuals to correspondence with these stereotypes. As in publicity, in general they produce a social stereotype and contribute to reinforcing the criteria offering models of identification and self-perception, pathologizing and medicalizing the physical aspect, and providing medical solutions for the aforementioned *pathology*.

Medical solutions reinforce the symptom. It is hoped to correct in the real body the dissatisfaction or distortion of the body image that corresponds to another order. Thus, the body becomes a screen concealing the conflicts of the subject.

The discourse of the achievable ideal has created a short circuit. In all manner of ways, they try to fill the gaps and block the conflicts inherent to human existence by creating an ideal image. The elaboration is substituted by the actual deed.

In opposition to the unity of the imaginary identity, the symbolic articulation introduces the recognition of the difference, not only between oneself and others, but also within the bosom of one's subjectivity.

With the collapse of this model, alienation is produced:

1. The organism turns transparent, potentially everything in the body can be seen, divided, and modified, and the body loses its organic unity in order to be transformed into a combination of organs without a body [47].
2. The corporality becomes disorganized as the subject does not recognize himself/herself in his/her image, nor in his/her body as a consequence.
3. Subjective models are lost, in a search for the ideal.
4. The self-image does not function with the perception, body experiences, and subjectivity, but is exalted and begins to occupy the place of the ideal of oneself, nullifying the ability to direct the activity, intellectual, ethical, and esthetic values.
5. Finally, we know that the relationship with the body is based on the external appearance; these short-circuits encourage the hope of obtaining the bonus of love and at the same time the bonus of pleasure in one's body.

This alienation supposes that there is a breeding ground for the occurrence of body image disorders and the risk of defective self-perception. Social and medical responses also come together with the pattern of symptomatic conduct, and trigger BDD.

9.6.2 Shame

> "The history of humanity is the long succession of synonyms for the same word. To contradict it is a duty." René Char

As we mentioned at the beginning, the BDD scheme is based on two aspects: defect and shame. In spite of being an omnipresent affect, the shame is barely described in books on psychology, psychopathology, and psychiatry. One of the earliest authors defines it as a feeling of insult directed at self-confidence and confidence in others [48]. Lewis described shame as a loss of self-esteem, which in the esteem of other people results in fury or anger that acts in order to regain the sense of being valued [49]. Wilson thought that shame is a strong feeling of being different and worth less than other human beings [50]. Tomkins described shame as one of the nine human affects [51], such as indignity, transgression, and alienation. He describes it as an impediment to the expression of interest, excitement or joy that interferes with the pleasure of an experience. Erikson developed the second evolutionary state centered on the autonomy versus shame and doubt. "The sense of self-control without a loss of self-esteem is the source of the sense of free will. From the inevitable sense of a loss of self-control and from the parental overcontrol comes a propensity for doubts and shame" [52]. Sullivan described the dynamics of shame with the term anxiety: "in the meaning that I use this term, shame is a sign of the fact that one's self-esteem is in danger. Anxiety is a sign of the danger for self-respect..." [53].

In addition to common usage, the Royal Academy of Spanish Language shows us different definitions of the word. On the one hand, the word's meaning varies from the discomfiture of mood, which turns the face red, caused by some misconduct, or by some dishonorable and humiliating act (their own or someone else's) as punishment for it. This would consist of exposing the accused to the affront and public confusion with some sign that would denote the crime: *put to shame*. On the other hand, shame can come from self-respect, an estimation of the own honor or dishonor, passing through the external parts of the generating organs [54]. The confusion concerning the term can be explained by the different-level analysis of the aforementioned affect.

Gershen Kaufman [55] realizes an analysis of shame on three levels:

First of all, shame is a moral feeling. An individual can feel ashamed of misbehaving, of diverging from the established norms of the environment. It refers to the ideal and to narcissism. This level is related to the previous chapter as a solution to the conflict, in the face of the organized and demanding ideal and an offer of solutions and methods for reaching the aforementioned ideal (gym, diet, surgery, creams, aesthetic treatments, etc.). The individual with damaged self-perception feels ashamed of himself/herself and tries to "behave in an appropriate way for the environment."

Second, shame is an existential feeling that concerns a person who is "feeling naked." Shame reveals the intimacy of every human being. Its deep subjectivity is related to self-esteem and the esteem of others. The feeling of shame comes from the relational experience where an individual feels himself exposed to other people looking.

The experience of the lack of a feeling of admiration is based on shame. Dysmorphophobia is a body phobia, a rejection of the own body, an external fear of not being accepted, in the face of which the individual responds with the shame of the body.

This is a kind of psychic suffering for someone who is trying to resolve his/her serious relational problems, because of the shame he/she conceals himself/herself behind *security systems*, which are directed toward "self-protection," such as image control. The disabling conviction in which the defect is inside of oneself forms the basis of dysmorphophobia. It is difficult that this conviction (of being someone defective) dissolves and passes to the acceptation and validation of one's own singularity. The recognition of the aforementioned singularity becomes more complicated when we deal with a woman who identifies herself as an object, as it is typical of her to validate her own wishes and recognize them without internalizing someone else watching. The antidote of shame is the acceptance, feeling accepted, but with our own specificity. What was considered a defect is transformed into the acceptation of one's singularity.

Velasco relates shame to initiative: daring to be myself, daring to question an ideal, what "I am supposed to be,", is always an experience that leads to "shame." Moreover, the belief of being flawed in the eyes of another individual, blocks any type of initiative (shame of being) [56]. The resignation of the subjective being, the resignation to daring and to disobeying or contradicting, as Char suggested, once again imply the confirmation of the norm and uniformity. It is in this field where male and female body ideals are located, and it is in this field, as well, where DBB hatches as hyperadaptation to the surrounding and to the ideal, to the detriment of intense suffering and resignation to subjectivity and difference.

Last, shame is a social feeling that involves the subject's identity. It is a feeling that possesses social control effects. It avoids the subject having to separate from norms and values that are inside the social contract fundaments; the main element is the need to belong to a community and to be recognized by it. English targeted shame and social control directly, describing shame as the price to pay for the child's internalization of a specific control message coming from his family and culture. Its effect consists of inhibition, limitation, and control of expanding curiosity [57].

From a sociological point of view, the post-modern society is defined as a risk society, based on the fact that contemporary society cannot rely on its legitimacy with regard to positivist goals, but by avoiding wrongness. It is in this new form of legitimacy where the emotional chain of horror–shame–worry acquires further importance and an indispensable social function [58].

There are not many reasons to discuss the idea that states that emotion generally starts from social interaction or that are social norms that dictate emotional answers in particular circumstances and for determinate groups of people. The role that the individual plays in society, as a vast array of psychological and anthropological studies proves, is also determinant in the experiencing of emotions [59–62].

Shame has also been defined in terms of a power relationship, in which the individual with tendency to suffer from shame finds himself/herself in a relatively weak position in comparison to the other individual. This is because, in order to feel shame, there is not only a negative evaluation of oneself, the influence of the vision of a third individual is also added. There are different ways through which culture and social environment can shape shame experiences, one of them being the development of what is and what is not shameful. Western societies build negative identities from those who are less competent, less productive, deformed or somehow considered unattractive or immoral. It seems reasonable to think that some negative identities are more susceptible to suffering these feelings [63].

Conclusion

Human beings need to join some of the identity categories in order to be recognized in our community. Male and female categorization could be listed amongst the simplest. These categories have varied historically, depending on their utility to the existing balance. Identification with uniform gender ideals narrows living spaces in the same manner as the concepts of unification and over-determination with regard to beauty and defect.

References

1. Morselli E. Sulla dismorfofobia e sulla tafetofobia. Bull Acad Med Genova. 1986;VI:110.
2. Berrios GE, Kan CS. A conceptual and quantitative analysis of 178 historical cases of dysmorphophobia. Acta Psychiatr Scand. 1996;94:1–7.
3. Berrios GE. The history of mental symptoms. Cambridge: Cambridge University Press; 1996. p. 263–8.
4. Tanzi E. A textbook of mental diseases. Robertson WF, Mckenzie TC (trans.) London: Rebman Limited; 1909.
5. Stutte H. Thersites-Komplex. A Criança Portuguesa. 1962–1963;21:451–456.
6. Fuentenebro de Diego F, Rojo A, Valiente C. Psicopatología y fenomenología de la corporalidad. Madrid: Feito; 2006. p. 249–65.
7. American Psychiatric Association. Diagnostic and statistical manual of mental disorders. 4th ed. Text rev. Washington, DC: American Psychiatric Association; 2000.
8. Phillips KA, Wilhelm S, Koran LM, Didie ER, Fallon BA, Feusner J, Stein DJ. Body dysmorphic disorder: some key issues for DSM-5. Depress Anxiety. 2010;27(6):573–91.
9. Phillips KA, Pope HG, McElroy SL, Hudson JI, Keck PE. Body dysmorphic disorder: symptom or syndrome. Or Phillips and colleagues reply (Letter). Am J Psychiatry. 1994;15t:461–2.
10. Thomas CS. Dysmorphophobia: a question of definition. Br J Psychiatry. 1984;144:513–6.
11. Andreasen NC, Bardach J. Dysmorphophobia: symptom or disease? Am J Psychiatry. 1977;134:673–6.
12. Bernad Polo JM, Pérez A. Trastorno dismórfico corporal. In: García-Campayo J et al., editors. Actualización en trastornos somatomorfos. Madrid: Médica Panamericana; 2001.
13. Conesa LL, Masanet MJ, Pérez JF, et al. Trastorno dismórfico corporal: una entidad nosológica debatida. An Psiquiatr (Madrid). 1996;12(2):76–84.
14. Jerome L. Body dysmorphic disorder: symptom or syndrome (Letter; comment). Am J Psychiatry. 1994;151:460–1.
15. Solyom L, Di Nicola VF, Phil M, Sookman D, Luchins D. Is there an obsessive psychosis? Aetiological and prognostic factors of an atypical form of obsessive compulsive neurosis. Can J Psychiatr. 1985;30:372–9.
16. Berrios GE. TOC y enfermedad neurológica: estado de la cuestión. In: Vallejo J, editor. Estados obsesivos. Madrid: Salvat; 1995.
17. Schachter M. Nervoses dysmorphiques (complexes de laideur) et delire ou conviction delirante de dysmorphie. Ann Med Psychol (Paris). 1971;129:723–45.
18. López-Ibor JJ, López-Ibor Aliño JJ. El Cuerpo y la Corporalidad. España: Gredos; 1974. p. 165–6.
19. Phillips KA. Body dysmorphic disorder: the distress of imagined ugliness. Am J Psychiatry. 1991;148:1138–49.
20. De-Leon J, Bott A, Simpson GM. Dysmorphophobia: body dysmorphic disorder or delusional disorder. Somatic subtype? Compr Psychiatry. 1989;30:457–72.
21. Neziroglu FA, Yaryura-Tobias JA. Exposure, response prevention and cognitive therapy in the treatment of body dysmorphic disorder. Behav Ther. 1993;24:431–8.
22. Phillips KA, McElroy SL. Insight, overvalued ideation, and delusional thinking in body dysmorphic disorder: theoretical and treatment implications. J Nerv Ment Dis. 1993;181:699–702.
23. McElroy SL, Phillips KA, Keck Jr PE, et al. Body dysmorphic disorder: does it have a psychotic subtype? J Clin Psychiatry. 1993;54:389–95.
24. Phillips KA, McElroy SL, Keck Jr P, Pope Jr H, Hudson JI. Body dysmorphic disorder: 30 cases of imagined ugliness. Am J Psychiatry. 1993;150:302–8.
25. Phillips KA, McElroy SL, Keck Jr PE, et al. A comparison of delusional and nondelusional body dysmorphic disorder in 100 cases. Psychopharmacol Bull. 1994;30:179–86.

26. Phillips KA. Gender differences in body dysmorphic disorder. J Nerv Ment Dis. 1997;185:570–7.
27. Phillips KA. Gender similarities and differences in 200 individuals with body dysmorphic disorder. Compr Psychiatry. 2006;47:77–87.
28. Perugi G. "Gender-related differences in body dysmorphic disorder" (dysmorphophobia). J Nerv Ment Dis. 1997;185:578–82.
29. Turner BS. Avances recientes en la teoría del cuerpo, en Carmen Bañuelos, (coord.) Monográfico sobre Perspectivas en Teoría del Cuerpo. REIS Revista Española de Investigaciones Sociológicas. Nº 58; Octubre–Diciembre 1994, p. 11–39.
30. Mauss M. Técnicas y movimientos corporales (1.ª ed. francesa 1936). Madrid: Sociología y Antropología, Tecnos; 1991. p. 335–356.
31. Douglas M. Símbolos naturales (1.ª ed. Inglesa, 1970; 1.ª ed. castellana, 1978). Madrid: Alianza Universidad.
32. Csordas TJ. Introduction: the body as representation and being-in-the-world. In: Csordas TJ, editor. Embodiment and experience. The existential ground of *culture and self*. Cambridge: Cambridge University Press; 1994.
33. Connell RW. Men's bodies. In: Connell RW, editor. Masculinities. Oxford/Cambridge: Polity Press; 1995. p. 45–67.
34. Esteban ML. Antropología del cuerpo. Barcelona: Bellaterra; 2013.
35. Wolf N. El mito de la belleza. Barcelona: Emecé; 1991.
36. Toro J. El cuerpo como delito. Anorexia, bulimia, cultura y sociedad. Barcelona: Ariel ciencia; 1996.
37. Gordon R. Anorexia y bulimia. Anatomía de una epidemia social. Barcelona: Ariel; 1994.
38. Martínez Benlloch I (coord). Género, desarrollo psico-social y trastornos de la imagen. Madrid: Instituto de la Mujer, Serie Estudios; 2001.
39. Butler J. Deshacer el género. Barcelona: Paidos; 2006.
40. Raich RM. Imagen corporal. Madrid: Pirámide; 2000.
41. Guimón J. Los lugares del cuerpo. Neurobiología y psicosociología de la corporalidad. Paidos: Fundació Vidal i Barraguer; 1999.
42. López-Ibor JJ, Ortiz T, López-Ibor MI. Percepción, Vivencia e Identidad Corporales. Actas Esp Psiquiatr. 2011;39:3–118.
43. Tulbert S. Culto a la imagen, sacrificio del cuerpo. [aut. libro] Mª Isabel Val del Valdivieso y Henar Gallego Franco. *Las huellas de Focault en la Historiografía.* Barcelona: Icaria Editorial; 2013. p. 73–99.
44. Berger J. Modos de ver. Barcelona: Gustavo Gili; 2000.
45. Lauretis T. Technologies of gender. Essays on theory, film and fiction. London: Macmillan; 1989.
46. Focault M. Tecnologías del yo y otros textos. Barcelona: Paidos; 1990.
47. Braidotti R. Des organes sans corps. Paris: Les Cashiers du Grif; 1987. p. 7–22.
48. Lynd HM. On shame and the search of identity. New York: Wiley; 1958.
49. Lewis HB. Shame and guilt in neurosis. New York: International Universities Press; 1971.
50. Wilson SD. Release from shame: recovery for adult children of dysfunctional families. Downers Grove, IL: Interuniversities Press; 1990.
51. Tomkins SS. Affect, imagery and consciousness, The negative affects, vol. 2. New York: Springer; 1963.
52. Erikson EH. Childhood and society. New York: Norton; 1950.
53. Sullivan HS. Problems of communication in the interview. [aut. libro] In: Perry H, Gawel M, editors. The psychoanalytic interview. New York: Norton; 1954. p. 206–226.
54. RAE. Diccionario de la lengua Española. Madrid: RAE; 2001.
55. Kauffman G. The psychology of shame. New York: Springer; 1989.
56. Velasco R. Dismorfofobia o verguenza del cuerpo. Clinica e Investigación Relacional. 2010;4:208–20.
57. English F. Shame and social control. Trans Anal J. 1975;5:24–8.
58. Alastuey B. El contenido emocional de la comunicación en la sociedad del riesgo. Reis. 1999;87:221–53.

59. Cash TF. Developmental teasing about physical appearance: retrospective descriptions and relationships with boy image. Soc Behav Pers. 1995;23:123–30.
60. Cash TF, Pruzinsky T. Body image: a handbook of theory, research, and clinical practice. New York: Guilford; 2002.
61. Veale D. Advances in a cognitive behavioural model of body dysmorphic disorder. Body Image. 2004;1:113–25.
62. Veale D. Mirror, mirror on the wall, who is the ugliest of them all? The psychopathology of mirror gazing in body dysmorphic disorder. Behav Res Ther. 2001;39:1381–93.
63. Leeming D, Boyle M. Shame as a social phenomenon: a critical analysis of the concept of dispositional shame. Psychol Psychother. 2004;77:375–96.

Eating Disorders

10

Margarita Sáenz-Herrero, Marta Zubia, Nuria Nuñez, and Josep Toro-Tralleras

The best was having nothing. No hope. No name in the throat.
And finding the breath in you, the body, to ask.
Tracy K. Smith

One cannot think well, love well, sleep well if one has not dined well.
Women have served all these centuries as looking glasses possessing the magic and delicious power of reflecting the figure of man at twice its natural size.
Virginia Woolf

Abstract

Eating disorders are highly important and affect women more frequently than men. This is because of their clinical severity, comorbidities, and increasing prevalence, as well as their social repercussions. It is impossible to deny that eating disorders are multidetermined conditions. Most of those who treat or research them are reconciled to the need to approach them broadly and flexibly. Implicating genetic factors in a disorder such as anorexia or bulimia nervosa is sensitive and the potential for misunderstanding and misusing gender theoretical concepts is very real. Psychiatry has a long, unfortunate history of

M. Sáenz-Herrero (✉)
University of the Basque Country UPV/EHU, Vitoria, Spain

Department of Psychiatry, Alava University Hospital, Vitoria, Spain
e-mail: margarita.saenzherrero@osakidetza.net

M. Zubia
Department of Psychiatry, Alava University Hospital, Vitoria, Spain
e-mail: marta.zubiamartin@osakidetza.net

N. Nuñez
Alava University Hospital, Vitoria, Spain
e-mail: Nuria.nunezmorales@osakidetza.net

J. Toro-Tralleras
University of Barcelona, Barcelona, Spain
e-mail: JTORO@clinic.ub.es

M. Sáenz-Herrero (ed.), *Psychopathology in Women*,
DOI 10.1007/978-3-319-05870-2_10

misconstructing and pathologizing female behavior. Only recently has there been broader theoretical appreciation of the power of gender differences in self-development and the adverse effects of stereotyping children too rigidly by sex or gender. This is our objective in this chapter. Clinicians have made an effort to create a multidimensional model for the explanation of eating disorders. However, this tends to omit the crucial dimension of culture, which includes the gender perspective.

10.1 Introduction

Hunger and appetite are bound together in the history of the world. Eating behavior communicates socially through the symbolic meaning that transcends the act of ingesting. From birth, we are prone to seeking relationships with others while simultaneously satisfying our hunger instinct. The body is the means of experiencing the world and it forms part of all our learning. Through our eating, we relate to the world. We see the world from our body and so the psychopathology of our eating behavior is closely linked to the psychopathology of our body image. Neuroscience has reached the same conclusions through its different methodologies toward phenomenology, psychiatric anthropology and philosophy. Mind, body, and the world interact in the way the individual adapts and survives. Identity is constituted around the physical body and the way we develop a feeling for what our body is like, as sensed by ourselves and as visible to others. This is very different for women and men. We require a relationship between body and culture with a gender perspective. Anorexia nervosa as a psychopathological condition that accords with our current criteria was first described in the nineteenth century, although Richard Morton had noted it two centuries earlier. Bulimia nervosa is a much more recent clinical condition: Gerald Russell first described it in the 1970s. Both pathologies are characterized by abnormalities in eating behavior and the need to control weight. This causes physical consequences and/or alteration of the individual's psychosocial functioning. The psychopathology that is most frequent in a clinical setting is anorexia nervosa (the restriction of food with considerable weight loss as well as body distortion and extreme fear of fatness) and bulimia nervosa (binging episodes and compensatory behaviors such as vomiting as well as fear of gaining weight). Pica, rumination, and sitiophobia are rarer. The incidence of binge eating disorder (BED) and obesity are increasing to pandemic proportions. There seems to be a connection with the cult of the body in Western society and the number of people on a diet, especially women and girls. Both are diagnosed in the *Diagnostic and Statistical Manual of Mental Disorders* (DSM-5).

10.2 Conceptual Aspects: Hunger and Appetite

Roland Barthes stated that "Feeding constitutes a means of communication with the rest" in *Pour une Psycho-Sociologie Contemporaine*, where he demonstrated the individual symbolic relationship maintained with everything involved in de facto nutrition [1].

Feeding has conditioned the evolutionary course of history. *Der Mensch ist, was er isst* (Man is what he eats). Human feeding is one of the basics of culture. However, feeding is not only eating. Food and the act of eating not only involve nutrition; they are also associated with multiple and various existential circumstances. "You are what you eat" cannot be distinguished from "you eat what you are."

The primitive relationship between women and men and food is related to the physiological sensation of hunger. Hunger, rather than appetite, is a biological need. It can cause an individual to die. In today's world, over 10 % of the world's population—or 800 million people—are starving. Hunger is a danger; it biologically limits our existence [2].

Hunger is described as the need for food as a physiological alarm. It is the urge to eat an amount of food to survive. Appetite is understood in a different way. It implies the preference or qualitative selection of what we are going to eat [3]. The difference is obvious: while hunger implies the urge, appetite is linked to the culture, society and customs in which it is immersed [4].

From birth, eating is a social act and a means of communication with others. When the mother breastfeeds she also speaks, looks at, and smiles at the baby. Breastfeeding serves as a bond and communication between them. The baby is designed to seek the relationship. There is a predisposition toward the relationship from birth. The neurologist Damasio saw this as a corporal disposition. Children up to 6 or 7 years old are asked what a mother is: for feeding us. In French, *mam-mam* means both "eating" and "mother" [5].

This is hunger as a vital feeling. In *The Life of Hunger*, Amélie Nothomb stated: "hunger is me."

"By hunger, I mean the terrible lack within the whole being, the gnawing void, the aspiration not so much to utopian plenitude as to simple reality: where there is nothing I beg for there to be something."

In the same way, food might be sad, exquisite nourishment that can be refused and even vomited in a conflicting or lived situation that threatens the individual. In a social psychology experiment, university students on campus were fed minced meat steak and then told that it had gone bad and that the infirmary would be open all night long. A significant percentage visited the infirmary showing typical symptoms of food poisoning.

The same happens with religious taboos. Mohamed, a 9-year-old boy who had recently arrived from Iran, was given pork by mistake at a Parisian school. Instantaneously, he ate it with pleasure. However, when informed of the mistake made by the canteen, with Islam prohibiting pork, the boy vomited the whole afternoon and needed to be taken home [6]. What was said had activated an area in the brain and when this reacted, it activated digestive motricity. Another experiment was performed using students on a university campus, adding caffeine to their milk and offering them caffeine-free coffee, which significantly altered the hours slept by the group who drank the coffee without caffeine [5].

We should not forget that there is nothing more threatening and intimidating than introducing something alien into the body. This happens every time we eat, when we use the mouth for nutrients to transact [7, 8]. By contrast, nourishment can be exquisite in satisfying situations.

The same happens in a religious sense. In Hebrew to eat is *A'hol*, which literally means unity-total. "Assimilate nutrients," do the same to yourself. Eating for Hebrews is to make a piece of the world a piece of oneself, a piece of God. In the case of Christians, it is the opposite. It is the piece of the world, a piece of God that will become a piece of oneself. "Take this, all of you and eat of it: for this is my body" [5].

Eating means coming into this world with your hands. Eating means knowing in which world you are living. When you make yourself the nourishment, in a way you organize the world, you make it coherent. One who eats calms the anger against the world and oneself while digesting the world of which one is a part.

The nourishment role is very diverse in different cultures and so is the social meaning linked to feeding and the ingestion of food. To Western societies like ours, food is basically what we find on our plates. Nowadays, we consume food that has been packaged in plastic and is decontextualized. There is no story behind it, where it comes from, who has made it, its symbolic value, and its meaning.

In Papua New Guinea, food is considered to have a "vital essence" known as ngaka. This is fundamental for the development and health of the members of that society. Moreover, vital essence is not only within one's body; it is also in the objects with which one makes any kind of contact, including food. One can acquire the properties of the person consuming the dishes that another person prepares ("you are what you eat"). Based on this principle, cannibalism is a common practice in these tribes. They eat their parents once they pass away, incorporating their virtues and abilities.

In the Hindi religion in India, food is shared in an intimate act of class-conscious solidarity. If someone belongs to a lower caste, she or he is rejected.

In their study, Baas and colleagues [9, 10] number the varied uses of food within societies and hence the different meanings that may be attributed to these uses (Table 10.1):

Food and sexuality are widely related in colloquial language and slang, as in words and phrases such as "juicy," "melons," and "forbidden fruit," together with the cherry and its associations related to virginity. "Getting your greens" refers not only to adequate consumption of vegetables but also a regular supply of sexual intercourse.

If eating can, and usually does, take on multiple meanings beyond merely nutritional aspects, the same may be said about a failure to eat or, more accurately, to eat "nothing," as with the first suffragettes whose hunger strikes had a political component: they refused the world in which they had found themselves living. With regard to hunger as an ideology, Susan Bordo analyzed the differences displayed by men and women when they were represented eating. A woman's appetite requires continence and control, while a man's appetite is legitimate and stimulated. "The man-eater" is seen as a dangerous image of female desire, "the temptress." These provocative bodies, "bodies that can talk," have enabled them to be viewed culturally as being responsible for the aggressive and sexual bodily responses of men. In industrialized societies, discipline, control, and the creation of "docile bodies" is a reality for women who receive greater gratification in nourishing and

Table 10.1 Varied uses of food within societies

1. To satisfy hunger and nourish the body
2. To start and maintain personal and business relationships
3. To prove the extension and nature of social relationships
4. To give chances for developing community activities
5. To express love and affection
6. To express individuality
7. To announce differences in the group
8. To prove group belonging
9. To face psychological and emotional stress
10. To indicate social status
11. For rewards and punishments
12. To reinforce self-esteem and merit social recognition
13. To practice political and economic force
14. To prevent, diagnose, and treat physical illnesses
15. To prevent, diagnose, and treat mental disorders
16. To symbolize emotional experiences
17. To manifest piety and devotion
18. To display confidence
19. To express moral feelings
20. To indicate wealth

feeding others than themselves. This underlines the gender divide of power: male public space and private female space.

In practice, there are no social or cultural groups without collective prohibitions with regard to the intake of certain foods. These are solidly established food taboos [11]. In fact, the principal taboos of our culture refer to food and sexuality: cannibalism and incest.

Anthropophagy, or cannibalism, was the most important consequence when the Australopithecus changed to a carnivorous diet. Both then and at any other time in history, cannibalism has appeared in its different forms [12].

Many peoples became cannibals because they lacked the proteins in meat and had no other way of finding them. Thus, the aborigines of Polynesia and Australia were habitual practitioners of anthropophagy until Captain James Cook introduced the pig to these lands. Cook himself fell victim to these practices when he was murdered and devoured by his enemies, who believed that they would acquire the manna, or extraordinary powers, that they attributed to the explorer.

In the sixteenth century, Sawney Bean, a highwayman in Angus (Scotland), held up travelers, killed them and ate them in his cave. Years later, his own daughter was burned alive on a bonfire when it was discovered that she had adopted the same practice. The search for both new food and hunger has been highly important in the development and dissemination of cannibalism. One example comes from Germany during the Thirty Years War (1618–1648), and recently, the tragedy experienced by the survivors of a plane crash in the Andes in the 1960s.

Art has never been far removed from this type of practice either. We only need to take a look at Goya's Black Paintings. The artist's inimitable style leads us to anthropophagy in his oil painting *Saturn Devouring His Son*, which may be viewed at the Prado Museum in Madrid.

10.3 Historical and Social Perspective of Eating Behavior

Historically, food has been closely linked to status and social prestige. The way we eat is a means of affirming and acquiring prestige with regard to others. The desire for social advancement has been a powerful driving force in the transformation of eating [10]. This manifests itself basically through the adoption of foods, dishes, and table manners inspired by those of a social stratum considered to be superior and for whom the aim was to equal or imitate. "I eat, therefore I am," Miguel de Unamuno said in an interesting prologue to the work by the biologist and philosopher, Ramón Turró, *Origins of Knowledge: Hunger* (1945).

10.3.1 Primitive Societies

The first references to body image date back to the Paleolithic era, 30,000–20,000 B.C. This was demonstrated by the discovery of the Venus of Willendorf, a statuette of a woman symbolizing fertility in a village on the banks of the Danube. Currently on show at the Vienna Natural History Museum, it is the image of a prehistoric woman.

Over all the cultures, the representation of the female body has been significantly larger in size than its male counterpart. In Paleolithic representations, female characteristics are unmistakable: adiposity of the torso, large buttocks and huge breasts, all of which underline the role of fertility and nutrition as a symbol of elevated social status.

It is unknown, however, whether the archeological Venuses are faithful representations tailored to the reality of what was observed or are an artistic and idealized vision that symbolizes the desire for abundance and fertility, particularly in a period of the history of humankind when hunger was a threat to human life.

Ford and Beach [13] studied 190 tribal societies and, as was observed in the Paleolithic figures, found in virtually all of them that obese women were considered more beautiful than their thinner counterparts owing to their greater procreative and feeding capacity. On the other hand, men's attractiveness lay rather in their skills and social standing.

Prehistoric sculpture representing the female prototype usually symbolizes female fecundity together with birth-giving and breastfeeding capacity. This was also contained in myths such as Hera's drop of milk, which gave rise to the Milky Way while she was suckling Hercules.

A large woman's body symbolized prosperity and luxury. It even suggested an abundant harvest. Both of these were necessary for group survival. Thinness signified sterility and penury. At a time of frequent famines, thinness was considered to be a messenger of death [14]. This evaluation of the physical attributes of females has never occurred in the animal kingdom, where the males possessing greater size and brighter colors (as well as other characteristics) conduct courtship.

10.3.2 From the Classical World to the Eighteenth Century

In Classical Greece, the attractiveness of the male body took precedence over that of the female. The cult of the male form, including being in good physical condition within the broader context of understanding the body–mind duality in this culture, represents a very different viewpoint from the subsequent concepts defended by Christianity [8].

In Ancient Greek, the word *limos* means "hunger." On adding the word *bou*, which means "a large amount," or *boul*, which means "ox," the resulting term may be translated as "voracious hunger" or "ravenous hunger."

In 970 B.C., Xenophon, in the *Anabasis*, described for the first time in Western culture what we now see as bulimic practices. This referred to the eating habits of some Greek soldiers who withdrew to the mountains of Asia Minor after mounting a campaign against Artaxerxes. It is interesting to note that these soldiers received only scant food rations [15]. Hippocrates distinguished *boulimos*, unhealthy hunger, from ordinary hunger. Aristophanes also used the same term in its meaning of "ravenous hunger."

For the Greeks, the measurement of beauty was the aureal proportion, a practical application of their cult of balance. Hippocrates defines in his work the functioning of the body according to physical elements and bodily humors. Health was synonymous with a state where there is proper balance between the humors, while illness appeared as an imbalance in the interaction between them. The female body is considered weaker and more prone to illness.

In the history of psychiatry, the pathological condition of the female body is a constant. For Greeks, hysteria is a word that means "uterus." Plato [56] in his text *Timaeus* (which has entered Western medical tradition through Galen and the Hippocratic writers) asserted that:

> . . . the matrix or womb in women, which is a living creature within them which longs to bear children. And if it is left unfertilized long beyond the normal time, it causes extreme unrest, strays about the body, blocks the channels of the breath and causes in consequences acute distress and disorders of all kinds. If it is not 'appeased by passion and love' the womb moved from its natural position within the body and, attaching itself to soft internal tissues, gave rise to a wide variety of symptomatic disturbances. (Plato 2005, p. 123)

Hippocrates identified the relevance for health of such factors as dietary restraint, an increase in exercise and a reduction in sleep. Hippocrates was the first to indicate the risk to health of obesity, which he associated with the existence of menstrual changes and infertility in women. He explained that infertility is a consequence of the fat accumulated in obese people, hindering intercourse, and closing the mouth of the womb. Hippocrates saw the therapeutic rules for combating obesity as: having a tough job, sleeping in a hard bed, eating only once a day and preferably food with a high fat content (in order to be satiated quickly), and walking naked as much as possible. More specifically, food needed to be taken soon after a hard day's work when the body was still tired and one had difficulty breathing.

Ancient Rome disagreed with Classical Greece in most of its body esthetic criteria. The Romans were more interested in the peculiarities of faces and people [8]. However, they produced a culture that valued thinness or at least tended to avoid excess weight. As they enjoyed copious banquets, they used vomiting as a means of regulating weight. Both bingeing and vomiting were socially accepted and therefore were integrated into their culture, especially in the middle and upper classes. Roman banquets could include over 20 courses. Whenever the stomach of the diners was full, they went to an adjoining room, the *vomitorium*, where vomiting enabled them to recommence their blow-out. In his treatise on morality, *Dialogi*, Seneca writes in *De consolatione ad Helvia* about Roman practices: "Vomunt ut edant, edunt ut vomant" (they vomit to eat and they eat to vomit).

Moreover, a woman was appreciated fundamentally for her role as mother in which she was obliged to present many children to a State that needed them to ensure its survival against the continuous threat of the intrigues of its enemies [16]. In return, this led some women to rebel against their fate, as was denounced in the writings of the philosopher Favorinus: "Not only do they refuse to breastfeed their children but they resort to a thousand tricks to avoid becoming mothers." Metrodora, a female physician of Greek origin who practiced in the Rome of the first century, wrote a treatise on female illnesses. In her chapter devoted to young women, she described *sitergia*, a Greek term whose literal meaning was "rejection of food."

Medieval cooking stems from a reaction to the banquets and abuse of wine that characterized the final days of the Roman Empire. Just like the Egyptian hermits and anchorites who barely ate enough to stay alive, the early Christians and some mystics interpreted food restraint from the religious viewpoint and practiced fasting as a penance (intensification of prayer, rejection of the world), and as a means of reaching the highest, purest spiritual state. "An emaciated body will pass more easily through the narrow gate of paradise; a light body will resurrect more quickly and a consumed body will be better preserved in the tomb" (Tertullian). Religious asceticism constituted a means of being above bodily needs and reaching a "pure" spiritual state.

In the Middle Ages, the reproductive woman and her figure were the predominant value on the esthetic scale. The female body had to denote corpulence, with a rounded belly as the symbol of fertility. It is significant that the ruling aristocracy were then generically called *popolo grasso*, (plump people), while the working classes are recognized as *popolo magro* (thin people) [10].

The appreciation of fatness implied the rejection of thinness, that is, a flight from hunger, illness, and poverty. The body and its functions were not hidden; everything was natural. It was possible even to defecate or have sexual intercourse in public without creating a scandal or a commotion [17].

For its part, Christian doctrine viewed the body as weak and sinful, requiring strict control and regulation by the mind. Ascesis was the path that led to perfection. Flesh needed to be overcome; the spirit had to triumph. Fasting was the ideal way to achieve this. Religious demands existed so that women would detest their bodies. The less their flesh was consented to, the holier they were. In this way, many women from comfortable classes left their homes and families for a religious life rather than marriage, the only way out for a woman; the convent also offered them the chance to receive an education which otherwise would have been impossible. We should remember that these were patriarchal societies where women were second-class citizens. (At the Council of Trent in 1563, the Inquisition established guidelines to be followed by women whose bodies did not belong to them. If they were virgins, they belonged to God who could call on them and, if not, they belonged to their husbands. If they were possessed, they belonged to the Devil and were persecuted and tortured; at prior Councils such as Nicea, it was discussed whether women had souls.)

Indeed, fasting was a symbol of medieval ascesis. But while monks fasted to purify their bodies and strengthen themselves before the temptations of the outside world, women sought the liberation of their own bodies, which were considered in Christian thought to be the true origin of sin. We should not forget that Christianity blamed original sin on Eve; she was the one to offer the apple to Adam, whose weakness was to accept it. Eve's original sin was in herself while for Adam sin was positioned in the outside world. It was in this context where "holy anorexia" (anorexia suffered by following God), appears, as noted by Rudolph Bell, a history professor at the University of Rutgers [18]. Bell reviewed the biographies of over 261 Italian nuns from the thirteenth century to the present day and found that many may have suffered anorexia nervosa. One was St. Liberata (St. Wilgefortis, a name that comes from Latin and means "strong virgin"). She challenged her father, the King of Portugal, by refusing to eat when he arranged her marriage. Asking God to take away her beauty, her body became hairy (lanugo, owing to malnutrition) and she even grew a beard. Her father decided to have her crucified rather than allowing her to enter a convent. Another example was St. Catherine of Siena. When she was 26, her idea of devoting her life to God clashed with her father's plan to marry her off. This situation led her to lock herself in her bedroom and refuse to eat. In the end, she entered the Dominicans' order, although she had lost half her body weight. Her head may be found in the church of Saint Domingo in Siena as a relic exhibited behind a glass urn; the rest of her body is buried in Rome and one of her feet is in Venice, as an example of holiness. She said in her final writings that she believed she was ill.

In the Renaissance, and principally in the various European courts, the body and overall appearance was granted a significance that was unknown in medieval Europe. In the court, food was usually guaranteed and habituation to it enabled it to be savored. Physical strength and the battle gave way to personal intrigues. The maintaining or improving of social status did not depend as much on fertility or body frame as on the social importance attributed to an individual, this being down to bearing, speech, manners and appearance [19]. The body became socialized.

From the fourteenth and fifteenth centuries, anorexia began to spread from the convents and the abbeys like an epidemic. This phase, called "secularization of anorexia," continued into the sixteenth and seventeenth centuries. The miraculous maidens appeared, most of them youngsters of humble origins who, by refusing food, attempted to attain the sublime, perfection and purity and, in the process, improve their social and economic standing.

Anorexia was progressively stripped of its religious background and moved to a more vulgar circle, with the appearance of so-called artists of hunger, who would exhibit at fairs and could even be seen in some cafés. Kafka described one of them in his story *An Artist of Hunger*." As Paul Auster asserted in his essay *The Art of Hunger* [20], these new, secularized anorexics did not fast in the same way or for the same reasons as the mystics of the past. Their rejection of food was not an attempt to reject earthly life in order to gain entry to heaven. It was simply a refusal to live of the life into which they had been born. The more prolonged their fasting, the greater the space that death occupied in their lives. Their fasting was a contradiction: to go on with it meant death, but death also ended fasting. Therefore, they needed to stay alive, but only to remain on the edge of the abyss, as reflected in the novel *Hunger* by the Nobel Prize winner, Knut Hamsun.

From the fifteenth to the eighteenth centuries, the large woman remained the model, however. This woman, even when obese, was considered to be attractive and elegant [8], like the fleshy women portrayed by the Italian Renaissance painter, Titian.

The history of the western world, and that of Europe in particular, is littered with characters, eras, and social groups in which bingeing and then vomiting was practiced assiduously. These vomiting individuals included England's Henry VIII and his closest subjects; Pope Alexander Borgia and his courtiers; Bruegel's playful Flemish peasants and Bosch's lacerating throngs; and, much more recently, Britain's King Edward VII of the UK or US President William Taft (all of them men) [21].

According to the Encyclopaedia Britannica of 1797, bulimia is defined as a disease in which the person is affected by a desire to eat insatiably and perpetually, and unless this is satisfied, it leads to fainting. Motherby, in 1785, had already described three types of bulimia: that characteristic of pure hunger; that where hunger ends in vomiting; and that associated with fainting.

We find the most complete reference to this disorder in James, who in 1743 devoted two pages to describing *boulimos* [6]. He noticed that while some patients experience the complication of vomiting after ingesting large amounts of food, others do not. He distinguished in this way between *boulimus* and *caninus apetitus*. Basing his approaches on Galen, he remarked that *boulimus* was caused by an acidic humor contained in the stomach, which produced intense but misleading indications of hunger.

At around the same time, the word "anorexia" was used in medical literature as a synonym for lack of appetite. The first medical approximation to the disorder came in 1689 from Richard Morton, the court physician of William II. In his work *Phthisiologia, seu Exercitationes de phthisi*, which is translated into English and subtitled *A Treatise of Consumptions*, he described a condition of anorexia nervosa with great accuracy. He related the condition of an adolescent boy of 16 and that of a young woman 18, of whom he said: "...I cannot recall in all my life anyone who was so involved with living and so consumed..." [22].

Subsequently, in 1764, Whytt described "nervous atrophy," based on the case of a boy of 14 who, after a period of loss of appetite and weight loss, went through a phase of impulsive ingestion, the symptoms not being attributable to any known pathology. In describing the case, Whytt referred for the first time to bradycardia as a symptom associated with cachexia.

In 1798 in France, Pinel published his *Nosographie Philosophique* [23] where he included anorexia, bulimia and pica in the chapter on digestive neuroses. The writer considered anorexia to be a frequently-presented gastric neurosis.

10.3.3 The Nineteenth Century: The Victorian Model

Many of our sociocultural values appeared to develop and become consolidated in this period, including the origin of slimming culture. Among them were: the existence of a growing bourgeoisie, the development of urban centers, the industrial revolution, and, subsequently, the development of the media [11].

In 1840, Imbert's *Traité Théorique et Pratique des Maladies de Femmes* was published. He included anorexia, bulimia and pica as stomach neuroses and distinguished gastric anorexia from anorexia nervosa, attributing the former to a digestive disorder of gastric origin and the latter to brain alterations. He also remarked on how patients with anorexia nervosa showed a loss of appetite and a great variety of neurotic signs, becoming melancholy, choleric, and fearful.

Two decades later, Marcé (1860), a physician from the University of Paris, described a form of hypochondriacal delirium that was consecutive to dyspepsia and was characterized by rejection of food. Patients, either because of a loss of appetite or discomfort caused by digestion, reach the crazed conclusion that they could not or must not eat.

It was in the midst of the Victorian Age when the contributions by William Gull and Ernest-Charles Lasègue appeared. These two authors began the scientific study of anorexia nervosa. Gull, Queen Victoria's physician, described "hysterical apepsia" in London in 1868. He said that this was a typical condition of young women that led to emaciation and that was initially felt to be of organic origin [24, 25].

Soon afterward in Paris, in 1873, Lasègue published the manuscript *De la Anorèxie Hysterique* where he described the cases of various patients aged between 18 and 22. He emphasized the emotional etiology of the disease, presenting it as a perversion or intellectual anomaly and indicating at its heart perturbed interpersonal relationships and, on occasion, unconscious desires as the basic personality traits of such patients [26].

In his description, Lasègue added something that we feel is important, bearing in mind subsequent interpretations of the anorexic syndrome: "fasting is not total and is completely unconnected with the rejection of foods practiced by the melancholy." As well as underlining emotional alterations resulting from the transition to an adult age in the etiology of the anorexic syndrome, he also indicated the existence of social aspects for the first time. He is probably the first doctor to consider the possibility of inter-family conflict between anorexic patients and their parents [27].

Six months later, Gull (in 1874) used the term "anorexia nervosa" for the first time. This was in an article in which he described the findings derived from the malnutrition of three anorexic patients, without paying attention to emotional aspects. This new name for the disease came about for two reasons: the rejection of the term "apepsia" as no alterations in digestion of food were observed and the rejection of the term "hysteria" on specifying that these patients did not present the clinical history of the typical hysteric. It recognized, however, the role of different psychological aspects that may well intervene in the etiopathogeny of the anorexic condition.

Gender perspective cannot be ignored in the genesis and maintaining of the eating behavioral disorders suffered mainly by women. Men and women have different ways of living in their bodies. At that time in history, women lacked the right to vote, they had no access to university, and they did not even have access to the inheritance of their parents unless they formed a good marriage. Hence, anorexia nervosa may be understood to be a challenge to the established order. It questions health criteria and questions the symptoms as social by incarnating a body exposed to the gaze. The appearance of the disease as a clinical diagnosis occurred at the same time as the appearance of novels written by women, such as Wuthering Heights (initially published under a male pseudonym as this was the only way to get published) by Emily Brontë (who was suspected to suffer from anorexia nervosa), and including the work of Jane Austen. All the female characters in literature up to that time had only been seen from the viewpoint of their relationship with the opposite sex. "And this is such a small part of the life of a woman" (as Virginia Woolf said). Love was the only role possible for women. Woolf [28] wrote that if in Shakespeare's tragedies men had been presented only as lovers of women and never as friends of men, as thinkers, as dreamers: "What few roles they could play! How literature would suffer!" This is how women have suffered in history, with the symptomatic expression of inequality and social unfairness frequently being anorexic symptoms. Many women allow themselves to be locked in the "prison of the body" represented by anorexia nervosa. "Hunger, insomnia, disease" were the three words Oscar Wilde used to describe his time in Reading prison in letters to friends and relatives. The problems of prison are also problems of the body and, in this case, prison became the body for these women.

The prestigious French physician Charcot, known for his study of hysteria at La Salpêtrière Hospital in 1889, proposed parentectomy (the isolation of the patient from her/his family) as a therapeutic formula for patients with anorexia nervosa. He was the first to indicate "fear of obesity" as a reason for refusing to eat.

Meanwhile, Lord Byron was the prototype of the romantic writer whose fame and literary prestige helped to publicize his ideas on the body and the mind. He fasted to clear his mind; he defined himself as "ascetic vegetable eater." He abhorred fatness as in his view it symbolized lethargy, clumsiness, and stupidity. His food restraint was accompanied by physical exercise: "I don't find it at all hard to fast for 48 h. Two years ago, I lived permanently on a diet of a thin slice of bread for breakfast, a dinner of fresh vegetables, only green tea and carbonated water in the interim. These days, when I start thinking that I am consuming, I chew tobacco, mastic gum or laudanum. . ." [29].

The first description of a diet was published in 1863. In it, a layman explained the way to reduce food ingestion with the aim of losing weight. This appeared in all the books that referred to food over subsequent years.

The image of women historically perceived and conceived in terms of their reproductive function started to show a clear change with the development of science. At this time, talk began of combating obesity by reducing food ingestion and increasing physical exercise. In fact, this was a return to Hippocratic advice.

In 1875, the concept of energy balance was described and it was postulated that a greater intake of the foods the body needed led to an excess of weight. Greed or gluttony emerged as the principal cause of obesity. It was also in this period that two causes of obesity were described. On the one hand, there was talk of obesity caused by a physical problem (with symptoms similar to Prader–Willi syndrome), and on the other, obesity due to hyperphagia secondary to a defect in the person's character (with symptoms resembling Pickwick syndrome).

It may be asserted that it was really in the nineteenth century that the first progress in the study of obesity was made, with an important role played by writers who worked almost simultaneously in Edinburgh, Paris, and, subsequently, Germany. In fact, the interest in obesity in the latter country gave rise to numerous physiological theories, some of which are discussed even today [30]. These include body composition, energy conservation, the excess of fat cells as a cause of obesity and the concept of family obesity. In late nineteenth century Belgium, Quetelet developed the Index that bears his name and that relates a person's weight in kilograms to the square of their height in meters. Subsequently, following the introduction of the Lavoisier calorimeter, it was suspected that obesity could well be a metabolic disorder.

10.3.4 Our Most Recent History: The Twentieth Century

In the twentieth century, a true explosion occurred and anorexia nervosa and bulimia nervosa increased to almost epidemic proportions. Specific intervention programs were created for these pathologies and there were major advances in research into obesity. Why was there such a large increase in the number of cases?

Psychopathology, as Jules Henry said, "is the final outcome of all that is wrong with a culture" [31]. Nowhere is this more strikingly true than in anorexia and bulimia, which were barely known two centuries ago, but which have reached epidemic proportions in the twentieth century. Far from being the result of a superficial fashion phenomenon, these disorders reflect our attention to some of the central ills of our culture, from our historical heritage of disdain for the body, to our modern fear of loss of control over our future, to the disquieting meaning of contemporary beauty ideals in an era of greater female presence and power than ever before" [32].

Changes in the incidence of anorexia have been dramatic. In 1945, when Ludwig Binswanger chronicled the now famous case of Ellen West, he said, "from a psychiatric point of view, we are dealing here with something new, with a new symptom" [33].

Anorexia nervosa is clearly, as Paul Garfinkel and David Garner have described it, a multidimensional disorder. It has familial, perceptual, cognitive, and biological factors that interact in varying combinations in different individuals to produce a final common pathway [34].

Bray [35] cited the principal areas connected with scientific developments over the century: the study of food intake and its control, and the use of behavioral measures for losing weight.

Habermas [36], who studied the historic concept of the voracious appetite (*Heisshunger*), saw bulimia nervosa as a much more recent disorder than anorexia nervosa and placed its origin at the start of the twentieth century. He also believed that pressure and the struggle of doctors against obesity originated in this phenomenon.

The contraceptive pill revolution allowed women to separate sex from procreation, as women on the pill could control their fertility. However, although it was acceptable for single men to have sex, when women showed the same attitude it proved disturbing for 1950s Western society. At that time, contrasting with the middle-class women who were once again out of the factories and safely immured at home, the dominant ideal of female beauty was exemplified by Marilyn Monroe. She was often described as femininity incarnate, femaleness embodied.

It is necessary to explore why it is that women who are more oppressed by what Kim Chernin calls "the tyranny of slenderness." This particular oppression is a post-1960s, post-feminist phenomenon.

Gerald Russell published a paper describing and naming bulimia nervosa in 1979. It was not long afterwards that the disorder was recognized as a common problem affecting young women in western societies.

In the early 1980s, attention began to turn to the significance of cultural factors in the pathogenesis of eating disorders. What we should ask is why our culture is so obsessed with keeping our bodies slim, pert, and young; when 500 people were polled about what they feared most in the world, 190 replied: "getting fat." This fear is more bizarre than the anorectic's misperceptions of her body image or the bulimic's compulsive vomiting. This is the desperate placing of our bodies into arenas of control, perhaps one of the few arenas of control that remained available to us in the twentieth century.

In the 1980s, a student of Bordo's described Marilyn Monroe as "a cow." Was this merely a change in what hip, breast and waist sizes were considered attractive? Or had the very idea of incarnate femaleness taken on a different meaning, different associations, the capacity to set up different fantasies and images for the culture of the decade? [37].

Psychopathologies that develop within a culture, far from being anomalies or aberrations, are characteristic expressions of that culture; indeed, they are the crystallization of much that is wrong with it. Every age, Christopher Lasch says, develops its own peculiar forms of pathology that express its underlying structure in an exaggerated manner.

The greater risk of women and girls developing eating disorders has been attributed to social pressure in a male-dominated world. Background cultural factors are often implicated, not only fashion, but also more relevant background structure and social norms.

In the 1980s, Bordo claimed that anorexia is the product of three cultural axes that mark the socially and culturally-mediated relationship that human beings have with their bodies and the way that, through this mediation, they are normalized. First, there is a dualistic axis upon which the body is felt to be separated from the experience of being a person and a mind (Descartes and his separation between mind and body). The second axis is body control, where the body is seen as a mute instrument to be controlled by the person. The third axis is gender/power in which women are subjected to images of female beauty that include youthfulness and slenderness. This is the ideal image of a woman who is not yet a woman, and the tendency of anorectics to retain their adolescence and to resist the more developed womanly form, which is often perceived as fatter and more curved.

Bordo remarked that the body of the anorectic is an illustration of how deeply power relations are etched on our bodies that serve them [38, 39].

Sheila MacLeod also wrote as a recovering anorectic a text that took an existential approach to anorexia nervosa. Female identity is seen as central to the state of anorexia nervosa, which MacLeod viewed as a manifestation of an existential crisis resulting from women's confusion about their being-in-the-world. She focused on the meaning of anorexia nervosa serving as a symbol for both, oppression and resistance, with starvation having its own esthetic.

MacLeod viewed anorexia nervosa as a particular existential dilemma facing women and a specific aspect of female identity. Anorexia nervosa is still constructed as a disease condition that is gendered.

Far from being fundamentally stable, a cultural constant with which we must contrast all culturally relative and institutional forms, the body is assumed to be constantly "in the grip," as Foucault put it, of cultural practices. There is no "natural body." Cultural practices are already and always inscribed, as Foucault underlined, on our bodies and their materiality, their forces, energies, sensations, and pleasures. Our bodies, no less than anything else that is human, are constituted by culture.

Women, besides having bodies, are also associated with the body, which has always been considered the sphere of women in family life, mythology and in scientific, philosophical, and religious ideology. This is related to the maintenance of power relations between sexes throughout history.

Anorexia is not a philosophical attitude but a debilitating affliction. It is quite often a highly conscious and articulate scheme of images and associations presented in these women. In this battle, thinness represents a triumph of the will over the body, and the thin body (that is to say, the non-body) is associated with absolute purity, hyper-intellectuality, and transcendence of the flesh. Fat is associated with the tainting of matter and flesh, wantonness, mental stupor, and mental decay.

"In early Christianity, individuals were exhorted to offset the threat raised by bodily appetites through fasting. Present-day societies have adopted a secular counterpart; it is called the diet. Lacking a moral vocabulary, contemporary societies have projected the notions of good and bad on the images of our own bodies: the idea of God (perfection, purity, and kindliness) is now enclosed in the image of thinness; while that of the Devil (sloth, corruption through appetite and avarice) is incarnated in fatness. We are certainly closer to puritanical tradition than to the early Christians, particularly in our fight for individual self-regulation and our devotion to the work ethic" [17].

Indeed, obesity and eating behavior disorders have an increasing impact on our culture with greater prevalence. There is no break in continuity between the attitudes and behaviors with regard to the body and the diet of the general population, sub-clinical eating disorders and actual clinical cases [11].

Nowadays, religion has lost its privileged position. Our dietary concerns are closely linked to two factors: aesthetics and death. To be "good-looking," "young," and "thin" is an imperious narcissistic necessity; quality of life, new social acquisition, overcoming ageing as a surrogate for immortality. Gaining weight is dangerous because it leads to death in the short or long term. There is now a dark and imperious need for health and beauty, gripped to the self of each individual, that has taken the place of ethics and religion [5].

People have grown increasingly self-centered in today's Western world. Wars may be declared, entire regions may be wiped away by earthquakes, unemployment is bellowing at the door, there is a global economic crisis, but what is most important for certain patients is whether they have been able to control their binges or the lack of control of various types of impulses. The cult of the self is characteristic of all eras but this way of making the body itself the center of everything may lead ethically and culturally to a cul-de-sac [5]. There is the socially transmitted belief that drinking abundant amounts of water is healthy "for internal cleansing" and this has a moral connotation. There is guilt in being fat. The only obsession is weight and the body aesthetic on which thinness and youth depend.

Moreover, we should not ignore the impact of globalization on the world food system. In a world where more food is produced than at any time in history, over 10 % of the population go hungry. The hunger of those 800 million people coincides with another historic record: "globesity," over a billion people are overweight. The obese and the hungry are interconnected. Hunger and obesity are symptoms of the same problem. The road that may lead to eradicating hunger would serve to prevent global epidemics of diabetes and heart complaints. There are moral excuses that act to calm a troubled conscience: the poor are hungry because they are lazy or the rich are fat because they eat fattening food. The prevalence of hunger and obesity affects people too often and in too many places for it to be the consequence of any personal defect. In Mexico, a developing country, there are more obese adolescents than ever, although the number of poor Mexicans is growing. The crucial factor is not economic revenue but the proximity to the border and the habits of their northern neighbors whose processed food is rich in fats and sugar [33].

The weight of sociocultural factors in the genesis of eating behavior disorders are a reality, as described in this historical introduction. So is the role of gender, the distribution of power, ethnicity and social class and wealth distribution at a global level. Everything influences what we eat. We are what we eat and we eat what we are, as we said at the start of this chapter.

10.4 Psychopathology of Eating Behavior

Eating disorders are the pathology most frequently presented by young people. Their medical complications, comorbidity and seriousness make them eligible for inclusion here.

We have divided this section into three parts. The first is devoted to the two syndromes that are most frequently presented in habitual clinical practice and that fundamentally affect women as often as they did two centuries ago: anorexia and bulimia nervosa. The second part discusses eating disorders that have been recently included in the DSM-5, such as bingeing disorder (which is also mostly presented by women) and childhood eating disorders such as pica and rumination (which are presented equally by both sexes). Finally, there are now new ways of presenting the psychopathology of eating behavior that still require a great deal more research in the future.

Epidemiological studies have found that anorexia nervosa and bulimia nervosa occur generally ten times more frequently in women than in men; thus the estimated female-to-male gender ratio would seem to be 10:1 [40].

10.5 Anorexia Nervosa

10.5.1 Epidemiological Data

The lifetime prevalence of anorexia nervosa almost doubled when the broad definition was used, 4.2 % (DSM-5) versus 2.2 % (DSM-IV). The crude mortality rate (CMR) was 5.1 deaths per 1,000 person-years [41].

10.5.2 Clinical Features

The distinguishing clinical feature of anorexia nervosa is extreme restriction of food intake, resulting in extensive weight loss (or a failure to gain weight during growth periods).

The refusal to maintain body weight at or above a minimal level for age and height has two fundamental aspects. First, individuals with anorexia nervosa, mostly women, are required to be significantly underweight, weighing less than 85 % of what is expected. The other essential aspect is that the individual wishes to be underweight and makes conscious attempts to avoid gaining weight.

Despite the fact that individuals with anorexia nervosa are by definition underweight, they are convinced that they will become substantially overweight if they cease their vigorous efforts to remain in control of their eating and exercising.

There is a disturbance in the way in which one's body weight or shape is experienced, an undue influence of body weight on self-evaluation, or a denial of the seriousness of the current low body weight.

Women with anorexia nervosa do not menstruate. Most women have progressed normally through pubertal development and have begun to menstruate before the onset of the eating disorder. However, some girls develop anorexia nervosa before the onset of menstruation.

Once anorexia nervosa has been diagnosed, the clinician is asked to classify the patient into one of two groups:

Restricting type: during the current episode of anorexia nervosa, the person has not regularly engaged in binge eating or purging behavior.

Purging behavior: during the current episode of anorexia nervosa, the person has regularly engaged in binge eating or purging behavior (i.e., self-induced vomiting or the misuse of laxatives, diuretics or enemas).

Individuals with anorexia nervosa usually perceive their size accurately. The problem lies more often in the judgment they make about the size they see. This is determined by socio-cultural factors and affects women more frequently.

It is also striking that this fear of becoming fat typically intensifies as more weight is lost.

The most powerful illustration of the effects of restrictive dieting and weight loss on behavior is an experimental study conducted in 1950 by Ancel Keys at the University of Minnesota. The experiment involved 36 carefully chosen, young, healthy, psychologically normal men who restricted their caloric intake for 6 months as an alternative to military service. What makes the study so important is that many of the experiences observed in the volunteers were the same as those patients with eating disorders. The question is that while anorexia nervosa is mostly presented by women, only men were used for this study. What does this mean? Table 10.2 shows the effects of starvation in the study.

Table 10.3 presents common reasoning errors among patients with eating disorders, as described by Garner and Garfinkel [42].

When a woman insists that the only way to succeed in our culture is to be thin, she could be described by clinicians as possessing distorted reasoning or a misperception of reality. But for most people in Western culture, especially women, slenderness is equated with competence, self-control, and intelligence. There is no firm demarcation between the normal and the pathological, as most women are affected in some way by the cultural construction of female beauty as involving slenderness. This means that most women have some sort of problem in relation to

Table 10.2 Effects of starvation

Attitudes and behavior toward food	
	Food preoccupation
	Collection of recipes, cookbooks, and menus
	Unusual eating habits
	Increased consumption of coffee, tea, and spices
	Gum chewing
	Binge eating
Emotional and social changes	
	Depression
	Anxiety
	Irritability, anger
	Lability
	Psychotic episodes
	Personality changes on psychological tests
	Decreased self-esteem
	Social withdrawal
Cognitive changes	
	Decreased concentration
	Poor judgment
	Apathy
Physical changes	
	Sleep disturbances
	Weakness
	Gastrointestinal disturbances
	Hypersensitivity to noise and light
	Edema (water retention, particularly in ankles)
	Hypothermia and feeling cold
	Paresthesia
	Decreased metabolic rate
	Decreased sexual interest
	Dry skin
	Hair loss

food consumption. There is a continuum of eating problems from dieting to the extremes of anorexia and bulimia nervosa.

Body image disturbance plays a prominent role in the psychopathology of eating disorders. Historically, either the perceptual or the cognitive-affective components of body image disturbance (body image distortion or body image dissatisfaction) have been incorporated into the diagnostic criteria for both anorexia nervosa and bulimia nervosa and focus on the influence of body shape and weight on self-evaluation.

Multiple factors of body image disturbance have been identified. These include body image distortion, body image dissatisfaction, and body image avoidance, which are all highly correlated. Patients with more severe body size distortion

Table 10.3 Reasoning errors

Selective abstraction, or basing a conclusion on isolated details while ignoring contradictory and more salient evidence
Over-generalization, or extracting a rule on the basis of one event and applying it to other dissimilar situations
Magnification, or over-estimation of the significance of undesirable consequent events. Stimuli are embellished with surplus not supported by an objective analysis
Dichotomous or all-or-none reasoning or thinking in extreme and absolute terms. Events can be only black or white, right or wrong, good or bad
Personalization and self-reference, or egocentric interpretations of interpersonal events or over-interpretations of events relating to the self
Superstitious thinking, or believing in the cause–effect relationship of noncontingent events (Garner and Garfinkel)

may benefit most from treatment that focuses on correction of size and weight overestimation. When body image dissatisfaction is more prominent, modifying negative and distorted thoughts and working toward acceptance of one's body may be indicated. Finally, treatment incorporating exposure to situations that provoke anxiety-provoking thoughts about appearance will be beneficial for those patients who exhibit extreme avoidance behaviors.

The anorectic's distorted image of her body, her inability to see it as anything but too fat, although more extreme, is not radically discontinuous, then, from fairly common female misperceptions [37].

Hilde Bruch reported that many anorectics talk of having a ghost inside them or surrounding them, "a dictator who dominates me," as one woman describes it; a little dictator, the "other self," was always reported by Bruch. The anorectic's other self, the self of the uncontrollable appetites, the impurities and taints, the flabby will, and the tendency to mental torpor is the body [37] but it is also the female self. These two selves are perceived as constantly being at war. But it is the male side, with the associated values of greater spirituality, higher intellectuality, and will-power that is being expressed and developed in the anorexic syndrome. For Bordo [37–39], there are two levels of meaning. The first concerns the fear and disdain for traditional female roles and social limitation. The other concerns a deep fear of the female, with all its more nightmarish archetypal associations of voracious hungers and sexual insatiability.

Adolescent anorectics express a characteristic fear of growing up to be mature, sexually developed, and potentially reproductive women. And indeed, as Bruch reports, many anorectics, when children, dreamt and fantasized about growing up to be boys.

Some authors interpreted these symptoms as a species of unconscious feminist protest, involving anger at the limitations of the traditional female role, rejections of values associated with it, and fierce rebellion against allowing their futures to develop in the same direction as their mothers'.

For women, the fatness that goes with normal adult body weight will always have had a sexual dimension, serving as it does both direct reproductive and related social and biological purposes, such as its attractiveness to men. The attempted regulation and control of weight and shape are commonplace among teenage girls searching for a greater sense of ownership of the body and its impulses; the success of such attempts leads to enhanced self-esteem.

The greater risk of women developing eating disorders has been attributed to social pressure in a male-dominated world. Background cultural factors are often implicated, not only fashion-related, but also more relevant background structure and social norms.

An explanation of a multidimensional model of anorexia nervosa should include the crucial dimension of culture and the construction of gender to understand the sociocultural analysis of the phenomenon. This is gender as primary and productive in the emergency of anorexia, rather than as merely a contributing factor.

10.6 Bulimia Nervosa

10.6.1 Definition

From *bous*, ox and *limos*, hunger, bulimia was used in Greece to define a devouring hunger. The term bolism (*bolisme*) appeared in all French medical treatises at least until the fourteenth century, although Pinel, in his *Nosographie Philosophique*, conceived of bulimia as a morbid type consistent with "hunger which is too intense and often insatiable" and included it in the "neuroses of the nutritional functions." During the nineteenth century, the term maintained a semiological meaning synonymous with terms such as *citorexia*, *hyperorexia*, *hyperphagy*, and *sitomania* [1]. In the latter half of the twentieth century, English literature established the nosological nature of bulimia nervosa, this being described by Russell as the appearance of recurring episodes of excessive voraciousness followed by inappropriate compensatory behavior. As in anorexia nervosa, there is both an irrational fear of gaining weight and severe alterations in the body image.

Epidemiologically, several community studies found that the prevalence of bulimia nervosa increased by 30 % when DSM-5 criteria were used, leading to a lifetime prevalence of around 2 % for women.

Mortality and suicide risk are elevated in bulimia nervosa as well, albeit not as markedly as in anorexia nervosa. CMR: 1.7 per 1,000 persons-years [41].

10.6.2 Clinical Features

The salient behavioral characteristic of bulimia nervosa is the frequent occurrence of binge eating episodes. A binge is defined on the basis of two elements: consumption of a large amount of food, and a sense of a loss of control during the eating episode (the feeling that one cannot stop eating or control what or how one is eating).

A second critical characteristic of bulimia nervosa is that following the eating binges, the individual engages in inappropriate attempts to rid her or himself of weight gain. In clinical samples, the most frequent inappropriate behavior is self-induced vomiting. Vomiting is often difficult to induce when the illness begins, but becomes less difficult and more habitual over time. Many individuals with bulimia nervosa eventually induce vomiting not only following binge episodes but also following the consumption of any meal, whether large or small. They also use utilize medications in an attempt to counteract the binges. Commonly, they use laxatives, diuretics, enemas and thyroid medication.

Bulimic episodes usually start from the afternoon and generally include every type of food. However, some studies have demonstrated that patients tend to ingest foods considered to be "taboo" for them, foods that they normally reject because they consider them to be high in calories, carbohydrates and fats. The manner of eating also tends to be altered, being rapid and voracious and mixing tastes, textures and foods. The binge frequency varies according to the seriousness of the disorder, morale, and finally becomes a routine act, without the existence of clear triggers.

Between binges, patients maintain a restrictive diet or even fast, which primes and facilitates the episodes of uncontrolled intake. Many patients find difficulty in feeling satiated at the end of a normal meal and may continue eating. This gives rise to continuous weight changes but without the notable weight loss of anorexia nervosa. Bulimic behavior begins after a period of dieting and there is a record of patients having previously suffered from anorexia nervosa in a significant percentage of cases.

The final aspect in the characterization of bulimia is persistent concern over figure and weight, with a morbid fear of weight gain. For many authors, this is the nuclear psychopathological aspect as it leads the patient to exclusive self-evaluation in terms of weight and figure.

Most bulimic patients present depressive symptoms such as sadness, guilt feelings, low self-esteem and suicidal thoughts.

High anxiety levels form an inseparable part of bulimic behavior. The moments prior to a binge are characterized by unease, excitation, tension and an imperious desire to eat. In this way, anxiety and dysphoria accompany and trigger most binges in bulimic patients. After the loss of control, anxiety may be reduced and subsequently there is an increase in guilt feelings, low self-esteem and fear of growing fat, leading the patient to cause her or himself to vomit. As well as the anxiety associated with the binge, high levels of anxiety between episodes are presented. Abuse of substances, mainly alcohol, together with kleptomania, are among the compulsive behaviors most frequently found in these patients. Many of them present borderline personality features and interpersonal relationship problems.

Complications result from purging and bingeing behaviors (as in the purging behavior of anorectics):

1. Electrolytic alterations such as dehydration and alkalosis as a consequence of vomiting. On occasions, there may be metabolic acidosis due to laxative abuse.
2. Cardiac alterations, with arrhythmias secondary to hypopotasemia and even sudden death.

10.6.3 Conclusion

Like patients with anorexia nervosa, those with bulimia nervosa are over-concerned with their body shape and weight and their self-esteem is regulated in the extreme by these aspects of their appearance. They feel under intense pressure to diet and avoid weight gain. This is more frequent in female patients.

As Bordo points out most women affected by eating disorders are pursuing today's boyish body ideal, which seems to be surrounded by an aura of freedom and independence. However, the body shape of most mature women does not fit the ideal and therefore they must either spend hours each day dieting and exercising or simply give up trying to attain it. In opposition to this, the bodies of mature women tend to have more body fat than the bodies of younger boys and are rounder and fuller. In turn, this "womanish fat" seems to symbolize women's supposedly voracious appetites, and also, for many women, the domesticity they associate with their mothers [37].

Thus, for many women, this appears to be a fight with their own bodies. This is not the pathological body. Instead, the average adult female body that is complexly and ambiguously symbolized is the problem for many women and not an internally distorted perception of their own body or cognitive malfunctions in the processing of information.

There is an embodied perception of the world. This is lived from a situated perspective that is both individual (the person's relation to the world and their experience of life events) and socio-historical. Behind this lies a culture that is driving more, and younger, girls and women into the regimes of rigorous dieting and exercise, largely by encouraging the fear of weight gain. This is normalizing images and ideologies of femininities and notions of female beauty (body image in men is muscular, fit and youthful; masculine beauty as the Grecian model or the David of Michelangelo). This will determine in some way how actual women are much more affected by these pathologies. People live in their bodies with the world, especially the social world. From this viewpoint, culture is seen as lived through the body.

10.7 Feeding and Eating Disorders Included in DSM-5

10.7.1 Pica

This is also known as "allotriophagy," which derives from Latin and refers to the magpie, a bird celebrated for its excessive appetite [43]. Pica is an extreme degree of dysorexia, that is, a severe disorder of the criteria of qualitative food selection.

The essential feature of pica according to DSM-5 is the eating of one or more non-nutritive, non-food substances on a persistent basis over a period of at least 1 month that is severe enough to warrant clinical attention. Typical substances ingested tend to vary with age and availability, and may include paper, soap, cloth, hair, string, wool, soil, chalk, talcum powder, paint, gum, metal, pebbles, charcoal or coal, ash, clay, starch, or ice. The term non-food is included because the diagnosis of pica does not apply to ingestion of dietary products that have minimal nutritional content. There is typically no aversion to food in general. The eating of non-nutritive, non-food substances must be developmentally inappropriate and not part of a culturally supported or socially normative practice. A minimum age of 2 years is suggested for a pica diagnosis to exclude the developmentally normal mouthing of objects by infants that results in ingestion. The eating of non-nutritive, non-food substances can be an associated feature of other mental health disorders (e.g., intellectual developmental disorder, autism spectrum disorder, schizophrenia). If the eating behavior occurs exclusively in the context of another mental disorder, a separate diagnosis should be made only if the eating behavior is sufficiently severe to warrant additional clinical attention in DSM-5. Pica occurs in both boys and girls. It can occur in women during pregnancy; however, little is known about the course of pica in the postpartum period.

In some populations, the eating of earth or other seemingly non-nutritive substances is believed to be spiritual, medicinal, or of another social value, or may be a culturally or socially normative practice. Such behavior does not warrant a diagnosis of pica. Some individuals may swallow potentially harmful items (e.g., pins, needles, knives) in the context of maladaptive behavior patterns associated with non-suicidal self-injury in personality disorders.

It has also been reported that there is an increase in the comorbidity of pica with other eating disorders (particularly bulimia nervosa), with obsessive–compulsive disorder, with the obsessive personality, and with the dysorexias that characterize pregnancy. With regard to the etiopathogeny of this disorder, this takes in cultural factors, psychological factors including those deriving from inadequate relationships between the child and her/his parents as well as factors that are characteristic of the family dynamic, this being more frequent in families that are seriously dysfunctional and with a greater prevalence of alcoholism, obesity and substance addiction.

The medical complications of pica, over and above those characteristic of the primary disorders that condition it, derive from malnutrition and the harmful nature of the substances ingested, with a frequency of poisoning, intestinal obstructive conditions due to bezoars or foreign bodies (phytobezoars, trichobezoars), perforations or processes of an infectious type.

Rumination (from the Latin *ruminare*, which means "chewing the cud") or mericism (a Greek term with same meaning) [4] is a disorder of low prevalence present in the early stage of life (between 3 and 12 months old). Its presence in adults is very unusual other than in severe cases of mental retardation. It was described by Fabricio d'Acquapendente in 1618 and included by Pinel under digestive neuroses in his *Nosographie Philosophique*.

Rumination consists of repeated and voluntary regurgitation of food ingested followed by new processing (mastication, salivation, swallowing) or expulsion from the oral cavity with the consequent reduction in intake and weight gain. This phenomenon occurs in those who previously presented a correct swallowing function and is therefore secondary. Despite being comparatively unusual, it has an elevated mortality rate, which is approximately 25 % of cases, due among other causes to the high risk of malnutrition or secondary complications in the form of food inhalation and the subsequent development of bronchopneumonia. Over and above the psychological factors involved in the origin of this disorder (almost always related to the mother-child relationship or to other learning aspects and psychomotor development), it is necessary to rule out possible organic causes of the anatomical and physiological aspects of the digestive function that may condition this process. Accordingly, the gastro-esophageal reflux is usually the most frequent cause of mericism [4].

The essential feature of rumination disorder in DSM-5 is the repeated regurgitation of food that occurs after feeding or eating over a period of at least 1 month. Previously swallowed food that may be partially digested is brought up into the mouth without apparent nausea, involuntary retching, or disgust. The food may be re-chewed and then ejected from the mouth or re-swallowed. Regurgitation in rumination disorder should be frequent, occurring at least several times a week, typically daily. The behavior is not better explained by an associated gastrointestinal or other medical condition (e.g., gastro-esophageal reflux, pyloric stenosis) and does not occur exclusively during the course of anorexia nervosa, bulimia nervosa, BED, or avoidant/restrictive food intake disorder. If the symptoms occur in the context of another mental disorder, they must be sufficiently severe to warrant additional clinical attention and should represent a primary aspect of the individual's presentation requiring intervention.

10.7.2 Selective Eating and Food Rejection

This condition is included in the section on ingestion and eating behavior disorders in the DSM-5. However, these are not accompanied by the symptomatic group of body image distortion, purging behavior or fear of getting fat [44] such as avoidant/restrictive food intake disorder.

This diagnosis replaces and extends the DSM-IVTR diagnosis of feeding disorder of infancy or early childhood. The main diagnostic feature of avoidant/

restrictive food intake is avoidance or restriction of food intake manifested by a clinically significant failure to meet requirements for nutrition or insufficient energy intake through oral intake of food. One of the following key features is present: significant weight loss, significant nutritional deficiency (or related health impact), dependence on enteral feeding or oral nutritional supplements, or marked interference with psychosocial functioning. The determination of whether weight loss is significant is a clinical judgment; instead of losing weight, children and adolescents who have not completed growth may not maintain weight or height increases along their developmental trajectory.

Determination of significant nutritional deficiency is also based on clinical assessment (assessment of dietary intake, physical examination, laboratory testing), and the related impact on physical health can be of a similar severity to that seen in anorexia nervosa (e.g., hypothermia, bradycardia, anemia). In severe cases, particularly in infants, malnutrition can be life-threatening. Dependence on enteral feeding or oral nutritional supplements means that supplementary feeding is required to sustain adequate intake.

This does not include avoidance or restriction of food intake related to lack of availability of food or to cultural practices (e.g., religious fasting or normal dieting), nor does it include developmentally normal behaviors (e.g., picky eating in toddlers, reduced intake in older people). The disturbance is not better explained by excessive concern about body weight or shape or by concurrent medical factors or mental disorders.

In some individuals, food avoidance or restriction may be based on the sensory characteristics of the qualities of food, such as extreme sensitivity to appearance, color, smell, texture, temperature, or taste. Such behavior has been described as restrictive eating, selective eating, choosy eating, perseverant eating, chronic food refusal, and food neophobia, and may manifest itself as a refusal to eat particular brands of foods or to tolerate the smell of food being eaten by others. Individuals with heightened sensory sensitivities associated with autism may show similar behaviors.

Food avoidance or restriction may also represent a conditioned negative response associated with food intake following, or in anticipation of, an aversive experience, such as choking: a traumatic investigation, usually involving the gastrointestinal tract; or repeated vomiting. The terms functional dysphagia and globus hystericus have also been used for such conditions.

It is equally common in boys as in girls in infancy and early childhood. If it is comorbid with autism spectrum disorder, it has a male predominance. Food avoidance or restriction related to sensory sensitivities can occur in some physiological conditions, most notably in pregnancy, but it is not usually extreme and does not meet the full criteria for the disorder.

The question is that feeding disorders presenting in childhood have equal prevalence in male and female patients. However, anorexia nervosa, bulimia nervosa, and BED are most frequent in the female population.

10.7.3 Binge Eating Disorder

To our knowledge, no incident studies on BED yet exist. The 12-month prevalence of BED among adult women is 1.6 % and among men it is 0.8 %. Data on the long-term outcome of BED, including mortality, are scarce. In a sample of 68 female in-patients with BED, CMR was 2.9 % after 12 years' follow-up [41].

This is a condition characterized by recurring food binges without the compensatory maneuvering typical of bulimia nervosa.

Binge eating disorder usually makes its appearance in late adolescence or young adulthood and most often affects women who have subjected themselves to strict diets to lose weight and have suffered relapses. The clinical condition is characterized by subjectively perceived recurring binges and behavioral manifestations, or a lack of control over them.

The delimitation of BED as a nosological condition is very recent: it arose as the result of a multicenter study published in 1992 by Spitzer [57]. This established the diagnostic criteria met by a group of individuals who presented recurring binge eating problems but without compensatory behaviors characteristic of bulimia nervosa, such as repeated vomiting or laxative abuse. It was observed in this study that this disorder could be diagnosed with a high index of reliability and that it was very frequent in hospital slimming programs, affecting 30 % of obese patients.

The key aspect of the psychiatric aspect of bingeing does not refer to the amount of food ingested but to the individual's lack of control over intake. This is the feeling the individual experiences on not being able to stop eating, or control what or how much she or he is going to eat. The manifestations of this lack of control are eating very quickly, eating so much that an unpleasant feeling of postprandial fullness is felt, the ingestion of a large amount of food, even though the individual is not hungry, and the feeling of disgust, guilt or depression after the episodes. According to the DSM-5 [45], for a diagnosis of the BED, the binges need to cause a clinically significant malaise, with dissatisfaction during and after the episodes and concern over its effects on weight and body image. The patient may obtain a degree of gratification while she or he is eating, but her or his experience after bingeing is always negative, with feelings of guilt, remorse, rage etc. After bingeing, the patient experiences a deep unease, but in general does not display the compensatory strategies of bulimia nervosa.

Differential diagnosis of BED therefore is made above all with atypical bulimia nervosa. However, the use of compensatory strategies characteristic of bulimia, such as fasting and excessive exercise, is not as frequent. Another difference between the two disorders is the degree of obesity. Indeed, patients with BED frequently present serious obesity (defined as a body mass index equal to or greater than 35) and greater weight fluctuations than patients with bulimia nervosa [46].

Some studies have suggested that "emotional eating" might exist. This affects a group of obese patients whose bingeing responds to emotional stress [45].

Patients with BED compared with other obese patients present a higher rate of personality and panic disorders [47], as well as family dysfunctions with abuse and emotional abandonment although not aggression or sexual abuse [48].

Environmental factors are essential in virtually all the patients in whom obesity develops. Epidemiological studies demonstrate that in the past 20 years the population of obese people in the USA and UK has doubled and this is increasingly affecting the child population. There is talk now of a pandemic and "globesity" [49]. The socio-cultural conditions of the population, the "consumer culture" and the "McDonaldization" of society, together with food technology, subject the public to a pressure that explains the increase in the prevalence of obesity [49], no matter how much the thin esthetic, of the slim body, is imposed. This causes in large sectors of the population, especially in women and girls, dissatisfaction with body image and an increase in the prevalence of eating behavior disorders in the female population.

Personality traits may play a major role in the development of this disorder through three possible mechanisms: first, they may show a predisposition to excessive eating; second, obesity itself, when it begins in the early stages of life, may affect personality development; and finally, the two mechanisms mentioned may act as a combination. The attitude to the body, the impulsiveness, and the relationship with food learned from young ages are key aspects in the genesis of obesity.

Classic literature has associated the passive-dependent personality with obesity, although this has not been demonstrated scientifically. However, it has been reflected in history and literature as in the character of Ignatius Reilly in the novel *A Confederacy of Dunces*. Specific aspects, such as insecurity, hypersensitivity and emotional instability, are more frequent than in the population as a whole; what is not clear is whether it is a prior disposition or a form of adaptation in a subject who finds difficulties in adapting to normality.

On the other hand, comorbidity with personality disorders such as borderline personality disorder is frequent. This suggests that a causal relationship exists between the two conditions, either with a common origin with a genetic and/or environmental basis, or because obesity is secondary to the alteration of the control of impulses that are so frequent in borderline personality disorder. In Western societies, thinness prevails as part of the present canons of beauty and obese people are aware of the social rejection and discrimination that they often receive, as well as suffering the limitations that their weight imposes on them in everyday life. This situation may produce dissatisfaction with their own body and with their body image. Their image becomes a principal source of their concerns and thinness takes top place in their scale of values, above everything else.

An example of the unease these people may experience is "mirror avoidance," which makes them travel large distances to avoid having to look at themselves in the mirror or in the reflection of a shop window. In fact, this suggests that these individuals present a body image disorder that is similar to what occurs in eating behavior disorders.

Body image disturbance that is not modified despite weight loss demonstrates to us the need to treat underlying psychological aspects such as body dissatisfaction and dysmorphophobic and alexithymic aspects.

Also, the anxiety secondary to the undertaking of slimming treatments comprising diets without psychotherapeutic support is often associated with this problem [50], above all in the female population.

The anxiety disorders most frequently associated with the severely obese are agoraphobia, simple phobia and post-traumatic stress syndrome, which is much more frequent than in the general population. It has been suggested that women with a background of violence and rape may seek relief in food [51].

Obesity in women is associated with a greater prevalence of depressive symptoms owing to a greater perception of social stigma, which is much more intense in women and girls. Corporality and body experience constitute a nuclear part of the female identity, as has been explained in previous articles.

10.8 New Conditions Related to the Psychopathology of Eating Behavior and/or Body Image

10.8.1 Orthorexia

This is an ill-defined and insufficiently studied spectrum at present. It consists of extreme concern over whether foods are healthy and contaminant-free. This condition may be related to obsessive health worries, to hypochondriacal fears of illness, and, to a certain extent, to cultural attitudes linked to diets and foods. It is true that restrictive diet anomalies and weight loss may be presented but these may not be considered as atypical or incomplete cases of anorexia nervosa [52]. This disorder may give rise to anemia or vitamin deficiencies and affect the health of children raised with this type of diet, leading to malnutrition. This has created raw vegans, who only eat uncooked vegetables. For example, *Rawer* (2012) is a Dutch documentary about 14-year-old Tom and his mother, Francis, who adhere to a strict diet of raw food (dairy, fish, meat, and eggs are also off limits). It is discovered that Tom is malnourished and not growing at the rate doctors think he should be and child welfare steps in. These are some of the controversial issues raised in the film. There are difficult questions that stem from conflict between health-care providers and families in a world where alternative nutritional practices continue to be viewed as oppositional to the logic of Western science.

10.8.2 Bigorexia

This condition is characterized by excessive concern over seeking bodily perfection through physical exercise. This leads to great dissatisfaction with self-image, exaggerated amounts of exercise, special diets and foods to a degree where there is dependence, and also the consumption of doping substances [53]. This condition is ill-defined at present and related to obsessiveness, perfectionism and dysmorphophobia. It is more frequent in men.

10.8.3 Night Eating Syndrome (Nocturnal Eaters)

Sleep is interrupted in those affected and in this situation/state they overeat. Whether these conditions are due to an eating behavior disorder or whether sufferers are individuals affected by primary sleep anomalies has not yet been defined [54, 55].

10.8.4 Ebriorexia (Drunkorexia)

Food restriction achieved through the ingestion of large amounts of alcohol with the aim of reducing food intake. This type of presentation is more frequent in young women.

10.9 Discussion

Young women present eating disorders more than any other pathology. The effects, complications and comorbidity of these disorders oblige us to assess why it is that they continue to affect women in similar proportions (10:1) to two centuries ago. We have chosen to ignore existing biological factors, studies of genetic factors with greater concordance between monozygotic twins, and the presence of alterations in neuropsychological aspects. Instead, we have focused on the sociocultural aspects that, to a certain extent, shape biology and make these disorders persist over time in a Western world where, owing to a lack of other ethical values, youth and thinness are what matter most.

An image of female thinness leads these dominant cultures to influence teenagers, who internalize these figures as personal values. It is a major achievement to be aware of this. In a society that emphasizes freedom, individual ability and free will and choice, awareness of the complexity and nature of the culture in which we are immersed is an advance with regard to those underlying aspects that condition our behavior, personal choices and even our professional vocations, according to Bourdieu's habitus model. One only achieves success by playing to the cultural norms. It is alienating that a woman feels "nothing" in this post-modern world unless she is slim, thin, unwrinkled, blemish-free, and fat-free (apart from her breasts). Literally a smaller body in the physical sense. We should remember that the ideal male figure has remained the same since the ancient Greeks and an athletic build has been the male beauty ideal throughout history. The post-modern discourse is disturbing, with fixed concepts such as "youth" or "old age" and their corporal expression becoming unstable, fluid, fragmented, and undetermined. They are dominated therefore by more sophisticated technologies that make us believe, for example, that any woman can become a mother after the menopause. "You only need an egg donor." The same happens with the gender paradigm. These discourses are altering the conception and experience of our bodies, encouraging us to imagine possibilities and to close our eyes to limitations and consequences. Anorexia nervosa and bulimia nervosa/binge eating reached epidemic proportions in the twentieth century. The prison of the body in which these patients' lives are transformed has become a clinical reality. New ways of addressing this problem are required. More research is needed to determine the role of gender in the construction of these symptoms. A failure to include the gender paradigm in clinical construction will make it impossible for us to practice good science.

References

1. Álvarez J, Esteban R, Sauvagnat F. Fundamentos de psicopatología psicoanalítica. Madrid: Editorial Síntesis; 2002.
2. Zutt J. Psiquiatría antropológica. Madrid: Gredos; 1974.
3. Alonso Fernández F. Trastornos de la afectividad. In: Compendio de Psiquiatría. 2nd ed. Madrid: Oteo; 1982. p. 217–27.
4. Segarra R. Psicopatología del instinto de nutrición. In: Eguiluz JI, editor. Introducción a la psicopatología. Madrid: IM&C; 2001.
5. Harrus-Révidi G. Psicoanálisis de la gula. Gijón: Trea; 2004.
6. James R. A medical dictionary. Londres: Osborne; 1743.
7. Rozin P. Social and moral aspects of food and eating. In: Rock I, editor. The legacy of Solomon Asch: essays in cognition and social psychology. Hillsdale, NJ: Lawrence Erlbaum Associates; 1990. p. 97–110.
8. Fallon A. Culture in the mirror: sociocultural determinants of body image. In: Cash TF, Pruzinsky T, editors. Body images: development, deviance and change. Nueva York: Guilford; 1990.
9. Baas MA, Wakefield LM, Kolasa KM. Community nutrition and individual food behavior. Minnesota: Burgess; 1979.
10. Contreras J. Antropología de la alimentación. Madrid: Eudema; 1993.
11. Toro J. El cuerpo como delito. Anorexia, bulimia, cultura y sociedad. Barcelona: Ariel Ciencia; 1996.
12. Carson IA. Ritchie. Comida y civilización. Madrid: Alianza; 1986.
13. Ford C, Beach R. Patterns of sexual behaviour. New Haven: Harper and Brothers; 1955.
14. Noordenbos G. Door dik en bun. In: Allagaert P, Cailleau A, editors. Vastenheiligen, wonder meisjes en hongerkunstenaars. Gante: Museum Dr. Guislain; 1991.
15. Stunkard AJ. A history of binge eating. In: Fairburn CG, Wilson GT, editors. Binge eating: nature, assessment and treatment. Nueva York Londres: Guilford; 1993.
16. Von Boehn M. La moda: historia del traje en Europa desde los orígenes del Cristianismo hasta nuestros días (edición española). Barcelona: Salvat; 1944.
17. Gordon RA. Anorexia and bulimia: anatomy of a social epidemic. Oxford: Blackwell; 1990.
18. Bell RM. Holy anorexia. Chicago: Universidad de Chicago Press; 1985.
19. Elias N. The court society. Oxford: Basil Blackwell; 1983.
20. Auster P. El arte del hambre. Ensayos. Barcelona: Edhasa; 1992.
21. Gianninni AJ. A history of bulimia. In: Gianninni AJ, Slaby AE, editors. The eating disorders. Nueva York: Springer; 1993.
22. Morton R. Phthisiolgia, or, a treatise of consumptions. Londres: Smith & Walford; 1694.
23. Pinel PH. Traité medico-philosophique sur l'alienation mental. 2nd ed. Paris: Brosson; 1809.
24. Gull WW. Anorexia nervosa. Trans Clin Soc Lond. 1874;7:22–8.

25. Gull WW. Anorexia nervosa. Lancet. 1888;i:516–7.
26. Lasègue C. De la anorexia hysterique. Archives Générales de Médecine. 1873;1:384–403.
27. Brumberg JJ. Fasting girls. The emergence of anorexia nervosa as a modern disease. Cambridge: Harvard University Press; 1988.
28. Wolf V. Una habitación propia. Barcelona: Seix-Barral; 2001.
29. Nye R. Las memorias de Lord Byron. Barcelona: Salvat; 1991.
30. Brownell KD. History of obesity. In: Brownell KD, Fairburn CG, editors. Eating disorders and obesity. Nueva York Londres: Guilford; 1995.
31. Henry J. Culture against Man. New York: Knopf; 1963.
32. Bordo S. The body and the reproduction of feminity. In: Unbearable weight: feminism, western culture, and the body. Chap. 5. Berkeley, CA: University of California Press; 1985.
33. Binswanger L. The case of Ellen West. In: May R, editor. Existence. New York: Simon and Schuster; 1958.
34. Garfinkel P, Gardner D. Handbook of treatment for Eating disorders. New York: The Guilford Press, 1985
35. Bray GA. Obesity: historical development of scientific and cultural ideas. Int J Obes. 1990;14:909–26.
36. Habermas T. Heisshunger: historische Bedingungen der bulimia nervosa. Frankfurt: Fischer; 1990.
37. Bordo S. Anorexia nervosa: psychopathology as the crystallization of culture. In: Diamond I, Quinby L, editors. Feminism and Foucault. Reflections on resistance. Boston: North East University Press; 1988.
38. Bordo S. Eating disorders: the feminist challenge to the concept of pathology. In: Leder D, editor. The body in medical thought and practice. The Netherlands: Kluwer; 1992.
39. Bordo S. Unbearable weight: feminism, western culture and the body. Berkeley, CA: University California Press; 1992.
40. Zanetti T, Strumia R. Epidemiology of eating disorders. Berlin: Springer; 2013.
41. Smink FR, van Hoeken D, Hoek HW. Epidemiology, course, and outcome of eating disorders. Curr Opin Psychiatry. 2013;26:543–8.
42. Garner D, Garfinkel P. Handbook of treatment of eating disorder. New York: Guildford; 1997.
43. Chatoor I. Feeding and eating disorders of infancy and early childhood. In: Sadock BJ, Sadock VA, editors. Comprehensive textbook of psychiatry. 7th ed. Philadelphia: Lippincott Williams & Wilkins; 2000.
44. Diagnostic and statistical manual of mental disorders. 5th ed. Arlington VA: American Psychiatric Association; 2013.
45. Telch CF, Agras WS. Obesity, binge eating and psychopathology: are they related. Int J Eat Disord. 1994;15:53–61.
46. APA. "Manual diagnóstico y estadístico de los trastornos mentales" DSM IVTR. Barcelona: Masson; 2002.
47. Yanowski SZ, Nelson JE, Dubbert BK, et al. Association of binge eating disorder and psychiatric comorbidity in obese subjects. Am J Psychiatry. 1993;150:1472–9.
48. Moyer DM, Di Pietro L, Berkowitz RI, Stunkard AJ. Childhood sexual abuse and precursors of binge eating in an adolescent female population. Int J Eat Disord. 1997;21:23–30.
49. Patel R. Obesos y Famélicos. Barcelona: Los Libros del Lince; 2008.
50. Organización Mundial de la Salud. CIE-10. Trastornos mentales y del comportamiento: descripciones clínicas y pautas para el diagnóstico. Madrid: Meditor; 1992.
51. Black DW, Goldstein RB, Masson E. Prevalence of mental disorder in 88 morbidly obese female candidates for gastric bypass. Am J Psychiatr. 1992;149:227–34.
52. Moore Jr DF, Sears DA. Pica, iron deficiency, and the medical history. Am J Med. 1994;97 (4):390–3.
53. Grupo de trabajo sobre guías de práctica clínica. Elaboración de Guías de Práctica Clínica en el Sistema Nacional de Salud. Manual metodológico. Madrid: plan de Calidad para el Sistema

Nacional de Salud del Ministerio de Sanidad y Consumo: Instituto Aragonés de Ciencias de la Salud-I + CS; 2007. Guías de Práctica Clínica en el Sistema Nacional de Salud: I + CS Nº2006/1.
54. Morgan JF. From Charles Atlas to Adonis complex—fat is more than a feminist issue. Lancet. 2000;356(9239):1372–3.
55. Striegel-Moore R, Dohm F, Hook J, Schreiber G, Crawford P, et al. Night eating syndrome in young adult women: prevalence and correlates. Int J Eat Disord. 2005;37:200–6.
56. Plato. Timaeus Dialogue. Stanford Encyclopedia of Philosophy; 2005.
57. Spitzer RL, Devlin M, Walsh BT, Hasin D. Binge eating disorder: a multisite field trial of the diagnostic criteria. Int J Eat Disord. 1992;11:191–203.

Paraphilic Disorders: Sexual Sadist and Masochistic Disorders

11

Rafael Segarra-Echebarría, Marta Crego-Meda, Aníbal Arrillaga-Trueba, and Margarita Sáenz-Herrero

Abstract

The paraphilia, or sexual perversion, is defined by a set of fantasies, needs, or unusual sexual behavior, generally repetitive, that produces sexual arousal in some people and that are clearly far away from "normal sexuality."

The term *paraphilia* denotes any intense and persistent sexual interest or interest other than sexual in genital stimulation or preparatory fondling with phenotypically normal, physically mature, consenting human partners. According to the *Diagnostic and Statistical Manual for Mental Disorders* (DSM-5), some paraphilias primarily concern the individual's erotic activities, and others the individual's erotic targets.

In the DSM-5 paraphilias are not ipso facto mental disorders. There is a distinction between paraphilias and paraphilic disorders. A paraphilic disorder is a paraphilia that is currently causing distress or impairment to the individual or one for which satisfaction has entailed personal harm or risked harm to others. A paraphilia is a necessary but not an adequate condition for having a paraphilic disorder, and a paraphilia by itself does not automatically justify or require clinical intervention.

R. Segarra-Echebarría (✉)
Cruces University Hospital, Bilbao, Spain

University of the Basque Country, UPV/EHU, Cruces, Spain
e-mail: rafaelsegarraechevarria@osakidetza.net

M. Crego-Meda • A. Arrillaga-Trueba
Cruces University Hospital, Bilbao, Spain

M. Sáenz-Herrero
Department of Psychiatry, Alava University Hospital, Vitoria, Spain

Araba University Hospital, Vitoria, Spain
e-mail: margarita.saenzherrero@osakidetza.net

M. Sáenz-Herrero (ed.), *Psychopathology in Women*,
DOI 10.1007/978-3-319-05870-2_11

Male gender and male domination paradigm is core to the construction of perversions, which are a predominantly male field, with the exception of masochism. In this way, sexuality becomes social, relational, determined and built by power. Sexuality becomes a factory of domination and passivity.

Finally, sadism and masochism cannot be separated because they are the two complementary sides of the same disease, the sadomasochistic disorder, as Freud enunciated back in 1905: a sadist is always a masochist at the same time.

"Vicious
You hit me with a flower
You do it every hour
Oh baby you are so vicious."
Lou Reed "Vicious"

11.1 Introduction

Sexual behavior has at least a double aspect: to obtain sexual pleasure and to carry out the reproductive function. In addition, such conduct is directed toward a particular object that can be autoerotic (masturbation) or aloerotic (homo- or heterosexual relationships).

Perversions, sexual inclination disorders, or paraphilias are a sexual, psychic, social, political, transhistorical, and structural phenomenon throughout all human societies and civilizations. In fact, all cultures share common elements: the prohibition of incest, the delineation of forms of dementia or mental insanity, and the description of what is accepted as monstrous or abnormal.

Although depraved people may be sublime when they turn their passions into art, creation, or mysticism (e.g. Sade, Sacher-Masoch, Mishima, Pasolini, etc.), or abject when they submit to their murderous or antisocial impulses, they are part of ourselves, part of our human condition, since they exhibit what we try to hide: our own negativity, our dark side [1].

Sexual perversions have been the subject of numerous works, including scholars' dictionaries of sexuality, eroticism and pornography. However, there is not a record of the "depraved" people. Michel Foucault had planned to include in his *Histoire de la Sexualité* a chapter devoted to the world of evil, that is, to those who have been described as such by a society concerned about dissociating themselves from their own dark side:

"Who are nowadays the depraved? And where does perversion begin? In a world where science has replaced divine authority, body has substituted the soul and aberration has substituted the evil, perversion remains regardless of what we think about it or what we don't, as a symptom of dehumanization, of annihilation" [1].

11.2 Historical Background

Before talking about paraphilias we should point out that although two genres coexist, most of the sexual perversions listed in psychopathology manuals have been conceptually developed by men. This is not a coincidence or a trivial fact if we consider the development of the history of human sexuality, especially from a gender perspective.

For centuries the idea of two genders has not existed, since male has prevailed over female throughout history, building the female figure into opposition to the male one, and even considering the vagina to be a reversed penis. Galen, whose works remained important until the Renaissance, believed that women were less complete than men in relation to the reproductive parts concerning reproduction. This author, based on the works of Aristotle and on the higher internal body temperature of men, argued that women had a natural disposition to submit and serve and considered them to be weak, crippled. According to Galen, the male fetus was able to turn his genitals out and thereby become a complete human being, while the female genitalia remained inverted and underdeveloped [2].

During the Middle Ages Alberto Magno went further, stating that if a girl originated during this process it was because of certain factors that have prevented the attachment to her body, hence the woman was not in her nature a human being, but a failed birth. In the eighteenth century the ovaries were considered to be female sperm ducts. While men had sexual attributes that can display and enhance, women were deprived of a place, and they were invested on a nonidentity, not only a physical one but also a linguistic deficiency, and consequently a social and cultural fault. The fact that women were derived from a proper and recognized denomination of their own sexual organs resulted in the separation of girls from their bodies and later in distancing them from their own sexual identity [2].

The lack of proper terminology establishes a difference between men who "have something" and women who do not. This certainly plays a role in the nuclear development of female sexuality, in how desire is outlined and how potential female perversions are subsequently established. The fear of daughters' sexuality is in fact greater than the fear that arises from their sexual health. How would girls describe what happens to them when they suffer sexual abuse if they do not even know how to name their own genitals?

Harriet Lerner, in an article published in 1970, mentions a well-known book, which explains: "a young woman has two ovaries, uterus and vagina. These are her sex organs. Young men's sex organs are the penis and testicles. One of the first changes in the body of the girl during puberty is the growth of pubic hair around the vaginal opening". In the face of this statement the author adds: "Such a partial and misleading name of the female genitalia can induce any young at puberty to sit on the floor of the bathroom with a mirror and come to the conclusion that it is a deformed creature" [3].

Young women cannot talk to each other about their genitals, and each reference to them remains reduced to the strictly private sphere, where no one speaks about it. What kind of perversion can women develop (with the exception of masochism, given the supposed willingness to submit postulated by Galen), if they lack even a name that identifies their genitals?

The repression of female sexuality in the western world, associated with the preponderance of the Christian religion, has been constant over time and history. This fact has a significant impact on both the oppression of women and the denial of their rights. The representations of hell and the jaws of depths in medieval painting are staged by obvious vaginal attributes. According to a famous saying (so widespread that it is collected in the *Malleus Maleficarum*, from the Latin "Hammer of the Witches") there are three insatiable things: the hell, the grave, and the vulva of women [1].

Thus, we should not forget that the original sin (ancestral sin) was committed by Eve (before her the snake, identified with the devil, also did it). As a result all Mankind was expelled from Paradise. By offering that apple to man, Eve becomes his guide. The idea of women being men's teachers is so threatening that Paul the Apostle prohibits them from any kind of verbal expression in public: "Women should listen to instruction in silence with all submission, and they should not be allowed to teach in public or over a man. I want them to remain silent, because God made Adam first, then Eve, and not Adam but Eve was deceived, and being deceived she felt into sin" [1].

If moderation in language is considered an ideal for all women, in the case of nuns this culminates in the requirement of tears instead of speaking. For art historian Silke Tammen, this fact has a direct effect on the distinction between femininity and passivity. Not only do female sexuality and legends about the *vagina dentata* sound threatening but so does the female voice, and legends speak about seafarers who, after listening to the sirens singing, lose their sanity and jump into the sea in search of them [1].

The archetypal fatal woman (femme fatale) who attracts men into the depths by revealing her body (such as Salome, the Jewish princess described in the Bible) has been a source of inspiration for writers, painters, and artists throughout history, especially in the nineteenth and twentieth centuries.

Women, who were considered to be impure by Christianity only because of their femininity, had to be purified. For this purpose in the Middle Ages mystic women organized sacrifice rituals that ranged from flagellation to devouring filth. The purpose of all these rituals is to destroy the physical body or expose it to the torments of the flesh, while they obtain some form of sexual satisfaction. The body, broken or bruised, fascinates the saints and holies. This particular relationship with the flesh is because Christianity is the only religion in which God is incarnated to live and die as a man, and incidentally as a victim. It is clear that this religion confers to the male body such a predominant status.

St. Margaret Mary Alacoque was so frail that the slightest piece of dirt made her stomach sick. However, when Jesus "called her to order" to clean the vomit from a sick patient, she could not think of anything but turning the vomit into her food. In another occasion she ate the excrement of a dysenteric woman, and she stated that the contact with excrement raised in her a vision of Christ that kept her lips close to his injury: “If I had a thousand bodies, a thousand loves, a thousand lives, I would sacrifice all of them for being submitted to you” [1].

St. Catherine of Siena came to declare that she had not eaten anything as delicious as the pus of cancerous breasts. Later she heard Christ speaking to her: “My beloved woman, you have experienced for me a hard battle and with my help you have been victorious. You’ve never been so dear to me and so pleasant as now” [1].

11.3 Definition and Conceptual Aspects

We understand perversion, paraphilia or sexual orientation disorder from a medical point of view, the deviation from the sexual act considered “normal” (see Table 11.1).

The paraphilia or sexual perversion is defined by a set of fantasies, needs or unusual sexual behavior, generally repetitive, that produce sexual arousal in some people, and that are clearly far away from the previous precepts.

In the past, a much more extensive view of perversion was held regarding the diagnosis of modern paraphilias. It is worth mentioning it because some doctors continue to have the same beliefs as before. This means that in some places we can still talk about perversion when orgasm is reached with different sex objects, with different parts of the body (not only the genitals), or when orgasm is subject to certain non-genital extrinsic conditions that cannot provide sexual pleasure by themselves.

These attitudes lead to a double view of sexuality among doctors: the “official” opinion, advocated by the scientific and research societies, defining paraphilias as very specific clinical situations, and another, “unofficial” view of some professionals still sticking to approaches of 40 or 50 years ago that leave a strong sociocultural and religious mark.

Laplanche and Pontalis [4] further extend the field to designate as perversions the whole range of psychosexual activities accompanying the previously explained atypia in obtaining sexual pleasure. According to Spanish psychoanalyst Coderch [5] perverse individuals exclude genital union with a person of the opposite sex from the fact of obtaining sexual pleasure, or they even subject it to certain acts that do not belong to sexual intercourse, such as the presence of a third individual, cruelty, harm to the couple, the use of a particular type of clothing to have sexual relations, sexual relations with minors or sexual relations related by blood.

Table 11.1 “Abnormal or deviant” sexual behavior

Destructive or damaging to the subject who displays it and to those who get involved in it
Not oriented to the other in a strict sense
Excludes the stimulation of the own genital organs and those of the partner
Is inappropriately associated with feelings of guilt and/or anxiety
Shows a repetitive nature of a compulsive kind

The main element for the diagnosis of a paraphilia is the presence in these individuals of specific and repetitive sexual fantasies with a double conscious and unconscious component, in which both excitation and sexual practice and attainment of orgasm are associated. The influence of these fantasies and of their behavioral manifestations are beyond strictly sexual arousal, and come to invade all spheres of an individual's living and fantasies, making them the preferred or the only ways of obtaining sexual satisfaction.

The presence of a sexuality that is called perverse based on the most classical psychopathological criteria is a constant in much of universal art and literature. For western civilization from Sade to Von Sacher-Masoch, from Henry Miller to Lucian Freud, from Robert Mapplethorpe to Helmut Newton, from Bernardo Bertolucci to Federico Fellini, from Pier Paolo Pasolini to Stanley Kubrick, sexuality often diverts from that ideal encounter that is considered to be "normal," and this also indicates the great variety of artistic evidence since the origins of humanity.

In fact, is art possible without violence or eroticism? Do sex and blood not form the basis of any artistic work? Camille Paglia [6], a specialist in art history and disciple of Harold Bloom, claims that sex and violence are always close to the social and personal surface. In her opinion all culture, even in the highest expression of art, is but a means by which the human being protects itself from nature, which is cruel and merciless. And nature is blood and semen, violence and sex, which hovers inevitably over every cultural product. For Paglia, "all the roads which arise from Rousseau take to Sade." Sexuality and eroticism are an inevitable result of the intersection between nature and culture.

11.4 Epidemiological Aspects

In a study in which 94 men are interrogated (a general, not a clinical population) about their sexual fantasies during masturbation or intercourse: 61.7 % say they fantasize about initiating a girl into sexuality; 33 % describe fantasizing about raping adult women; 11.7 % describe masochistic fantasies; 5.3 % fantasize about having sex with animals; and 3.2 % describe fantasies about initiating a boy [7].

Meanwhile, another study on a non-clinical population comprising 60 male college students shows that 42 % admits having practiced voyeurism; 35 % frotteurism; 8 % have made obscene phone calls; 5 % have participated in coercive sexual practices; 3 % have had sexual contact with girls under 12; and 2 % has practiced exhibitionism. In total, 65 % say that they have participated in some form of paraphilic behavior. In this same group 54 % recognize that they have an interest in practicing voyeurism; 7 % want to practice exhibitionism, and 5 % crave sexual contact with children under 12 years of age [8].

With regard to clinical populations, the data collected over 90 treatment programs in the United States relating to 2,129 cases of individuals seeking psychiatric evaluation, we can conclude the following: 37.1 % have been involved in child abuse; 20.2 % in voyeurism; 13.8 % in indecent exposure; 13.3 % in fetishism; 11.2 % in frotteurism; and 10.7 % in public masturbation [7].

Meanwhile another study of 561 paraphilic people (mostly men) who have committed more than 291,000 such acts against more than 195,000 victims, indicates that 37.3 % were victims of exhibitionism; 28.6 % of frotteurism; 13.6 % of voyeurism; 11.8 % of child abuse outside of the home; 3.5 % of public masturbation; 2.3 % of abuse of girls outside of the home; 1 % were victims of obscene phone calls; 0.9 % of bestiality; 0.5 % of the rape of adult women; 0.2 % of child abuse at home; another 0.2 % of urophilia; and 0.1 % of sadism, fetishism, masochism or coprophilia [7].

The true prevalence of sexual perversions is unknown to us. The best estimations derive from cases of legal claims, according to which the most widespread paraphilia is pedophilia [9]. Such disorders are practically confined to the male sex. Half of them have symptoms before they are 18 years old, and decline significantly (at least from a criminal point of view) past the 50s. Frequently, the same individual of up to three or four different paraphilias, depending on the biographical timeline considered. In the latter case the adjective "polymorphous perverse" is applied to describe the coexistence of multiple sexual deviations in the same person [10].

According to new edition of the American Psychiatric Association's DSM-5 [11]:

"Voyeuristic acts are the most common of potentially law-breaking sexual behaviors. The population prevalence of Voyeuristic Disorder is unknown. However, based on voyeuristic sexual acts in nonclinical samples, the highest possible lifetime prevalence for Voyeuristic Disorder is approximately 12 % in males and 4 % in females (ratio male–female 3:1).

"The prevalence of Exhibitionistic Disorder is also unknown. However, based on exhibitionistic sexual acts in nonclinical or general populations, the highest possible prevalence for Exhibitionistic Disorder in the male population is 2–4 %. The prevalence of this disorder in females is even more uncertain, but it is generally believed to be much lower than in males.

"The prevalence of frotteuristic acts, including the uninvited sexual touching of or rubbing against another individual may occur in up to 30 % of adult males in the general population. Approximately 10–14 % of adult males seen in outpatient settings for Paraphilic Disorders and hypersexuality have a presentation that meets diagnostic criteria for Frotteuristic Disorder. Hence, whereas the population prevalence of Frotteuristic Disorder is unknown, it is not likely that it exceeds the rate found in selected clinical settings.

"The population prevalence of Sexual Masochism Disorder is once again unknown. In Australia, it has been estimated that 2.2 % of males and 1.3 % of females had been involved in bondage and discipline, sadomasochism, or dominance and submission in the past 12 months. Community individuals with paraphilias have reported a mean age at onset for masochism of 19.3 years, although earlier ages, including puberty and childhood, have also been reported for the onset of masochistic fantasies. Very little is known about persistence of this disorder over time.

"The population prevalence of Sexual Sadism Disorder is equally unknown and it is largely based on individuals in forensic settings. Depending on the criteria for sexual sadism, prevalence varies widely from 2 to 30 %. Among civilly committed sexual offenders in the United States, less than 10 % have sexual sadism. Among individuals who have committed sexually motivated homicides, rates of sexual sadism disorder range from 37 to 75 %. Individuals with sexual sadism in forensic samples are almost exclusively male, but a representative sample of the population in Australia reported than 2.2 % of men and 1.3 % of women said they had been involved in bondage an discipline, sadomasochism, or dominance and submission in the previous year. Information on the development and course of Sexual Sadism Disorder is extremely limited. One study reported that females became aware of their sadomasochistic orientation as young adults, and another reported that the mean age at onset of sadism in a group of males was 19.4 years. Whereas sexual sadism is probably a lifelong characteristic, Sexual Sadism Disorder may fluctuate according to the individual's subjective distress or his or her propensity to harm nonconsenting others. Advancing age is likely to have the same reducing effect on this disorder as it has on other paraphilic or normophilic sexual behavior.

"The population prevalence of Pedophilic Disorder is once again unknown. The highest possible prevalence for Pedophilic Disorder in the male population is approximately 3–5 %. The population prevalence of Pedophilic Disorder in females is even more uncertain, but it is likely a small fraction of the prevalence in males.

"The population prevalence of Fetishistic Disorder is unknown, and in clinical samples this disorder is nearly exclusively reported for males. Usually paraphilias have an onset during puberty, but fetishes can develop prior to adolescence. Once established, Fetishistic Disorder tends to have a continuous course that fluctuates in intensity and frequency of urges or behavior.

"The prevalence of Transvestic Disorder is unknown. Transvestic Disorder is rare in males and extremely rare in females. Fewer than 3 % of males report having ever been sexually aroused by dressing in women's attire. The percentage of individuals who have cross-dressed with sexual arousal more than once or a few times in their lifetimes would be even lower. The majority of males with Transvestic Disorder identify themselves as heterosexuals, although some individuals have occasional interaction with other males, especially when they are cross-dressed. In males, the first signs of Transvestic Disorder may begin in childhood, in the form of strong fascination with a particular item of women's attire. Prior to puberty, cross-dressing produces generalized feelings of pleasurable excitement. With the arrival of puberty, dressing in women's clothes begins to excite penile erection, and in some cases, leads directly to first ejaculation. In many cases, cross-dressing elicits less and less sexual excitement as the individual grows older. Eventually it may produce no discernible penile response at all. The desire to cross-dress, at the same time, remains the same or grows even stronger. Individuals who report such a diminution of sexual response typically report that the sexual excitement of cross-dressing has been replaced by feelings of comfort or well-being. In some cases, the course of Transvestic Disorder is continuous, and in others is episodic. Some cases of transvestic disorder progress to Gender Dysphoria. The males in these cases, who may be indistinguishable from other with Transvestic Disorder in adolescence or early childhood, gradually develop desires to remain in the female role for longer periods and to feminize their anatomy. The development of Gender Dysphoria is usually accompanied by a self-reported reduction or elimination of sexual arousal in association with cross-dressing." This topic will be widely examined in the correspondent chapter on this book.

It is important to emphasize the fact that these data should be understood with considerable caution and as a mere orientation toward reality for several reasons. Surveys attempt to capture behaviors considered to be negative by society, and sometimes clearly criminal cases, which must be clarified and not obscured. There are behaviors in certain situations and with certain intensity and frequency that cannot be classified as paraphilias in a clinical sense. Normal sexuality includes partial aspects that overlap with what we call perversions, differing only by the context, intensity, exclusivity, compulsion or other aspects. The young man or woman who enjoys watching the naked body of his/her partner is not a voyeur in the clinical sense; the boy or girl picking sexy lingerie for his/her partner is not an exhibitionist, and so on. Sexual behaviors that include some specific aspects of paraphilias should be distinguished from other behaviors that meet the diagnostic criteria.

11.5 Etiopathogenesis

Among the main hypothesis about the origin of disorders of sexual preferences there are biological factors involved, such as alterations in the neurodevelopment, in the levels of sexual hormones in plasma, mild neurological symptoms, certain chromosomal abnormalities, electroencephalographic alterations, epilepsy and mental impairment [9]. In general, all are extremely unspecific and inadequate from an epistemological point of view.

This group of disorders has been associated with a higher prevalence of severe psychiatric pathology as well as with cluster B Personality Disorders [11]. Also, the influence of the social and cultural environment of the individual, as well as his particular biographical moment, must not be ignored as a clear role in its sexual preferences.

Paraphilic disorders have also been related to childhood sexual abuse, substance misuse and sexual preoccupation/hypersexuality as risk factors, although the causal relationship with paraphilias is uncertain and the specificity unclear.

Male gender and the male domination paradigm is core to the construction of perversions, which are a predominantly male field, with the exception of masochism. In this way, sexuality becomes social, relational, determined and built by power. Sexuality becomes a factory of domination and passivity.

Pornography is a clear example of an exercise of domination. It makes women become objects for sexual use and transaction, and makes its potential consumers desire them as objects but also crave to possess or dominate them, often in a cruel and ruthless way. Gender inequality, submission, the hierarchical position and the objectification that results from an explicit denial of self-determination and the apparent consent of sexual desire, are the most appealing traits of these object-women.

Andrea Dworkin claims that the main subject of pornography is male power. In general terms, the role of a woman in pornography is to be raped and possessed by men, either through a camera or a script, always in the name of the watcher. This sexuality of observation, of visual intromission, of domination and access, of entertainment, turns sex into a kind of sport for its audience [12].

11.6 The Dynamics of Perversion: Origin and Development

Over the past few years the term "sexual perversion" has been substituted for others such as "paraphilia" (which etymologically has its origin in Greek: "further" and "love") [11], disorder of sexual behavior or disorders of sexual preferences (International Classification of Diseases version 10 [ICD-10]) [8], with a more sociological than a clinical base, given that these disorders suppose a behavioral deviation from statistical normality. The main point is to avoid moral judgments regarding the pathological origin of these aforementioned disorders.

Coderch claims that traditionally and from a clinical point of view the term "perversion" has been used to define any function or instinct that deviates from its natural goal (for example, pica can be considered a perversion of the instinct of nutrition). That a certain phenomenon may not be in line with the statistical norm does not necessarily bestow upon it a pathological nature (for example, the influenza infection is a pathological phenomenon from a medical point of view, although it may be considered normal from a statistical point of view during certain seasons of the year; running 100 m in 10 s is also a deviation of the statistical norm, although it has no medical pathological connotation by any means) [5]. This author defends preserving the term "perversion" to refer to this kind of disorders.

Castilla del Pino [13], another Spanish psychiatrist, considers that physicians in their daily routine either openly or covertly corrupt their medical judgments with their own moral judgments: men (and women) are social beings, with their own problems regarding themselves and their relationships (dependence on social class, group, personal expectations) and therefore they are often tendentious concerning the direction of their own moral, religious, political or cultural convictions. This author criticizes the evolution of these medical and psychopathological concepts, as he claims that the substitution of moral/immoral for normal/abnormal is nothing but a deletion of terms with no changes in the hidden attitude toward the concepts they represent. He adds that no action can be considered inherently moral or immoral, mainly because it is its application within a context that confers the said quality upon the action. Empathizing with the context of the individuals in their relationships, not in our own context, that is the key. This fact becomes decisive in judging our own or other people's sexual behaviors.

The concept of "perversion," semantic traits aside, has been modified through time owing to the contributions granted by psychoanalysis. Before Freud, and throughout the twentieth century, research carried out by several authors on deviations of sexual behavior was focused on descriptive and nosological contributions.

Freud [14] considers that the main aspects of pathological sexual behavior consist in the exclusivity, repetitive and persistent substitution of adult genital sexual relationships for other activities with an infantile and pre-genital nature, as a result of a defensive mechanism toward the unbearable castration anxiety experienced during the "Oedipal period." This author places perversions as the reverse of neurotic disorders, with infantile drives surpassing the defense mechanisms of the Ego and transforming them into neurotic symptoms.

Freud interprets perversions as the product of a fixation that results in a disorder of the maturative evolution of normal sexual impulses. He later changes his point of view, giving perversions a more defensive (and therefore neurotic) connotation, in which regression and repression play a determinant role against a conflictive "Oedipus complex" [15].

In the specific case of Leonardo Da Vinci, a Renaissance figure whose "pure homosexuality" Freud has no doubt about, the father of psychoanalysis thinks that the accidental circumstance of his illegitimate birth and the excessive tenderness of his mother had a decisive influence on the development of his personality and his consequent fate, which led his libido to be sublimated into a desire to know, determining the sexual inactivity of his life [15].

However, precautions must be taken with the creation of myths (and the "Oedipus complex" represents one of them). From a psychoanalytical perspective we find authors who demonstrate that self-awareness and other-awareness evolve through the possibility that separate minds may implicate sharing feelings and intentions within a process of mutual recognition. This recognition may be established in a mother/son dyad, or father/daughter, or in any other asymmetrical relationship, as long as there is no falsification of the other person's needs through fabrications or representations that justify or hide domination [16].

Robert Graves dissects the double function of the myth: on the one hand, its attempt to give sense to the enigmas of life; on the other one, the concealment of violence to justify a certain social system. This author also remarks on its power, which becomes part of the same definition of myth: allegoric fiction that contains a creative or even magical force in which the people that created it are included, ruling their lives and behavior [17].

The Oedipus complex is a myth built from psychoanalytical theory. It excludes the concealment, the masking of a relationship of power, and participates in its dilution. Historically, adults have not been conscious of the generational transmission of the drama that results from the father–mother/son–daughter relationships. What is being hidden in the theory that portrays Oedipus as a representation of the recognition of the difference between the two sexes? Basically, Oedipus is not a normal child, but someone who has suffered extreme parental violence. Son of Laius and Jocasta, Oedipus lacks parents as he is abandoned (by them) in the mountains. In the play by Sophocles the chorus says: "Is he son of Pan, of Apollo, of Hermes, of Bacchus, of one of Helicon's nymphs?" [18]. The abandoned boy may become everything or nothing. He is an enigma. A naked man, alone, and nobody knows how he came into the world. He is the most intimate essence of a man, even lacking the social shield that should protect him (his parents). His only protection comes from the mercy of a man, a stranger, a shepherd that decides to nurture him. A defenseless child, saved from doom. We already have a naked man introduced into the world of humanity. What will become of him? Because the loneliness of a man is, in Oedipus' case, notable because of his irregular family situation: a birth that should not have been, parents who should not have been parents, and conflict and constant risk for everyone.

Oedipus does not really represent any children. The androcentrism of the psychoanalytical theory about differences between the sexes starts here, in the double absence of the father toward the mother and daughter, thus, they both find the path to developing their own subjectivity [16].

Femininity and masculinity are not roles or intended behaviors, but an organizing principle of the whole subjectivity: ego, super-ego, and sexual desire. The object of desire is not an anatomical body, but a body built by all the inter-subjective thoughts and practices. Both boys and girls organize themselves through their relationships with other objects (for example, their mother), which are not just objects as both boys and girls can recognize those objects as different from them and similar to them at the same time. This way, inter-subjectivity has an effect in the structuration of the psyche.

The application of a sexual double standard on women leads them to find it increasingly difficult to achieve a mental balance because they only find admiration and recognition through their physical appearance, and their psyche endures extra effort to reconcile the multiple requests of their motivational systems [19].

Since these fantasies and behaviors are not shared with other people and are kept secret for fear of reprisal or punishment, they remain in time until the individual becomes aware of the incompatibility of his (her) interests with the social and cultural rules and conditions of the times in which he (she) lives. Once this moment arrives, those activities have already become a repetitive and compulsive personality pattern with an effect on the basic needs of the individual, who is unable to discard them [9].

McDougall [20] and Chasseguet-Smirgel [21, 22] agree with regard to pointing out the importance of perversion as a creation of a new reality in which the barriers between generations and sexes are removed, providing an escape from anguish with a new reality. Both authors consider perversion to be an individual's reaction to a narcissistic injury connected to the "primary scene" and the perception of the difference between the two sexes.

With his viewpoint, Stoller keeps a distance from this classical approach to perversion to remark on an alternative origin of this narcissistic injury: questioning sexual identity during childhood. As a reaction, the adult develops a sexual relationship defined by a need to control the object, and therefore with a sadomasochistic trait regardless of the final form of the perverse behavior. Stoller considers aggression to be the common basic factor among all perversions, which allows revenge for all the pain suffered during childhood. In some of these behaviors the aggression is expressed in a conscious and direct way, as in sadomasochistic practices [23].

One of the most relevant authors with the current psychoanalytical outlook, Otto Friedemann Kernberg [24], agrees with Stoller on targeting sadomasochistic traits as the basis for all perversions, and even for "normal" sexual relationships. Kernberg points out the existence of different dynamics depending on the expression of perversions in the context of the different organization of personality. He retains the basic concept for stable perversions that appear within a neurotic structure. He assigns a dynamic such as that described by the British object relations school to perversions that are found in borderline organizations of personality. And he considers Chasseguet-Smirgel's concepts appropriate for their application to perversions that appear within a narcissistic structure, especially when applied to a malignant narcissism.

According to Kernberg [25] the core affect of severe psychopathological conditions (that include perversions) is hatred, an aggressive, complex, chronic, and stable affect with regard to its cognitive component, with a powerful characterological basis, accompanied by a rationalizing habit and severe distortions of personality concerning the function of the Ego and the Superego of the individual. Hate, intensified by some unconscious motivations (such as a search for revenge rooted in early affective experiences) claims to destroy of the object, both as an unconscious fantasy and in its conscious dimension. However, paradoxically the object that the individual wants to destroy is also needed and desired, which results in a circular dynamic of perversion.

According to González Torres [26], the most significant contribution by Otto Kernberg in this field is based on his opinion that polymorphic perverse sexuality plays a necessary role in the normal sexual relationships. He retains the inquisitiveness set by Stoller years before in this field. Kernberg states that the perverse traits of a normal sexual life assume a way to express aggressive impulses within a couple, avoiding the progression from what is strictly sexual toward a mechanic and unpleasant activity. The capability to unconsciously integrate love and hatred into a polymorphous sexual behavior provides a way of allowing the "use" or "exploitation" of the partner within sex play, safeguarding the object-relation at the same time. This supposes a "splitting" or duplication of sex play, in which the reality of the object-relation is sustained while the other reality of the object, regressive and fantastic, is performed playfully as part of sexual desire and arousal.

In reference to this last point, it should be mentioned that authors such as Oyebode [10] reserve the term "polymorphous perverse" for those people who show all deviations of sexual behavior or paraphilias, while from a psychoanalytical perspective the approach is different, and perverse and polymorphous sexuality are inseparable parts of the sexual life of boys and girls in the early stages of their libidinal development, establishing a basis for the integration of the said behaviors into normal sexual relationships, affective relationships and fantasies in adulthood, in a pleasant way.

Castilla del Pino suggests that a large part of the prodromal behavior of normal sexual activity, and even a greater share in the case of pathological activity, is demonstrated by rituals that reveal the existence of traces of fixations that took place before the stages of libidinal development, making kisses or bites "benign" oral expressions. Even keeping the focus strictly on genital sexual relationships with the desired object, a sublimation of pre-genital object-relationships appears frequently, granting a significant role to hidden fantasies [13].

Kernberg [25] states that the body of the beloved becomes a geography of personal meanings, so that the fantasized early polymorphous perverse relations to the parental objects are condensed in the admiring and invasive relationship with the lover's body parts. Erotic desire is rooted in the pleasure of unconsciously enacting polymorphous perverse fantasies and activities, including symbolic activation of the earliest object relations of the infant with the mother and of the small child with both parents. All this is expressed in the perverse components of intercourse and sexual play (fellatio, cunnilingus, anal penetration, and in exhibitionistic, voyeuristic, and sadistic sexual play). All of them, by the way, are sexual perversions that are almost exclusive to the male gender.

The study of perversions within the male gender, although still scanty, contrasts with the absence of studies about perversions and sexuality, both normal and pathological, in the female population. In addition, there is a current lack of appropriate vocabulary to refer to the external female genitals, using, for example, "vagina" and "vulva" as if they were synonyms, as if using these terms incorrectly were harmless to the sexual and psychological development of women.

Psychoanalyst Harriet Lerner claims that naming female genitalia incorrectly is almost as surprising in its consequences as it is regarding the silence that surrounds this. It is true that in the USA female genitalia are not mutilated, the clitoris and labia are not amputated, as is performed in countless girls and women in other cultures. Here, the job is carried out not with a knife but with words: the result is a psychological genital mutilation. Language can be as sharp and fast as a surgical scalpel blade. What is not named does not exist [3].

Psychoanalysis intends to monopolize the true discourse about female sexuality. A discourse that is apparently true upon the logic of this truth: precisely, that femininity only has a place within the models and laws that have been promulgated by men. This means that only one sex exists, not two. One single practice and portrayal of sexuality, with its history, its needs, its reverses, its flaws, its negative or negatives, which are supported by the female sex.

Following the theory of psychosexual development published in 1908 by Freud, 3- to 5-year-old girls discover they lack a penis, and conclude that they are missing something, that they have been castrated. This concept of "penis envy," joined by the "fear of castration" that children endure, performed on both an individual level and on the collective consciousness of sexuality, with obvious negative consequences due to denying women a sexuality determined by themselves, depriving them of their creative skills, even of their potential perversions [19].

Furthermore, Freud claims that the greatest wish of every girl, and later on of every woman ("penis envy") is the desire to have a phallus, and that desire can only be replaced by the desire to conceive a baby. Irigaray agrees by stating that the woman can only be completed when she becomes a mother, by bringing into the world a child who becomes a "substitute for the penis," and with some luck the baby will have one himself. According to Freud, the perfect fulfillment of becoming a woman consists of creating a male sex while neglecting her own sex [19].

With the imaginary lack of existence of female genitalia other non-existences are approached. Jacques Lacan claims: "A woman can but be excluded by the nature of things, which is the nature of words and it must be said that if there is something that women themselves complain about enough for the time being, that's it. It's just that they don't know what they're saying—that's the whole difference between them and myself" [16]. Isn't this an aberration from an intellectual point of view?

In psychoanalysis rivalry between sexes has been approached mainly in genital terms, confusing the shape with what it represents, confusing genitality with the broad spectrum of human action that masculinity symbolizes. Psychoanalysis aspires to provide a scientific explanation, while it merely strengthens a circular myth. Women and men inserted into this cultural and para-scientific discourse continue to conceive the creativity and potential of the woman, in traditionally non-female areas, as some kind of misappropriation or transgression: phallic women, men threatened by mutilation.

The hierarchical order between genders is still being masked and emphasized through the constant appeal to the difference between sexes, reducing the complexity of the conflicts that are inherent to human otherness and inequality [16].

11.7 Paraphilic Disorders According to the DSM-5

Paraphilic disorders included in the new DSM-5 edition (American Psychiatric Association, 2014) are [11, 27–34]:

Voyeuristic disorder—spying on others in private activities.
Exhibitionistic disorder—exposing the genitals.
Frotteuristic disorder—touching or rubbing against a nonconsenting individual.
Sexual masochism disorder—this is undergoing humiliation, bondage or suffering.
Sexual sadism disorder—inflicting humiliation, bondage or suffering.
Pedophilic disorder—sexual focus on children.
Fetishistic disorder—using nonliving objects or having a highly specific focus on nongenital body parts.
Transvestic disorder—engaging in sexually arousing cross-dressing.

These eight disorders have traditionally been selected for specific listing and assignment of explicit diagnostic criteria in the DSM for two main reasons:

They are relatively common.
Some entail actions for their satisfaction that, because of their noxiousness or potential harm to others, are classed as criminal offenses.

These eight disorders listed above do not exhaust the list of possible paraphilic disorders. In fact many dozens of distinct paraphilias have been identified and named, and almost any of them could, by virtue of its negative consequences for the individual or for others, rise to the level of a paraphilic disorder. The diagnoses of the other specified and unspecified paraphilic disorders are therefore indispensable and will be required in many cases.

The term paraphilia denotes any intense and persistent interest other than sexual in genital stimulation or preparatory fondling with phenotypically normal, physically mature, consenting human partners. In some circumstances the criteria intense and persistent may be difficult to apply, such as in the assessment of persons who are very old or medically ill and who may not have real intense sexual interest of any kind. In such circumstances the term paraphilia may be defined as any sexual interest greater than or equal to normophilic sexual interests. There are also specific paraphilias that are better described as preferential sexual interests than as intense sexual interests.

According to DSM-5 some paraphilias primarily concern the individual's erotic activities, and others the individual's erotic targets. In DSM-5 paraphilias are not ipso facto mental disorders. There is a distinction between paraphilias and paraphilic disorders. A paraphilic disorder is a paraphilia that is currently causing distress or impairment to the individual or a paraphilia whose satisfaction has entailed personal harm, or risked harm to others. A paraphilia is necessary but not a sufficient condition for having a paraphilic disorder, and a paraphilia by itself does not automatically justify or require clinical intervention. The distinction between paraphilias and paraphilic disorders was implemented in the DSM-5 without making any changes to the basic structure of the diagnostic criteria, as they have existed since DSM-III-R.

The change proposed for the DSM-5 is that individuals who meet both criterion A (which specifies the qualitative nature of the paraphilia) and criterion B (which specifies the negative consequences of the paraphilia) would now be diagnosed as having a paraphilic disorder. A diagnosis would not be given to individuals whose symptoms meet criterion A but not criterion B, which is given to those who have a paraphilia but not a paraphilic disorder.

An overarching change in the DSM-5 (compared with DSM-IV) is the addition of the course specifiers "in a controlled environment" and "in remission" to the diagnostic criteria sets for all the paraphilic disorders. These specifiers are added to indicate important changes in an individual's status.

It has already been said that it is not rare for an individual to manifest two or more paraphilias. In some cases, the paraphilic foci are closely related. In other cases, the connection between the paraphilias is not obvious, and the presence of many paraphilias may be coincidental or else related to some generalized vulnerability to anomalies of psychosexual development.

One last consideration: the most widely applicable framework for assessing the strength of a paraphilia itself is one in which the examinees' paraphilic sexual fantasies, urges, or behaviors are evaluated in relation to their normophilic sexual interests and behaviors. Not only the distress and impairment stipulated in criterion B but also the possibility of a reactive depression, anxiety, guilt, poor work story and impaired social relations among others must be clinically evaluated.

11.8 Sadism and Masochism

Sadism and masochism cannot be separated as they are the two complementary sides of the same disease, the sadomasochistic disorder, as Freud enunciated back in 1905: "A sadist is always at the same time a masochist" [14].

According to Freud, masochism is not the manifestation of an instinct, but derives from sadism and invariably appears to be intensively associated with it. Subsequently, the pages of the psychoanalytical literature are flooded with sadomasochism, as it includes one of the most basic human drives and in its extended form, aggressiveness, which is involved in many of our behaviors.

Ey infers that sadistic and masochistic movements form a dialectical couple, being linked in the same way as activity and passivity, pleasure and pain, tension and relaxation. This author also reflects the relationship among sadomasochism, death drive and its role in the so-called "repetition automatism," of which perversion is a prominent example [35].

Castilla del Pino [13] believes that sometimes sadistic or masochistic behavior constitutes part of the rituals of normal sex foreplay. Many of these rituals are connected with the identification of the male and female roles by the boy and girl mainly through linkage to the "primal scene," parental intercourse, which is ambivalently portrayed as a scene of aggression but rather voluptuously.

However, as Butler says the boy gets easily separated from the mother and identifies with the father, who has the power, but the girl always maintains ambivalence toward the mother figure, who carries less sociocultural weight [36].

11.8.1 Sadism

Sadism is the search for and provocation of moral or physical damage to the couple as a way of obtaining sexual pleasure and satisfaction. It may be expressed at different levels in the form of murder, rape, harassment, beating, pinching, flagellation, burns, bites, chains, and torture.

All these practices are part of the sexual and literary Donatien Alphonse François de Sade repertoire, the man who obtained both success and scandal when he wrote "Justine," and who marked the birth of the sadistic mythology. The same man who back in 1780, imprisoned and in the middle of his life, wrote to his wife [37]: "my way of thinking, you say, cannot be approved. And who cares? A man who acquires a way of thinking for others is crazy! My way of thinking is the result of my reflections; it is part of my existence, of my organization. I'm not anybody to change that, and if I were, I would not do it. This mindset that you reproach me is the only comfort of my life, relieves all my pains in prison, composes all my pleasures in the world and I need it more than life. It is not my way of thinking that has brought misfortune to me, but other people's."

Sade continues to be a tragic author, with more of a pariah existence than a marquis, who spends half of his life locked between inmates and crazy people, in prison or in Charenton's asylum, where he wrote an unclassifiable work defined as "gospel of evil", "a sudden abyss" or "subversion of the difference between vice and virtue". His stories encourage people to take up the revolutionary act to deflagration, thinking that this way, in a destructive fantasy, the transition between the old and the new society is precipitated. Later, he was considered to be a precursor of sexology, or an heir of Satanism. Sade also makes evil desirable through his writings [1].

Obviously, actions of a sadistic nature and individuals that perpetrate them have provided multiple diagnostic interpretations, within an overall perverse behavior scheme. In this context a careful differential diagnosis should be made, as the motley quality of them sometimes denotes the performance of schizophrenic patients, feeble-minded, insane, or people affected by dissociative episodes, impulse control disorder or organic personality disorder.

Sadism has undergone numerous etiopathogenic interpretations. These include alterations in the child's early learning, a result of the manifestations of sexual aggression directed toward him during his childhood by parents or alternative figures, perceived changes in the parental image and models, hormonal, neuropsychiatric or genetic alterations, all plausible but inadequate when considered separately [9].

For psychoanalysis, sadism is connected to other forms of perverse behavior, in the sense that it is a defense against castration anxiety (again the myth loop). Thus, the sadistic sexual pleasure is only felt when the individual does to others what he fears to have done to himself; thus, weakening and subjecting his partner exorcises the fear of being punished and dominated himself.

Coderch [5] makes a distinction between erotic sadism and criminal sadism:

"In the first, the behaviour of the sadistic individual exceeds the defense against castration anxiety, and provides a defense against the self-destructive impulses of thanatic origin (death drive), which he avoids directing them towards others.

"In the erotic sadism, sadistic behaviors are more fictitious than real, this is false and agreed with their victims, which fail to feel a true physical or moral harm. The objective here is to lose his fears verifying that, in the end, the punishment inflicted on his partners (the same that he avoids) is not as bad as a real castration but only some suffering and symbolic amputations that seem tolerable."

In those cases when real damage to the couple is caused (without reaching the extreme of criminal sadism) the role played by the individual's superego is determinant; in these cases, the purpose of the sadistic act is to make the victim love and forgive the offender, so that he can be free of his fantasy of guilt, which deprives him of sexual satisfaction.

According to psychoanalytic theory fantasies of being beaten up and punished by the father are the regressive expression of the desire to be sexually loved by him, in a passive feminine kind of relationship on the individual's part and supplemented with masochistic fantasies, as will be exposed later.

According to Castilla del Pino [13] the incidence of the superego appears in the playful trait that sadistic behavior appears to have; in other words, in not taking seriously the aggression produced. From here it is inferred that, with few exceptions (discussed below), the sadist imposes a limit on his aggression toward the sexual object, and rarely culminates in total destruction.

Regarding criminal sadism, it can be said that it expresses an extreme cruelty that can reach the homicide stage without any apparent justification (absence of self-defense, hatred toward the victim, or profit), or complicity or physical intimacy between the sadist and his victim, which allows us to consider the practiced violence (unjustified) as part of a sexual activity.

The person responsible for sending millions of Jewish people to the gas chamber in World War II, Adolf Eichmann, was not a sadist, a psychopath, a pervert, a monster, nor was he suffering from some visible mental illness. He was normal, horrifyingly ordinary. After sending millions of individuals to the gas chamber, he stated that he had just been following orders, even denying being anti-Semitic. It would have been comforting to think that Eichmann was a monster. From the point of view of our legal institutions and our moral standards, his normality is much more terrifying than all the atrocities he committed, because it implies that this new kind of offender commits his crimes under circumstances that almost prevent him from knowing or guessing that he is performing acts of evil [1].

In her reporting of the 1961 Adolf Eichmann trial for *The New Yorker*, which evolved into *Eichmann in Jerusalem: a Report of the Banality of Evil*, the philosopher and political theorist Hannah Arendt coined the phrase "the banality of evil" to describe Eichmann. She raised the question of whether evil is radical or simply a function of thoughtlessness, a tendency of ordinary people to obey orders and conform to mass opinion without a critical evaluation of the consequences of their actions and inaction. As she was also critical of the way the trial was conducted in Israel, and of the way that some Jewish leaders acted during the Holocaust, Arendt was criticized by many Jewish public figures, who charged her with a coldness and lack of sympathy for the victims of the Holocaust [38].

The Nazi regime based on its own criteria reaches the extreme threshold to decide not only that certain groups of people do not deserve to live in the country of residence, but also decide the place and time of their extermination. Indeed, what is striking in the testimonies of the Nazi mass murderers is the terrifying normalcy they show, which is not the symptom of a perversion in the clinical sense of the term (sexual), but an adherence to a perverse system as a way of undergoing an extreme dehumanization of man toward man, which can only be invented by mankind, since the animal kingdom never finds joy in evil, and is not perverse or criminal.

The criminal in the sense of Sade submits to a wild nature that defines him, but does not accept submission (unlike the Nazi war criminal) to the power of a State that leads him to obey a law of crime: "The executioners have no voice" said Bataille, and "if they had one, it'd be the voice of the State" [1].

In fact, Sade remarks that since human nature is essentially criminal, the abolition of the capital punishment must be unconditional: "Capital punishment is pointless. Not only does it not repress crime, which is natural to man, but adds one crime to another by causing the death of two men instead of one" [37].

This kind of sadism, according to Coderch [5], should not be included within perversions, because the existence of a certain degree of sexual arousal in this kind of crimes is possible, then taking a different path and being led to serve a destructive instinct (the aggressive instinct), rendering, therefore, the initial excitation merely a trigger.

A different way of expressing the sadistic behavior is called moral sadism [39], in which sadism can be degraded or diluted toward symbolic behavior in which the sexual component is not experienced by the individual as such. Among its methods of expression we find the unjustified verbal violence that some people display, abuse of authority, corporal punishment and even the declaration and practice of war. The confessions of children who are victims of sexual abuse, also reveal, as Shengold points out, mental torture in which hatred and indifference, silence and masked madness are necessary conditions [40].

Radical Islamists consider women as objects of desire, as the ultimate expression of perversion, even more than the homosexuals, who just disguise their masculinity. Thus, when the woman escapes from voluntary servitude, seeks to run away from slavery as her only destiny, they consider that she should be battered, bruised, tortured, stoned, and murdered. By embodying a form of radical impurity, she is permitted to choose between the concealment of her body and the death of his identity [1].

11.8.2 Masochism

Masochism can be defined as an opposite to sadism, that is, the search and provocation of a person's own suffering as a way of obtaining sexual pleasure.

According to Laplanche and Pontalis [4] masochism is a sexual perversion in which sexual satisfaction is linked to the suffering or humiliation suffered by the subject: "Actually what defines this behavior is more a scene of humiliation than a real appetite for pain: the masochistic partner requires staging, this is really a ritual, a form of contract" [35].

In masochism the fantasy of being humiliated and subjected plays a key role; thus, imagination gets imposed to more active behaviors, typical of sadism. Masochistic people have a recurring obsession with sexual fantasies and impulses related to their submission to humiliation, corporal punishment, or any other activity that results in pain or degradation. However, up to 30 % of them have concurrently sadistic fantasies [9], which once again links the two concepts together.

This sexual behavior deviation owes its name to the detailed practices by Leopold von Sacher-Masoch, famous Austrian novelist of the nineteenth century whose characters reached their sexual pleasure by being abused and dominated by certain women, having previously and solemnly signed different contracts in which the rules of behavior of both signatories [41] were collected.

From a cognitive perspective and learning theories it is postulated that masochist individuals may have experienced situations in which they have been subjected to intense suffering during their childhood, or may have observed such situations in their closest people's lives; thus, they finally become convinced that suffering and pain are necessary requirements for achieving sexual pleasure [9].

Castilla del Pino argues that we must look for the origin of secondary masochism in a mother who frustrates the "oedipal expectations" of the child. The child attempts aggression against her, but he experiences guilt and thus the need to be punished, hence, the feeling of being rewarded for the pain. From here, a model of gratification that plays through a sadistic sexual partner [13] is produced. This author argues that masochistic fantasies are frequent during masturbation and intercourse, and during homosexual anal intercourse.

Regarding feminine masochism, also derived from a psychoanalytical point of view from the "Oedipus conflict," like the previous one, it is not exactly a defense against castration anxiety but a real desire to be castrated by the father and loved by him, as the mother is. According to Melanie Klein the primary origin of masochism in women stems from the oral-sadistic period and the desire to incorporate the father's penis, which subsequently and once inside her body is experienced as bad, destructive, and aggressive, targeting it with a whole group of sadistic impulses with the help of her partner, typically a sadist, who through another evil penis destroys all the harmful objects inside her [5].

Even if in this chapter we continue to discuss sadomasochism from a psychodynamic perspective (after all psychoanalysis is the theory that has devoted more research to these aspects of the human psyche), it is evident that psychoanalytical jargon regarding psychosexual development and the perverse behavior of individuals tends to make us blush for being unscientific, interpretative, outdated, and sexist.

Celia Amorós, Spanish philosopher and first female winner of the Spanish National Essay Prize in 2006, states that the relationship between feminism and psychoanalysis has been and continues to be paradoxical, given that feminism emerged and developed denouncing the subordinate role that culture has built for women, while psychoanalysis is one of the institutions that has helped to raise representations of women as subordinates. Feminism believes that Freudian positions are essentialist, and condemn femininity to the fate that anatomy has provided it with, to be considered a deviation, a reproduction or a flaw in the pattern that works as a standard of development [42].

Returning to the previous focus, facing these forms of masochism allegedly secondary to castration anxiety, Coderch [5], quoting Freud's opinion, speaks of a primary erogenous masochism, in which the pain, far from avoiding greater suffering (castration), provides pleasure. The explanation of these cases is once again related to the early affective experiences during the "summit affective states" [13], in which a sharp rise in tension (including that produced by displeasure) is a source of sexual arousal, and it becomes fixated as such for the rest of the individual's life.

During the libidinal development of the baby a basic conflict between the life instincts (Eros) and death (Thanatos) arises. The libido, the representative of the instinct of life, is projected outwardly as a method of defense against self-destruction, part of the death instinct, placing the management of this on sexual function and thus embodying the sadistic impulses. However, another part of the death instinct is inside the individual and results in the primary or erogenous masochism, representative of the death instinct, and from this moment it is linked to the libido being itself a source of pleasure. The part of the thanatic instinct projected outward may in certain circumstances be internalized again, returning regressively to the primary object and producing the secondary masochism. This will be more evident and intense, the higher the erogenous or primary masochism, and will perform as a defensive mechanism against castration anxiety, allowing sexual pleasure to be obtained, while the primitive erogenous masochism is a source of pleasure in itself [5].

As in the case of sadism, masochism exists in multiple forms of degradation, including the moral masochism concept developed by Freud and coming to determine the pattern of constant failure of certain individuals, as well as the polysymptomatic courtship typical of some forms of neurosis. In this form of masochism the suffering of the individual appears seemingly detached from any erotic situation or sexual pleasure, and he experiences severe punishment and pain derived from the multiple circumstances of vital events. This applies to people who leave an existential disgrace and quickly get into another that may even be worse, being a slave to some form of repetition compulsion.

In moral masochism it is the Ego of the individual that requires punishment, either by his Superego (in the shape of an excess of pressure, coercion, and moral stiffness) or from external circumstances that are symbolically represented by the superior power of fate [5]. If we say of the Superego of these people that it is very punitive, inflicting an unconscious sense of guilt on them, resulting in an active search for suffering, which although unpleasant is preferred and produces some relief of an intolerable guilt. This kind of masochism is also reflected in the "negative therapeutic reaction," which consists of the individual's resistance to the psychoanalytical cure because the psychic suffering deeply satisfies the masochistic needs.

The alleged de-linkage between moral masochism and sexuality is misleading: being punished by the Superego or external factors means to be punished for the father because the Superego is, primarily, the internalized image of the parental couple, the male parent being the main representative of the external force that has power to command, enforce, and punish. Later, that power is transferred to authority figures or to the impersonal forces of destiny [5]. Once again, we observe the gender discourse within androcentric psychoanalytical theory, and also the loop of the Oedipal myth.

According to Kernberg, we all pay a price with minor manifestations of masochistic pathology as a precursor step to the normal integration of the Superego functions in our psychic apparatus "masochism cannot be understood without taking into account the vicissitudes of libidinal and aggressive impulses, the development and pathology of the Superego, the Ego levels of organization, the pathology of internalized object relations and the extent to which normal or pathological narcissistic features predominate" [25].

For instance, the sublimatory ability to withstand pain or hard work as a way to bolster success and future achievements is rooted in this universal masochistic predisposition.

Meanwhile, in those aspects related to "normal" sexuality, the adult capacity to preserve and maintain certain aspects of the polymorphous perverse infantile sexuality includes the possibility of sexual arousal with fantasies and masochistic and sadomasochistic experiences.

Finally, the sadomasochistic aspects of infantile sexuality play in the adult a key role in maintaining the balance between libidinal drives (Eros) and the aggressive impulses (Thanatos), and that basically represents a primitive synthesis between love and hate.

11.8.3 The "Masochistic Syndromes": Towards a New Nosology of Masochism

Kernberg proposes a clustering called "masochist syndromes" within two blocks, considering the level of personality structure. As we move forward in this proposed scheme the severity of the symptoms increases.

11.8.3.1 Neurotic Level of Personality Structure

Within the so-called senior figures, i.e., those with a well-defined Ego identity, a good tolerance to anxiety and frustration, good impulse control, adequate sublimatory capacity, and definitely a strict but well-integrated Superego, we distinguish different types of masochist expression. These include:

The depressive-masochistic personality disorder

This group includes the so-called moral masochism discussed earlier, i.e., that kind of masochism in which the subject, as a result of an unconscious sense of guilt, seeks a victim position with no (apparent) sexual pleasure involved.

The depressive-masochistic personality disorder is defined by three major characterological traits: those that reflect an intransigent Superego, those that reflect an overdependence on the love, support, and acceptance of others, and those that reflect difficulties in expressing aggressiveness.

The masochistic infatuation

According to Freud, during a normal crush the Self is empty of libidinal cathexes, which are invested in the loved object, which replaces the ideal Ego (an integral part of the Superego).

Chasseguet Smirguel (as Kernberg) [25] believes that this is not exactly true, since if love is reciprocated the self-esteem of both partners is enhanced, thus enriching the libidinal investment of the Self of the one who loves. In other words, this is a two-way interactive process.

Masochistic love is characterized by the unconscious choice of certain objects that are either unable to respond to love, or are unwilling to do so. In this context the individual subjects all the other aspects and aspirations of his life to the pursuit of an inaccessible and idealized love object. Slavery regarding an inaccessible object reveals a sense of narcissistic gratification in these people, who pride themselves on being "the greatest sufferers on earth," an image dynamically linked to other forms of narcissistic gratification as being "the biggest sinner" or "the worst victim."

This kind of pathological love represents submission to certain aspects of the Ideal Ego projected on the object; thus, this painful and unsatisfactory love fills the individual with pride and emotional intensity. For Kernberg this way of "suffering love" reflects a primitive infantile narcissism that makes the experiences of the masochistic patient adhere to the strict scope of suffering love and not to other areas of his life, which does not happen in the structures of borderline personalities.

In these more severe cases, narcissism extends to all the object-relations of the individual and permeates all his life. We are no longer talking about the projection of a normal Ideal Self on an inaccessible love object but about a pathological and grandiose Self that makes a considerable effort to establish an affective relationship that unconsciously reaffirms his own grandeur.

These masochistic love relationships in narcissistic personalities represent an unconscious effort to consolidate a symbolic integration within the great Self of the subject of the characteristics of both sexes, thus trying to establish a symbolic union with the idealized object. In these cases it is typical that the relationship with the idealized loved object reflects a condensation of oedipal and pre-oedipal issues: the positive, idealized oedipal love object and the negative, sadist pre-oedipal love object, which is necessary nonetheless. This is definitely a combination of narcissistic and masochistic characterological traits.

The masochistic perversion

It is at the neurotic level of the personality structure that the masochistic sexual perversion occurs in the way it has been previously described. Here, sexual masochism takes the shape of a predetermined and performed script in the context of an object relationship experienced as safe.

We will see later how as the individual progresses through the analyzed pathological level, both eroticism and sex drive associated with masochistic behavior disappear, self-injurious behaviors and mutilation increase, and confusion and diffusion about the individual's sexual identity increases.

11.8.3.2 Boundary or Border Level of Personality Organization

Here, we are facing different personalities characterized by the presence of overt signs of Ego weakness (lack of tolerance to distress and frustration, poor impulse control, poor sublimatory capacity), predominance of partial and incomplete object relations, prevalence of primitive defense mechanisms (splitting, projective identification, primitive idealization, omnipotent control, devaluation), progressive fading of eroticism or sexual drive and increased confusion and diffusion in terms of sexual identity.

In this group, Kernberg distinguishes three alternative forms of expression of masochism.

The sadomasochistic personality disorder

These people usually feel victims of aggression themselves and complain bitterly of being abused, obstinately justifying their own attacks against people they depend on, on the basis of this perception of being attacked.

These are highly dependent personalities, on whose psychodynamic traits we find severe oedipal and pre-oedipal conflicts, as well as an intense internal dependence on certain maternal images experienced as sadistic, dishonest, and controlling. These images influence the development of severe behavioral disorders that are not observed in the depressive-masochistic disorder, which depends more on the Oedipal conflict period.

The projection of the primitive precursors of the Superego onto other people, appearing as paranoid traits, and the tendency of these people to defend their contradictive behaviors through rationalization (i.e., aggressiveness) illustrate the failure of the functions of the Superego at the psychic integration of these individuals, unlike what is observed in the depressive-masochistic disorder, ruled by a rigid and dominating Superego.

Sexual masochism with self-destructive traits

These people have in common the following characteristics: strong and primitive aggressive impulses, a severe pathology in the field of object relations, a predominance of oedipal conflicts and goals in the masochistic sexual script, a lack of Superego integration, and finally a confusion about their sexual identity, in order that the homo- and heterosexual interactions are part of his daily life along with sexual masochism, which represents its primary organizer feature.

Extreme forms of mutilation and self-sacrifice

Otto Kernberg framed individuals with extreme self-destructive behavior around three possible psychic structures:

Histrionic personality disorder. It fits within the borderline personality disorder proposed by the DSM-5 [11] (and personality traits included in the dimensions of antagonism, disinhibition, and negative affectivity), and the emotional instability personality disorder described by ICD-10 [8]. In this group the self-destructiveness arises at moments of intense anger, sometimes mixed with depressive feelings. Self-injurious behaviors represent an unconscious effort to reassert control over the surrounding environment, causing guilt feelings in others (i.e., when someone opposes the desires or does not obey patient expectations).

Malignant narcissism. It represents a step forward in severity over the previous group. Here, there are no manifestations of dependence as before. These are distant individuals, with a lack of commitment with other people. Their self-destructive behavior occurs when their pathological grandiosity is challenged, which induces in them a traumatic sense of humiliation or defeat, often accompanied by sadistic behavior. The grandeur of these individuals is satisfied with a sense of triumph over the fear of pain and death, and a sense of superiority over other people, who will feel shocked or angry at their behavior. According to the DSM-5 [11] the dominant personality dimension of these individuals would be antagonism.

Atypical psychosis. When we face grotesque and unusual suicide attempts with regard to their particularity and cruelty (self-castration, enucleation of both eyes, lingual tearing), we attend the staging of individuals affected by certain atypical psychotic conditions. The main difference in this group compared with the previous ones lies in the quality of repetitive behavior of self-mutilation. Thus, the eroticism of pain and mutilation seem to have acquired the meaning of a triumph over life and death, pain and fear, and unconsciously mainly over the world of object relations [25]. Needless to say, that from the prognostic standpoint this is the group with poorest therapeutic expectations.

In his book *Pain and Passion*, Stoller [43] goes through a psychoanalytical–anthropological tour of the sadomasochistic clubs of Los Angeles' surrounding area, interviewing clients and professionals trying to understand what motivates them, what it is that makes those activities pleasant, and what these people are like in their everyday lives. Stoller ends his journey by passing on more questions than answers, and shows the huge variety of personality structures and ways of life in which these deviations from the norm do occur. Therefore, there is no definitive psychoanalytical formulation that can be applied to all patients with such material. Which leaves us with a more open and exploratory attitude: in this patient, what function does this fantasy or behavior have? What is the patient defending himself from? How does he find enjoyment in it?

Depending on the authors we consult, the origins of masochism can be traced to libidinal and aggressive derivatives of the Id, feelings of guilt, and needs for punishment with their origin in the Superego, or can be considered as a way of having a relationship with internal or external objects, trying to avoid feared situations and object relations [44, 45].

Contemporary proposals (Soccarides, Brenner) support a more integrated perspective with a multiple function connected with the Id, the Ego, and Superego to serve both defensive and adaptive goals. Stolorow [46], following this conciliatory point of view, states that masochistic activities may represent sometimes fruitless efforts (sometimes primitively sexualized) to restore and maintain positive structural cohesion, temporal stability, and positive affective coloring of a poor representation of the crumbling Self. This author also points out that the masochistic self-abasement attempting to extol the object maintains a symbiotic or dependant object relation, illusory but vital, and discards the aggression and damage that would result from the loss of the object if the patient accepted (instead of denied) the hateful and hostile aspects of the object.

Sometimes people (especially women) construct object relations in which the perverse has a relevant weight, as a defense against situations of personal distress related to aggression and social violence, added to personal experiences. In pornography, for instance, the sexualization of gender inequality, the violence against women, abuse and multiple variations of male dominance and female submission can be identified. To the extent that the more unequal, the more sexual. It is a reflection of our society. It is not just that women are the main targets of rape, nor that they are the main group that suffers sexual abuse by family members, friends or authority figures within an early interpersonal sexual encounter. Not even that, being adults, they can be more vulnerable to acts of physical violence by their male partner, nor that they more frequently suffer sexual harassment at work. The key is that this all documents the degree and the extent of abuse, of systematic sexual assault, which suggests the clear permissibility of such a structure based on power.

Perversions appear to be a phenomenon with multiple meanings and can simultaneously cover several defensive lines. In contrast, queer theory, for example, not only tries to fully deconstruct the sexual difference but also embodies a project that seeks to abolish the idea that perversion is necessary for civilization. This theory rejects both biological sex and social gender, and believes that each individual is free to take at any time the role of either of the sexes, their clothes, their behaviors, and their own delusions. Hence, the assertion that the transgressive sexual practices, nomadism, porn, escapism, fetishism, voyeurism, are just the equivalent of the rules issued by the self-proclaimed heterosexual society [1].

To Roudinesco, discourse of the queer theory is nothing but the puritanical continuation of the sadistic utopia. However, while Sade justifies crime, incest, and sodomy as the foundations of an imaginary society centered on an inversion of law, the queer theory transforms human sexuality into a domesticated eroticism, in which any reference to love and hatred has been evacuated. Actually, this theory seeks to erase borders and deny perversion its transgressive power dealing with human sexuality, to the point that erasing its name is equal to converting what has been erased in a variation of normality [1]. Since this area is very complex, and initiatives or innovative contributions do not abound, any constructive effort is welcomed.

References

1. Roudinesco É. Our dark side, a history of perversion. Cambridge: Polity Press; 2009. Spanish translation: Roudinesco É. Nuestro lado oscuro. Una historia de los perversos. Barcelona: Anagrama; 2009.
2. Sanyal MM. Vulva: Die Enthüllung des unsichtbaren Geschlechts. Berlin: Wagenbach; 2009. Spanish translation: Sanyal MM. Vulva. Barcelona: Anagrama; 2012.
3. Lerner H. Was Frauen verschweigen. Warum wir täuschen, heucheln, lügen müssen. Frankfurt: Fischer; 1996. Spanish translation: Lerner H. Por qué fingimos las mujeres? Verdad y mentira en la vida de las mujeres. Barcelona: Círculo de Lectores; 1995.
4. Laplanche J, Pontalis JB. Vocabulaire de la psychoanalyse. Paris: Presses Universitaires de France; 1967. Spanish translation: Laplanche J, Pontalis JB. Diccionario de Psicoanálisis. Barcelona: Paidós; 1996.
5. Coderch J. Trastornos del carácter. Continuación. In: Coderch J, editor. Psiquiatría Dinámica. 5th ed. Barcelona: Herder; 1991.
6. Paglia C. Sexual personae. Art and decadence from Nefertiti to Emily Dickinson. New Haven, CT: Yale University Press; 1990.
7. American Psychiatric Association. Paraphilias: prevalence, characteristics, evaluation and cognitive-behavioral treatment. In American Psychiatric Association: Advanced selected topics in Psychiatry. Washington, DC: American Psychiatric Publishing; 2004
8. International Statistical Classification of Diseases and Health Related Problems. Geneva: The ICD-10. World Health Orgnization; 1992. Spanish translation: Trastornos Mentales y del Comportamiento, CIE 10. Madrid: Meditor; 1992.
9. Sorrentino RM. Paraphilias. In: Sadock BJ, Sadock VA, Ruiz P, editors. Comprehensive textbook of psychiatry. 9th ed. Philadelphia: Lippincott Williams & Wilkins; 2009.
10. Oyebode F. Disorders of gender and sexuality, Sims' symptoms in the mind. An introduction to descriptive psychopathology. 4th ed. London: Saunders; 2008.
11. APA. Diagnostic and statistical manual of mental disorders, DSM 5. 5th ed. Arlington, VA: American Psychiatric Association; 2013.
12. Dworkin A, MacKinnon CA. Pornography and civil rights. A new day for women's equality. Originally published and distributed by Organizing Against Pornography, a Resource Center for Education and Action based in Minneapolis; 1998.
13. Castilla del Pino C. Conductas paradigmáticas sexuales. In: Castilla del Pino C, editor. Introducción a la Psiquiatría. Tomo I. Problemas generales. Psico(pato)logía. 4th ed. Madrid: Alianza Editorial, S.A.; 1993.
14. Freud S. Three essays on the theory of sexuality. Spanish translation: Freud S, editor. Tres ensayos para una teoría sexual. In: Freud S, editor. Obras completas. Tomo II. 4th ed. Madrid: Biblioteca Nueva; 1981.
15. Freud S. Leonardo da Vinci, a memory of his childhood. Spanish translation: Freud S. Un recuerdo infantil de Leonardo de Vinci. In: Freud S, editor. Obras completas. Tomo II. 4th ed. Madrid: Biblioteca Nueva; 1981.
16. Dio Bleichmar E. La sexualidad femenina. Barcelona: Paidós; 1997.
17. Graves R. The Greek myths. London: Penguin; 1981.
18. Sophocles. Oedipus the King. London: The University of Chicago Press; 2010.
19. Irigaray L. Das Geschlecht das nicht eins ist. Berlin: Merve Verlag; 1979. Spanish translation: Ese sexo que no es uno. Madrid: Akal; 2009.
20. McDougall J. The anonymous spectator-a clinical study of sexual perversión. Contemp Psychoanal. 1974;10:289–310.
21. Chasseguet-Smirgel J. Reflexions on the connexions between perversion and sadism. J Psychoanal. 1978;59:27–35.
22. Chasseguet-Smirgel J. Perversion and the Universal Law. Int R Psychoanal. 1983;10:293–301.
23. Stoller RJ. Hostility and mystery in perversión. Int J Psychoanal. 1974;55:425–34.

24. Kernberg OF. Sadomasochism, sexual excitement and perversion. J Am Psychoanal Assoc. 1991;39:333–62.
25. Kernberg O. Love relations: normality and pathology. Yale University Press, New Edition; 1998. Spanish translation: Kernberg, O. Relaciones amorosas. Normalidad y patología. Buenos Aires: Paidós; 1995.
26. González Torres MA. Transsexualism: some considerations on aggression, transference and countertransference. Int Forum Psychoanal. 1996;5:11–21.
27. Blanchard R. The DSM, diagnostic criteria for transvestic fetishism. Arch Sex Behav. 2010;39 (2):363–72.
28. Kafka MP. The DSM, diagnostic criteria for fetishism. Arch Sex Behav. 2010;39(2):357–62.
29. Långström N. The DSM, diagnostic criteria for exhibitionism, voyeurism and frotteurism. Arch Sex Behav. 2010;39(2):317–24.
30. Krueger RB. The DSM, diagnostic criteria for sexual masochism. Arch Sex Behav. 2010;39 (2):346–56.
31. Krueger RB. The DSM, diagnostic criteria for sexual sadism. Arch Sex Behav. 2010;39 (2):325–45.
32. Hucker SJ. Hypoxyphilia. Arch Sex Behav. 2011;40(6):1323–6.
33. Stern P. Paraphilic coercitive disorder in the DSM: the right diagnosis for the right reasons. Arch Sex Behav. 2010;39(6):1443–7.
34. Kafka MP. The DSM, diagnostic criteria for paraphilia not otherwise specified. Arch Sex Behav. 2009;39(2):373–6.
35. Ey H, Bernar P, Brisset Ch. Manuel de Psychiatrie. Spanish translation: Las perversiones sexuales. In: Ey H, Bernard P, Brisset Ch. Tratado de Psiquiatría, 8ª Ed. Barcelona: Masson; 1978.
36. Butler J. Undoing gender. London: Routledge Chapman & Hall; 2004.
37. Lever M. Donatien, Alphonse, François, marqués de Sade. Barcelona: Seix Barral; 1994.
38. Arendt H. Eichmann in Jerusalem: a report of the Banality of Evil. London: Penguin; 1977.
39. Abel GG, Osborn CA. Paraphilias. In: Gelder MG, López-Ibor Jr. JJ, Andreasen N. editor. Spanish translation: Tratado de Psiquiatría. Barcelona: Ars Medica; 2003.
40. Shengold L. Meurtre d'âme. New Haven, Paris: Le destin des enfants maltraités; 1989.
41. Sacher-Masoch L. Venus in furs. Spanish translation: La venus de las pieles. Madrid: Alianza Editorial; 1973.
42. De Miguel A, Amorós C. Teoría feminista. Minerva, Madrid: De la Ilustración a la globalización; 2005.
43. Stoller RJ. Pain & passion. New York: Plenum; 1991.
44. Reich W. Charakteranalyse. Technik und Grundlagen für studierende und praktizierende Analytiker; 1933. Spanish translation: Reich W. Análisis del character. Buenos Aires: Paidós Ibérica; 2005.
45. Horney K. The problem of feminism masochism. Psychoanal Rev. 1935;22:241–57.
46. Stolorow R. The narcissistic function of masochism (and sadism). Int J Psychoanal. 1975;56:441–8.

Gender Dysphoria 12

Rafael Segarra-Echebarría, Beatriz Rodríguez-Paz, Arantzazu Zabala-Rabadán, and Margarita Sáenz-Herrero

One day I'll grow up, I'll be a beautiful woman.
One day I'll grow up, I'll be a beautiful girl.
But for today I am a child, for today I am a boy ...
Antony and The Johnsons, For today I'm a boy

Abstract

Individuals with gender dysphoria (GD) have a marked incongruence between the gender they have been assigned (usually at birth, referred to as natal gender) and the gender they have experienced/expressed. This discrepancy is the core component of the diagnosis. There must also be evidence of distress about this incongruence. Experienced gender may include alternative gender identities beyond binary stereotypes. Consequently, the distress is not limited to a desire to simply be of the other gender, but may include a desire to be of an alternative gender, provided that it differs from the individual's assigned gender.

The debate about whether GD should be in the *Diagnostic and Statistical Manual of Mental Disorders* has been going on for decades. As psychiatry's professionals, we are sure that being transsexual, transgender, or gender nonconforming is a matter of diversity, not necessarily pathology. The World Professional Association for Transgender Health released in May 2010 a

R. Segarra-Echebarría (✉)
Cruces University Hospital, Bilbao, Spain

University of the Basque Country, UPV/EHU, Cruces, Spain
e-mail: rafaelsegarraechevarria@osakidetza.net

B. Rodríguez-Paz
Lucus Augusti University Hospital, Lugo, Spain

A. Zabala-Rabadán
University of the Basque Country, UPV/EHU, Leioa, Spain

M. Sáenz-Herrero
University of the Basque Country, UPV/EHU, Araba, Spain

Araba University Hospital, Vitoria, Spain

M. Sáenz-Herrero (ed.), *Psychopathology in Women*,
DOI 10.1007/978-3-319-05870-2_12

statement urging the de-psychopathologization of gender nonconformity worldwide. This statement noted that the expression of gender characteristics (including identities) that are not stereotypically associated with one's assigned sex at birth is a common and culturally diverse human phenomenon that should not be judged as inherently pathological or negative.

Only some gender-nonconforming people experience GD at some point in their lives. Treatment is available to assist people with such distress to explore their gender identity and find a gender role that is comfortable for them.

12.1 Introduction: Gender Dysphoria and the So-Called Third Sex—The Crying Light

Gender dysphoria (GD) is a new controversial diagnostic class in the American Psychiatric Association's (APA) *Diagnostic Statistical Manual of Mental Disorders* (DSM) 5 [1], and it reflects a change in the conceptualization of the disorder's defining features, emphasizing the phenomenon of "gender incongruence" rather than cross-gender identification per se, as was the case in DSM-IV: gender identity disorder (GID) [2].

DSM-5's GD includes separate sets of criteria for children and for adults and adolescents. For the adolescent and adult criteria, the previous criterion A (cross-gender identification) and criterion B (aversion toward one's gender) are merged. In the wording of the criteria, "the other sex" is replaced by "the other gender" (or "some alternative gender") [1]. This change may not be much, but it can be considered a starting point.

Gender instead of sex is used systematically because the concept "sex" is inadequate when referring to individuals with a disorder of sex development. In the children's criteria, a "strong desire to be of the other gender" replaces the previous "repeatedly stated desire to be the other sex" to capture the situation of some children who, in a coercitive environment, may not verbalize the desire to be of another gender.

For children, criterion A1 ("a strong desire to be of the other gender or an insistence that he or she is the other gender") is now necessary but not sufficient, which makes the diagnosis more restrictive and conservative. The subtyping on the basis of sexual orientation is removed because that distinction is no longer considered clinically useful [1].

A post-transition specifier has been added to identify individuals who have undergone at least one medical procedure or treatment to support the new gender assignment (i.e., cross-sex hormone treatment). Although the concept of post-transition is modeled on the concept of full or partial remission, the term *remission* has implications in terms of symptom reduction that do not apply directly to GD [1].

That is the APA's proposal. Now we go further into controversy: Matt Kailey is an award-winning author, blogger, professor, and transgender community activist. He began his transition from female to male in 1997, and since then he has educated, enlightened, and entertained audiences across the USA and the world through his writing and presentations focusing on transgender issues. He has appeared in five documentary films and is the recipient of four community awards for activism. His book *Just Add Hormones: An Insider's Guide to the Transsexual Experience* was a Lambda Literary Award finalist, and his short story *Cam's Decision* was the recipient of the Poets & Writers Inc. Writers Exchange Award for fiction. Matt's latest book, *Teeny Weenies and Other Short Subjects*, is a collection of humorous essays about his life before and after transition. He's also working on a series of short books offering 10 tips for those involved with "trans" people. He's also a part-time college-level psychology instructor and teaches his own class, *Writing Your Gender*, offering college students a chance to explore their own gender through the art of personal essay.

With reference to Matt Kailey's Tranifesto blog (transgender and transexual issues, information, advice, and opinion) we take a look at his opinion posted 16 April 2012 (http://tranifesto.com/2012/04/16/ask-matt-should-gender-dysphoria-be-in-the-dsm/), just a year before DSM-5 was published:

> The debate about whether or not GID (or some other language that represents a similar "condition") should be in the DSM (Diagnostic and Statistical Manual of Mental Disorders) has been going on for at least as long as I have been in the community. I first learned of the debate when I began transition fifteen years ago.
>
> The DSM-5 is scheduled to be released in May of 2013, and at this point, it appears that GID will now be called Gender Dysphoria (GD), but I don't think it's as simple as a name change. There are various pieces of the diagnosis that have been changed or moved to different categories within the DSM-5, and there have been other changes in language.
>
> Some people feel that these changes are positive, while others want certain categories out of the DSM altogether. However, my understanding is that it will appear as GD in the DSM-5.
>
> But in the limited space of a blog, with the knowledge that I have, we can look at your question: is it good or bad to remove ourselves from the DSM at this point in time?
>
> It turns out to be a moot point, because GD will be in the DSM-5. However, the arguments at their most basic level are:
>
> We should be in the DSM, because if we are not, we will not be seen as having a legitimate condition that requires medical intervention. We will be seen as "choosing" transition, and we will not be taken seriously. Any strides that we have made with regard to insurance paying for transition procedures will stall. We need the backing of the medical and psychiatric communities in order to realize full rights and full equality.
>
> We should not be in the DSM, because we do not have a mental health disorder. If anything, we have a medical condition that was present at birth and is possibly due to hormonal fluctuations during pregnancy or we do not have any kind of "condition" at all, and we are simply one of many ways to be as human. By virtue of our humanity, we are equal to all other humans, and by virtue of a strongly demonstrated need to align our body with our gender identity, we should be able to transition with informed consent and with the understanding from insurance companies and medical professionals that transition is a medical necessity.
>
> My own opinion is that I would like to see GID, GD, or whatever psychiatric label comes about for people whose gender identity does not align with their physical sex (or sex assigned at birth) removed from the DSM. I don't think that my "condition" is a mental health issue.

> Research has demonstrated that transition, a series of medical procedures, can reduce or eliminate the suicidal ideation and other emotional difficulties that many trans people experience. Therefore, I believe that this is a medical issue and should be treated as such. However, there are some trans people who think that even that is too pathologizing, and that transition procedures should be available as on-demand procedures, with the idea that we know our own bodies and minds and should have the right to make our own decisions about care.
>
> I agree with this as well, and this is where I am torn. I believe that I am responsible for my own body, and that I am capable of making decisions about it. I don't think that I should have to jump through a bunch of someone else's hoops to do what is best for me. But if gender issues are not part of either a psychiatric or a medical diagnosis, and transition procedures can be issued upon request, then transition becomes a series of "elective" procedures, not considered medically necessary, not covered by insurance or other medical programs, and not recognized as a life-saving intervention.
>
> A quick aside about language: I generally say "we are in the DSM" or "I am in the DSM" simply for ease of communication. The truth is that we are not in the DSM and I am not in the DSM. I am diagnosed with a "condition" that appears in the DSM. I think it's an important distinction, at least when thinking about yourself as a trans person. We are not our diagnosis".

Certainly it seems difficult to disagree whith his first-person point of view. Moreover, after 15 years of revision, the American Psychiatric Association's board of trustees approved the changes, including the removal of the term GID. Simultaneously, the term GD will be used to diagnose the distress occurring over a marked incongruence between a person's experienced gender and their assigned gender.

Although linguistically subtle, the difference between "disorder" and "dysphoria" should have a huge impact on the outlook and treatment of transgendered individuals.

According to the National Institute of Mental Health (NIMH), disorders are thought of as a clinically significant behavior, psychologically syndrome, or a pattern that occurs in an individual typically associated with distress, painful symptomology, disability or impairment.

Dysphoria, on the other hand, is a psychological state that causes one to experience feelings of anxiety, restlessness, and depression. It is not necessarily diagnosable, or something that would be identified in the DSM, but it is more a state of being, a feeling of unpleasantness or discomfort.

The previous diagnosis of GID implied that the problem might lie within the client, further suggesting that the client might need to be cured or somehow mentally and emotionally fixed. The pending reclassification speaks to the mental state that accompanies being transgendered within this society.

Rather than indicating that a person needs to be fixed, the diagnosis indicates that the issues that need to be addressed lie outside the individual. Kelly Winters, from the group GID Reform Advocates, believes that the change in diagnosis signifies that "the problem to be treated is not the person's identity, but rather the distress that is often experienced by those who need access to medical transition care" (http://dot429.com/articles/2125-from-disorder-to-dysphoria-transgender-identity-and-the-dsm-v).

Although transgender individuals are still dependent upon these institutions, the removal of GID is compared with the organization's declassification of homosexuality as a mental disorder in 1973. Prior to its removal, homosexuality was a reason for therapy and institutionalization.

Although the social climate and treatment of mental health patients have changed since gays and lesbians could be deinstitutionalized for their diagnosis, transgendered individuals who were diagnosed with GID were still left potentially vulnerable to medical and mental health workers.

Winters further states that the change in the diagnosis signals a change of attitude within the APA that our gender identities are no longer considered the focus of pathology (http://dot429.com/articles/2125-from-disorder-to-dysphoria-transgender-identity-and-the-dsm-v).

But the fact remains that trans and especially transsexual people needing hormonal or surgical transition care are still classified as having a mental disorder.

Although this keeps the relationship between the transgendered community and health institutions strong, because of the need for hormones and surgeries, it does show a cultural shift in acceptance and understanding.

Prior to the change, the term "disorder" gave the impression, both socially and psychologically, that there was something damaged or dangerous about transgendered individuals, much like a mood disorder would make someone feel that he or she was unstable or unable to function in society.

Removing the stigma is the first step in social change, taking the transgender community out of the mental health field toward an accepting society.

It is time to write about biopolitics, 30 years afters Michel Foucault's death. This French philosopher, social theorist, and philologist's works remain among the most important writings for understanding the relationship between society and mental disorder. According to Foucault, madness, crime or sexual deviance categories are constructed according to political discourses to normalize them. From this perspective, it is necessary to note that being different is not being sick. The main question formulated by Foucault (it must be highlighted that it came about when he was still a young student who was completing his training at the Hospital of Sainte Anne in Paris) could hardly be more clear and was aimed at the root of the issue, "I had also followed psychopathology studies, an alleged discipline that didn't teach too much. Then I raised the question: how a little knowledge can drag so much power?" [3].

Foucault contemplates why society delegates such great power to mental health professionals, and wonders whether it will be because they fulfill the specific function of social control to serve the interests of the system, and not by the value of their scientists' knowledge, scarce in some historical periods, as he stated in his works, without diminishing his power at all. For Foucault psychiatric diagnosis is not something objective or neutral, but is linked to what he called biopolitics, which would be an attempt by the authorities to control the health, hygiene, power, sexuality, and birth since they are political issues, mainly from the eighteenth century. Also, Foucault introduces the concept of *episteme*, which would be the thought structure of each historical period [3].

Thus, according to Foucault, psychiatry is not an exact science, but it is conditioned by the historical moment *episteme*. In itself, as transcultural psychiatry demonstrates (and as already raised with great acuity by Karen Horney in the 1950s) [4], we have not even yet had a definition of what mental health and mental disorder are, because they depend on the social and cultural contexts, which are obviously linked to power relations. In one of his first books, *Madness and Civilization: a History of Insanity in the Age of Reason* [5], Foucault notes that in medieval times madness was considered a sacred mystery that was part of the vast field of human experience. Also, in the Renaissance, madness was seen as a special kind of ironic reason to show this ridiculous world. Insanity was tragic and comic at once. This image crystallizes in the "ship of fools," a group of people who stood outside of society, but they were also considered pilgrims searching for reason and by extension, the reason of the world, representing the connection between order and chaos.

As Lisa Downing points out [6], Foucault argues that in the Middle Age and in the Renaissance, madness was seen as an integral human phenomenon. Madness opposed reason, but as an alternative mode of human existence, not as its simple rejection. He understands *The Praise of Folly* by Erasmus or the tragedies of Shakespeare in this way. Until the Enlightenment, madness was seen as an imaginary place, a crossing between the world and what is behind it, between life and death, between the tangible and the sacred.

In the Classical Period (1700s and 1800s), the great change takes place, and insanity becomes unreason, something linked to the inhumane, opposed to the rational in the Cartesian approach. With the advent of the modern therapeutic, the madman returns to the society again but is subjected to a moral therapy. Foucault criticizes Pinel, much admired in the history of psychiatry, because he freed the patients from their chains at Bicêtre in 1793; or Samuel Tuke in England who founded a Quaker asylum for the alienated. As Downing points out, to Foucault, neither one nor the other was a proper philanthropist, or introduced a humanitarian twist to the insanity treatment, as the history of psychiatry has shown us. Actually, he considers that Tuke's treatment had a strong component of bourgeois morality because it sought that alienated behavior did not disturb the morals of society. According to Foucault, Tuke replaced the terror of madness with the anguish of bourgeois morality. As it is known, Tuke organized "tea parties" where he taught insane people to be polite and to behave according to established social norms. Foucault maintained that Tuke did not leave mad people to express themselves. Meanwhile, regarding Pinel, Foucault considered that the asylum still maintaining the insane is also an authority system. The alienated is now free of his chains, but is a prisoner of bourgeois morality [5].

At the end of the Enlightenment another important change occurs, the madman becomes "mentally ill." But the authority of the physician is not scientific; it is the authority conferred by society. Thus, the use of the term disease legitimates the physician's work. As Dawning argues, to Foucault, and since the Enlightenment, the new social area of madness has become an object of knowledge. The character of the doctor, psychiatrist, psychologist, becomes the subject of that knowledge [5].

Coming back to the topic of GD, we can assure that being transsexual, transgender, or gender nonconforming is a matter of diversity, not necessarily pathological. The World Professional Association for Transgender Health (WPATH) released a statement in May 2010 urging the de-psychopathologization of gender nonconformity worldwide. This statement noted that “the expression of gender characteristics, including identities, that are not stereotypically associated with one’s assigned sex at birth is a common and culturally diverse human phenomenon [that] should not be judged as inherently pathological or negative” [7].

Unfortunately, there is a stigma attached to gender nonconformity in many societies around the world. Such a stigma can lead to prejudice and discrimination, resulting in “minority stress.” Minority stress is unique (additive to general stressors experienced by all people), socially based, and chronic, and may make transsexual, transgender, and gender-nonconforming individuals more vulnerable to developing mental health problems such as anxiety and depression. In addition to prejudice and discrimination in society at large, stigma can contribute to abuse and neglect in one’s relationships with peers and family members, which in turn can lead to psychological distress. However, these symptoms are socially induced and are not inherent to being transsexual, transgender, or gender-nonconforming.

Incidentally, gender nonconformity refers to the extent to which a person’s gender identity, role, or expression differs from the cultural norms prescribed for people of a particular sex. GD refers to the discomfort or distress that is caused by a discrepancy between a person’s gender identity and that person’s sex assigned at birth (and the associated gender role and/or primary and secondary sex characteristics). Only some gender-nonconforming people experience GD at some point in their lives [7].

Treatment is available to assist people with such distress to explore their gender identity and find a gender role that is comfortable for them. Treatment is individualized: what helps one person alleviate GD might be very different from what helps another person. This process may or may not involve a change in gender expression or body modifications. Medical treatment options include, for example, feminization or masculinization of the body through hormone therapy and/or surgery, which are effective in alleviating GD and are medically necessary for many people. Gender identities and expressions are diverse, and hormones and surgery are just two of many options available to assist people with achieving comfort with self and identity.

Gender dysphoria can largely be alleviated through treatment. Hence, while transsexual, transgender, and gender-nonconforming people may experience GD at some point in their lives, many individuals who receive treatment will find a gender role and expression that is comfortable for them, even if these differ from those associated with their sex assigned at birth, or from prevailing gender norms and expectations [7].

This may be the starting point that leads us to consider the “third sex.” Australia and Germany have recognized gender-neutral, while the intersex community begins to organize to fight for their rights. In the book “Evolution’s Rainbow” [8] the American biologist, Joan Roughgarden, reveals how half of all species on earth, whether animal or vegetable, could not be included in the classification of male or female. Most plants are hermaphrodites and some animals, such as barnacles, snails, starfish, and many fish, begin their life as males and then become females or vice versa.

Humans have always been very clear about the sexual binary scheme; however, this is not always the case, and many begin to question this model. In 2013, Australia and Germany recognized gender neutral, i.e., the possibility that a citizen of these countries should not be necessarily registered as male or female, but leave the box for sex unchecked. Germany is the first European country to approve this initiative and it seems that in the coming years we will see others join in with this policy.

For many, this decision sets the stage for combat, so far the usual habit of practicing genital surgeries in neonates when their sexual organs are not clear, or when they present physiological characteristics of both sexes. The boy/girl child has to be defined as a man or woman to enroll in the registry and, in most cases, it is decided by the doctor, who chooses to give priority to the more developed or visible organs, removing the smaller ones. Thus, the anguish of uncertainty is settled and the child grows up with a definite gender.

The cases of hermaphroditism or androgyny intersex individuals, as they have started to be called, are not as isolated as we think. Statistics conclude that there is a case for every 250 people, and according to the World Health Organization, this affects 1 % of the world's population. In Germany, each year, 400 children are born without a defined sex and in the USA, every day, five surgical sex assignment operations are performed in newborns. These kinds of operations are not harmless, endanger the patient's health, and may damage the genitals or decrease sensitivity. Supporters of this surgery claim that sex-role assignment prevents the baby from suffering future discrimination and relieves the emotional stress experienced by the parents [8].

Intersex conditions include a variety of syndromes in which persons have gross anatomical or physiological aspects of the opposite sex [9]:

> Congenital virilizing adrenal hyperplasia was formerly called the adrenogenital syndrome. An enzymatic defect in the production of adrenal cortisol, beginning prenatally, leads to overproduction of adrenal androgens and virilization of the female fetus. Postnatally, excessive adrenal androgen can be controlled by steroid administration. The androgenization can range from mild clitoral enlargement to external genitals that look like a normal scrotal sac, testes, and a penis, but hidden behind these external genitals are a vagina and a uterus. The patients are otherwise normally female. At birth, if the genitals look male, children are assigned to the male sex and so reared; the result is usually a clear sense of maleness and unremarkable masculinity. If the children are assigned to the female sex and so reared, a sense of femaleness and femininity usually results. If the parents are uncertain about the sex of their child, a hermaphroditic identity results. The resultant gender identity usually reflects the rearing practices, but androgens may help determine behavior. Children raised unequivocally as girls have a more intense tomboy quality than that found in a control group. The girls most often have a heterosexual orientation. Some of these children experience gender identity conflicts and do not feel comfortable in the sex of assignment. Higher rates of bisexual or homosexual behavior in adulthood have been reported.

Androgen insensitivity syndrome was formerly called testicular feminization. In these persons with the XY karyotype, tissue cells are unable to use testosterone or other androgens. Therefore, the person appears to be a normal female at birth and is raised as a girl. She is later found to have cryptorchid testes, which produce the testosterone to which the tissues do not respond, and minimal or absent internal sexual organs. Secondary sex characteristics at puberty are female because of the small, but sufficient, amount of estrogens, which results from the conversion of testosterone into estradiol. The patients usually sense themselves as females and are feminine. However, some experience gender conflicts and distress.

Turner's syndrome, in which one sex chromosome is missing, such that the sex karyotype is simply X. Children have female genitalia, are short, and, possibly, have anomalies such as a shield-shaped chest and a webbed neck. As a consequence of dysfunctional ovaries, they require exogenous estrogen to develop female secondary sex characteristics. Gender identity is female.

Klinefelter's syndrome, in which an extra X chromosome is present in Klinefelter's syndrome, such that the karyotype is XXY. At birth, patients appear to be normal males. Excessive gynecomastia may occur in adolescence. Testes are small, usually without sperm production. Such persons are tall, and body habitus is eunuchoid. Reports suggest a higher rate of GID.

5-α-Reductase Deficiency in which, an enzymatic defect prevents the conversion of testosterone to dihydrotestosterone, which is required for prenatal virilization of the genitalia. At birth, the affected person appears to be female, although some anomaly is visible. In earlier generations, before childhood identification of the disorder was common, these persons, raised as girls, virilized at puberty and changed their gender identity to male. Later generations were expected to virilize and, thus, may have been raised with ambiguous gender. Recently, there are reports of a small number of patients for whom early removal of the testes and socialization as girls have resulted in a female gender identity.

Pseudohermaphroditism: infants born with ambiguous genitals are pseudohermaphrodites. True hermaphroditism is characterized by the presence of both testes and ovaries in the same person. It is a rare condition. Sex assignment based on the genitals' appearance at birth determines gender identity, which is male, female, or hermaphroditic, depending on the family's conviction about the child's sex. Recently, treatment has changed, postponing sex assignment based on the appearance of the genitalia at birth to adolescence, when the child is included in the decision-making process. Male pseudohermaphroditism is incomplete differentiation of the external genitalia even though a Y chromosome is present; testes are present but rudimentary Female pseudohermaphroditism is the presence of virilized genitals in a person who is XX, the most common cause being the adrenogenital syndrome described previously.

Because intersex conditions are present at birth, treatment must be timely, and some physicians believe the conditions to be true medical emergencies. The appearance of the genitalia in diverse conditions is often ambiguous, and a decision must be made about the assigned sex (boy or girl) and how the child should be reared.

Problems should be addressed as early as possible, so that the entire family can regard the child in a consistent, relaxed manner. This is particularly important because intersex patients may have gender identity problems because of complicated biological influences and familial confusion about their actual sex. When intersex conditions are discovered, a panel of pediatric, urological, and psychiatric experts usually determines the sex of rearing on the basis of clinical examination, urological studies, buccal smears, chromosomal analyses, and assessment of the parental wishes.

Education of parents and presentation of the range of options open to them is essential because parents respond to the infant's genitalia in ways that promote the formation of gender identity. One option is for parents to decide against immediate surgery for ambiguous genitalia, but assign the label of boy or girl to the infant on the basis of chromosomal and urological examination. They can then react to the child according to sex-role assignment with leeway to adjust the sex assignment should the child act definitively as a member of the sex opposite to the one designated.

If the parents decide on surgery to normalize genital appearance, it is generally undertaken before the age of 3 years. It is easier to assign a child to be female than male because male-to-female genital surgical procedures are far more advanced than female-to-male procedures. This is an inadequate reason, however, to assign a chromosomal male to be female.

Some groups oppose surgical interventions on principle. Some advocate that the US Congress pass laws prohibiting doctors from performing such surgery, especially because the infant cannot consent. The goal standard of treatment, however, is to have genitals concordant with chromosomal, biological, physiological, and other genetic antecedents, thus allowing the development of a person with a healthy gender identity. If this cannot be determined with certainty, then treatment can and should wait.

The voices of the intersex community are beginning to rise and there are organizations that look after their rights such as OII (Organisation Intersex International) or the ISNA (Intersex Society of North America) in the USA, and that are against the sexual identity of the newborn belonging to this group being decided in an operating room by the medical team. They advocate that the decision should be taken later by the individual, who must decide whether to have surgery or not. The question then is, and until that time comes, how do we educate that person, as a man, a woman, or obscure? The ISNA is always in favor of giving the child a genre, although this may be modified in adulthood or puberty, independently of their genitalia, as the classification of "neutral" will only label the individual as a stranger or outsider. In the article *How Can You Assign a Gender (Boy or Girl) without surgery?*, the ISNA explains how this will be based on hormonal and genetic tests, in addition to the experience and opinion of the physician, who can somehow predict with which of the two sexes the baby will feel more comfortable. The ISNA is not against the surgery, if the aim is to improve the physical health of the child or help him to meet their physiological functions, for example, making a hole in the penis to urinate when the child does not have one (http://www.isna.org/faq/gender_assignment).

The case of the intersex community opens another debate that focuses on the fact that being male or female is sometimes independent of the sex organs possessed, as demonstrated in the case of transsexuals. Transsexuals are becoming more visible, and some are beginning to choose not to undergo operation, regardless of their sexual orientation, because the genitals, among other things, serve to give pleasure. However, there is still a long way to go before intersex admission begins.

Although it may seem a big step forward for equality, most intersex organizations reject the "third gender" proposed by Germany and Australia because they think it can stigmatize children. An article published on the OII website (http://www.oiiinternational.com) by the philosopher, activist, cultural worker, and magazine publisher Antke Engel, director of the Institute for Queer Theory in Hamburg and Berlin, entitled *About the Violent Construction of Sex as Binary* can give us an idea of its position, seemingly contradictory: to highlight the fact that this has not yet been even considered a possibility, it can be concluded that the regulations governing sexual ambiguity are not made at all in the interest of those affected, but rather in the interest of those who wish to keep intact the present hierarchy of sex, in order to prevent any uncertainty.

Now, we will extract some paragraphs from a recent interview by Fiona Sturges (*The Independent*, 15 July 2012) with Antony Hegarty, vocalist and composer from Antony and the Johnsons (http://www.independent.co.uk/news/people/profiles/antony-hegarty-it-takes-nerve-to-get-through-your-sense-of-shame-on-stage-7939045.html):

> "As a transgender person it's shocking to find out how many people in the press are willing to euphemistically or directly try to talk about your anatomy, in a way that you never would another person, in this really degrading way" (...) "Sometimes, I have fallen under the illusion that the writer wants to conspire with me to say something that's meaningful. But often, when you're trying to put a point across, they're more interested in framing you as the source of all these eccentric ideas. Actually, my thought with journalists is, why don't we take this opportunity to have a platform to express ourselves and our concerns. A lot of writers are throwing that [opportunity] away".

And he goes on:

> "The systems that ensure the subjugation of the feminine are the same systems that have divorced people from nature and from a sense that nature is our creator. Everyone is so hypnotised by religion that they don't even belong to the Earth. Half of them are waiting for an apocalypse as a climax to their experience. It's that bonkers! We're dealing with a lot of people who are fast asleep" (...) "Especially because my situation is ambiguous because I haven't transitioned from male to female. My experience as a transgender person has been to become comfortable expressing my sense of difference within the identity of being trans. For a lot of people, that's not their experience at all. They don't want to be trans, they want to be the opposite sex. I have so much love for those people because their condition is very real. It's almost like a sacred condition. Kids experiencing that are in a sacred crisis. They have all these gifts that boys and girls don't have" (...) "But they don't feel it like, of course not. For a lot of kids it feels like an absolute curse and it's very painful. And, in fact, a lot of that experience of alienation is part of the reason that people become so tremendous. It's growing through the pain of that experience".

Next summer, we will go to Madrid to listen again to Antony Hegarty. We think of him as a true visionary, highly aware of the artistic legacy to which he is connected and the political future of which he dreams. We recommend that you read the transcript of this fascinating monologue below, *Future Feminism*, which included in his/her album *Cut the World* and represents Antony's singular way of seeing and singing the world:

"I've been thinking all day about the moon. Like, is it an accident that women menstruate once a month and that the moon comes once a month? Are other animals synchronized in this way with the moon? You know, my brother works in mental health and he says that there's a lot more hospitalizations and periods of activity during the full moon. It's a known fact in mental health that people are more excitable around the full moon.

And then, what about the fact that we're made of 70 % water? And then the whole ocean reacts to the full moon, right? In a serious way. Everything's ticking around that moon and if we're 70 % water I must be having some—at least homeopathic—relationship with the changing cycles of the moon.

I can't escape my obsession with the idea that I'm made out of this place, because I was raised to believe that I fundamentally was constituted of spiritual matter that was from somewhere else like Heaven or from a Sky God. Like Gore Vidal talks about Sky Gods and I really picked up that language because in patriarchal monotheisms we all worship a God elsewhere who has a plan for us in a paradise elsewhere: After we die there will be a paradise waiting for us and this place is like a kind of work station where we sort of get all our 'T's crossed and our 'I's dotted before we go off to a real spiritual dimension.

But I'm a witch. I actually de-baptised myself. And what's great about being transgender is you're born with a natural religion. It applies almost across the board no matter what culture or economic group or nation that you're from—you're almost automatically a witch. None of the patriarchal monotheisms will have you. It's very clear that in most of those religions you'd be put to death. In many parts of the world you still are put to death.

Did you hear what the Pope said a couple years ago on Christmas? He said that the marriage of gays and lesbians was as much a threat to the future of our world as the collapse of the rain forests. So, that gives you a sense—just an inkling of his approach to the homosexual question. And that's just the homosexual question. He didn't even address the transgender question. God knows what we've caused. All sorts of wars and strife—all manner of hurt.

I'm worried about that the ecology of the world is collapsing and that I won't have anywhere to be reborn because I actually believe, like, where is any of us going? Where have any of us ever gone? We've come back here in some form. Did you know that whales were once land roaming mammals? And then they crawled back into the ocean trying to find something to eat? And then eventually they got rid of their hands and legs.

I've been searching and searching for that little bit of my constitution that isn't of this place and I still haven't found it. Every atom of me, every element of me seems to resonate, seems to reflect the great world around me. So, I've come to the conclusion that this is God's best idea—that this manifest world is the frontier of his dream, or her dream in my opinion. So, that's just my point of view from where I can start to establish a new way to value the world that I'm a part of. Cause if I'm not heading off to paradise elsewhere when I die then I have more of a vested interest in observing a sustainable relationship with this place.

It's a very indigenous idea that the Earth is a female, that the Earth menstruates, that the water of the world is the blood of a woman's body and that's what we crawled out of just in the same way that we crawled out of our mother's wombs. It's the most basic idea; any child could come up with it and it's so obvious. And yet we've been straining for these Sky Gods for a couple thousand years now. And I remember praying to God when I was like six years old. I was raised Catholic and I prayed really hard, and I waited and waited to hear that summons. I think in a funny way, a lot of my music I'm listening for that response still.

I've heard two rumors about the Dalai Lama. One is that he said he wasn't going to be reincarnating because the world was going to be too dangerous and that's probably just a rumor. But then I heard a far more interesting new rumor, which is that the Dalai Lama said the next time he incarnates it will be as a girl, which will be the first in the history of Buddhism. But I think that that is the most revolutionary thing he could possibly do and the most helpful spiritual gesture that he could make. And I'm very interested in the feminization of the deities. I'm very interested in Jesus as a girl. I'm extremely interested in Allah as a woman. And contrary to popular opinion, it's not bad to say that—you can say it. I mean you might get a little letter in the mail but I'm probably due a hundred letters in the mail already, so . . . It's a wonderful day to die.

But nonetheless, Allah as a woman is a critical threshold and Buddha as a mother is another one because I truly believe that unless we move into feminine systems of governance we don't have a chance on this planet. And there's no one else that can lead the masses to do that except for, like, the major religious institutions. And I'm someone who's looking for a reason to hope, and for me hope looks like feminine systems of governance being instated in, like, the major religious institutions and throughout corporate and civil life. And it might sound far-fetched, but if you look at your own beliefs, just imagine how quickly you've accepted the idea that the ocean is rising and the ecology of our world is collapsing. We can actually imagine that more readily than we can imagine a switch from patriarchal to matriarchal systems of governance—a subtle shift in the way our society works.

It's obviously a very broad statement—and of course Sarah Palin exists so don't bother me with that. But, Sarah Palin is working very much within patriarchal systems. I just love that moment when Benazir Bhutto was being interviewed and she just talked about motherhood and daughters and how she wished she'd had done more for the girls of her country. For as problematic as she was, she was an exciting forerunner".

Isn't it impressive? We think definitely it is.

Finally, we will dedicate some words to the punk-rock band called Against Me!, originally formed in Gainesville, Florida, in 1977, by the singer and guitarist Laura Jane Grace, who publicly came out transgender, beginning a transition toward living as a woman and dropping the name Tom Gabel. The band finished recording their sixth studio album, *Transgender Dysphoria Blues*, during the summer of 2013, and released it on 21 January 2014. It contains 11 songs: *Transgender Dysphoria Blues*; *True Trans Soul Rebel*; *Unconditional Love*; *Brinking with the Jocks*; *Osama Bin Laden as the Crucified Christ*; *Fuck My Life 666*; *Dead Friend*; *Two Coffins*; and *Paralytic States*; *Black Me Out*.

Let's take the track 2 and listen to *True Trans Soul Rebel*:

"All dressed up and nowhere to go/You're walking the streets all alone/Another night to wish that you could forget/Making yourself up as you go along/Who's gonna take you home tonight?/Who's gonna take you home?/Does god bless your transsexual heart?/True trans soul rebel/Yet to be born, you're already dead/You sleep with a gun beside you in bed/Follow it through to the obvious end/Slit your veins wide open, you bleed it out/Who's gonna take you home tonight?/Who's gonna take you home?/Does god bless your transsexual heart?/True trans soul rebel/You should have been a mother/You should have been a wife/You should have been gone from here years ago/You should be living a different life/Who's gonna take you home tonight?/Who's gonna take you home?/Does god bless your transsexual heart?/True trans soul rebel".

Do you know? Some days it is so difficult for us to not feel ourselves, like menstruating moons, men and women, just like people at last. These are the real days, the good ones.

12.2 Some Definitions

The area of sex and gender is highly controversial and has led to a proliferation of terms whose meanings vary over time and within and between disciplines. An additional source of confusion is that in English "sex" connotes both male and female sexuality.

As we understand sex and sexual refer to the biological indicators of male and female (understood in the context of reproductive capacity), such as in sex chromosomes, gonads, sex hormones, and non-ambiguous internal and external genitalia [1].

Disorders of sex development denote conditions of inborn somatic deviations of the reproductive tract from the norm and/or discrepancies among the biological indicators of male and female.

The need to introduce the term gender arose with the realization that for individuals with conflicting or ambiguous biological indicators of sex (i.e., intersex), the lived role in society and/or the identification as male or female could not be uniformly associated with or predicted from the biological indicators and, later, that some individuals develop an identity as a female or male at variance with their uniform set of classical biological indicators. Thus, gender is used to denote the public (and usually legally recognized) lived role as boy or girl, man or woman, but, in contrast to certain social constructionists theories, biological factors are seen to be contributing, in interaction with social and psychological factors, to gender development.

Terminology in the area of health care for transsexual, transgender, and gender-nonconforming people is rapidly evolving. New terms are being introduced, and the definitions of existing terms are changing. Thus, there is often misunderstanding, debate, or disagreement about language in this field. Many terms used in relation to this population are not ideal. For example, the terms transsexual and transvestite—and, some would argue, the more recent term transgender—have been applied to people in an objectifying fashion. Yet such terms have been more or less adopted by many people who are making their best effort to make themselves understood. By continuing to use these terms, World Professional Association for Transgender Health (WPATH) proposals are only to ensure that concepts and processes are comprehensible, in order to facilitate the delivery of quality health care to transsexual, transgender, and gender-nonconforming people. The WPATH remains open to new terminology to further illuminate the experience of members of this diverse population and lead to improvements in health care access and delivery [7].

Sex is assigned at birth as male or female, usually based on the appearance of the external genitalia. When the external genitalia are ambiguous, other components of sex (internal genitalia, chromosomal and hormonal sex) are considered in order to assign sex. For most people, gender identity and expression are consistent with their sex assigned at birth. For transsexual, transgender, and gender-nonconforming individuals, gender identity or expression differs from their sex assigned at birth.

Gender assignment refers to the initial assignment as male or female. This occurs usually at birth and, thereby, yields the "natal gender."

Gender-atypical refers to somatic features or behaviors that are not typical (in a statistical sense) of individuals with the same assigned gender in a given society and historical era. For behavior, gender-nonconforming is an alternative descriptive term.

Sex reassignment surgery (gender affirmation surgery) refers to surgery to change primary and/or secondary sex characteristics to affirm a person's gender identity. Sex reassignment surgery can be an important part of medically necessary treatment to alleviate GD. Moreover, cross-sex hormone treatment denotes the use of feminizing hormones in an individual assigned male at birth based on traditional biological indicators or the use of masculinizing hormones in an individual assigned female at birth.

Gender reassignment denotes an official (and usually legal) change of gender.

Gender identity refers to the sense one has of being male or being female, which corresponds, normally, to the person's anatomical sex. The text revision of the fourth edition of the Diagnostic and Statistical Manual of Mental Disorders (DSM-IV-TR) defines GID as a group whose common feature is a strong, persistent preference for living as a person of the other sex. The affective component of GID is gender dysphoria (discontent with one's designated birth sex and a desire to have the body of the other sex and to be regarded socially as a person of the other sex). GID in adults was referred to in early versions of the DSM as transsexualism. In DSM-IV-TR no distinction is made for the overriding diagnostic term GID as a function of age. In children, it can manifest as statements of wanting to be the other sex and as a broad range of sex-typed behaviors conventionally shown by children of the other sex. Gender identity crystallizes in most persons by the age of 2 or 3 years [9].

Transsexual is an adjective often applied by the medical profession to describe individuals who seek to change or who have changed their primary and/or secondary sex characteristics through femininizing or masculinizing medical interventions (hormones and/or surgery), typically accompanied by a permanent change in gender role in order to live entirely as permanent, full-time members of the gender other than that they were assigned to at birth. The term was used in the title of a 1949 article by D. O. Caldwell, *Psychopathia transexualis*, but it was popularized by Dr Harry Benjamin in the 1950s and became widely known as a result of the spectacular publicity given to the 1952 surgical sex change of Christine Jorgensen, a former photographer and film editor from the Bronx whose genital conversion operation made headlines around the world. The term transsexual was introduced to draw a distinction between those transvestites who sought medical interventions to change their physical bodies (that is, their sex) and those who merely wanted to change their gendered clothing (the vestments at the root of transvestism). Historically, the practice of transsexuality has involved surgical modifications of the reproductive organs and chest, hormone use to change secondary sex characteristics, and permanent removal of facial and body hair for individuals moving from male embodiment toward social womanhood. These medical procedures have then been the basis for legal or bureaucratic changes in gender designation. More recently, people who do not consider themselves to be transsexual are increasingly continuing to use the same body modification practices, and they may do so without trying to change their legal gender. For example, a person born with a female body may use testosterone or have mastectomies, but still live legally or socially as a woman with traditionally masculine attributes. The result of such practices is another layer of human-generated complexity on top of already complicated biological sex differences and cultural gender categories. The breakdown in familiar distinctions between who is a transsexual and who is not, and who (based on diagnosis with GID) is considered an acceptable recipient of medicalized body modification procedures, is another hotly debated topìc. The rapid evolution of new motives for changing one's embodiement (for example, a woman with a known genetic risk for breast cancer opting for a preventive mastectomy, or a professional athlete taking performance-enhancing drugs, neither of whom may consider themselves transgender, but who do some of the same things to their bodies that transgender people do, coupled with new biomedical possibilities for doing so, is part of what drives the rapid developing terminology in the transgender field [10].

Transition is the period of time when individuals change from the gender role associated with their sex assigned at birth to a different one. For many people, this involves learning how to live socially as a person of that gender. For others this means finding a gender role and expression that is most comfortable for them. Transition may or may not include feminization or masculinization of the body through hormones or other medical procedures. The nature and duration of transition is variable and individualized.

Gender dysphoria (GD) as a general descriptive term used in the APA's new publication, the DSM-5, refers to an individual's affective/cognitive discontent with the assigned gender, but is more specifically defined when used as a diagnostic (clinical) category. In this case, it refers to the distress that may accompany the incongruence between one's experienced or expressed gender and one's assigned gender. Although not all individuals will experience distress as a result of such incongruence, many are distressed if the desired physical interventions by means of hormones and/or surgery are not available. The current term is more descriptive than the previous DSM-IV term GID, and focuses on dysphoria as the clinical problem, not identity per se [1].

Gender-nonconforming is another adjective used to describe individuals whose gender identity, role, or expression differs from what is normative for their assigned sex in a given culture and historical period.

Gender role or expression appeals to the characteristics in personality, appearance, and behavior that in a given culture and historical period are designated as masculine or feminine (that is, more typical of the male or female social role). While most individuals present socially in clearly masculine or feminine gender roles, some people present in an alternative gender role such as genderqueer or specifically transgender. All people tend to incorporate both masculine and feminine characteristics in their gender expression in varying ways and to varying degrees.

Genderqueer is the identity label that may be used by individuals whose gender identity and/or role does not conform to a binary understanding of gender as limited to the categories of man or woman, male or female.

Internalized transphobia implies some kind of discomfort with one's own transgender feelings or identity as a result of internalizing society's normative gender expectations.

Transvestite is a word coined in 1910 by the German sexologist Magnus Hirscheld [10]. He used it to describe the erotic urge for disguise that it shows, as he understood the motivation that led some people to wear clothing generally associated with a social gender other than that assigned to them at birth. For Hirchfield, "transvestites" were one of many different types of sexual intermediaries, including homosexuals and hermaphrodites, who occupied a spectrum between "pure male" and "pure female." Initially, this term was used in much the same way that transgender is used now, to convey the sense of a wide range of gender variant identities and behaviors. During the course of the last century, however, to the extent that it has not fallen entirely out of favor, it refers primarily to people who wear gender atypical clothing, but do not engage in other kinds of body modification. It usually carries with it the association of cross-dressing for erotic pleasure. Transvestism is also called cross-dressing.

Transgender implies movement away from an initially assigned gender position. It generally refers to any and all kinds of variation from gender norms and expectations. Gender varies through the place and time, defining transgender in this way inevitably brings up the related questions of which norms and expectations? And whose norms and expectations? What counts as transgender varies as much as gender itself, and it always depends on the historical and cultural context. The gender identity of transgender people differs to varying degrees from the sex they were assigned at birth [10].

Disorders of sex development are congenital conditions in which the development of chromosomal, gonadal, or anatomical sex is atypical. Some people strongly object to the "disorder" label and instead view these conditions as a matter of diversity, preferring the terms "intersex" and "intersexuality."

12.3 Epidemiology

Formal epidemiological studies on the incidence and prevalence of transsexualism specifically or transgender and gender-nonconforming identities in general have not been conducted, and efforts to achieve realistic estimates are fraught with enormous difficulties [11].

Even if epidemiological studies established that a similar proportion of transsexual, transgender, or gender-nonconforming people existed all over the world, it is likely that cultural differences from one country to another would alter both the behavioral expressions of different gender identities and the extent to which GD—distinct from one's gender identity—is actually occurring in a population. While in most countries, crossing normative gender boundaries generates moral censure rather than compassion, there are examples in certain cultures of gender-nonconforming behaviors (i.e., in spiritual leaders) that are less stigmatized and even revered [7].

For various reasons, researchers who have studied the incidence and prevalence have tended to focus on the most easily counted subgroup of gender-nonconforming individuals: transsexual individuals who experience GD and who present for gender-transition-related care at specialist gender clinics [12].

De Cuypere and colleagues reviewed the specific literature and concluded that the prevalence figures reported range from 1:11,900 to 1:45,000 for male-to-female individuals (MtF) and 1:30,400 to 1:200,000 for female-to-male (FtM) individuals [13].

Nevertheless, the prevalence may be much higher depending on the methodology used in the research. Direct comparisons across studies are near impossible, as each differed in their data collection methods and in their criteria for documenting a person as transsexual (i.e. whether or not a person had undergone genital reconstruction, versus whether they had initiated hormone therapy, versus whether they had come to the clinic seeking medically supervised transition services). The trend appears to be toward higher prevalence rates in the more recent studies, possibly indicating increasing numbers of people seeking clinical care [14].

The numbers yielded by studies such as these can be considered minimum estimates at best. The published figures are mostly derived from clinics where patients met criteria for severe GD and had access to health care at those clinics. These estimates do not take into account that treatments offered in a particular clinical setting may not be perceived as affordable, useful, or acceptable by all self-identified gender dysphoric individuals in a given area. By counting only those people who present at clinics for a specific type of treatment, an unspecified number of gender dysphoric individuals are overlooked.

Other clinical observations (not yet firmly supported by any systematic study) support the likelihood of a higher prevalence of GD [7]:

Previously unrecognized GD is occasionally diagnosed when patients are seen with anxiety, depression, conduct disorder, substance abuse, dissociative identity disorders, borderline personality disorder, sexual disorders, and disorders of sex development.

Some cross-dressers, drag queens/kings or female/male impersonators, and gay and lesbian individuals may be experiencing GD.

The intensity of some people's GD fluctuates below and above a clinical threshold.

Gender nonconformity among FtM individuals tends to be relatively invisible in many cultures, particularly to western health professionals and researchers who have conducted most of the studies on which the current estimates of prevalence and incidence are based.

Overall, the existing data should be considered a starting point, and health care would benefit from more rigorous epidemiological study in different locations worldwide.

According to the APA's new DSM-5, for natal adult males the prevalence of GD ranges from 0.005 % to 0.014 %, and for natal females from 0.002 % to 0.003 %. Since not all adults seeking hormone treatment and surgical reassignment attend specialty clinics, these rates are likely modest underestimates. Sex differences in the rate of referrals to specialty clinics vary by age group. In children, sex ratios of natal boys to girls range from 2:1 to 4.5:1. In adolescents, the sex ratio is close to parity. In adults, the sex ratio favors natal males, with ratios ranging from 1:1 to 6.1:1. In two countries the sex ratio appears to favor natal females (Japan 2.2:1, Poland 3.4:1) [1].

Most children with GD are referred for clinical evaluation in the early grade school years. Parents, however, typically report that the cross-gender behaviors were apparent before 3 years of age. Among a sample of boys younger than age 12 years referred for a range of clinical problems, the reported desire to be the opposite sex was 10 %. For clinically referred girls younger than age 12 years, the reported desire to be the opposite sex was 5 %. The sex ratio of referred children is four to five boys for each girl [9].

The best estimate of GD or transsexualism in adults comes from Europe, with a prevalence of 1 in 30,000 men and 1 in 100,000 women. Most clinical centers report a sex ratio of three to five male patients for each female patient. Many adults with GD may well have qualified for GD in childhood. Most adults with GD report having felt different from other children of the same sex, although, in retrospect, many could not identify the source of that difference. Many report feeling extensively cross-gender identified from the earliest years, with the cross-gender identification becoming more profound in adolescence and young adulthood [9].

12.4 Etiopathogenesis

As von Goethe points out "there's nothing more frightful than ignorance in action."

The development and maintenance of GD is held to be a multifactorial pathological process, in which individual psychological factors exert their effects in concert with biological, familial, and sociocultural ones.

It would be wrong to imagine that patients with GD constitute a homogeneous group with a uniform pathogenesis. Different theoretical conceptions imply different—complementary, not necessarily contradictory—notions of the possible causes of GD. In view of the still unsatisfactory state of the data, any generalizations should be made with caution.

12.4.1 Biological Factors

For mammals, the resting state of tissue is initially female (see the corresponding chapter of this book). As the fetus develops, a male is produced only if androgen (coded for by a region of the Y chromosome, which is responsible for testicular development) is introduced. Without testes and androgen, female external genitalia develop. Thus, maleness and masculinity depend on fetal and perinatal androgens. The sexual behavior of animals lower on the evolutionary tree is governed by sex steroids, but this effect diminishes as one ascends the evolutionary tree. Sex steroids influence the expression of sexual behavior in mature men and women. That is, testosterone can increase libido and aggressiveness in women, and estrogen can decrease libido and aggressiveness in men. However, masculinity, femininity, and gender identity more frequently result from postnatal life events than from prenatal hormonal organization [9].

The same principle of masculinization or feminization has been applied to the brain. Testosterone affects brain neurons that contribute to the masculinization of the brain in such areas as the hypothalamus. Whether testosterone contributes to so-called masculine or feminine behavioral patterns in gender identity disorders remains a controversial issue [9].

Neurobiological genetic research has not yet convincingly shown any predominant role for genetic or hormonal factors in the etiology of GD. Some studies' findings were originally thought to suggest a possible effect of sex steroids in utero and an inadequate masculinization or defeminization of hypothalamic nuclei ("gender role centers") because of pathologically altered maternal hormone levels. Nevertheless, these findings are now viewed more critically [15].

Some studies have also supported the hypothesis of a strong heritable component to GID, in as much as gender identity may be much less a matter of choice and much more a matter of biology. But once again, these data are as yet inconclusive [16].

In addition, neuroanatomical findings in the dichotomous brain nuclei of transsexual patients may provide further evidence for a biological component in the complex etiology of GD. Some studies have also proposed not only that the bed nucleus of the stria terminalis (BSTc) is female in size and neuron number in male-to-female transsexual people, but also that the hypothalamic uncinate nucleus, which is composed of two subnuclei; namely, the interstitial nucleus of the anterior hypothalamus (INAH) 3 and 4, is altered in post-mortem brain material obtained from GD subjects: the INAH3 volume and number of neurons of male-to-female transsexual people is similar to that of control females; the female-to-male transsexual subjects have an INAH3 volume and number of neurons within the male control range, even though treatment with testosterone had been stopped 3 years before death; the castrated men have an INAH3 volume and neuron number that was intermediate between males and females; and there is no difference in INAH3 between pre-and post-menopausal women, either in the volume or in the number of neurons, indicating that the feminization of the INAH3 of male-to-female transsexuals is not due to estrogen treatment. The authors conclude that the sex reversal of the INAH3 in transsexual people is at least partly a marker of an early atypical sexual differentiation of the brain and that the changes in INAH3 and the BSTc may belong to a complex network that may be structurally and functionally related to gender identity [17].

Cerebral responses to putative pheromones and objects of sexual attraction were recently found to differ between homo- and heterosexual subjects. Although this observation may merely mirror perceptional differences, it raises the intriguing question as to whether certain sexually dimorphic features in the brain may differ between individuals of the same sex but different sexual orientation. In another study the authors addressed this issue by studying hemispheric asymmetry and functional connectivity, two parameters that in previous publications have shown specific sex differences. Ninety subjects (25 heterosexual men [HeM] and women [HeW], and 20 homosexual men [HoM] and women [HoW]) were investigated with magnetic resonance volumetry of the cerebral and cerebellar hemispheres. Fifty of them also participated in PET measurements of cerebral blood flow, used for analyses of functional connections from the right and left amygdalae. HeM and HoW showed a rightward cerebral asymmetry, whereas volumes of the cerebral hemispheres were symmetrical in HoM and HeW. No cerebellar asymmetries were found. Homosexual subjects also showed sex-atypical amygdala connections. In HoM, as in HeW, the connections were more widespread from the left amygdala; in HoW and HeM, on the other hand, from the right amygdala. Furthermore, in HoM and HeW the connections were primarily displayed with the contralateral amygdala and the anterior cingulate, in HeM and HoW with the caudate, putamen, and the prefrontal cortex. The present studies shows sex-atypical cerebral asymmetry and functional connections in homosexual subjects. The results cannot be primarily ascribed to learned effects, and they suggest a linkage to neurobiological entities [18, 19].

Savic and Lindström describe sex-atypical cerebral asymmetry and functional connections in homosexual subjects that cannot be primarily linked to reproduction and suggest a link between sexual orientation and neurobiological entities. Further research is needed on the putative influence of testosterone on the same parameters (i.e., in individuals with complete androgen-insensitivity syndrome). Neurobiological research related to sexual orientation in humans is only just gathering momentum, but the evidence already shows that humans have a vast array of brain differences, not only in relation to gender, but also in relation to sexual orientation [20].

Studies of GD in patients with various types of intersex syndrome (i.e., complete versus partial androgen receptor defects) have led to the formulation of a biological hypothesis for the etiology of GD, in which these are caused by hormone resistance restricted to the brain. Contrary to earlier assumptions, gender identity cannot be changed by external influences alone, i.e., attempts at so-called "re-education," even when these attempts are begun as early as the first year of life. This implies an early, somatic determination of gender identity. Moreover, because bodily and genital sensations exert a major effect on psychosexual and gender-identity development, it must be assumed that the overall process involves an interaction of biological and psychosocial factors [21].

Etiological and pathological influences should thus be sought in both areas, taking into account some key issues such as the geometric structure of the brain fiber pathways or the hierarchical genetic organization of the human cortical surface area [22, 23].

12.4.2 Psychosocial Factors

Children usually develop a gender identity consonant with their sex of rearing (also known as "assigned sex"). The formation of gender identity is influenced by the interaction of children's temperament and parents' qualities and attitudes. Culturally acceptable gender roles exist: boys are not expected to be effeminate, and girls are not expected to be masculine. There are boys' games (e.g., cops and robbers) and girls' toys (e.g., dolls and dollhouses). These roles are learned, although some investigators believe that some boys are temperamentally delicate and sensitive and that some girls are aggressive and energized—traits that are stereotypically known in today's culture as feminine and masculine respectively. However, greater tolerance of mild cross-gender activity in children has developed in the past few decades [9].

The quality of the mother–child relationship in the first years of life is paramount in establishing gender identity. During this period, mothers normally facilitate their children's awareness of, and pride in, their gender: children are valued as little boys and girls, but devaluing, hostile mothering can result in gender problems. At the same time, the separation–individuation process is unfolding. When gender problems become associated with separation–individuation problems, the result can be the use of sexuality to remain in relationships characterized by shifts between a desperate infantile closeness and a hostile, devaluing distance.

Some children are given the message that they would be more valued if they adopted the gender identity of the opposite sex. Rejected or abused children may act on such a belief. Gender identity problems can also be triggered by a mother's death, extended absence, or depression, to which a young boy may react by totally identifying with her—that is, by becoming a mother to replace her.

The father's role is also important in the early years, and his presence normally helps the separation–individuation process. Without a father, mother and child may remain overly close. For a girl, the father is normally the prototype of future love objects; for a boy, the father is a model for male identification [9].

Multiple publications have concerned a possible traumatic etiology of gender identity disorders and an overlap of the psychopathological findings in GID with those of borderline personality disorder, although there is some controversy on the latter point. A profound disturbance of the mother–child relationship can often be empirically demonstrated and is postulated to be a causative factor. The desire to belong to the opposite sex is held to be a compensatory pattern of response to trauma. In boys, it is said to represent an attempt to repair the defective relationship with the physically or emotionally absent primary attachment figure through fantasy; the boy tries to imitate his missing mother as the result of confusion between the two concepts of having a mother and being one. In girls, the postulated motivation for gender (role) switching is the child's need to protect herself and her mother from a violent father by acquiring masculine strength for herself [21, 24].

Other authors, in line with psychoanalytical theory, do not attribute the desire to belong to the opposite sex to any prior trauma. Rather, they postulate the formation of a classic neurotic compromise, in which the child symbolically achieves a symbiotic fusion with the beloved parent by switching genders [25].

Excessive identification with the opposite sex is said to help affected boys cope with fears of loss of maternal attention, while affected girls are said to identify with their fathers in order to compensate for a relationship with their mothers that they perceive to be deficient [26–28].

From the perspective of developmental psychology, psychopathology, and psychiatry, such maladaptive reactions can be seen as failed attempts to fulfill particular developmental tasks: separation from parents, establishment of an individual identity, and attainment of sexual maturity. Some adolescents, meanwhile, seem to view a gender switch as a universal problem-solving strategy when confronted by other, totally different developmental tasks, bearing no relation to the establishment of sexual identity, that they perceive as insurmountable. It seems clear that the manner of psychological processing of conflicts and traumatic experiences can be expected to vary greatly from one child or adolescent to another, depending to a major extent on temperamental factors and on the developmental stage that the individual's cognitive, emotional, and social skills have reached [21].

Learning theory and concepts derived from it tend to favor a causative model in which the primary attachment figure(s) is (are) postulated to exert an exogenous-reinforcing, active-manipulative effect on the development of features typifying the opposite sex. This explanatory approach ascribes primary importance to a desire on the parent's part for the child to be of the opposite sex. A high rate of psychological abnormalities in the parents of children with GID has been reported in more than one study [29, 30].

Schema-focused theory was developed for the treatment of personality disorders and has been applied to many different forms of psychopathology, but there has been little published research investigating the relevance of this theory for GD. A recent study concludes that the psychological evaluation of individuals with GD can be effective in its prevention, diagnosis, and treatment. It may be a relationship between defense mechanisms and early maladaptive schemas in individuals with GD, based on a positive significant relationship between the disconnection and rejection domain and early maladaptive schemas and inmature style of the defense mechanisms, and in a negative significant relationship between them and mature style; there is no statistically significant relationship between them and neurotic style [30].

It is essential, therefore, to explore thoroughly the psychopathology of the child's attachment figures and their "sexual world view," including any sexually traumatizing experiences they may have undergone, in order to discover any potential "transsexualogenic influences." The same holds for overarching sociocultural variables. Presentations currently appearing in the mass media of ever younger patients describing their treatment in euphoric terms are a cause for concern. Two further reasons for the rising demand for sex changes among minors would appear to be the "feasibility delusion"—the notion that modern medicine can effect a sex change with no problem at all—and a tendency to view the choice of one's own sex as a type of fundamental right.

Finally, in a recent work, Ramachandran working on the conscious self points out that it seems to arise from a small set of brain areas connected in a surprisingly powerful network. This author also includes a curious aspect of the as yet unexplained apotemnophilia with his model: the sexual orientation tendencies associated with some of these individuals are directed toward intimacy with another amputee subject. Perhaps the sexual esthetic preference for certain body morphology is dictated in part by the shape of the body image displayed in the right sensorial parietal lobe (SPL) and/or in the insular cortex. Thus, there may be a genetically specified mechanism, that allows the template body image (in SPL) of a person to be transcribed in their limbic circuits, thus determining the visual esthetic preference [31]. Moreover, there are certain similarities among somatoparaphrenia, anosognosia, and the Capgras delusion. And in a riskier conceptual leap it can also be assumed that the conscious Self has sex. As with somatoparaphrenia, certain distortions or disparities in the SPL may partly explain the symptoms of transsexuals, in which the discrepancy between sexual body image internally specified, including details of the sexual anatomy, and external anatomy causes a profound malaise, and a yearning to reduce the disparity.

We ask the reader not to be impatient in this regard, as it is a hypothesis, and as such, it must be subjected to verification and validation processes. But it is still an interesting proposal from an epistemological point of view.

12.5 GD: Clinical Features, Diagnostic Criteria, Comorbidity, and Differential Diagnosis

Individuals with GD have a marked incongruence between the gender they have been assigned to (usually at birth, referred to as the natal gender) and their experienced/expressed gender. This discrepancy is the core component of the diagnosis. There must be also evidence of distress about this incongruence. Experienced gender may include alternative gender identities beyond binary stereotypes. Consequently, the distress is not limited to a desire to simply be of the other gender, but may include a desire to be of an alternative gender, provided that it differs from the individual's assigned gender.

The main diagnostic criteria of DSM-5 [1] are shown in Tables 12.1 and 12.2.

At the extreme of GID in children are boys who, by the standards of their cultures, are as feminine as the most feminine of girls, and girls who are as masculine as the most masculine of boys. No sharp line can be drawn on the continuum of GID between children who should receive a formal diagnosis and those who should not. Girls with the disorder regularly have male companions and an avid interest in sports and rough-and-tumble play. They show no interest in dolls or playing house (unless they play the father or another male role). They may refuse to urinate in a sitting position, claim that they have or will grow a penis and do not want to grow breasts or to menstruate, and assert that they will grow up to become a man (not merely to play a man's role).

Table 12.1 Gender dysphoria criteria in children according to the DSM-5

DSM-5 gender dysphoria in children. 302.6 (F64.2)	
A.	A marked incongruence between one's experienced/expressed gender and assigned gender, of at least 6 months' duration, as manifested by at least six of the following (one of which must be Criterion A1):
1.	A strong desire to be of the other gender or an insistence that one is the other gender (or some alternative gender different from one's assigned gender)
2.	In boys (assigned gender) a strong preference for cross-dressing or stimulating female attire; or in girls (assigned gender) a strong preference for wearing only typical masculine clothing and a strong resistance to the wearing of typical feminine clothing
3.	A strong preference for cross-gender roles in make-believe play or fantasy play
4.	A strong preference for the toys, games, or activities stereotypically used or engaged in by the other gender
5.	A strong preference for playmates of the other gender
6.	In boys (assigned gender), a strong rejection of typically masculine toys, games, and activities
7.	A strong dislike of one's sexual anatomy
8.	A strong desire for the primary and/or secondary sex characteristics than match one's experienced gender
B.	The condition is associated with clinically significant distress or impairment in social, school, or other important areas of functioning
Specify if:	With a disorder of sex development (e.g., a congenital adrenogenital disorder such as 255.2 [E25.0] congenital adrenal hyperplasia or 259.50 [E34.50] androgen insensitivity syndrome
Coding note:	Code the disorder of sex development as well as gender dysphoria

Boys with the disorder are usually preoccupied with stereotypically female activities. They may have a preference for dressing in girls' or women's clothes or may improvise such items from available material when the genuine articles are not available (the cross-dressing typically does not cause sexual excitement, as in transvestic fetishism). They often have a compelling desire to participate in the games and pastimes of girls. Female dolls are often their favorite toys, and girls are regularly their preferred playmates. When playing house, they take a girl's role. Their gestures and actions are often judged to be feminine, and they are usually subjected to male peer group teasing and rejection, a phenomenon that rarely occurs with boyish girls until adolescence. Boys with the disorder may assert that they will grow up to become a woman (not merely in role). They may claim that their penis or testes are disgusting or will disappear or that it would be better not to have a penis or testes. Some children refuse to attend school because of teasing or the pressure to dress in attire stereotypical of their assigned sex. Most children deny being disturbed by the disorder, except that it brings them into conflict with the expectations of their families or peers.

Children with a gender identity disorder must be distinguished from other gender-atypical children. For girls, tomboys without gender identity disorder prefer

Table 12.2 Gender dysphoria criteria according to the DSM-5 in adolescents and adults

DSM-5 gender dysphoria in adolescents and adults. 302.85 (F64.1)	
A.	A marked incongruence between one's experienced/expressed gender and assigned gender, of at least 6 months' duration, as manifested by at least two of the following:
1.	A marked incongruence between one's experienced/expressed gender and primary and/or secondary sex characteristics (or in young adolescents, the anticipated secondary sex characterisitics)
2.	A strong desire to be rid of one's primary or secondary sex characteristics because of a marked incongruence with one's experienced/expressed gender (or in young adolescents, a desire to prevent the development of the anticipated secondary sex characteristics)
3.	A strong desire for the primary and/or secondary sex characteristics of the other gender
4.	A strong desire to be of the other gender (or some alternative gender different from one's assigned gender)
5.	A strong desire to be treated as the other gender (or some alternative gender different from one's assigned gender)
6.	A strong conviction that one has the typical feelings and reactions of the other gender (or some alternative gender different from one's assigned gender)
B.	The condition is associated with clinically significant distress or impairment in social, school, or other important areas of functioning
Specify if:	With a disorder of sex development (e.g., a congenital adrenogenital disorder such as 255.2 [E25.0] congenital adrenal hyperplasis or 259.50 [E34.50] androgen insensitivity syndrome
Coding note:	Code the disorder of sex development well as gender dysphoria
Specify if:	*Post-transition*: The individual has transitioned to full-time living in the desired gender (with or without legalization of gender change) and has undergone (or is preparing to have) at least one cross-sex medical procedure or treatment regimen—namely regular cross-sex hormone treatment or gender reassignment surgery confirming the desired gender (e.g., penectomy, vaginoplasty in a natal male; mastectomy or phalloplasty in a natal female)

functional and gender-neutral clothing. By contrast, gender identity-disordered girls adamantly refuse to wear girls' clothes and reject gender-neutral clothes. They make repeated statements of being or wanting to be a boy and wanting to grow up to be a man, along with repeated cross-sex fantasy play, so that, in mother–father games or other games imitating characters from the mass media, they are male. This accompanies a marked aversion to traditionally feminine activities.

For boys, the differential diagnosis must distinguish those who do not conform to traditional masculine sex-typed expectations, but do not show extensive cross-gender identification and are not discontent with being male. It is not uncommon for boys to reject rough-and-tumble play or sports and to prefer non-athletic activities or occasionally to role play as a girl, to play with a doll, or to dress up in girls' or women's costumes. Such boys do not necessarily have a GID. Boys who do have a GID state a preference for being a girl and for growing up to become a woman, along with repeated cross-sex fantasy play, as in mother–father games, a strong preference for traditionally female-type activities, cross-dressing, and a female peer group.

Because the diagnosis of GID excludes children with anatomical intersex, a medical history needs to be taken, with the focus on any suggestion of hermaphroditism in the child. With doubt, referral to a pediatric endocrinologist is indicated [9].

Similar signs and symptoms are seen in adolescents and adults. Adolescents and adults with the disorder manifest a stated desire to be the other sex; they frequently try to pass as a member of the other sex, and they desire to live or to be treated as the other sex. In addition, they find their genitals repugnant, and they desire to acquire the sex characteristics of the opposite sex. This desire may override all other wishes. They may believe that they were born the wrong sex and may make such characteristic statements as "I feel that I'm a woman trapped in a male body" or vice versa.

Adolescents and adults frequently request medical or surgical procedures to alter their physical appearance. Although the term transsexual is not used in DSM-5 [1], many clinicians find the term useful and will probably continue to use it. In addition, transsexualism appears in the tenth revision of International Statistical Classification of Diseases and Related Health Problems (ICD-10) [32], and such persons refer to themselves as transsexuals.

Most retrospective studies of transsexuals report gender identity problems during childhood, but prospective studies of children with GID indicate that few become transsexuals and want to change their sex. The disorder is much more common in men (1 per 30,000) than in women (1 per 100,000) [9].

Men take estrogen to create breasts and other feminine contours, have electrolysis to remove their male hair, and have surgery to remove the testes and the penis and to create an artificial vagina. Women bind their breasts or have a double mastectomy, a hysterectomy, and an oophorectomy. They take testosterone to build up muscle mass and deepen the voice and have surgery in which an artificial phallus is created. These procedures may make a person indistinguishable from members of the other sex.

Gender identity disorder can be associated with other diagnoses. Although some patients with GID have a history of major psychosis, including schizophrenia or major affective disorder, most do not. When a diagnosis of GID is made, as well as another DSM Axis I diagnosis, it is necessary to consider whether the diagnoses are distinct. A variety of Axis II personality disorders may be found in patients with gender identity disorder, particularly borderline personality, but none is specific. A proportion of nonhomosexual men with GID report a history of erotic arousal in association with cross-dressing, and some would still qualify for a concurrent diagnosis of fetishistic transvestism. Some are more sexually aroused by imagining themselves with a female body or by seeing themselves cross-dressed in a mirror (autogynephilia) than by items of women's clothing per se.

12.5.1 Differential Diagnosis

Nonconformity to Gender Roles. Gender dysphoria should be distinguished from simple nonconformity to stereotypical gender role behavior by the strong desire to be of another gender than the assigned one and by the extent and pervasiveness of gender-variant activities and interests. The diagnosis is not meant to merely describe noncomformity to stereotypical gender role behavior. Given the increased openness of atypical gender expressions by individuals across the entire range of the transgender spectrum, it is important for the clinical diagnosis to be limited to those individuals whose distress and impairment meet the specified criteria.

Transvestic Disorder. The DSM-IV-TR lists cross-dressing—dressing in clothes of the opposite sex—as a GID if it is transient and related to stress. If the disorder is not stress-related, persons who cross-dress are classified as having transvestic fetishism, which is described as a paraphilia in the DSM-IV-TR. An essential feature of transvestic fetishism is that it produces sexual excitement. Stress-related cross-dressing may sometimes produce sexual excitement, but it also reduces a patient's tension and anxiety. Patients may harbor fantasies of cross-dressing but act them out only under stress. Male adult cross-dressers may have the fantasy that they are female, in whole or in part.

Cross-dressing is commonly known as transvestism and the cross-dresser as a transvestite. Cross-dressing phenomena range from the occasional solitary wearing of clothes of the other sex to extensive feminine identification in men and masculine identification in women, with involvement in a transvestic subculture. More than one article of clothing of the other sex is involved, and a person may dress entirely as a member of the opposite sex. The degree to which a cross-dressed person appears as a member of the other sex varies, depending on mannerisms, body habitus, and cross-dressing skill. When not cross-dressed, these persons usually appear to be unremarkable members of their assigned sex. Cross-dressing can coexist with paraphilias, such as sexual sadism, sexual masochism, and pedophilia. Cross-dressing differs from transsexualism in that the patients have no persistent preoccupation with getting rid of their primary and secondary sex characteristics and acquiring the sex characteristics of the other sex. Some persons with the disorder once had transvestic fetishism, but no longer become sexually aroused by cross-dressing. Other persons with the disorder are homosexual men and women who cross-dress. The disorder is most common among female impersonators.

Body Dysmorphic Disorder. An individual with body dysmorphic disorder focuses on the alteration or removal of a specific body part because it is perceived as abnormally formed, not because it represents a repudiated assigned gender. When an individual's presentation meets criteria for both GD and body dysmorphic disorder, both diagnoses can given. Individuals wishing to have a healthy limb amputated because it makes them feel more complete usually do not wish to change gender, but rather desire to live as an amputee or a disabled person.

Schizophrenia and Other Psychotic Disorders. In schizophrenia there may rarely be delusions of belonging to some other gender. In the absence of psychotic symptoms, insistence by an individual with GD that he or she is of some other gender is not considered a delusion. Schizophrenia and GD may co-occur.

Other Clinical Presentations. Some individuals with an emasculinization desire who develop an alternative, nonmale, nonfemale gender identity do have a presentation that meets the criteria for GD. However, some males seek castration and or penectomy for esthetic reasons or to remove psychological effects of androgens without changing male identity. In these cases the criteria for GD are not met.

12.5.2 Comorbidity

Clinically referred children with GD show elevated levels of emotional and behavioral problems (most commonly anxiety, disruptive and impulse-control, and depressive disorders). In prepubertal children, increasing age is associated with having more behavioral or emotional problems. This is related to the increasing non-acceptance of gender-variant behavior by others. In older children, gender-variant behavior often leads to peer ostracism, which may lead to more behavioral problems. The prevalence of mental health problems differs among cultures. These differences may also be related to differences in attitudes toward gender variance in children. Anxiety has been found to be relatively common in individuals with GD, even in cultures with accepting attitudes toward gender-variant behavior.

Autism spectrum disorder is more prevalent in clinically referred children with GD than in the general population [33]. Clinically referred adolescents with GD appear to have more comorbid mental disorders, with anxiety and depressive disorders being the most common. As in children, the autism spectrum disorder is more prevalent in clinically referred adolescents with GD than in the general population. Clinically referred adults with GD may have coexisting mental health problems, most commonly anxiety and depressive disorders [34].

12.6 Course and Prognosis

Boys begin to have the disorder before the age of 2–4 years, and peer conflict develops during the early school years, at about the age of 7 or 8 years. Grossly feminine mannerisms may lessen as boys grow older, especially if attempts are made to discourage such behavior. Cross-dressing may be part of the disorder, and 75% of boys who cross-dress begin to do so before the age of 4 years. The age of onset is also early for girls, but most give up masculine behavior by adolescence.

In both sexes, homosexuality is likely to develop in one third to two thirds of all cases, although, for reasons that are unclear, fewer girls than boys have a homosexual orientation. Follow-up studies of gender-disturbed boys consistently indicate that homosexual orientation is the usual adolescent outcome [9].

A small minority of children express discomfort with their sexual anatomy or will state the desire to have a sexual anatomy corresponding to the experienced gender (anatomical dysphoria). Expressions of anatomical dysphoria become more common as children with GD approach and anticipate puberty.

Rates of persistence of GD from childhood into adolescence or adulthood vary. In natal males, persistence has ranged from 2.2 % to 30 %. In natal females, persistence has ranged from 12 % to 50 %. Persistence of GD correlates modestly with dimensional measures of severity ascertained at the time of a childhood baseline assessment [1].

For both natal male and female children showing persistence, almost all are sexually attracted to individuals of their natal sex. For natal male children whose GD does not persist, the majority are androphilic (sexually attracted to males) and often self-identify as gay or homosexual (ranging from 63 % to 100 %). In natal female children whose GD does not persist, the percentage who are gynephilic (sexually attracted to females) and self-identify as lesbian is lower (ranging from 32 % to 50 %) [1].

Adult male patients who are GD and sexually attracted to male partners may have a continuous development of GD from childhood. Some manifestations of their GD may be driven underground, however, in an effort, during their teens and, perhaps, early 20s, to merge with the larger community. They may also hope or think that their GD will disappear. Sexual interest in male partners begins in early puberty, and some may consider themselves to be homosexual. They find, however, that they do not integrate effectively into the gay community. Approximately two thirds of adult men with GD are sexually attracted to men only.

Gender dysphoria in men sexually attracted to female partners may be characterized as a more progressive disorder with insidious onset. The course is fairly continuous in some cases. In others, the intensity of symptoms fluctuates. Some experience a lifelong struggle with feminine identification that changes in intensity from time to time and may temporarily recede in the face of conflicting desires, such as those for marriage and family. In most cases, the first outward manifestation is cross-dressing in childhood—dressing in mother's or sister's clothing—and many patients report that they first began wishing to be female during that period. The extent of their cross-gender behavior in childhood does not usually warrant diagnosis of GID, however.

Female patients may experience adolescence in which they initially consider themselves lesbian because of sexual attraction to female partners. They come to define themselves as distinct from lesbians, however, because they consider themselves to be men in their relationships with women. They insist that their partners treat them as men and that the partners are heterosexual women. Female patients are often, more often than male patients, in a romantic or sexual relationship at the time of initial clinical assessment.

In earlier clinical experience, it was the rare female-to-male transsexual who reported sexual attractions to male partners. This has changed. Some gender identity clinics report that approximately one tenth of patients born female have a sexual orientation toward men and consider themselves to be gay men [9].

12.7 Treatment

We want to start this topic remembering Matt Kailey's words (http://tranifesto.com/2012/04/16/ask-matt-should-gender-dysphoria-be-in-the-dsm/):

> "When I first started transition, I was pretty anti-therapy, even though I loved my own therapist. I did not, and still don't, like the "oversight" component of therapy with regard to transition. I think that therapy can be very helpful, and I think that it can be especially beneficial when dealing with the "reality checks" that I think are necessary for transition, as well as offering support and ideas with social-role and adjustment issues that can come with transition.
>
> I've always thought that the "gatekeeper" aspect of the therapist's role with regard to approval for hormones and surgery can interfere with a truly beneficial therapeutic relationship. On the other hand, a good therapist, working with a healthy trans person with realistic expectations, can result in a positive experience.
>
> Unfortunately, a lot of trans people have suffered at the hands of ill-prepared, misinformed, or just plain uncaring therapists who have required a lot of jumping through unnecessary hoops, which does not bode well for a valuable relationship. And there are a lot of therapists out there who still believe that gender issues can be "cured", particularly in childhood (one of the concerns of the community was that one of the doctors on the DSM-5 revision committee was known for "treating" children who exhibited gender issues by forcing them into stereotypical gender roles associated with their birth sex).
>
> My own opinion is that I would like to see GID, GD, or whatever psychiatric label comes about for people whose gender identity does not align with their physical sex (or sex assigned at birth) removed from the DSM. I don't think that my "condition" is a mental health issue.
>
> Research has demonstrated that transition, a series of medical procedures, can reduce or eliminate the suicidal ideation and other emotional difficulties that many trans people experience. Therefore, I believe that this is a medical issue and should be treated as such. However, there are some trans people who think that even that is too pathologizing, and that transition procedures should be available as on-demand procedures, with the idea that we know our own bodies and minds and should have the right to make our own decisions about care.
>
> I agree with this as well, and this is where I am torn. I believe that I am responsible for my own body, and that I am capable of making decisions about it. I don't think that I should have to jump through a bunch of someone else's hoops to do what is best for me. But if gender issues are not part of either a psychiatric or a medical diagnosis, and transition procedures can be issued upon request, then transition becomes a series of "elective" procedures, not considered medically necessary, not covered by insurance or other medical programs, and not recognized as a life-saving intervention".

In the second half of the twentieth century, awareness of the phenomenon of GD increased when health professionals began to provide assistance to alleviate GD by supporting changes in primary and secondary sex characteristics through hormone therapy and surgery, along with a change in gender role. As the field matured, health professionals recognized that while many individuals need both hormone therapy and surgery to alleviate their GD, others need only one of these treatment options and some need neither [35].

Often with the help of psychotherapy, some individuals integrate their trans or cross-gender feelings into the gender role they were assigned at birth and do not feel the need to feminize or masculinize their body. For others, changes in gender role and expression are sufficient to alleviate GD. Some patients may need hormones, a possible change in gender role, but not surgery. Others may need a change in gender role along with surgery, but not hormones. In other words, treatment for GD has become more individualized.

As a generation of transsexual, transgender, and gender-nonconforming individuals has come of age—many of whom have benefitted from different therapeutic approaches—they have become more visible as a community and demonstrated considerable diversity in their gender identities, roles, and expressions. Some individuals describe themselves not as gender-nonconforming, but as unambiguously cross-sexed (i.e., as a member of the other sex). Other individuals affirm their unique gender identity and no longer consider themselves to be either male or female. Instead, they may describe their gender identity in specific terms such as transgender, bigender, or genderqueer, affirming their unique experiences, which may transcend a male/female binary understanding of gender [35].

They may not experience their process of identity affirmation as a "transition," because they never fully embraced the gender role they were assigned at birth or because they actualize their gender identity, role, and expression in a way that does not involve a change from one gender role to another. For example, some young people identifying as genderqueer have always experienced their gender identity and role as such (genderqueer). Greater public visibility and awareness of gender diversity have further expanded options for people with GD to actualize an identity and find a gender role and expression that are comfortable for them [7].

Health professionals can assist gender dysphoric individuals with affirming their gender identity, exploring different options for the expression of that identity, and making decisions about medical treatment options for alleviating gender dysphoria.

For individuals seeking care for GD, a variety of therapeutic options can be considered. The number and type of interventions applied and the order in which these take place may differ from person to person. Treatment options include the following [7]:

Changes in gender expression and role (which may involve living part time or full time in another gender role, consistent with one's gender identity).

Hormone therapy to feminize or masculinize the body. Persons born male are typically treated with daily doses of oral estrogen. This may be conjugated equine estrogens or ethinylestradiol or estrogen patches. These hormones produce breast enlargement, the amount being largely determined by genetic predisposition, which continues for approximately 2 years. Other major effects of estrogen treatment are testicular atrophy, decreased libido, and diminished erectile capacity. In addition, a decrease occurs in the density of body hair and, perhaps, an arrest of male pattern baldness. Side effects of endocrine treatment can be elevated levels of prolactin, blood lipids, fasting blood sugar, and hepatic enzymes. Patients should be monitored with appropriate blood tests. Smoking is a contraindication of endocrine treatment because it increases the risk of deep vein thrombosis and pulmonary embolism. There is no effect on voice. Facial hair removal is required by laser treatment or electrolysis. Biological women are treated with monthly or three-weekly injections of testosterone. Because the effects of exogenous testosterone are more profound than those of estrogen, clinicians should be more cautious about commencing female patients on hormone treatment. The pitch of the voice drops permanently into the male range as the vocal cords thicken. The clitoris enlarges to two or three times its pretreatment length and is often accompanied by increased libido. Hair growth changes to the male pattern, and a full complement of facial hair may grow. Menses cease. Male pattern baldness may develop, and acne may be a complication. Ethinylestradiol in male-to-female transsexuals increases regional fat depots and thigh muscle mass. Conversely, female-to-male transsexuals receiving testosterone may have increased thigh muscle and reduced subcutaneous fat deposition. Thus, cross-sex steroid hormones affect general body fat and muscle distribution, as well as promote breast development in patients born male [9].

Surgery to change primary and/or secondary sex characteristics (e.g. breasts/chest, external and/or internal genitalia, facial features, body contouring). Sex-reassignment surgery for a person born anatomically male consists principally in removal of the penis, scrotum, and testes, construction of labia, and vaginoplasty. Some clinicians attempt to construct a neoclitoris from the former frenulum of the penis. The neoclitoris may have erotic sensation. Postoperative complications include urethral strictures, rectovaginal fistulas, vaginal stenosis, and inadequate width or depth. Some male patients who do not have adequate breast development from years of hormone treatment may elect augmentation mammoplasty. Some also have thyroid cartilage shaved to reduce the male-appearing thyroid cartilage. Patients need to undergo vocal retraining, and those who do not have a fully effective response may undergo a cricothyroid approximation procedure, which can raise vocal pitch. The results of these operations are variable. Female-to-male patients typically may undergo bilateral mastectomy and construction of a neophallus. Because of increased technical skills in phalloplasty, more female-to-male patients are now electing these procedures. Uncertainty and controversy exist with respect to the capacity for sexual arousal by the patient postsurgery. Some patients maintain that they are orgasmic. They describe the sensation of orgasm as more gradual and attenuated than their orgasms preoperatively. On the other hand, some patients report little sexual responsivity postsurgery. No adequate assessments have been made of the physiological functioning of postoperative male-to-female transsexuals with respect to the human sexual response cycle. Many patients, however, report satisfaction with being able to have vaginal intercourse with a male partner [9].

Psychotherapy (individual, couple, family, or group) for purposes such as exploring gender identity, role, and expression; addressing the negative impact of gender dysphoria and stigma on mental health; alleviating internalized transphobia; enhancing social and peer support; improving body image; or promoting resilience.

Options for Social Support and changes in gender expression. In addition (or as an alternative) to the psychological and medical treatment options described above, other options can be considered to help alleviate GD, for example: in person and online peer support resources, groups, or community organizations that provide avenues for social support and advocacy; in person and online support resources for families and friends; voice and communication therapy to help individuals develop verbal and nonverbal communication skills that facilitate comfort with their gender identity; hair removal through electrolysis, laser treatment, or waxing; breast binding or padding, genital tucking or penile prostheses, padding of hips or buttocks; changes in name and gender marker on identity documents.

No convincing evidence indicates that psychiatric or psychological intervention for children with GID affects the direction of subsequent sexual orientation. The treatment of GID in children is directed largely at developing social skills and comfort in the sex role expected by birth anatomy. To the extent that treatment is successful, transsexual development may be interrupted. The low prevalence of transsexualism in the general population, however, even in the special population of cross-gender children, thwarts the testing of this assumption.

No hormonal or psychopharmacological treatments for GID in childhood have been identified.

Adolescents whose GID has persisted beyond puberty present unique treatment problems. One is how to manage the rapid emergence of unwanted secondary sex characteristics. Thus, a new area of treatment management has evolved with respect to slowing down or stopping pubertal changes expected by the anatomical birth sex and then implementing cross-sex body changes with cross-sex hormones.

Young persons whose previous GID has remitted may experience new conflicts should homosexual feelings emerge. This may be a source of anxiety in the adolescent and may cause conflict within the family. Teenagers should be reassured about the prevalence and nonpathological aspects of a same-sex partner preference. Parents must also be informed of the nonpathological nature of same-sex orientation. The goal of family intervention is to keep the family stable and to provide a supportive environment for the teenager [36].

Adult patients coming to a gender identity clinic usually present with straightforward requests for hormonal and surgical sex reassignment. No drug treatment has been shown to be effective in reducing cross-gender desires per se. When patient GD is severe and intractable, sex reassignment may be the best solution.

12.7.1 Evidence for Clinical Outcomes of Therapeutic Approaches

One of the real supports for any new therapy is an outcome analysis. Because of the controversial nature of sex reassignment surgery, this type of analysis has been very important. Almost all of the outcome studies in this area have been retrospective.

It is difficult to determine the effectiveness of hormones alone in the relief of GD. Most studies evaluating the effectiveness of masculinizing/feminizing hormone therapy on GD have been conducted with patients who have also undergone sex reassignment surgery. Overall, studies have been reporting a steady improvement in outcomes as the field becomes more advanced. Outcome research has mainly focused on the outcome of sex reassignment surgery. In current practice there is a range of identity, role, and physical adaptations that could use additional follow-up or outcome research [11].

For more in-depth information about these topics (the treatment options and clinical outcome of therapeutic approaches in GD) we recommend reading the *WPATH Standards of Care for the Health of Transsexual, Transgender and Gender-Nonconforming People*, seventh version, 2011 [7].

Finally, as health professionals, we must be aware of the corresponding protocols for hormone therapy and surgeries, the informed consent forms, and the biosanitary and bioethical aspects surrounding this topic.

References

1. APA. Diagnostic and statistical manual of mental disorders, DSM 5. 5th ed. Arlington, VA: American Psychiatric Association; 2013.
2. Byrne W, et al. Report of the American Psychiatric Association Task Force on treatment of gender identity disorder. Arch Sex Behav. 2012;41(4):759–96.
3. Foucault M. Surveiller et punir. Paris: Gallimard; 1975.
4. Horney K. The unknown Karen Horney essays on gender, culture and psychoanalysis. New Haven: Yale University Press; 2000.
5. Foucault M. Folie et déraison: histoire de la folie á lâge classique. Paris: Union Gènerále d'Éditions; 1961. English translation: Madness and civilization: a history of insanity in the age of reason. New York: Vintage books edition; 1998.
6. Downing L. The Cambridge introduction to Michel Foucault. Cambridge: Cambridge University Press; 2008.
7. Coleman E, Bockting W, Botzer M, Cohen-Kettenis P, DeCuypere G, Feldman J, Fraser L, et al. Standards of care for the health of transsexual, transgender, and gender-nonconforming people, Version 7. Int J Transgenderism. 2011;13:165–232.
8. Rough garden J. Evolution's rainbow. Berkeley: University California Press; 2004.
9. Sadock BJ, Sadock VA, Ruiz P. Gender identity disorders. 9th ed. Philadelphia: Lippincott Williams & Wilkin; 2009.
10. Strynker S. Transgender history. Berkeley: Seal Press; 2008.
11. Institute of Medicine. The health of lesbian, gay, bisexual, and transgender people: building a foundation for better understanding. Washington, DC: National Academies Press; 2011.
12. Zucker KJ, Lawrence AA. Epidemiology of gender identity disorder: recommendations for the standards of care of the World Professional Association for transgender health. Int J Transgenderism. 2009;11(1):8–18.
13. De Cuypere G, Van Hemelrijck M, Michel A, Carael B, Heylens G, Rubens R, Monstrey S. Prevalence and demography of transsexualism in Belgium. Eur Psychiatry. 2007;22(3):137–41.
14. Reed B, Rhodes S, Schofield P, Wylie K. Gender variance in the UK: prevalence, incidence, growth and geographic distribution. 2009. http://www.gires.org.uk/assets/Medpro-Assets/GenderVarianceUK report.pdf
15. Wallien MS, Zucker KJ, Steensma TD, Cohen-Kettenis PT. 2D:4D finger-length ratios in children and adults with gender identity disorder 2008. Horm Behav. 2008;54:450–4.
16. Coolidge FL, Ll T, Young SE. The heritability of gender identity disorder in a child and adolescent twin sample. Behav Genet. 2002;32(4):251–7.
17. García-Falgueras A, Swaab DF. A sex difference in the hypothalamic uncinate nucleus: relationship to gender identity. Brain. 2008;131:3132–46.
18. Savic I, Berglund H, Lindström P. Brain response to putative pheromones in homosexual men. Proc Natl Acad Sci USA. 2005;102:7356–61.
19. Savic I, Lindström P. PET and MRI show differences in cerebral asymmetry and functional connectivity between homo- and heterosexual subjects. http://dx.doi.org/10.1073/pnas.0801566105
20. Swaab DF. Sexual orientation and its basis in brain structure and function. Proc Natl Acad Sci USA. 2008;105(30):10273–4.
21. Korte A, Goecker D, Krude H, Lehmkuhl U, Grüters-Kieslich U, Beier KM. Gender identity disorders in childhood and adolescence. Dtsch Arztebl Int. 2008;105(48):834–41.
22. Wedeen VJ, Rosene DL, Wang R, Dai G, Mortazavi F, Haggman P, Kaas JH, Tseng WI. The geometric structure of the brain fiber pathways. Science. 2012;335(6076):1628–34.
23. Chen CH, Gutierrez ED, Thompson W, Panizzon MS, Jernigan TL, Eyler LT, Fennema-Notestine C, Jak AJ, Neale MC, Franz CE, Lyons MJ, Grant MD, Fischl B, Seidman LJ, Tsuang MT, Kremen WS, Dale AM. Hierarchical genetic organization of human cortical surface area. Science. 2012;335(6076):1634–6.

24. Bradley SJ. Female transsexualism—a child and adolescent perspective. Child Psychiatry Hum Dev. 1985;11:12–8.
25. Meyer JK. The theory of gender identity disorders. J Am Psychoanal Assoc. 1982;30:381–418.
26. Silvermann MA. The prehomosexual boy in treatment. In: Socarides CW, Volkan VD, editors. The homosexualities. Reality, fantasy, and the arts. Madison: International University Press; 1990.
27. Haber CH. The psychoanalytic treatment of a preschool boy with a gender identity disorder. J Am Psychoanal Assoc. 1991;39:107–29.
28. Gilmore K. Gender identity disorder in a girl: insights from adoption. J Am Psychoanal Assoc. 1995;43:39–59.
29. Zucker KJ, Bradley SJ, Ben-Dat DN, Ho C, Johnson L, Owen A. Psychopathology in the parents of boys with gender identity disorder. J Am Acad Child Adolesc Psychiatry. 2003;42: 2–4.
30. Samkhaniyani E, Khalatbari J, Arkiyan F. The relationship between disconnection and rejection domain on early maladaptive schemas with defense mechanisms in individuals with gender identity disorder. Life Sci J. 2013;10(1s):436–40.
31. Ramachandran VS. The Tell-Tale brain. London: WW Norton & Company; 2011.
32. International statistical classification of diseases and health related problems. The ICD-10. World Health Organization, Geneva, 1992. Spanish translation: Trastornos Mentales y del Comportamiento, CIE 10. Madrid: Meditor; 1992.
33. de Vries ALC, Noens ILJ, Cohen-Kettenis PT, Berckelaer-Onnes IA, Doreleijers TA. Autism spectrum disorders in gender dysphoric children and adolescents. J Autism Dev Disord. 2010; 40(8):930–6.
34. Hoshiai M, Matsumoto Y, Sato T, Ohnishi M, Okabe N, Kishimoto Y, Terada S, Kuroda S. Psychiatric comorbidity among patients with gender identity disorder. Psychiatry Clin Neurosci. 2010;64(5):514–9.
35. Bockting WO. Psychotherapy and the real-life experience: from gender dichotomy to gender diversity. Sexologies. 2008;17(4):211–24.
36. Cohen-Kettenis PT, Gooren LJ. Transsexualism: a review of etiology, diagnosis and treatment. J Psychosom Res. 1999;46:315–33.

Life Instinct and Gender

13

Olatz Napal and Aitor Francos

> *"The irony of man's condition is that the deepest need is to be free of the anxiety of death and annihilation; but it is life itself which awakens it, and so we must shrink from being fully alive." [1]*
>
> *"Every existing thing is born without reason, prolongs itself out of weakness, and dies by chance. . . . The contradiction of our existence as for-itself is that our essence only becomes complete when our existence is no more." [2]*

Abstract

The instinct for survival or self-preservation represents the most relevant tendency of the human being, as the development of other instincts and vital functions depends on it.

Life and death are interdependent; they exist simultaneously and not consecutively and they exert an enormous influence on experience and behavior.

Our life and hence our experience, behavior, and identity (including gender) are related to experiences of change, pain, risk, symptoms, ambivalence, loneliness, the experience of "the other," grief, anxiety before death, and the perception of the meaning of life.

Based on Pierre Bourdieu's model, through his work *Masculine Domination*, we conduct an analysis of how culture and society interfere/interact in our behavior, and therefore in our lifestyle and our identity (from a gender perspective), to the extent that we unconsciously add incorporations (from that culture/society) and subsequently assume them as "natural," "immovable" aspects that are determined by our sex ("biologically").

However, things are not as simple as that because, if so, we would not feel disagreement with those behaviors/manifestations/ways of feeling that are given to us "naturally," and that is where the human being (regardless of sex/gender) makes an effort to "take the reins" of what belongs to him: his life, his body. We

O. Napal (✉) • A. Francos
Alava University Hospital, Vitoria, Spain
e-mail: olatz.napalfernandez@osakidetza.net; AITOR.FRANCOSAJONA@osakidetza.net

M. Sáenz-Herrero (ed.), *Psychopathology in Women*,
DOI 10.1007/978-3-319-05870-2_13

thus approach the subject of suicide, as well as the subject of self-harm, specifically self-mutilation, from some different theoretical perspectives and models and conclude by providing our own reflections.

13.1 The Instinct for Survival

Instinct is a pattern of inherited behavior, characteristic of the animal species, which varies little from one individual to another. It develops according to a temporal sequence that is slightly susceptible to being disturbed and seems to answer a purpose. The instincts constitute biological impulses, inherited and intermittent, that are likely to be activated by physiological or environmental factors.

The instinct for survival or self-preservation represents the most relevant tendency of the human being, as the development of other instincts and vital functions depends on it. The drive is a dynamic process consisting of a thrust that makes the organism tend to come to an end. It arises from a state of tension and tends to suppress it. The term *drive* is a limited concept between what is psychic and what is somatic; it involves a representative that is sent from the soma to the psyche. Drives are responsible for the psychological motivation of human behavior, and they act in a constant and non-intermittent manner.

Freud organized the drives into a duality that showed mutual opposition: drives of self-preservation (protective of the individual), which were quickly subjected to the reality principle; and sexual drives (imperative of the species), intended to be operated according to the pleasure principle and only late and laboriously reproduced their adaptation to reality.

In the second stage of his theory, the so-called second topic (1920), Freud includes both the life drive and the death drive (or self-destruction):

Life drive (Eros): The libido is home to both the self-preservation drive and the sexual drive.

Death drive (Thanatos): Prone to unbinding, it constantly tries to simplify the complex on a quest to reduce tensions, until it returns the living being to the absolute inorganic stability, ergo death. The death drive primarily operates inside the individual, and only secondarily is is directed to the outside as a destructive instinct. The concept of death drive was originally described by Sabina Spielrein. It is noteworthy that Freud only refers to his predecessor in this concept, Sabina Spielrein, in a footnote of his essay "Beyond the Pleasure Principle" (1920).

Sabina Spielrein played an especially significant role in the development of Freud's theory on death drive, presenting her work in 1912 (after obtaining her Doctorate in Medicine with a case of schizophrenia the previous year) with the title *Destruktion als Ursache des Werdens* (Destruction as a Cause of Coming into Being).

The novelty in Sabina Spielrein's theory is that it links death drive with life drive. She holds that not only are these two forces balanced, but they are a condition of each other, both of them are primary. Thus, the existence of one of them is inconceivable without the other. It is remarkable that Sabina Spielrein, before all else, shows how myths, legends, and sacred texts of different cultures interrelate death with birth. There is some logical connection, she says, between the return to the original material and rebirth. She also shows how the same myths and legends reveal knowledge of the aggressive and destructive element in the erotic and how self-destruction is within us as an instinct because it both opens the way to what is new and is related to the feeling of pleasure.

In her work, Sabina Spielrein believes: "You feel that the enemy is within (. . .) Its characteristic ardour compels you, with inflexible urgency, to do what you do not want to do; you feel the end, the transient, before which you vainly may attempt to flee to an uncertain future."

In the twentieth century other psychoanalysts, such as Karen Horney, denied that there was a death drive, or Thanatos, but wrote that adverse situations in the society would create the drive against the person itself in every individual. Others argue, following Winnicot, that there is only one life drive, with two roots (erotic and aggressive) that should remain integrated [3].

From the most existentialist point of view, death is a fact that always hurts; our attitudes toward it have an influence on our way of living and growing, our hesitations, and our diseases. Life and death are interdependent; they exist simultaneously and not consecutively and they exert an enormous influence on experience and behavior [4].

Heidegger argued that there are two fundamental ways of being in the world: the state of self-neglect (immersed in the routine, lost from "others"), and the state of care for the self, not marveling at the routine itself, but because it exists (transcendental). In general, we live in the routine, but there are experiences (which Jaspers called "limit" [5]) that move us and take us out of that state to take us to the "superior" condition, death being one of them, that allows us to live life authentically [4]. Denying death in any way is to deny the basic nature of the human being, which would restrict consciousness and experience more and more. "Though the physicality of death destroys us, the idea of death can save us."

The awareness of change often breaks the certainty of an "organized" life that has up to then been a referent of identity. Change is transformation, metamorphosis, the process and assimilation of which is the founding of the sense of identity. Changing is experiencing satisfaction and suffering. The anxiety that appears when we "intuit" the change is linked to the feeling of identity loss. In cases where this occurs, it is intended that nothing is changed. This is to avoid recognizing a discontinuous temporality, the difference between past and future, despite the fact that those changes mean success or progress for the individual. This can be experienced as an approach to death. The transformation, as Hegel says, starts as an antithesis. We are ourselves as we become a combatant against our dependency without forgetting that we ourselves are also the dependency that we fight against. So that the transformation is authentic, it has to go through our process of identifying what we reject. Everything that has a negative result also involves our human condition [6].

"Who is not, cannot release from any pain." (Améry)

Pain is inevitable in the experience of change. There is no change without pain, but with only pain there is no change either. When there is no tolerance for change, whether internal or external, the sense of identity tends to be unstable. Thus, the tendency to avoid change may sometimes cause a high level of pathology, leading to the repetition, to the compulsion, in order to preserve, at any cost, the aspects of reality or oneself that we do not want to be exposed to transformation. The identity of the individual that rejects change is mortgaged and alienated in the object. This individual is denying that, as Yalom says: "We are time."

The awareness of change is the process by which we can recognize our crisis as emerging from our identity and not as the antithesis of it. That awareness is the awareness of the future too, that is to say, of the reparative dimension of change [6]. But for this we need to go through the experience of risk. Because risk exists. It is an inevitable feature of life that is not only taken before the unknown and unpredictable, but also when we are about to get trapped, or when we are already trapped, in the hands of the known.

The symptom is a crack, malady, or an expression of needs. Its presence disorganizes the chronic present. It not only talks about itself, but it is itself. It is an expression of needs, the individual feels placed between two opposing realities: an identity that is already losing and another that is not yet in sight, but threatens with its indetermination. Many times, the symptom is the expression that ambivalence assumes through the body.

The ambivalence is the experience in which the subject lives simultaneously with its hope and frustration. It is the possibility of oscillating between the parts of a whole, identifying them as interrelated and complementary. The emphasis, in the ambivalence, falls in the middle, that is to say, at the point of convergence of the extremes. In duality, the emphasis falls on the opposition, not on the convergence. Accepting ambivalence means accepting, inside oneself, two aspects first experienced as contradictory rather than complementary: "I am the love and the hate," "I am a man and a woman," or better said, "I am masculine and feminine," "I am life and death." To accept both aspects as equally constituent parts of the personal identity opens up the possibility of a dialogue link that is not antagonistic, between the two parts, which places the subject in a different perspective to deal with the change from a reality of internal and external knowledge.

To accept the ambivalence means to accept the other, not only the other as a different and separate fellow, but to "the other self." It means accepting the proper limits of the human condition. The greater the acceptance of ambivalence, the greater the authenticity and the greater the wealth before the difficulty of accepting death.

The awareness of one's own death does not appear to be a biological fact, but an experience of the limits of the possibilities of development of the self. By understanding the limits of our development, we understand the possibilities.

It is true that the duality of gender may seem inevitable at first sight, as it is generally interpreted that sex and the gender role ascribed in birth remains throughout the life of any person. However, there is not necessarily continuity in the subjective experience of the gender identity, as this is *dynamic* (i.e., more or less masculine, more or less feminine, more or less androgynous, etc. depending on our references, feelings, contexts, etc.).

Within what we culturally "incorporate" (Bourdieu's "habitus") as feminine, the woman insists on believing that the symptoms through which she tries to communicate are not directly related to the environment that she is involved in. There is fear of posing problems, the personal dissatisfaction within a social model into which she does "not fit," so that she is trapped in a perspective that is insufficient for understanding her own pain, the guidelines of the conventional system that she belongs to, which are in part the guidelines of the person itself.

As Jean Amery believes: "Identity is not given by being a coherent person suffering from contradictions, but a contradictory someone because of his human nature who seeks certain coherence in his contradictions."

From our cultural perspective, loneliness is emptiness, isolation, abandonment or deterioration. It is, fundamentally, privation.

Loneliness implies impoverishment. It is equated with the loss of the self. Loneliness involves failure because being alone is to be lost. Being alone is identified as "not to be." The assumed proof of one's existence comes when we have someone else next to us. I can only be when someone else next to me confirms my existence with their presence. This happens to the human being regardless of gender.

In solitude, time consciousness is visceral: "In my solitude, I become aware of my finitude. If I can build my self is because I am going to die. I am not a once and forever something, I am in permanent evolution. Only what can die, can change."

Spinoza stated that every human being seeks to persist in its own being and Hegel, claiming that wish is always a wish for recognition, suggests that we can only keep our own self if we commit ourselves to receiving and providing recognition from the others. In our own ability to persist, we depend on whatever is outside of us, a wider sociality, and this dependence is the basis for our resistance and our ability to survive (Butler)

The relationship with the Other determines the constitution of our "self."

A woman who is alone breaks an established order, both objective and subjective [7]. She transgresses ideological guidelines and traditional values, she has supposedly failed and has been unable to consummate her femininity, as she is exposed to the "elements," she cannot be a complete woman and she is forced "to be a man."

According to Mitzrahi, the dissociation that leads to the absolute inconsistency of the person with itself, results in and feeds back to the practice of rejection to the self. The woman, apparently more often, moves between disassociation and symbiosis so as not to remain or be left alone. Depression becomes a way of confession and denouncement of sadness in fear behaviors, which are the expression of a deep dependence and the absence of a reflective consciousness. Sadness is useful in realizing and making contact with aspects of one's personality that we try to keep aside.

It is through the body that gender and sexuality are exposed to others and become involved in social processes that are registered by cultural rules and apprehended in their social meanings (Bordieu's "habitus"). To be a body is to be given to others, despite the fact that as a body, I am deep down, "my embodied-self."

As Esteban holds [8], "identity, besides being constructed through interaction, is embodied: the corporal image and the individual and social body are fundamental in the construction of one's identity and the belonging to different groups. In our society, the person is constituted by an individual entity whose borders lie on the surface of the body." We are given to another: this makes us vulnerable to violence, but also to another set of contacts, contacts ranging from the eradication of our self at one end, to the physical support of our lives at the other.

Therefore, the experience of the loss of someone (the Other) in mourning provokes shock and confusion. There are feelings of confusion and emptiness, feelings of depersonalization can be described, and there is a tendency to deny that the loss has happened [9]. In this experience, the bonds between us and others are revealed. These relationships constitute our sense of the self so that, when we lose them, we lose our self in a fundamental sense: we don't know who we are or what we do. The social relationship that constitutes our self exposes us [10].

The fear of death is permanent and of such a size that an important part of the vital energy itself is consumed in the act of denying death. One of the basic desires of the human being is to try to transcend it. According to Freud, the basic human group (the core of social life) is formed around the fear of death: the first humans settled together driven by the fear of separation since they were unaware of whatever stalked them in the dark. We perpetuate the group to perpetuate ourselves.

To give meaning to life by devoting oneself to one cause can take various forms:

(a) Altruistic: to find meaning in contributing to the good of others.

Irvin Yalom, in a text from his work *Existential Psychotherapy*, adds: "Much developmental research has dealt primarily with the male life cycle and has not taken special circumstances in the lives of women sufficiently into consideration. Middle-aged women, for example, who earlier in their lives devoted themselves to marriage and motherhood, seek different meanings to fulfill than their middle-aged male counterparts. Traditionally women have been expected to meet the needs of others before their own, to live vicariously through husbands and children, and to play a nurturing role in society as nurses, volunteers, and purveyors of charity. Altruism has been imposed upon them rather than freely chosen. Thus, at a time when their male counterparts have achieved worldly success and are ready to turn to altruistic considerations, many middle-aged women are, for the first time in their lives, concerned primarily with themselves rather than with others." Those who *can* (both by internal and external factors), we dare to say.

(b) Creativity

"Creativity is a 'natural' process implying pain and ambivalence, as the procreation" [11]. Some authors define creativity as the quality of the human being through which something new takes place transcending the existing one, which requires (i) an exercise of association between the outer and the inner world (subjectivity), and to be cognizant of it; (ii) an elaboration; and (iii) a communication with the outer, the latter two overlapping [12]. We must note that "to fantasize" is not "to create" [13]. The fantasy is a subset of the creative process that occurs in the inner world before manifesting it to the outer world. The creation, as a whole, requires activity, an exposure outside, an "externalization," "arting out" as Feder mentions (1998) [11]. Therefore, the fantasy (staying inside, without getting outside) would be more related to women, to the waiting, to "not acting-out." It is a shelter without reaching the "arting out" (or with higher difficulty than men, at least) as in the creativity, since the product is publicly exposed and is "visible," it is likely to be damaged [14],

and because the public space continues to be mainly masculine. The public art space is mostly occupied by men, as the *Guerrilla Girls* report.

This movement has been concerned with upsetting fictions like artistic genius and masterpiece. which sustain a concept of art that presents itself as independent of its historical and social context. Remaining anonymous, behind gorilla masks and adopting the names of iconic dead female artists, they focus on the political dimension of art and denounce the way women are systematically overlooked in contemporary society. Forged in the nineteenth century, this concept continues in force today.

(c) Hedonistic solution

The purpose of life is to live with plenitude, to seek the pleasure in the deepest sense of the term. Hedonists believe that pleasure itself is a satisfactory and sufficient explanation of human behavior. Even the behavior that leads to pain, contempt or self-sacrifice, can be considered hedonistic, as it is an investment in future pleasure. The pleasure principle surrenders to the reality principle: temporary discomfort may produce future dividends in the form of differed pleasure.

(d) Self-actualization

Maslow states that the person has inside a propensity toward development and unity of the personality, and toward a type of inherent pattern that consists of a unique set of characteristics and an automatic impulse to self-expression. We have a hierarchy of inherent motivations. Maslow considers society as an obstacle for self-actualization, because it usually forces the individual to abandon the development of its unique personality, to accept inappropriate roles and paralyzing conventions. In terms of gender, Maslow would refer to Bourdieu's concept "objective domination," which we will refer to later.

The latter two concepts (hedonism and self-actualization) differ from former two (altruism and creativity) because they take responsibility for oneself, while the others reflect a "basic impulse" to transcend the interest of the self in order to try to achieve something external and "superior" to oneself. In the first two, we could include the concept of father/motherhood (within creativity, procreativity), but we will not explain this now as the topic will be addressed in another chapter of the book).

The transcendence of the self is the main feature that Viktor Frankl gives to the question of *meaning* [15], stating that "one of the constitutive features of the human being is always pointing and addressing something beyond himself," taking care to differentiate the impulses (sexual or aggressive, for instance) that *push* the person from the inside, and the meaning that *pulls* the person from the outside. The difference is similar to the one between *impulse* and *effort*, so that in our most essential being, in those features that make us more humans than animals, we do not feel ourselves to be driven, but we actively make an effort to achieve a goal. The effort, in contrast to the drive, means that we are facing something outside our self (i.e., we are transcendent) and moreover, we are free to accept or deny the goal that invokes us. It also means an orientation toward the future: what will be attracts us and pulls us, instead of letting us be influenced by the past and the present.

"I sleep badly again and I have decided to rip everything I wrote and start again. I am sure this is the best. This misery of mine persists and I am absolutely crushed under its burden. If I could ever write again with my former fluency, the spell would be broken. It is the continuous effort, the slow creation of an idea, and then, before my eyes and out of my control, its slow dissolution." (Mansfield, 1987)

13.2 Life with Gender

Social psychology has taken an interest in studying how the process of gender self-construction is made in relation to the dominant roles and stereotypes in the *social environment*. More specifically, we will refer to the sociologist Bourdieu and his work *Masculine Domination* [7].

Bourdieu believes that the "domination" processes in a society are produced through a dual mechanism:

(a) Objectively, referring to social phenomena (through separate places, spaces where some people remain excluded. . .) that, whether or not are standardized by law, are produced, as it happens with certain professions in which women or men are not represented (in the case of women, in terms of authority, leadership, either by representing a smaller number or by differences in the wage. . . in the case of men, in terms of cleaning. . .).
(b) Subjectively, as a "principle of vision," as a mental structuration that is gradually incorporated and integrated from the objective space, in an "unconscious" manner, from society, in what the author calls "habitus," and is gradually assumed and perpetuated through the "patterns of perception, appreciation and action." It refers to the incorporation of opposites as public/private, coffee or chat/home, word or expression or policy/feeling, privacy, psychology, care, reproduction. . . the former attributed to men and the latter to women.

The combination of these objective and subjective "dominations" will lead to "everything appears to be given," to a something that is natural, and therefore immovable. He presents, as a model, the concept "*vocation*" (example: women for more human and caring areas, men for the most technical ones). Bourdieu found vocation to be one of the great differential "principles of elimination" between men and women: "those eliminated are unconsciously eliminated, women (and also men) lean toward that for which they were made," while thinking that they choose it freely. It would be the incorporation ("somatization") of objective structures in the subjective that will result in a series of categories, thoughts, perceptions, actions, and judgments through which we interpret the reality (he calls it "*habitus*"). There is an objective difference and it is incorporated. Men and women are unconsciously involved in it.

Within the outer space, which we have previously indicated corresponds to men, the woman finds her place through the body, the esthetic, the cosmetic, the elegance...The specialization attributed (socially constituted) to women with regard to the outside world would be through the esthetic, the taste, the decoration...Here, the author goes back to Simone de Beauvoir's concept "trophy wife," but with a different meaning, as a bearer of the man's social condition (i.e., if she wears jewelry, etc.), the woman more as an object than a person, which also occurs in the labor market, where we find that there is a predominance (although that is changing) of women in professions where the manner, the clothing, the appearance, of hostesses prevail. However, the dominant and dominated cannot be "blamed" as this is an "accomplice" domination. "Dominants can also be dominated by their domination," which can lead men, 'to come up to what society has imposed on me," and to self-impose sacrifices (up to the ultimate sacrifice of life, as happens with the absurdity of wars, etc.).

Bourdieu thus indicates to us that "symbolic violence" is a powerful foundation of the social order.

Despite all of that, there is often space for resistance and change (in both men and women) since, as Maslow says, the person has inside a propensity toward the development and unity of the personality; thus, we sometimes feel that we do not fit or identify "with what we are supposed to be/do", and a cognitive–emotional struggle takes place in which there is recognition of the double imposition lived (subjective and objective), which would sometimes give rise to a kind of "revenge" that may take different shades (empowerment, rebellion, self-assertion, crisis... or all of them) [7].

13.3 Suicide

13.3.1 Epidemiological Data

> "Suicidology is right. Except that for suicides and potential suicides what it says is empty. For what it comes to for them is the total and unmistakable singularity of their situation, the *situation vecue* (lived situation) that can never be completely communicated, so that therefore every time someone dies by his or her own hand or even just tries to die, a veil falls that no one can lift again, which in the best of cases can only be illuminated sharply enough for the eye to recognize as a fleeting image." (Améry, p. 19)

It has been estimated that suicide is responsible for one million deaths per year, with the rate of 14.5 deaths per 100,000 deceased subjects. Globally, suicide constitutes 1–5 % of all deaths [16–18]. Suicidal behavior not only involves complete suicide, but it ranges from presenting ideas of death or uncommitted suicidal thoughts, to suicide attempts of varying degrees of medical severity, to fatal suicide.

In response to suicidal behavior, we find that literature provides results in terms of gender differences: women have higher rates of suicidal ideation and behavior than males, while suicide mortality is typically higher in men [19–21]. The suicide ratio male:female ranges from 2 (Western Europe) to 4 (USA) to 1 [18], and this differentiation seems to increase [17]. Asian countries, however, show lower ratios of men:women [22], while in China more women than men die by committing suicide [23]. In the West, while the ratio of committed suicide is higher in men, suicidal ideation, as well as nonlethal suicidal behavior, is more common in women [19, 20, 24]

This striking difference in the suicidal behavior (i.e., the higher prevalence of women in the non-lethal suicidal behavior, and the hyper-representation of men in the committed suicide) has been called "the gender paradox of suicidal behavior" [19]. Several authors emphasize that the concept of "gender paradox" refers not only to the biological differences between males and females but also to the social standards and cultural expectations that vary between the two genders [25, 26].

We could mention here what Aurelia Martin [27] calls "gender stratification," referring to the inequality between men and women, which reflects the social hierarchization and the existing male domination in most societies. This means that, even within the issue of committing suicide, the final decision-making and the process from the step to the act are in the hands of men. However, in the "fantasy," "in the inside" in terms of Bourdieu, it would predominate in women, without reaching the final step of "acting out" and therefore remaining at the "limits" of both the inner–outer body and the life–death (self-injuries such as superficial cuts, nonlethal drug poisoning, etc.). It would be a kind of "suffocated or muted cry."

However, we observe that this "paradox" is absent in India and China, where women and men have similar ratios of suicide [22, 28, 29], to the point that the prevalence is higher in young women in rural areas [30, 31].

Several authors refer to the existing chronological relation between suicidal ideation and the suicidal act itself, to what they call the "suicidal process" considering that it begins with the presentation of ideas of death, hence passing to suicidal ideation and later involving progression to suicidality, consisting in the ideation and planning to take control of life and the communication of it, and the increase in all this through recurrent suicide attempts, with a progressive rise in lethality and suicidal intention, which ends in fatal suicide [32, 33]. Once a person is introduced to the suicidal process, he or she becomes more vulnerable to showing future suicidal behavior. Depending on what stage of the "suicidal process" the person is at, the impact of various factors (such as life stress, socio-economic conditions or mental illness, etc.) on suicidal behavior may vary [34, 35].

13.3.2 Stages of the Suicidal Process

Ideation stage: Initially, the individual considers the possibility of committing suicide to be a solution, for instance, to specific problems on a real or imaginary basis. This is an ideational or imaginative stage in which the desires and fantasies of escaping from an adverse situation, guilt, claiming self-punishment (according to Grinsberg, a persecutory guilt that better appertains to melancholic conditions), hostility and revenge with the expectation of exercising control over others beyond death, renascence to a new way of life, ecstasy, and meeting with the deceased loved one, or masochistic submission linked to a strong erotic desire and pleasure-seeking, prevail.

Ambivalence stage: The ideational or imaginative stage is followed by another stage in which the struggle between the life drive (Eros) and death drive (Thanatos) predominates. In this struggle, the role of the individual self, as an integrator of the other psychic instances of the life of the subject, is essential. If this self is in a situation of weakness, as a result of a personality structure with a more impulsive component, a somatic or mental illness, or the toxic effects of consumption, this stage may be brief and culminates in a *short-circuited suicide*, impulsive and poorly planned. On the contrary, if the self accomplishes the assignment in this period, it can be extended in time and the individual may show signs of suicidal thoughts or intentions to those around him, with the consequent possibility of acting preventively.

Decision-making: The individual finally makes the decision to commit suicide and, at this time, seems to relax and a huge burden is relieved. Externally, this stage is crucial and indicative signs of it (by bringing the will or legal matters up-to-date, attempts at reconciliation, etc.) may be identified. These indirect ways of communicating an imminent suicide add up to the most direct ones, in which the patient verbalizes or shows signs in advance of his intentions, which is crucial to aborting the attempt. As Jean Amery believes, "The bravery of the potential suicide is certainly not arrogance. There always dwells within it an additional trace of shame that, derived from the logic of life, makes the person standing before the leap ask why it is specifically he or she that can't stand it, can't stick it out, when the others still...."

The suicidal process can take many years or be extremely short, like just a few minutes, during which the intensity of the suicidal ideation may vary considerably. Generally, the duration of the suicidal process is shorter in men than in women: once the process has begun, men commit suicide much more quickly and successfully than women [32, 35].

We find authors who believe that the "intention," the message, is different between men and women, women showing more suicide attempts with the aim of a cry for help, signalization of the suffering they are going through (we do not like to say "attention-seeking" owing to the usually negative connotation). This suggestion seems to be supported by the evolution of frequently used psychotropics over a period of decades: 40 years ago, "toxic" agents (barbiturates and tricyclic antidepressants) were widely prescribed, whereas nowadays safer products such as low-dose benzodiazepines and selective –serotonin reuptake inhibitors are mostly used [20]. Owing to the disappearance of these toxic psychotropics, it was expected that the women's methods of suicide would shift from intoxications with safe products to the more "fatal" methods. However, no substantial increase in suicide or change in suicide methods has been reported in women; thus, the lower suicide ratio in women is not just a consequence of the method, but this could—at least in part—also be a reflection of the suicidal intention [20]. However, a growing number of women use more violent methods, especially younger women [26].

Given that, apparently, the "suicidal process" in women is longer, it can lead to the possibility of applying wider therapeutic interventions in this group and thus reducing the rate of committed suicides [36].

Some authors consider that another difference in the duration of the "suicidal process" would be related to the fact that men find it more difficult to withdraw their decisions, while women are more likely to reconsider the decisions they made. Moreover, most women do not regard asking for help as something negative when they do not feel good, while men have a tendency to think that asking for help is a sign of weakness [37, 38].

13.3.3 Stress Factors

13.3.3.1 Psychosocial

The literature refers to stress factors such as separation of the couple, troubled relationships, economic problems (finances, unemployment, etc.), immigration, gender identity or somatic disease. The first two (separation of the couple and troubled relationships) have been considered to have the greatest influence on suicidal behavior, regardless of sex and gender [36].

With respect to age, suicide in childhood is very uncommon. The literature reflects the emergence of the gender paradox in children at the ages of 10–19. Adolescent girls at the age of 13 show a sharp increase in suicidal ideation, planning, and attempts [39]. Young men (aged under 25 years) with major depressive disorder (MDD) show a far higher risk of suicide than adult men with MDD [40], considering separation, unemployment, and financial problems to be the most influential stress factors in this cohort of young men [36]. There is a higher risk of suicide in separated men than in separated women, regardless of age; thus, factors such as a history of previous suicide attempts or mental health problems, a lower level of education or financial problems, significantly raise the risk [41]. Furthermore, the ratio of suicide in white men increases after the age of 65, while the opposite occurs in women after the age of 55 [37]. The arguments given for these differences lean toward socio-professional issues, and states of life: most men retire from professional life at the age of 65, thus drawing apart from most of the contacts, interpersonal relationships, and friendships they have, especially in the work environment. Moreover, they consider that their "masculine self-esteem" is damaged as they stop being the provider or primary breadwinner of the family. These authors consider that retirement does not have the same effect on women, as throughout their entire professional life, they have combined it with the majority of the housework [37, 42], which they will continue with after retirement.

In addition, marriage is considered by several authors to be a protective factor against suicide, which implies that widowhood increases the risk of suicide, especially in men [37, 42, 43]. Having a child under the age of 2 years is a greater protective factor against suicide for women than for men [20, 37, 42, 43].

13.3.3.2 Sexual Abuse

Sexual abuse is more prevalent in women than in men. However, the fact that men show a greater reluctance and difficulty to relate these experiences [44] may have an influence on the lower ratio of men, as (in terms of Bourdieu's "habitus") they would not "live up to what society has imposed on them as men," but quite the opposite, they would be the "dominated" within the "masculine dominance." Needless to say, if the authorship of such abuses belonged to women...

Given the relation between sexual abuse in childhood and the subsequent suicidal behavior, we find a direct association between the two in men. Thus, suicide risk becomes 4–15 times higher in men who suffered from sexual abuse in childhood than in men who have not suffered from it [45–47]. In the case of women, this linkage has also been described, but appears amongst other factors such as depressive symptoms, hopelessness, and the level of family functioning, in which case the risk of suicide is three times higher than in women who have not undergone such abuse [45, 46].

13.3.3.3 Psychiatric Comorbidity

There is a clear association between suicide and psychopathology. Some authors note that over 80 % of suicides were previously diagnosed with a mental illness [48], and a history of hospitalization for mental illness has been found to be a significant risk factor for suicide in both men and women [42]. More specifically, a strong association has been demonstrated between the major depressive disorder or the borderline personality disorder and suicidal behavior; more women are diagnosed with such disorders than men [49–52]. Personality disorders, use of substances, and attention deficit hyperactivity disorder are related to an increased risk of suicide in men [18, 37, 43, 48, 53]. In this context, the literature mentions that some personality traits such as impulsiveness, hostility, or aggressiveness (also related to these disorders) are more prevalent in men, raising the emergence of suicidal behaviors, and especially, committed suicides [54, 55]. The majority of patients with schizophrenia who commit suicide are men [56]. In the case of affective conditions, suicide risk increases in men when it is associated with an anxiety disorder and a consequent worsening of depressive conditions, while in the case of women, the presence of affective conditions is only related to a high suicide risk [48, 57, 58].

Some authors have noted that in the presence of psychiatric illness, the differences in the male:female suicide ratio decrease, contemplating whether this may be due to the devastating impact of psychiatric illness, regardless of gender [59], or that the high male:female suicide ratio in nonclinical populations is due to a high prevalence of undiagnosed psychiatric disorders in men [59]. Furthermore, it has been demonstrated that, in clinical populations, there is a higher "over-diagnosis" of depression in women and/or under-diagnosis of the said clinical in men, which has been denominated "machismo-factor" [40, 60]. This has been associated with the fact that men show more difficulty to seek help from family, friends or professionals when they don't feel good [37, 61].

Compared with women, men who commit suicide are under-represented in the psychiatric clinical population and over-represented in terms of contacts with government services because of substance abuse and antisocial behavior [40, 62].

Gender differences have been considered regarding the "interiorization" of some disorders such as anxiety and depression, which could be related to this difference in rank in the male:female suicide rate. The fact that women better assimilate suffering from these disorders is reflected in a higher rate of suicidal ideation and attempts ("self-aggression"), while in men we would find more phenomena of "externalization," that is to say, antisocial behaviors, violence, use of substances, impulsiveness, etc., resulting in a larger number of lethal suicides.

In fact, some authors refer to the "male depressive syndrome," characterized by an increased externalization of symptoms such as anger, aggressiveness, irritability, and hostility [40, 62, 63].

13.3.3.4 Methods and Statements of Suicide

Several studies report that men show a greater tendency to perform suicide attempts that involve a more immediate lethality than those methods chosen by women, because men use more violent or faster-acting methods, such as hanging, carbon monoxide poisoning (the poet Anne Sexton used this method to commit suicide) or firearms. Women, on the other hand, tend to use voluntary poisonings that may involve a high toxicity, but are usually associated with a lower mortality rate and a slower-acting mechanism [19, 20, 57]. It is important to note that the methodology used for suicide not only depends on its accessibility to the future suicidal victim, but also on those specific cultural, religious, and social factors of the region where the suicide victim is situated [64–66]. It is also important to emphasize that the type of method used may influence the classifications and statements of suicide, depending on the sex of the suicidal victim (and yes, here it refers to gender): on the one hand, many of the suicides committed by women may be under-registered compared with those committed by men, and on the other, nonfatal suicidal behaviors in men may also be under-registered [19, 20, 40, 67]. In many (Western) cultures, suicides committed by women are more disapproved of than those committed by men, which results in the suicide records being biased [20]; while in some Asian countries like China, there is an opposing cultural belief, thus showing the reverse trend in male:female suicide rates compared with the Western ones [64–66].

Deaths by poisoning are often unreported as suicides, which results in many suicides committed by women not being recorded as such, while the most violent methods used by men are rarely reported as accidental deaths. On the other hand, it is considered that men are more aware of the social disapproval of their suicidal behaviors and thoughts, as they might be considered as "unmanly," which may provoke nonlethal suicidal behaviors not being reported as such in men. They may occur in male-dominated contexts such as prisons, where they could be marginalized [19].

13.3.3.5 Cultural Beliefs and Social Attitudes

As previously mentioned, the "gender paradox" in terms of suicide primarily occurs in Western countries, while in Asian countries (China, rural areas of India, Sri Lanka, Japan, etc.) we see that the male:female suicide rate tends to be 1:1. Actually, in some of these places, the suicide rate of women is higher [26], and more violent suicide methods are used (i.e., in China, insecticides in rural areas; in India or Sri Lanka, self-immolation by gas cooker or kerosene; "self-immolation of the widow"—*suttee* or *sati*—recognized and institutionalized by Hinduism until very recently, in which the widow had to throw herself into the funeral pyre of her deceased husband to atone for his sins and ensure the eternal blessings of both) [68].

Nowadays, isolated events in Indian rural communities are still found in the press: "A 65 year old woman burned to death in the funeral pyre of her husband in the village of Tamoli Patna (in Madhya Pradesh, 415 km far from Bhopal, in central India). The incident corresponds to a *sati* (ritual suicide of widows, banned since 1829). The woman, Kuttu Bai, sat on the pyre that burned the corpse of her husband, and two policemen who tried to take her out of there were deterred with stones by some 1,000 people. One of the agents, Nari Shankar Ghosh, recounted the rescue attempt and the hostile attitude of the horde. 'It is not clear if the woman did so voluntarily or was forced,' Gosh stated, adding that both Kuttu's children did nothing to prevent the incident" [69].

The situation of women in India once their husbands die is dramatic; being widowed is a "social death." In many cases, women are disowned by their family or ravaged by poverty so that they end up in the city of Vrindavan, called the "city of widows," a place that seems to be forgotten by time and is only 150 km from New Delhi and 70 km from Agra, where the Taj Mahal is located, which was ironically built because of the love of a woman. This is the situation of women in India today. They make up a third of the Vrindavan population, and they roam the city living on alms and awaiting purification through their prayers.

13.3.4 Theories of Suicide

Contemporary psychological conceptions of suicide share an eclectic position and tend to integrate psychodynamic, sociocultural, cognitive, and biological aspects. Suicidal impulses are not necessarily linked to certain specific psychopathological or personality structures. Notable is Mann's diathesis-stress model [70], which understands suicidal behavior to be a clinical syndrome, influenced by some biological traits that are dependent on a number of genes, and by the psychosocial environment. The suicide risk increases if there is a psychiatric disorder (preferably depressive conditions) or a chronic and disabling medical condition, if there are adverse life events, and if there are structures of borderline personality in which there is an objectified increase in the feelings of impulsivity or hopelessness and a tendency to pass from the step to the act, low self-esteem, and a lack of psychological and adaptive resources.

13.3.4.1 Psychodynamic Theories

For Freud, suicide represents the expression of aggressive impulses that address the introjected and emotionally inverted objects in a narcissistic and ambivalent manner. This hostility represents the primitive reaction of the self against the objects of the external world.

Menninger talks about retroflexed suicide, which can be addressed outward in the form of open aggression, or inward as a self-destructive tendency, based on the extreme child abandonment that we are born with and on the functioning of group institutions (family, civilization, perhaps gender) that require a moral response from each member of the group).

From the perspective of Melanie Klein, that self-destructiveness should be placed within the permanent failure to elaborate the paranoid–schizoid position, owing to a massive presence of the persecutory bad object, which would impede the passage to the second depressive and reparative position. Grinsberg, in the same vein, alludes to an unbearable and persecutory guilt, located in body or mind, on which the suicidal individual focuses his aggressive pulsions in order to, through self-destruction, get rid of it. ("It's not fair to be the one to bear this guilt. Since you have not understood and helped me to get rid of it, I kill myself for you to be now who owe bear it"). According to the psychiatrist Castilla del Pino: "Suicidal attitude connotes self-destructive requests for the individual that are inhibited to be projected outward. Many melancholic individuals have, along with fantasies of self-destruction, fantasies of destruction and repulsion of the world, which are very active in the fantastic plane. There is also the fantasy… also exists the fantasy of reconciliation, achieved after the suicide or precisely by the suicide, so that the fantasies of self-accusation would disappear."

From a dynamic perspective, Hendin proposes suicide as a form of expressions for different conflicts (Table 13.1).

13.3.4.2 Cognitive Theories

Cognitive theories have concentrated on styles of thinking that lead to an increased risk of self-harm. Cognitive studies have found that people who self-harm have more passive problem-solving styles than others, with solutions being less versatile and less relevant to the problem [71]. Poor problem-solving leads to hopelessness and/or helplessness, which increases the risk of self-harm [72]. Hopelessness and poor problem-solving ability may, however, act independently of each other to increase risk. There is no evidence that any of these cognitive styles is sex-specific.

We could refer here to the term "learned helplessness," by Seligman, as behavioral conditioning, and associate it with Bourdieu's "habitus." The helplessness does not occur immediately, but requires a learning process, in which the information of the relation between a given response and some reinforcement is assimilated. It is

Table 13.1 Types of suicides according to Hendin

	Conflict expresses
As retaliation or revenge after abandonment	Illusion of being able to control a situation of rejection, feeling of omnipotence by means of death
As retroflexed murder	"Acting" of a violent individual that reflects, through suicide and self-punishment, an internal struggle against the desire to kill or attack others
As meeting	After the death of a significant figure from an emotional point of view
As rebirth	As a preliminary step or initiation rite to access a new way of life, in which the failures and frustrations of the previous one are deleted, and an everlasting union with the lost object occurs
As punishment	From the most intense guilt—sometimes delirious—combined with melancholic manifestations.
Psychotic suicide	Typical of melancholic depression with psychotic symptoms, and schizophrenia. Known under the eponym "Cotard's syndrome." The patient has the delirious belief of being dead

based on the consequences of perceiving a lack of correlation between the objectives proposed and the objectives achieved, causing feelings of helplessness and lack of control. The individual adapts his behavior to a situation of non-control, so motivational, cognitive, and emotional deficits are generated in him. For Seligman, a body becomes defenseless before a certain consequence when it occurs independently of all its voluntary responses. Abramson, Seligman, and Teasdaler reformulated the theory in terms of attributional processes. According to them, a negative event by itself is not sufficient to acquire learned helplessness. It would also be necessary for it to be perceived as an uncontrollable, not contingent, event.

In the theory of hope, Abramson argues that there are different attributional styles. Suicidal behavior has been associated with cognitive alterations such as rigidity, defined as difficulty in developing positive alternatives to emotional problems. Aspects such as personality or self-worth could be related to the inferences taking place about the consequences of different events.

13.3.4.3 Social Theories

Durkheim believes that suicide is the result of the influence and control exerted by society. He proposes two variables to consider: a) the degree of social integration of the individual and b) the degree of social regulation of the individual desires (quote).

For Durkheim, suicide, from the cultural point of view, arises from four different categories:

Egoistic suicide: in individuals who, for various reasons, are not steadily and bindingly integrated into a particular social group, and act based on individual and not collective interests (for existentialists, the "earthly meaning").

Altruistic suicide: opposite of the above, in individuals that are excessively linked to the social group they belong to, with a notable absence of individual criteria (die for the cause, religious faith, politics, etc.).

Anomic suicide: practiced by those who are excluded from the group they belong to, either because they have suffered an economic setback and a loss of status and social recognition, or because they have been deprived of their liberty, or because they have been imprisoned for some type of crime. What brings these people to kill themselves is the feeling of non-acceptance and of irretrievably losing their previous social position.

Fatalistic suicide: occurs in those individuals who do not resist the pressure derived from the strict conditions and regulations to which they are subjected by the social environment in which they live.

"*. . .someone who was banned from another language. . .*" (J. Amery).

Queer[1] researchers claim that heterosexuality is approved in the dominant ideology of the "natural" sexual identity. Kosofsky considers that this belief leads to suicide in people who do not identify with these symbolic forms of expression of personal identity. He argues that *queer* teenagers are two or three times more likely to attempt suicide and commit it than other young people, and that in the USA, almost 30 % of young people who commit suicide are gay or lesbian [73].

13.3.4.4 Existentialist Theories

"*There is but one truly serious philosophical problem and that is suicide*" (*The Myth of Sisyphus*, Camus, 1942).

"Each of us has the plague within him." (*The Plague*, Camus, 1947)

The "plague" that Camus suggests is what Kierkegaard called "feeling of anxiety" in 1844, and was later called "existential anxiety" by the humanistic–existential stream, and consists of the fear of death. It is strange then that the suicidal candidate comes to embrace what he fears the most. What happens, therefore? The suicidal individual eliminates the self-preservation instinct conclusively. Suicide affects the two essential dimensions involved in our "being-in-the-world." The term "being" corresponds to the very existence, and the term "in-the-world" refers to our place, to what happens, to what occurs. Both terms within the expression "being-in-the-world" are fused or homogenized by the problem of meaning. And this is precisely what the suicidal subject eliminates all at once.

Irvin D. Yalom refers to the variety of "suicide as a magical act," in which there is no thought of death, but rather the contrary, suicide as a means of defeating death

[1] The **queer theory** is a hypothesis about gender affirmation implying that sexual orientation and sexual or gender identity of people are the results of a social construction and that therefore, there are no essential or biologically registered sex roles in human nature, but socially variable forms of performing one or more sex roles.

"The subject decides for itself in its full sovereignty. That doesn't mean 'against society.' The individual can destroy what he or she own, which never really was one's own, for the sake of an authenticity about which one is anxious. One lays hands on oneself." (Améry)

Table 13.2 Types of suicide according to Schneider

	Characteristics
Rational suicide	Derives from an objective and detailed analysis of a limited and insolvable existential situation. The psychotic subject can sometimes face, as a person, psychosis
Short-circuited suicide	Arises from a primitive impulsive discharge before an acutely stressful situation. It appears as a reflex action that escapes from the psychic processing or mental development. According to the author, it is more common in women
Theatrical suicide	It comes with an exhibitionist courtship, whose primary objective is to draw the attention of those people close to the patient, rather than cause death itself. It arises from a form of parasuicide or parasuicidal behaviors. However, sometimes we can come across truly committed suicides within this group. In these cases, the lack of impact and consideration generated from their actions, usually repetitive and clearly blackmailing to those who, powerless, face them (family, partner, friends), leads them to force their exhibitionist behavior or to demonstrate their anger and helplessness, increasing the lethality of their actions, with the consequent risk of death

by thinking that others will remember him for a long time, the belief in continuing to live if he exists in the consciousness of another person [74].

The "moral or social suicide" [75] is where the person looks for long-term self-destruction, by living a degrading way of life that excludes him from social intercourse.

The "epicurean suicide" is where death is considered rationally and dispassionately, as Lucretius explained: "Where death is, I am not; where I am, death is not," or in the words of Epicurus: "Death is nothing to us, since when we are, death has not come, and when death has come, we are not."

13.3.4.5 Classic Theories

The classic theories are summarized in Table 13.2.

13.4 Self-Harm and Gender

> "The relationship of body and ego is perhaps the most mysterious complex of our lived existence or, if one prefers, of our subjectivity of our being-for-itself. We are not aware of our body during everyday existence. To our being-in-the-world our body is what Sartre called '*le negligé*,' '*le passé sous silence*,' neglected, one scarcely speaks of it, doesn't think of it. We are our body: we do not have it. [. . .] however, we become conscious of it as a foreign body only when we see it with the eyes of the other [. . .] or when it becomes a burden." (Améry)

> "I hurt myself today
>
> To see if I still feel
>
> I focus on the pain
>
> The only thing that's real."

(*Hurt* written by Trent Reznor of Nine Inch Nails, sung by Johnny Cash)

Nonsuicidal self-injurious behaviors refer to deliberate self-injuries without a suicidal intent [76]. Examples of this could be cutting, burning, scratching the skin, hitting or biting oneself.

Conventionally, the term excludes harm resulting from drug or alcohol use or from eating disorders. Self-harm involves either self-poisoning or self-injury. Self-poisoning is synonymous with taking a drug overdose or ingesting substances never designated for human consumption, and self-injury refers to any form of intentional self-inflicted damage including cutting the skin, self-immolation, swallowing objects, hanging or jumping off buildings without (usually) ever compromising the patient's life.

We want to review now the concepts of "transference" and "acting-out" that we often find in the literature as synonyms, while some authors distinguish between them. Bernard, using the description given by Laplanche and Pontalis, argues that "transference" can take all kinds of forms (sometimes very discreet, he says) with the proviso that it holds that impulsive character, poorly motivated in the eyes of the same individual, but breaking with the usual behavior, even if the action in question is secondarily rationalized. He notes that "transference" can be differentiated from "acting-out" (of the subject has difficulty fantasizing) in that the latter arises in a more or less symbolic form in the course of analytical psychotherapy, in which the subject "leaves" the psychic material of the fantasy and the mental world to perform it before the psychotherapist with an aggressive character of varying severity.

The relationship between body and language is established by the cut, which is what writes, what engraves the writing of suffering on our flesh. It is, like Pane says, what the body will make memory of. The possibility that these cuts might be "read" by others overshadows the pain, time itself can deal with them because the body has the ability to heal. The flesh has the property of self-sealing (healing) and not remaining open. "Physical suffering is not merely a personal problem but also a problem of language. The act of self-inflicting wounds upon myself represents a temporary gesture, a psychovisual gesture that leaves marks" [77].

As Bataille believes, "The urges of the flesh pass all bounds in the absence of controlling will. Flesh is the extravagance within us set up against the law of decency" (Western flesh is Christian, as Michel Onfray argues). "Flesh is the born enemy of people haunted by Christian taboos, but if as I believe an indefinite and general taboo does exist, opposed to sexual liberty in ways depending on the time and the place, the flesh signifies a return to his threatening freedom" [78].

Christian iconography emphasizes the role of flesh and its transgression by marking its limits as the boundary that merges the flesh with the world by means of gashes, sores, cuts, decapitations, etc. This would cause horror in contemporary art, as with the photographs of David Nebreda (a photographer diagnosed with paranoid schizophrenia who uses his own self-portraits. In them, he is subjected to all kinds of lacerations, fasting in the place in which he is confined, because this is his way of expressing the pain). However, indoctrination and repetition for centuries make Christian iconography assume these cuts, wounds, and sores to be nonquestionable beauty since it is transcendent, and is built on beliefs through the centuries, following the direction of Bourdieu's "habitus." Thus, the infringed body is promoted by the ecclesiastical power and, far from being repudiated (as with Marina Abramovic's performances) by some sectors of our society, it is valued for its beauty.

A wounded body is a crossed frontier beyond which we go. Body art represented a barrier that some women artists crossed by using their body as a canvas to denounce their submission, their social under-representation, and their performatively marked sexuality. As Kruger shouts: "My body is a battleground". Body art is not only practiced by women, but by all those artists who consider it a form of social and gender protest.

The way in which sex and the role of women have been introduced in our society has been denounced by numerous artists, from Frida Kahlo to Louise Bourgeois, one of the first artists who used the female body to denounce the traditional role attributed to women.

Also, the artist Ana Mendieta, through *Mutilated Body on Landscape* (1973) and *Tied-up Woman*, where she appears naked, tied and humiliatingly immobilized, denounces the situation of women. Orlan, at the same time, did so through her works, such as *Le Baiser de l'Artiste* (The Artist's Kiss, 1977), performance with the slogans "art and prostitution."

Artists such as Pane, Carole Scheenemann, Kiki Smith, Cindy Sherman, Barbara Kruger or Linda Benglis should be added to this list. The last three highlight the role of the media and Western consumer society on their way to publicizing female imaginary, reporting the imposed media violence and making the imposed sex roles problematic [79].

In Table 13.3, we can see a classification of the different terms used for "nonfatal self-inflicted harms" by Skegg, in 2005 [80].

Casadó Marín [81] classifies self-harm according to the scenario; thus she elaborates this classification by oppositions:

- Standardized self-harm/Stigmatized self-harm
- Public self-harm/Private self-harm

Standardized self-injuries are those involving body art, body modification processes (diets, aesthetic care/Botox, surgeries, tattoos, piercings, scarifications), self-injuries in the ritual context—flagellations, fasting, crucifixions—also those that take place in penitentiary contexts—hunger strikes—and primarily in religious contexts.

Public self-injuries are those that occur in the ritual context.

Private self-harm occurs in situations of armed conflict (self-injury to avoid the front), in the working environment (in the face of certain working conditions), as a sign of identity among "emos" and "gothic"[2] young people, and in situations where self-injuries are interpreted under a diagnostic criterion of mental illness.

[2] The dark-gothic movement became relevant in the mid- to late 1970s, while the "emo" movement took place in the 1980s. Both styles included a philosophy and a way of conceiving the world

Table 13.3 Modified table on nonfatal, self-inflicted self-harm terminology. [80]

Terms for nonfatal, self-inflicted harm
ATTEMPTED SUICIDE Used widely (especially in North America) for episodes where there was at least some suicidal intent, or sometimes without reference to intent. Repetitive bodily harm may be excluded
DELIBERATE[a] SELF-HARM Used in the UK for all episodes survived, regardless of intent North American usage refers to episodes of bodily harm without suicidal intent, especially if repetitive. Usually excludes overdoses and methods of high lethality
PARASUICIDE Episodes survived, with or without suicidal intent (especially in Europe) or episodes without intent. Repetitive bodily harm may be excluded
SELF-POISONING OR SELF-INJURY Self-harm by these methods regardless of suicidal intent
SELF-MUTILATION Serious bodily mutilation (such as enucleation of an eye) without suicidal intent Repetitive superficial bodily harm without suicidal intent (synonymous with the North American term deliberate self-harm). Also known as self-injurious behavior, self-wounding Sometimes the term is used to describe both the above meanings and also stereotypical self-harm in intellectually disabled people

[a]The adjective “deliberate” is not favored now by patients in the UK

Through this classification, the author wants to draw our attention to the fact that self-harming actions must not only be rethought in exclusively pathological terms, but as a practice that can be interpreted and lived in different ways depending on the context, which legitimizes or stigmatizes it. Thus, she brings out the importance of the *social* aspect when it comes to attributing meaning to the act.

The mortification of the body in relation to the atonement of sins, or the compliance of promises or vows, has to do with the fact that, at the base of Catholicism, the body was a part of the human nature that limited the perfection of the soul, as well as the instrument through which the sin materialized. The disciplines and rules that mortified the body are those that managed to control the sinful nature of men and women and that constantly reminded us of our sinful essence.

13.4.1 Epidemiological Data

Although the estimated prevalence of self-harm varies depending on definitions and methodology, it is clear that it is highest during adolescence [82]. Theoretically, self-injurious behaviors can differ from suicide attempts in three basic aspects: intention, repetition, and lethality [83–87].

---

that went beyond the musical style and the clothing. Suicide and death are recurrent in the sense that gothic people are given to self-harm, while for “emo” people (the name is an abbreviation of emotional), self-injuries tend to be less aggressive, but rather superficial cuts [81].

Hawton estimates that, during the year after someone inflicts self-harm, the suicide risk is 60 times higher than in the general population [87]. Despite self-harm predicting future suicide attempts, suicide attempts do not predict future self harm.

In the general population, the prevalence of self-harm in adolescents is 5–37 %, compared with 4 % [84] in the adult population [88]. In the clinical population, we found a prevalence of self-harm in adolescence of 61.2 %, with regard to cuts [89, 90]. Most studies report that self-harm is more common in girls than boys, in ratios ranging from 20.3 % vs 8.5 % [91] to 45.2 % vs 38.1 % [92]. However, it seems that the prevalence in children has been increasing in recent years [82].

The greatest risk of hospital presentations in the WHO/EURO Study was in women aged 15–24 years and men aged 25–34 years [93]. Older people are at a much lower risk, and when they do self-harm they are much more likely to commit suicide later [94].

Although being male is an important risk factor for suicide, presentations of self-harm to health agencies are generally more common in women [93].

There are differences in sex distribution between self-cutting and overdose, with intentional overdose presentations involving a preponderance of women and self-cutting presentations displaying a more even gender distribution [95–97].

Past literature has often emphasized self-cutting as the main method of self-harm for women, but more recently research has shown a significantly higher proportion of women self-poisoning compared with men [98, 99]

However, compared with poisonings, cuts (with or without poisonings) are more common in men than in women, mainly in men under the age of 35 years [100]. Some studies [101] show that self-injurious behavior begins in early adolescence, with an increase in frequency and intensity in its evolution, and being more prevalent in women. The underlying factors include being a victim of sexual abuse and alexithymia.

In other research [102], we found significant correlations between self-injurious behaviors or self-mutilation and eating disorders, borderline personality disorder, post-traumatic stress disorder, and dissociative disorders. There is also a relationship between the extremely high rates of self-harm and suicide attempts in girls with ADHD, being associated with inattention, hyperactivity and impulsivity, and a history of trauma in childhood, such as abuse [103].

Between 70 and 80 % of patients who meet the DSM-IV criteria for borderline personality disorder (BPD) do self-inflict injury [104]; the DSM-IV shows that 75 % of BPD is diagnosed in women. Some studies show that between 35–80 % of individuals who self-inflicted injury also suffered from disordered eating behaviors [105]. For them, self-harm and eating disorders should be considered the desire to end with the body.

Recent studies suggest that there are different patterns in terms of self-directed violence in men and women [106], and that women with antisocial traits have a higher prevalence of self-harm and of being diagnosed with BPD than men with antisocial traits [107, 108]. However, it seems that the repetition of self-harm, when there is a history of such behavior, is almost equal in men and women [109].

Some authors say that men and women with gay, lesbian or bisexual orientation are more likely to self-harm than are heterosexuals [110, 111], although there have been conflicting results for teenage girls [112]. High risks have been identified in men who described their orientation as bisexual or who had experienced only minor same-sex attraction [110, 111]. The risk in gay, lesbian or bisexual youth could not be attributed to exposure to some risk factors, including depressed mood, substance abuse, pubertal timing, in fact, most self-harm occurred after or around the time that participants realized that they were not exclusively heterosexual [112]; thus, we can deduce that the social impact (acceptance) has a great influence on these behaviors.

13.4.2 Self-Injuries as a Separate Category

In the DSM-IV, nonsuicidal self-injuries were only mentioned as a diagnostic criterion for BPD, and described as suicidal behaviors, gestures, threats or self-mutilating behaviors [113], in autism, mental retardation, and factitious disorders. In the DSM-IV, self-injury is not considered a disorder in itself.

In the DSM-5, the nonsuicidal self-injury (NSSI) disorder as diagnostic entity was proposed as "conditions for further study." They insist on differentiating it from BPD, although they recognize the high existing comorbidity with both the said disorder and the eating disorders or the use of substances. They report that, although both diagnoses (along with BPD) are frequently associated, BPD does not invariably appear in all self-injurers. The difference between the two entities is that BPD often shows hostile and aggressive behaviors, while NSSI disorder is associated with situations of closeness, intimacy, collaborative behaviors, and positive social relationships. They also allege differences in the neurotransmitter systems.

The first case of self-harm without suicidal intent was described by L. Eugene Emerson in the *Psychoanalytic Review*, published in 1913. He talked about the case of Miss A[3] and proposed the challenge to understand why a person like her could come to self-inflicting injury when "this patient was not insane." It was a 23-year-old woman who had self-inflicted injuries in different parts of her body, one of them a "w" on her calf . Throughout therapy, Miss A relates that she was sexually abused in childhood by her uncle and subsequently her father. The particularity of Emerson consisted in investigating the experience of the symptoms, considering that the classification was less important than the causation and its manifestation through the body. For Emerson, there was a relationship between abuse and self-harm, highlighting the sexual nature of the act [114].

Other authors have called a combination of behaviors, including self-mutilation, substance abuse, and abnormal eating, often with a history of childhood sexual

[3] Miss A explained to Emerson that she self-inflicted that injury when a man she was in love with, and with whom she had had an affair, rejected her when she proposed to him and he called her "whore." She drank alcohol, took a blade, and marked the letter "w" (for whore) on her calf. For Emerson, Miss A felt that her past did not make her suitable for marriage, an idea that she could not stand; thus, she hurt the part of herself that represented a symbolic embodiment of her torment.

abuse, "trauma re-enactment syndrome," with women seen to be doing to their bodies something that represents what was done to them in childhood [115].

Miller described four common characteristics in these women: the feeling of struggling with their own body (the body as an enemy), the excessive discretion as a principle of life, the inability to protect themselves, and a certain dissociation of consciousness, where thoughts take three roles: the bully, the victim, and the witness who does not protect.

Pattison and Kahan supported the idea of a *deliberate self-harm syndrome* and described establishment in late adolescence, the episodes being recurrent and multiple, the low-lethality, the production of deliberate injuries to the body, and the tendency toward chronicity being major characteristics.

13.4.3 "The Portrait of the Typical Self-Injurer"

Favazza argued that self-injury affects 1 % of US population, and that 97 % of these are women [116]. This author defined "The portrait of the typical self-injurer" as a "white woman, in her late twenties, who began hurting herself at the age of fourteen. She had injured herself at least 50 times, usually by cutting but also by other methods, including burning or self-hitting."

Galley [117] defines self-injurers as: "Bright, sensitive, helpful to others, caretakers of their friends and family, good listeners, above average students, and invisible. They are very creative, artists and neat kids, but ones who do not make their needs well known."

Craigen [118] considers self-harm to be the "new anorexia" affecting young women.

Froeschle and Moyer consider that there are gender differences in terms of self-harm. For men, self-injury is a rite of passage, while for women, the actions are more private and emotionally charged [119], which confirms Bourdieu's model of "masculine domination." It is also necessary to note that, in the case of men who self-harm, we find a double stigma, since they perform an action that is considered "feminine," which jeopardizes their masculine identity, and that, as a practice, it is considered a diverted behavior, which often leads them to remain in anonymity.

13.4.4 Comprehensive Approach of the Motivations for Developing Self-Injurious Behaviors

Klonsky summarizes the main biopsychosocial models proposed by other authors [120]. These functions are not mutually exclusive; thus, it is common for several of them take place at once.

1. **Affect regulation model**
   It is suggested that self-injury might be a strategy to alleviate acute and intense negative affects [121, 122]. From the systemic and cognitive perspective, it is

postulated that early disabling environments hinder the development of appropriate strategies for coping with emotional stress. The individuals that have grown up in these environments and are vulnerable to emotional instability, can find useful means in self-injurious behaviors to regulate and express (to others and oneself, as it brings emotional distress to consciousness itself) intolerable negative affects. Sometimes, people who self-injure state that self-injury is a way of expressing the pain that they cannot put into words. They refer to emotions that combine pain, sadness, anger, and emotional numbing with feelings of guilt, desires for abstraction, self-punishment, loneliness and emptiness. Injuries become the text that gives us access to the emotional universe, the universe of experience through carnal registration. The body is the vehicle for what. The body is the vehicle for what we cannot put into words. As Nietzsche, in *Thus Spoke Zarathustra*, wrote: "Of all that is written, I love only what a person hath written with his blood. Write with blood, and thou wilt find that blood is spirit."

2. **Anti-dissociation model**

   This includes self-harm as a response to states of dissociation, depersonalization, and/or derealization. Gunderson proposes that some temperamentally vulnerable subjects may be precipitated in states of dissociation when they are far from a loved object. This unpleasant state can trigger injurious behavior with the aim of reconnecting with the sense of "ownliness" and body property through the pain, allowing them to feel real and revitalized. This model is more frequently seen in women [101].

   The dissociation model can be linked with the affect regulation model. Some people who self-harm report feelings of dissociation from their environment; a feeling of separateness or a lack of self. The function of self-harm is often to end that dissociation [109]. Other authors suggest that self-harm can also function as a means of becoming dissociated, so as to escape overpowering emotion [123]. What the authors believe with this is that, in an episode of dissociation, the cuts allow a reconnection with the world through the pain (seen and interpreted pain that returns to reality), while in the episode of depersonalization, the blood pouring from the wound would be what allows reconnection with the body.

3. **Anti-suicide model**

   Self-injurious behavior appears to be an adaptive mechanism for resisting the genuine desire to kill oneself. Self-inflicting a skin injury is an alternative way of expressing self-destructive thoughts and feelings, without the direct risk of dying [124]. Early childhood experiences of neglect, abuse or abandonment lead to low self-esteem. Self-harm allows the person to partially self-destruct without the finality of suicide and without dealing with unresolved issues from childhood. Partial self-destruction helps the subject to maintain a "recovery envelope" and carry on living.

4. **Interpersonal influence model**

   Self-injurious behavior would be used to influence behavior, emotions, and decisions of other significant people. Self-harming should be understood to be an alarm, a means of avoiding abandonment or an attempt to be valued. Here, once again referring to Bourdieu's "masculine domination" model, we find that this is one of the models more frequently shown by women than men in the context of the difficulty of "externalization" of distress, of expression of the message. In this attempt, the message is on the boundary between the "self" and the outer, in the body.

5. **Interpersonal boundaries model**
   It is believed that the individual who has not developed an integrated sense of identity, experiences a painful difficulty in individuating and separating from significant objects. Self-injuring the skin as an organ that physically separates the individual from its environment and others, would allow him/her to specifically distinguish his/her physical identity to support his/her autonomy [125, 126]. " [. . .] My body becomes my protest. My body is my protest against the great expectations of my parents, against the big and stupid expectations of the world. My body is my protest. My body is my action. My abnormal decision is my action. In short, my life is my action [. . .]," as referred to by Angélica Liddell in *La desobediencia hágase en mi vientre. Pliego de teatro y danza (*Disobedience is made in my belly. Sheets of theater and dance) [127].
6. **Self-punishment model**
   Marsha Linehan suggests that subjects who grew up in early unfavorable environments learn that punishment and invalidation are acceptable and even necessary to shape behaviors. Self-injury is ego-harmoniously lived, becoming a self-control conduct aimed at encouraging and maintaining collectively desirable behaviors [128].
7. **Sensation-seeking model**
   Includes self-injury as a way of generating excitement or joy in an individual who is in need of intense emotions to feel connected with life. It is suggested that, biologically, they would have a basal hypo-hedonic state, which would boost them to the active pursuit of limits sensations: pleasurables and painfuls. These behaviors are characterized because they are addictively repeated, favoring the production of novelty over the avoidance of self-harming [129–131].
   When studying the neurobiochemical systems and processes affected in traumatic situations [132], it has been proved that a high level of emotional excitement interferes with the normal brain functions of experience processing. It has also been speculated that there are brain mechanisms that act as regulators of both pain and affect (i.e., the endogenous opioid peptides system and the serotonergic systems [133] when it comes to analyzing symptoms of acute pain in patients with BPD). The participation or discharge of endogenous opioids at moments of self-harming (Bessel Van der Kolk's hypothesis; 1989) would determine, on the one hand, a degree of addiction, and would explain why, in individuals with mental retardation or neurological and genetic abnormalities, pharmacological interventions focused on the endogenous opioid system reduce and sometimes eliminate self-injurious behaviors in a significant proportion of individuals [134].

13.4.5 Classification of Clinical Presentations

One of the most useful classifications in clinical practice is proposed by Simeon and Favazza in 1995 (Table 13.4).

13.4.5.1 Self-Mutilation

Self-mutilation constitutes a more advanced degree of the expression of self-injuries. It consists of amputating some part of the body, sometimes with "some symbolic value" (enucleation of the eye, castration, lingual mutilation), in order to self-inflict a punishment as a result of some intense experiences of guilt, or unconsciously wanting to hurt an internalized "object" in anger. It appears in various clinical conditions such as melancholic depression, schizophrenia, mental retardation, in intermittent explosive disorder or post-traumatic stress disorder, usually in the context of added substances use (usually alcohol) or in unstable personalities from the emotional point of view (borderline or antisocial) [3].

Higher rates of sexual abuse, as well as child abuse, have been described in these patients, both men and women, in addition to a greater tendency to show high levels of dissociation during their mutilating actions [138].

There is a rare disease, called apotemnophilia, or body integrity identity disorder (BIID), which is defined as a syndrome in which the sufferer is concerned about the desire to self-amputate a healthy limb. It seems to be related to an alteration in the perception of identity, where limb amputation can temporarily relieve the patient's feeling of pain, adjusting to their own misperception of the identity of the person [139].

Within self-mutilation, genital self-mutilation should be mentioned, which has traditionally been associated with psychotic processes (mainly schizophrenia). However, more recent reviews report that more than 60 % occur in gender identity disorder in men [140, 141]. Despite genital self-mutilations being less common in women [140, 142], when they occur, they have been associated with personality disorders and Münchausen syndrome [143]. There are a few cases in women regarding a background psychosis [144].

13.4.5.2 Reflection

The Western tendency to think in the form of binary oppositions, and therefore conceptualize the world into masculine and feminine, life drive/death drive, good/bad, etc., excluding other possibilities of identity (gender among them), greatly affects the perception of the human essence.

One of the great risks of binarism is projecting, dually and contrastively, the human identity in the form of male/female categories [145], because it seems that disparities between women and men lie in something stable, "immovable," such as sexual differentiation, and not cultural issues, as the gender category highlights. As Martin Casares argues, the fear of change and destabilization of the gender representation system is at the root of discrimination and difficulties in creating neologisms that account for the new realities [27].

Table 13.4 Classification of self-injurious behaviors clinical conditions according to Simeon and Favazza (1995) [101, 135–137]

Self-injurious behaviors	Characteristics	Associated pathological symptoms
Major	Severe tissue damage (castration, enucleation of the eye, amputation of limbs, etc.) Sudden, impulsive, and bloody apparition	75 % psychotic episodes (schizophrenia, ½ in the first psychotic episode) [135] Severe affective disorders Intoxications Encephalitis Severe personality disorders [136, 137] Transsexualism
Stereotyped	Moderate severity of damage Repetitive, rigid, and inflexible pattern of presentation	Autism Severe mental retardation Neurological pathology (Lesch Nyhan, Cornelia de Lange and Prader Willi syndromes)
Compulsive	Mild to moderate damage severity (scratching skin and producing excoriations, nail biting, hair pulling) Repetitive, compulsive pattern, sometimes even experienced as automatic acts	Neurotic symptoms Mental retardation Trichotillomania
Impulsive	Mild-moderate severity (cutting, burning skin, inserting sharp objects in subdermal space, producing even cavities in tissues). Episodic or repetitive Episodic: • Fear for self-harm (ego-dystonia) • Stress prior to self-harm/posterior relief Repetitive: • Certain obsessive–compulsive predisposition • High frequency (could be daily) • No external or internal precipitant • Compulsive–addictive pattern. • Usually starts in pre-adolescence (or before) • Could last throughout life • More common in women	More common in women Personality disorder (limit) PTSD Dissociative disorders Eating disorder Mood disorders Antecedents of sexual abuse in childhood (especially) [101]

Another of the great risks is the conception of life drive/death drive as antagonistic and mutually incompatible entities. We are both, we are life and death, construction and destruction, ambivalence, the self and the others, and our body becomes the contact between the two poles, the interlocutor, the paper on which history and time are written, where change is continuous; what we are now, we will never be again, and neither were before. We cannot, therefore, cling to immovable, static "identities" as, although this was possible, it would produce "symptoms." This awareness of change, this modification over time, counteracts the concept of "natural" as "what is given to us." Awareness of change is also related to the concept of effort, because of that heading to the future. And here is where the essence of the human being is settled, the eternal ambivalence, the status between hope and frustration. We move from one to another, and there is a range of possibilities in-between, or we live with both at once, as they are relative and complementary to each other. Accepting ambivalence is to accept the Other, not only other people but also the "other self," it is to accept the limits of the human condition, and at the same time, its possibilities.

Throughout the text, we have referred to "feminine" and "masculine" conditions that we consider as our own, when what we really did was to incorporate them from the environment (Bourdieu's "habitus"), but nevertheless cause us acute discomfort. Examples of this would involve the "gender paradox of suicidal behavior," where parasuicidal behavior is more common in women as a means of "expression" of certain emotions that otherwise they find impossible to "externalize." However, we see that this is not a constant paradox in all cultures, considering that in China the percentage of women who commit suicide is higher, especially young women. With regard to men, we found the "male depressive syndrome" with more "externalizing" characteristics such as anger, aggressiveness, irritability, and hostility rather than expression of sadness and mourning, as these are considered "unmanly" behaviors.

In relation to the body, we want to allude to the concept "biopower," described by Foucault to refer to the practice by modern countries in the exploitation of numerous and diverse techniques to control both body and society, and this is what we may find today in what we called "standardized" self-harm, such as diets, Botox, esthetic surgery, implants, muscle-building, etc.

We consider it necessary to highlight the multidimensionality/complexity of the self-harm phenomenon with the aim of achieving the cultural and symbolic dimensions found in the meanings of self-harm. It is necessary to understand self-harm in its context, where the body becomes profound through the skin, and through cuts, signs, and inscriptions, transmits a message. The body becomes a "*speaking body*" (following Foucault's idea); thus, we consider it essential to address the self-injuries experience not as a sign of specific diagnosis, but as a way of being-in-the-world and in-between-the-world (body in suffering). A proven fact is that self-harm is more frequent in women. Here, we may consider two aspects:

(a) Based on Bourdieu's model, revealing how the "only" public space granted to women corresponds to the "exposure" of their body. Therefore, we see how women resort to this more frequently as a means of expressing their discomfort, emotion, disagreement, etc., anything that is "banned" in terms of public expression

(b) There is a higher prevalence of self-harm than that registered in men, but they keep it "hidden" because of the discomfort, feelings of shame, etc. since it is considered a more "feminine" action and therefore inferior

In any case, self-harm is the means of expressing an inexpressible emotion (indicating that a clear component of cultural construction is perceived and that it comes from what is and what is not emotionally appropriate to express), and we want to highlight how, in modern times, there are other areas (specifically, pro-self-harm virtual communities), where through forums, videos, blogs, etc., bodily self-harm is exhibited, claiming a space that has been denied, expropriated in real life.

We have addressed different concepts already revealed by the Queer theory [146, 147], like destabilizing the concepts of sex, gender, and sexuality. We join this movement considering how necessary it is that bodies are identified, not as men or women, but as speaker bodies that grant themselves the ability to access all signifying practices, as well as the ability to be enunciated, as subjects, in all the positions that history has determined as masculine, feminine, perverse, etc. This means not only renouncing a closed-minded and naturally determined sexual identity, but also (as Butler [10]and Preciado [147] argue), to renounce the benefits they could obtain from a naturalization of the social, economic, and legal effects of their signifying practices.

References

1. Becker E. Denial of death. New York: Simon & Schuster; 1973. p. 66.
2. Sartre JP cited in Hepburn R (1965) Questions about the meaning of life. Relig Stud 1: 125–140
3. Erroteta JM, Rodrigo I (2013) Pulsión de vida. En Introducción a la Psicopatología, una visión actualizada. Segarra R, Eguíluz I. 3ª ed. España. Ed. Panamericana
4. Yalom ID (2011) Psicoterapia existencial. Herder, p 47
5. Jaspers K cited in Choron J (1963) Death and Western thought. Collier Books, New York, p 226
6. Mitzrahi L (1992) La mujer transgresora. Emecé
7. Bourdieu P (2012) La dominación masculina. 7ª edición. Anagrama, Barcelona
8. Esteban ML. Los estudios de salud y el género: las ventajas de un enfoque antropológico y feminista. Salud Colect Buenos Aires. 2006;2(1):9–20.
9. Sims A (2003) Affective and emotional disorders. En Symptoms in the mind. An introduction to descriptive Psychopathology. Andrew CP Sims. 3ª ed. Elsevier, Oxford
10. Butler J. Undoing gender. New York: Routledge; 2006.
11. Feder (1998) Cuadernos de Psicoanálisis. Asociación Psicoanalítica Mexicana. Plaza Valdés
12. González de Chávez MA. Feminidad y masculinidad. Madrid: Biblioteca Nueva; 1999.
13. Chasseget-Smirgel J (1999) "El poeta y los sueños diurnos: un comentario" y de EMDE, R. N., "La fantasía y más allá de la fantasía" en "En torno a Freud: "El poeta y los sueños diurnos", Fonagy y otros, Biblioteca Nueva, Madrid
14. López Mondéjar L. La quietud de Penélope: sublimación, creación y feminidad. Murcia: Ad Hoc, CENDEAC; 2002. 2009.
15. Frankl V. El hombre en busca de sentido. Barcelona: Herder; 1984.
16. WHO. World health statistics. Geneva: World Health Organization; 1989.
17. WHO. World report on violence and health. Geneva: World Health Organization; 2002.

18. Hawton K, Van Heeringen K. Suicide. Lancet. 2005;373:1372–81.
19. Canetto SS, Sakinofsky I. The gender paradox in suicide. Suicide Life Threat Behav. 1998;28:1–23.
20. Beautrais AL. Gender issues in youth suicidal behaviour. Emerg Med (Fremantle). 2002;14:35–42.
21. Henderson JP, Mellin C, Patel F. Suicide-a statistical analysis by age, sex and method. J Clin Forensic Med. 2005;12:305–9.
22. Yip PSF. Suicide in Asia. Causes and prevention. Hong Kong: Hong Kong University press; 2008.
23. Philips MR, Li X, Zhang Y. Suicide rates in China 1995-99. Lancet. 2002;359:835–40.
24. Van Rijsselberghe I, Prtzky G, Van Heeringen C. Zelfbeschadigend gedrag bij adolescenten in Vlanderen. Tijdschr Psychiatr 51:629-640.
25. Möller-Leimkühler AM. The gender gap in suicide and premature death or: why are men so vulnerable? Eur Arch Psychiatry Clin Neurosci. 2003;253:1–8.
26. Schrijvers DL, Bollen J, Sabbe BGC. The gender paradox in suicidal behavior and its impacto n the suicidal process. J Affect Disord. 2012;138:19–26.
27. Martín Casares A (2012) Antropología del género: culturas, mitos y estereotipos sexuales. 3ªedic. Ediciones Cátedra, Madrid, p 51
28. Philips MR, Cheng HG. The changing global face of suicide. Lancet. 2012;379(9834): 2318–9.
29. Soman CR, Safraj S, Kutty V, Vijayakumar K, Ajayan K. Suicide in South India: a community-based study in Kerala. Indian J Psychiatry. 2009;51(4):261–4.
30. Sudhir Kumar CT, Mohan R, Ranjith G, Chandrasekaran R. Gender differences in medically serious suicide attempts: a study from South India. Psychiatry Res. 2006;189:465–6.
31. Yip PSF, Liu KY. The ecological fallacy and the gender ratio of suicide in China. Br J Psychiatry. 2006;189:465–6.
32. Van Heeringen K. The suicidal process and related concepts. In: Van Heeringer K, editor. Understanding Suicidal behaviour. The suicidal process approach to research, treatment and prevention. Chichester: Wiley; 2001. p. 3–15.
33. Runeson BS, Beskow J, Waern M. The suicidal process in suicides among young people. Acta Psychiatr Scand. 1996;93:35–42.
34. Arensman E, Kerkhof JF. Classification of attempted suicide: a review of empirical studies, 1963–1993. Suicide Life Threat Behav. 1996;26:46–67.
35. Neeleman J, de Graaf R, Vollebergh W. The suicidal process; prospective comparison between early and later stages. J Affect Disord. 2004;82:43–52.
36. Cupina D. Life events, gender and suicidal behaviours in the acute community setting. Australas Psychiatry. 2009;17:233–6.
37. Murphy GE. Why women are less likely than men to commit suicide. Psychiatry. 1998;39: 165–75.
38. Möller-Leimkühler AM. The gender gap in suicide and premature death or: why are men so vulnerable? Eur Arch Psychiatry Clin Neurosci. 2003;253:1–8.
39. Eaton DK, Kann L, Kinchen S. Youth risk behavior surveillance- United States, 2007. Morb Mortal Wkly Rep Surveill Summ. 2008;57(4):1–131.
40. Blair-West GW, Cantor CH, Eyeson-Annan ML. Lifetime suicide risk in major depression: sex and age determinants. J Affect Disord. 1999;55:171–8.
41. Kölves K, Ide N, De Leo D. Suicidal ideation and behaviour in the aftermath of marital separation: gender differences. J Affect Disord. 2010;120:48–53.
42. Qin P, Agerbo E, Westergard-Nielsen N, Eriksson T, Mortensen PB. Gender differences in risk factors for suicide in Denmark. Br J Psychiatry. 2000;177:546–50.
43. Hawton K. Sex and suicide. Gender differences in suicidal behaviour. Br J Psychiatry. 2000;177:484–5.

44. Bebbington PE, Cooper C, Minot S, Brugha TS, Jenkins R, Meltzer H, Dennis M. Suicide attempts, gender and sexual abuse: data from the 2000 British Psychiatric Morbidity Survey. Am J Psychiatry. 2009;166:1135–40.
45. Molnar BE, Berkman LF, Buka SL. Psychopathology, childhood sexual abuse and other childhood adversities: relative links to subsequent suicidal behaviour in the US. Psychol Med. 2001;31:965–77.
46. Martin G, Bergen HA, Richardson AS, Roeger L, Allison S. Sexual abuse and suicidality: gender differences in a large community simple of adolescents. Chil Abuse Negl. 2004;28: 491–503.
47. Olshen E, McVeigh KH, Wunsch-Hitzig RA, Ricket VI. Dating violence, sexual assault and suicide attempts among urban teenagers. Arch Pediatr Adolesc Med. 2007;161:539–45.
48. Arsenault-Lapierre G, Kim C, Turecki G. Psychiatric diagnoses in 3275 suicides: a meta-analysis. BMC Psychiatry. 2004;4:4–37.
49. Kessler RC, McGonable KA, Swartz M. Sex and depression in the National Comorbidity Survey; lifetime prevalence, chronicity and recurrence. J Affect Disord. 1993;29:85–96.
50. American Psychiatric Association. Diagnostic and statistical manual of mental disorders. 4th ed. Washington, DC: APA; 2000.
51. Skodol AE, Bender DS. Why are women diagnosed borderline more that men? Psychiatr Q. 2003;74:349–60.
52. Paris J. Gender differences in personality traits and disorders. Curr Psychiatry Rep. 2004;6: 71–4.
53. Oquendo MA, Bongiovi-García ME, Galfalvy H, Goldberg PH, Grunebaum MF, Burke AK, Mann JJ. Sex differences in clinical predictors of suicidal acts after major depression: a prospective study. Am J Psychiatry. 2007;164:134–41.
54. Brezo J, Paris J, Turecki G. Personality traits as correlates of suicidal ideation, suicide attempts, and suicide completions: a systematic review. Acta Psychiatr Scand. 2006;113: 180–206.
55. Strüber D, Lück M, Roth G. Sex, aggression and impulse control: an integrative account. Neurocase. 2008;14:93–121.
56. DeHert M, McKenzie K, Peuskens J. Risk factors for suicide in Young people suffering from schizophrenia: a long-term follow-up study. Schizophr Res. 2001;47:127–34.
57. Bjerkeset O, Romundstad P, Gunnell D. Gender differences in the association of mixed anxiety and depression with suicide. Br J Psychiatry. 2008;192:474–5.
58. Bradvik L, Mattisson C, Brogen M, Nettelbladt P. Long-term suicide risk of depression in the Lundby cohort 1947-1997-severity and gender. Acta Psychiatr Scand. 2008;117:185–91.
59. Liu KY, Chen EY, Cheung AS, Yip PS. Psychiatric history modifies the gender ratio of suicide: an East and West comparison. Soc Psychiatry Psychiatr Epidemiol. 2009;44:130–4.
60. Chang CM, Liao SC, Chiang HC, Chen YY, Tseng KC, Chau YL, Chang HJ, Lee MB. Gender differences in healthcare service utilisation 1 year before suicide: national record linkage study. Br J Psychiatry. 2009;195:459–60.
61. Bjerkeset O, Romundstad P, Gunnell D. Gender differences in the association of mixed anxiety and depression with suicide. Br J Psychiatry. 2008;192:474–5.
62. Rutz W, von Knorring L, Pihlgren H, Rihmer Z, Walinder J. Prevention of male suicides: lessons from Gotland study. Lancet. 1995;345:524.
63. Cochran SV, Rabinowitz FE. Men and depression. Clinical and empirical perspectives. San Diego: Academic; 2002.
64. Kanchan T, Menezes RG. Suicidal hanging in Manipal, South India victim profile and gender differences. Forensic Leg Med. 2008;15:493–6.
65. Kanchan T, Menezes RG. Suicidal poisoning in Southern India: gender differences. Forensic Leg Med. 2008;15:7–14.
66. Kanchan T, Menon A, Menezes RG. Methods of choice in completed suicides: gender differences and review of literature. J Forensic Sci. 2009;54:938–42.

67. Cooper PN, Milroy CM. The coroner's system and underreporting of suicide. Med Sci Law. 1995;35:319–26.
68. Baca García E, Ceverino Domínguez A, Pérez Rodríguez MM, Saiz Ruiz J (2007) Aspectos diferenciales en la conducta suicida. En Salud Mental y género en la práctica clínica. Ferrando Bundío Ed. Barcelona. Ars Médica
69. Reportaje: Una viuda en la pira. Periódico El País. 8 de agosto, 2002. Sociedad
70. Mann JJ, Waternaux C, Haas GL, Malone K. Toward a clinical model of suicidal behavior in psychiatric patients. Am J Psychiatry. 1999;156(2):181–9.
71. Orbach I. Styles of problem-solving suicidal individuals. Suicide Life Threat Behav. 1990; 20:56–64.
72. Schotte D, Clum G. Suicide ideation in a college population: a test of model. J Consult Clin Psychol. 1982;50:690–6.
73. Kosofsky Sedwick E (2002). A(queer) y ahora. En Mérida Jiménez R (ed) Sexualidades transgresoras. Una antología de estudios queer. Barcelona, Icaria, pp 29–54
74. Yalom ID (1984) Psicoterapia existencial. Herder, Barcelona, p 451
75. Rojas Montes (1996). En Compendio de Psicopatología. López Sánchez JM, Higueras Aranda Ed. .4ª ed. Granada, España. Círculo de estudios psicopatológicos
76. Nock MK, Favazza AR. Nonsuicidal self-injury: Definition and classification. In: Nock MK, editor. Understanding nonsuicidal self-injury. Origins, assessment and treatment. Washington, DC: American Psychological Association; 2006. p. 9–18.
77. Pane G (2006) En El arte en acción, Aznar Almazán, S. 2ºEd. San Sebastián. Ed. Nerea, pp 67–68
78. Bataille G. L'erotisme. France: Unione Generale d'éditions; 1974.
79. Aguilar T. Cuerpos sin límites. Madrid: Casimiro Ed; 2013.
80. Skegg K. Self-harm. Lancet. 2005;366:1471–83.
81. Casadó Marín L (2013) Antropología de las autolesiones corporals: cuerpo, identidad, género y emociones. Alemania. Editorial Académica Española. OmniScriptum Gmbh & Co. KG
82. Rodham K, Hawton K. Epidemiology and phenomenology of nonsuicidal self-injury. In: Nock MK, editor. Understanding nonsuicidal self-injury. Origins, assessment and treatment. Washington, DC: American Psychological Association; 2009. p. 9–18.
83. Guertin T, Lloyd-Richardson E, Spirito A, Donaldson D, Boergers J. Self-mutilative behavior in adolescents who attempt suicide by overdose. J Am Acad Child Adolesc Psychiatry. 2001;40:1062–9.
84. Muehlenkamp JJ, Gutiérrez PM. An investigation of differences between self-injurious behavior and suicide attempts in a sample of adolescents. Suicide Life Threat Behav. 2004; 34:12–23.
85. Patton GC, Harris R, Carlin JB, et al. Adolescent suicidal behaviours: a population-based study of risk. Psychol Med. 1997;27:715–24.
86. Brown MZ, Comtois KA, Linehan MM. Reasons for suicide attempts and nonsuicidal self-injury in women with borderline personality disorder. J Abnorm Psychol. 2002;111:198–202.
87. Harriss L, Hawton K. Suicidal intent in deliberate self-harm and the risk of suicide: the predictive power of the Suicide Intent Scale. J Affect Disord. 2005;86:225–33.
88. Muchlenkamp JJ, Claes L, Havertape L, Plener PL. International prevalence of non-suicidal self-injury and deliberate self-harm. Child Adolesc Psychiatry Ment Health. 2012;6:10.
89. Briere J, Gil E. Self-mutilation in clinical and general population samples: prevalence, correlates, and functions. Am J Orthopsychiatry. 1998;68:609–20.
90. DiClemente RJ, Ponton LE, Hartley D. Prevalence and correlates of cutting behavior: risk for HIV transmission. J Am Acad Child Adolesc Psychiatry. 1991;30:735–9.
91. Laye-Gindhu A, Schonert-Reichl KA. Nonsuicidal self-harm among community adolescents: understanding the "whats" and "whys" of self-harm. J Youth Adolesc. 2005;34:447–57.
92. Lundh LG, Wangby-Lundh M, Bjärehed J. Deliberate self-harm and psychological problems in young adolescents: evidence of a bidirectional relationship in girls. Scand J Psychol. 2011;52:476–83.

93. Schmidtke A, Bille-Brahe U, DeLeo D, et al. Attempted suicide in Europe: rates, trends and sociodemographic characteristics of suicide attempters during the period 1989–1992. Results of the WHO/EURO Multicentre study on parasuicide. Acta Psychiatr Scand. 1996;93: 327–38.
94. Hepple J, Quinton C. One hundred cases of attempted suicide in the elderly. Br J Psychiatry. 1997;171:42–6.
95. Harriss L, Hawton K, Zahl D. Value of measuring suicidal intent in the assessment of people attending hospital following self-poisoning or self-injury. Br J Psychiatry. 2005;186:60–6.
96. Hawton K, Harriss I, Simkin S. Self-cutting: patient characteristics compared with self-poisoners. Suicide Life Threat Behav. 2004;34:199.
97. Lilley R, Owens D, Horrocks J. Hospital care and repetition following self-harm: multicenter comparison of self-poisoning and self-injury. Br J Psychiatry. 2008;192:440–5.
98. Horrocks J. Attendances in the accident and emergency department following self-harm: a descriptive study. Leeds: Academic Unit of Psychiatry and Behavioural Sciences, University of Leeds; 2002.
99. Hawton K. Self-harm in England: a tale of three cities. Soc Psychiatry Psychiatr Epidemiol. 2007;42:513–21.
100. Arensman E, Larkin C, Corcoran P, Reulbach P, Perry IJ (2013) Factors associated with self-cutting as a method of self-harm: findings from the Irish National Registry of Deliberate Self-Harm. Eur J Public Health:1–6
101. Favazza AR, Conterio K. Female habitual self-mutilators. Acta Psychiatr Scand. 1989;79: 283–9.
102. Zlotnick C, Shea MT, Pearlstein T, Simpson E, Costello E, Begin A. The relationship between dissociative symptoms, alexithymia, impulsivity, sexual abuse and self mutilation. Compr Psychiatry. 1966;37(1):12–6.
103. Hinshaw SP, Owens EB, Zalecki C, Huggins SP, Montenegro-Nevado AJ, Schrodek E, Swanson EN. Prospective follow-up of girls with attention-deficit/hyperactivity disorder into early adulthood: continuing impairment includes elevated risk for suicide attempts and self-injury. J Consult Clin Psychol. 2012;80(6):1041–51.
104. Mendoza Y, Pellicer F. Percepción del dolor en el síndrome de comportamiento autolesivo. Salud Ment. 2002;25(4):10–6.
105. Austin L, Kortum J. Self-injury: the secret language of pain for teenagers. Educ Comm Tech J. 2004;124:517–27.
106. Sadeh N, Javdani S, Finy MS, Verona E. Gender differences in emotional risk for self- and other-directed violence among externalizing adults. J Consult Clin Psychol. 2011;79:106–17.
107. Jordan BK, Schlenger WE, Fairbank JA, Caddell JM. Prevalence of psychiatric disorders among incarcerated women: II. Convicted felons entering prison. Arch Gen Psychiatry. 1996;53:513–9.
108. JI W, Burnette ML, South SC, Chauhan P, Bale R, Friend R, Van Patten I. Psychopathy in women: structural modeling and comorbidity. Int J Law Psychiatry. 2003;26:223–42.
109. Horrocks J, House A. Self-harm and suicide in women. In: Kohen D, editor. Oxford textbook of women and mental health. Oxford: Oxford University Press; 2010.
110. Skegg K, Nada-Raja S, Dickinson N, Paul C, Williams S. Sexual orientation and self-harm in men and women. Am J Psychiatry. 2003;160:541–46.
111. Jorm AF, Korten AE, Rodgers B, Jacomb PA, Christensen H. Sexual orientation and mental health: results from a community survey of young and middle-aged adults. Br J Psychiatry. 2002;180:423–27.
112. Wichstrom I, Hegna K. Sexual orientation and suicide attempt: a longitudinal study of the general Norwegian adolescent population. J Abnorm Psychol. 2003;112:144–51.
113. American Psychiatric Association. Diagnostic and statistical manual of mental disorders. 4th ed. Washington, DC: American Psychiatric Association; 1994.

114. Caryn L. The construction of female sexual trauma. In: Micale M, Lerner P, editors. Traumatic pasts history, psychiatry and trauma in the modern age (1870–1930). Cambridge: Cambridge University Press; 2001.
115. Miller D. Women who hurt themselves. New York: Basic Books; 1994.
116. Favazza A. What we know about affective disorders? Am J Psychiatry. 1988;143(10):1328.
117. Galley M. Student self-harm: silent school crisis. Educ Week. 2003;23:14–6.
118. Craigen LM, Foster V. It was like a partnership of the two of us against cutting: investigating the counseling experience of young adult women who self-injure. J Ment Health Couns. 2009;31:76–94.
119. Froeschle J, Moyer M. Just cut it out: legal and ethical challenges in counseling students who self-mutilate. Prof Sch Couns. 2004;7:231–5.
120. Klonsky ED. The functions of deliberate self-injury: a review of the evidence. Clin Psychol Rev. 2007;27:226–39.
121. Favazza AR, Rosenthal RJ. Diagnostic issues in self-mutilation. Hosp Community Psychiatry. 1993;44:134–40.
122. Gratz KL. Risk factors for deliberate self-harm among female college students: the role and interaction of childhood maltreatment, emotional inexpressivity, and affect intensity/reactivity. Am J Orthopsychiatry. 2006;76:238–50.
123. Suyemoto KL. The functions of self mutilation. Clin Psychol Rev. 1988;18:531–54.
124. Haines J, Williams CL, Brain KL, Wilson GV. The psychophysiology of self-mutilation. J Abnorm Psychol. 1995;104:471–89.
125. Chowanec GD, Josephson AM, Coleman C, Davis H. Self-harming behavior in incarcerated male delinquent adolescents. J Am Acad Child Adolesc Psychiatry. 1991;30:202–7.
126. Carroll J, Schaffer C, Spensley J, Abramowitz SI. Family experiences of self-mutilating patients. Am J Psychiatry. 1980;137:852–3.
127. Liddell A (2008) In: Disobedience is made in my belly. Sheets of theater and dance. Aflera Producciones SL, Madrid
128. Friedman M, Glasser M, Laufer E, Laufer M, Wohl M. Attempted suicide and self-mutilation in adolescence: some observations from a psychoanalytic research project. Int J Psychoanal. 1972;53:179–83.
129. Klonsky ED, Oltmanns TF, Turkheimer E. Deliberate self-harm in a nonclinical population: prevalence and psychological correlates. Am J Psychiatry. 2003;160:1501–8.
130. Nixon MK, Cloutier PF, Aggarwal S. Affect regulation and addictive aspects of repetitive self-injury in hospitalized adolescents. J Am Acad Child Adolesc Psychiatry. 2002;41: 1333–41.
131. Osuch EA, Noll JG, Putnam FW. The motivations for self-injury in psychiatric inpatients. Psychiatry. 1999;62:334–46.
132. Yehuda R. Biological factors associated with susceptibility to posttraumatic stress disorder. Can J Psychiatr. 1999;44:34–9.
133. Symons 2002; Russ et al. 1992. Simons DG, Hong C-Z, Simons, LS, PT. Endplate potentials are common to midfiber myofacial trigger points. Am J Phys Med Rehabil 81(3):212–222
134. Sandman CA, Touchette P. Opioid and the maintenance of self-injurious behavior. In: Schoeder SR, Oster-Granite ML, Thompson T, editors. Self-injurious behavior: gene-brain-behavior relationships. Washington, DC: American Psychological Association; 2002. p. 191–204.
135. Large M, Babidge N, Andrews D, Storey P, Nielssen O. Major self-mutilation in the first episode of psychosis. Schizophr Bull. 2009;35:1012–21.
136. Cleveland SE. Three cases of self-castration. J Nerv Ment Dis. 1956;123:386–91.
137. Kushner AW. Two cases of auto-castration due to religious delusions. Br J Med Psychol. 1967;40:293–8.
138. Zlotnick C, Mattia JI, Zimmerman M. Clinical correlates of self-mutilation in a simple of general psychiatric patients. J Nerv Ment Dis. 1999;187(5):296–301.

139. Bou Khalil R, Richa S. Apotemnophilia or body integrity identity disorder: a case report review. Int J Low Extrem Wounds. 2012;11(4):313–9.
140. Eke N. Genital self mutilation: there is no method in this madness. BJU Int. 2000;85(3): 295–8.
141. Catalano G, Catalano MC, Carroll K. Repetitive male genital self-mutilation: a case report and discussion of possible risk factors. J Sex Marital Ther. 2002;28(1):27–37.
142. Millán-González R (2010) Genital mutilation in a transsexual patient: is it an indication of an imprecisely defined pathological spectrum? Revista Colombiana de Psiquiatría 39(3)
143. Ajibona O, Hartwell R. Feigned miscarriage by genital self-mutilation in a hysterectomised patient. J Obstet Gynaecol. 2002;22(4):451.
144. McGuire BE, Ahmed SN. Genital self-mutilation: a literature review and case report. Sex Marital Ther. 1998;13(2):201–5.
145. Reiter R. Toward and anthropology of women. Nueva York: Monthly Review Press; 1975.
146. Kosofsky Sedgwick E (1993) Identidades, minorías, comunidades. Construir significados queer. Non grata. Madrid (3)
147. Preciado B (2002). Manifiesto contrasexual. Prácticas subversivas de identidad sexual. Madrid. Pensamiento-Opera prima

Use, Misuse, and Gender Differences 14

Carmen Meneses and Iñaki Markez

Abstract

The use of drugs in Western societies has been associated with male gender roles and behaviors and is poorly regarded in female behavior. For men, drug use has most often been regarded as a risk behavior, a deviation, or an illness when serious consequences for health arise. On the other hand, for women, drug use has been viewed as a vice, a disease, a response to female problems or disorders, and, above all, as a transgression of women's traditional roles.

The vulnerability of women is exacerbated by their invisibility: few resources are allocated to cover the needs of female drug users; there is a shortage of staff trained on gender matters; treatments begin at a late stage; a growing number of women are imprisoned in men's prisons; few if any women hold responsible positions in drug user associations, etc. Thus, the invisibility that exacerbates their vulnerability results in complete exclusion in some cases. At the same time, the invisibility of female drug users is not only obvious when they are the object of policies but also when they are the subject.

We can foresee that as a gender approach is incorporated into the policy guidelines designed and issued by the various organizations dedicated to drafting drug policies in the European Union, and as these guidelines are effectively applied by the member States, we will be able to obtain clearer information about the problematic uses and the contexts in which drugs are used and about the treatment programs and accessibility by all the people who need such programs, which also cover women's needs, with their strategies and resources.

C. Meneses (✉)
Comillas Pontifical University, Madrid, Spain
e-mail: cmeneses@upcomillas.es

I. Markez
Advanced Medical Psychiatrist (AMSA), Bilbao, Spain

Basque Institute of Psychotherapy, Bilbao, Spain
e-mail: imarkezalonso@gmail.com

M. Sáenz-Herrero (ed.), *Psychopathology in Women*,
DOI 10.1007/978-3-319-05870-2_14

14.1 Introduction

Throughout the twentieth century, drug use has varied according to the social, political, and legal context particular to each moment in Western society. The use of tobacco, alcohol, and other drugs has been socially accepted to varying degrees depending on the gender roles specific to the historical moment. In the first half of the twentieth century, practically all nontherapeutic consumption of psychotropic substances was tolerated and accepted among men but not among women. Female participation in drug use increased gradually from the 1960s onward, as the use of legal and illegal drugs started to spread in the population and as women's social participation increased.

The spread of drug use would be conditioned by the social roles and stereotypes attributed to each sex. Thus, women participated in drug use as drugs became more socially accepted and tolerated, keeping away from those drugs that are criminalized or stigmatized for women. Therefore, we can talk of two types of drug use patterns [1]. On the one hand, legal drug use: tobacco, alcohol, and psychotropic drugs. There is a greater female presence in the use of these substances, as we subsequently show. Meanwhile, men were most highly represented in the use of illegal drugs, with women remaining a minority in these cases. In the first decade of the new century, there seemed to be a certain convergence of drug use among the youngest population groups; furthermore, in some cases, as we show later on, young girls are the biggest users, especially of the most socially accepted drugs.

What lies behind these differences between boys and girls, men and women, in drug use and abuse? To answer this question, we must return to the gender approach, in other words, we must consider the cultural lines that are drawn between male and female gender roles, relationships, and representations [2].

The use of drugs in Western societies has been associated with masculine roles and behaviors and is poorly regarded in feminine behavior. For men, drug use has most often been regarded as risky behavior, a deviation, or an illness when serious consequences for health arise. On the other hand, for women, drug use has been viewed as a vice, a disease, a response to female problems or disorders, and, above all, as a transgression of women's traditional roles [3].

Women have remained invisible because of the small extent to which they initially participated in drug use, with the consequence that they received insufficient attention in studies of drugs and in the various proposals for intervention and prevention [4]. As the female presence in drug use has grown, drugs have become increasingly criminalized and stigmatized for women, associated with prostitution and with the neglect of their responsibilities as mothers. The supremacy of men and the invisibility of women has led to differences in their behaviors and women's subordination to men, overlooking the different power relations between the sexes.

The type of drug use helps us to classify the pattern of use and the problems associated with drug use. Therefore, the experimental use and intensive use of a drug should not be evaluated in the same way, although, depending on the substances used and the circumstances, either of them may present great risks to user health. Using drugs is not synonymous with drug dependency or drug-related problems. Thus, the evaluation of dependency or problematic use may vary depending on the outlook of the users, of the professionals, of the social representations and their cultural contexts. Therefore, and according to Camí, the distinction between drug use and abuse is a value judgment that refers to the ingestion of psychotropic drugs using parameters determined by a culture's social and medical use of drugs [5].

14.2 Addiction Pattern and Gender Differences

In the explanation we make about patterns of drug use among women, we will present, on the one hand, comparative data for both sexes, which will allow us to show the differences, and, on the other hand, we will differentiate between the data obtained on drug use[1] and that covering drug problems or dependency.[2]

14.2.1 Alcohol and Tobacco Use

Since 1975, the number of liters of pure alcohol consumed per capita has dropped from 14.2 in that year to 9.5 in 1995. In other words, in general terms the Spanish population consumes fewer liters of alcohol per capita each year. Also, men are generally the biggest consumers of alcohol, and suffer most frequently from alcohol poisoning and other problems related to this substance. On the other hand, a pattern of use started to appear in the 1990s that was different to that of the previous decade and is more closely related to its use in Central Europe. We are referring to a more intensive use, centered around leisure and the weekend, outside of the family setting and starting at an earlier age. The female presence in this type of consumption has been increasing, especially among adolescents.

Traditionally, the public use of alcohol centered on males, whilst any type of consumption by women took place mainly in a private or domestic setting. Nevertheless, the greater possibilities of social participation for many social groups, including women, and the social acceptance of alcohol, for which a strong tradition exists in our country, has eliminated or reduced the stereotypes and prejudices that

[1] In the surveys, drug use is associated with a temporal frequency: use in the last month, use in the last year and use at some point in one's life or so-called lifetime prevalence. In this work we will look at annual frequency as these data are available to us in various works.

[2] Various sources and approximative data are available for estimating the problems associated with drugs and drug dependency. In this case, we will use an indirect indicator, the request for treatment from SEIT, the Government System of Information on Drug Addicts of Spain's National Drug Strategy (PNsD). We understand that a drug user who requests treatment does so because s/he has a problem with the use of one or more psychotropic substances. We are aware of the limitations of this indicator, as not all the people who use drugs and have problems with drugs, or feel dependent upon them, seek treatment.

Table 14.1 Alcohol consumption (last 12 months, General Directorate of the National Drug Strategy, DGPNsD)

AGES (15–64 years)	Males (%)	Females (%)
1997	86.4	70.5
1999	83.2	67.2
2001	85.2	70.9
2003	84.5	68.4
2005	84.0	69.2
2007	80.4	66.4
2009	84.4	72.7
Binge drinking 2009	21.0	8.6
Government Survey on the Use of Drugs in Secondary Education (ESTUDES; 14–18 years)		
1994	82.4	82.4
1996	81.4	82.0
1998	80.7	83.1
2000	74.8	75.8
2002	74.3	75.3
2004	79.0	80.5
2006	78.4	80.7
2008	80.8	81.7
2010	74.9	75.2
Binge drinkers 2010	52.2	53.5

women suffered for this type of consumption. In Table 14.1, we have collated the percentages of alcohol use for men and women in the last 12 months from the two main surveys, as this is the most stable measurement. The Survey of the General Directorate of the National Drug Strategy (DGPNsD) and the Government Survey on the Use of Drugs in Secondary Education (ESTUDES) found that the annual prevalence of alcohol use is higher among men than women, except in schools, where it is slightly higher among girls than boys.

The percentages for are also higher than those for women with regard to excessive alcohol consumption. The consumption of five or more alcoholic drinks at a single event (binge drinking) is higher among men, whose pattern of alcohol consumption is of a higher intensity and frequency than that of women. In this sense, the Spanish data are no different to the European context [6]. Among school-goers, there are slightly more binge-drinkers among girls, reversing the relationship that occurs in the general population. It has been observed that, as age increases, alcohol consumption decreases, becoming more moderate [7].

As for tobacco use, as Table 14.2 reveals, it is the adult men who smoke most in general terms, whilst in other age groups we can find equality between the sexes. On the other hand, school-girls smoke more than school-boys, with significant differences between the two. It is possible that the smoking of tobacco has been influenced by transition from junior school to secondary school, as the age for this

Table 14.2 Tobacco use (last 12 months, DGPNsD)

AGES (15–64 years)	Males (%)	Females (%)
1997	55.0	38.7
1999	50.3	39.2
2001	51.5	40.5
2003	53.0	42.6
2005	47.2	37.5
2007	46.0	37.6
2009	48.4	37.0
Daily 2009	36.2	27.2
ESTUDES (14–18 years)		
2008	36.0	40.1
2010	28.1	36.4
Daily 2010	11.0	13.6

has lowered, with its consequent effects on the rites of passage and cultural meanings associated with tobacco use [8].

That female school-goers drink and smoke more than their male counterparts may be related to various factors. First, female adolescents today share the same spaces and participate in the same leisure rites as their male counterparts. In previous decades, the leisure environments and times were different for both sexes and the acceptance of women's incorporation in all social settings and scenes has been gradually increasing. Second, there are few studies that approach the relationship between female tobacco and alcohol use and advertising in detail, although there is no doubt that it has a strong impact on adolescents. For example, women and adolescent girls are major users of the light cigarettes and the tobacco companies are aware of this fact, incorporating the female image into their advertising campaigns. In the same way, alcohol advertising is associated with images of its social and public use, in which women are highly represented. In other words, the slogan of one alcoholic drink that says "it's a man's thing" is no longer an advertising device, as it would exclude female adolescents and young girls, who are important customers for the alcohol industry. Third, legal or illegal drugs can be a substitute for or an inhibitor of food consumption, as are alcohol, tobacco, and psychotropic substances, leading to lower food consumption and therefore becoming a means of weight control [9,10]. The image of the female body is an important advertising device, and establishes standards of identification. Fourth, it is likely that female adolescents and girls find themselves in a dilemma regarding a conflict of roles: the traditional female role models are not relevant to the new generations in which gender roles are being redefined. Finally, drugs, as we will subsequently discuss, are a source of pleasure, fun, and a search for new sensations, which are motivations not previously associated with women [11].

14.2.2 Psychotropic Drug Use

When we talk of psychotropic drugs, we are referring to a series of pharmaceutical products that are used for a wide range of mental health disorders or illnesses, ranging from stress to personality disorders. In our explanation of this pattern of use we will focus on those drugs that are used to treat anxiety, stress or other psychological illnesses, such as tranquillizers and sedative–hypnotics.

We find two types of psychotropic drug use in the general population: first, that prescribed by GPs or mental healthcare doctors as a treatment for some psychological disorders or illnesses; and second, personal use without medical prescription for similar reasons or circumstances. In both cases, women predominate.

In a study about the use of psychotropic substances among women [12, 13] it became evident that women are prescribed with psychotropic drugs twice as frequently as men when they attend GPs or mental health care services. Alongside gender, age is another key variable. The prescription of psychotropic drugs to women is related to a series of characteristics:

- More women than men attend health consultations in which they discuss their illnesses. In other words, they are frequent attenders, meaning that they are more likely to be medicated.
- Psychiatric morbidity associated with women oscillates between 20 % and 34 % compared with men, for whom the percentages vary between 8 % and 22 %.
- A higher number of women are diagnosed with anxiety and depressive disorders, while personality and substance abuse disorders prevail among men. In other words, more anxiety, depression, and insomnia problems are diagnosed in women than in men.
- Around 50 % of patients who visit GPs have a psychosocial-related query, and this is higher among women than men.
- There is a tendency to treat as illnesses and medicate those disorders that are associated with the various life stages of women (premenstrual syndrome, postnatal depression, menopause, etc.). In other words, the tendency is to classify a female's subjectivity as pathological when its origin lies in the specific biological characteristics of the woman's body.
- Many psychological illnesses that are treated with psychotropic drugs are related to the development of the women's gender roles, these being the origin or cause of their illnesses, and which lead to the medication or prescription of psychotropic drugs.

As Goudsmit [14] suggested from a female-centered perspective, there is a supposition among medical professionals that women exaggerate their complaints and express their illnesses externally, thus generating stereotypes of women as hypochondriacs. Any errors or gender biases in the diagnosis lead to two outcomes: on the one hand, no other factors that may be causing the woman's illness are reviewed or investigated, with important repercussions for women's health. On the other hand, as we have already said, the medication of women's psychosocial illnesses, not considering alternative treatments when the source is the living conditions or social situations.

The medication or self-medication processes for psychotropic substances are not recent; we can trace their origins back to the 1950s and 1960s when the Spanish people had extensive healthcare coverage and the healthcare processes were more clearly defined in the medical community. Together with this situation, the growth and advance of the drug industry made numerous products available on the market to mitigate the illnesses and disorders of the Spanish people.

Thus, surveys carried out in the 1980s were already revealing a higher prevalence in the use of psychotropic drugs by women [15]. We may say that these concern the psychotropic substances most frequently used in the last 40 years, mainly by women and about which there are very few single-subject studies. It may be that the secondary role given to women's illnesses, how they are deemed to be of little severity and women's disorders being deemed psychological issues, has led us to ignore one of the biggest uses of psychotropic drugs in Spain.

We have extracted data about the use of tranquillizers and hypnotics without medical prescription from the two PNsD surveys, which we show in Table 14.3:

The differences found in the PNsD's home-based surveys are similar between sexes, but for school-goers, again, the percentages are higher among girls.

The survey on drug use among the female population carried out in 2000 by EDIS for the Women's Institute of Spain (Instituto de la Mujer de España), indicated that users of tranquillizers were 35 years of age and over, with a low level of education, usually married or widows, and were pensioners, housewives, unemployed, and professionals of all social classes. For hypnotics, some older ages were recorded, of 50 years and over; these were separated women and widows, also with a low level of education, professionals, housewives, and pensioners. These characteristics tally with those recorded in other studies [12].

14.2.2.1 Reasons for and Circumstances of Use

The reasons for taking psychotropic drugs are essentially related, as we have previously mentioned, to psychosocial disorders experienced by women and that may be different depending on the moment or stage of their life they are at. Thus, stress faced with entering the job market and professional development, together with a lack of female role models to replace the traditional ones may be a triggering factor among younger women; an overload of work outside and inside the home, playing the role of carer and mother, plus other social demands that hinge on them may be the cause of disorders among middle-aged women; finally, their traditional role as housewives and the loneliness they faced when their children leave home may lie behind the illnesses and disorders of older women [12]. Ultimately, the conflict of gender roles, the absence of new female role models, and the lack of public acknowledgement of the traditional roles played contribute toward the dissatisfaction, illnesses, and conflicts that women experience and that they mitigate with psychotropic drugs, whether self-medicated or by prescription.

Thus, the work of the EDIS, the Sociological Research Team, clearly indicated how women acquire psychotropic substances from medical professionals or family

Table 14.3 Use of psychotropic drugs without prescription (last 12 months, DGPNsD)

AGES (15–64 years)	Males (%)	Females (%)
2005	1.1	1.3
2007	1.2	1.4
2009	1.9	1.9
ESTUDES (14–18 years)		
2008	7.7	11.0
2010	8.4	12.3

members. The guidelines for self-care at home and the current self-medication processes lead to the transmission of knowledge about pharmaceutical products for treating various ailments among members of the family group, for example, a female transmission from mother to daughter. Therefore, the doctor was specified as the source for obtaining tranquillizers and hypnotics by the female group that the EDIS studied (96 %), but the PNsD surveys revealed how it is not difficult for women and school-goers to receive or access these pharmaceutical products.

Some risk factors have been related to the use of psychotropic drugs among women [12, 16]. Of these, we highlight the following: the double working day, as a result of not only having a job, but also responsibilities in and out of the home, financial insecurity, conflicts with partners, stress, personal insecurity and dissatisfaction, work conditions and future expectations, the care of sick older and younger family members, which falls upon the women, the crisis of identity in the balance of the gender roles played, or situations of dependency and subordination to the husband. Not forgetting the relationship between the methods learnt for dealing with conflict in gender socialization and the use of psychotropic drugs [17, 18].

Ultimately, women are the biggest users of psychotropic drugs, via both medical prescriptions and self-medication, and this use is greatly linked to the gender stereotypes projected around female health by both the prescribers and the rest of society [13].

14.2.3 Opiate Use

In this section on the use of opiates, will we will focus on heroin, bearing in mind that the users of this substance are usually multiple substance users. Other opiates such as methadone or morphine are mainly used in a therapeutic context, without ruling out that these may be subject to different uses.

The prevalence and incidence of heroin use has been dropping over the last two decades. The same does not apply to requests for treatment for the dependency on illegal drugs which, as we will see later, has a greater presence, and in recent years it has been taken in combination with cocaine and other drugs.

Since it erupted onto the national scene and its subsequent expansion in the late 1970s, heroin use has been concentrated among men, with female users being in the minority, especially in the early days [19]. The first groups of users of this substance determined its pattern of use, partly imported from other countries where its use previously began and spread. Afterward, some changes were observed to this pattern of use that were related to new social circumstances, such as AIDS, the type of heroin on the black market or the social representation of its compulsive users.

14.2.3.1 Data on Use

Before heroin use spread, the data we have on the use of opiates are scarce, dispersed, and barely accurate. However, some works [20–22] have indicated that heroin use was preceded by the use of morphine. According to the cases analyzed by González Duro [20] this concerned middle-aged women, who started taking morphine by medical prescription or who were related to medical professionals. They were women from a well-off social class, whose intravenous use was integrated, concealed, self-controlled, and not socially relevant. The censuses of morphine addicts treated and supplied with morphine during the dictatorship era also revealed similar characteristics. This high feminine presence in the use of morphine greatly contrasted with the subsequent use of heroin in which women would be in the minority. We will most probably find the reasons behind this if we compare the two sociocultural contexts, and analyze the woman's role in each.

The prevalence of heroin use in the surveys on this subject show very small percentages compared with other illegal drugs. This situation is evident in all the surveys, from the first to the current ones. Thus, quoting one of the surveys from the 1980s, by the Spanish General Directorate of Public Health in 1984 [15], 0.9 % of people had taken heroin in the last year (1.6 % of the men and 0.3 % of women). In the home-based surveys on drugs from 1995 to 2009 by the PNsD we also observe very low prevalence, between 0.1 % and 0.8 %, which continues to drop among both men and woman (Table 14.4).

The data obtained from the surveys in the last two decades does not reflect the impact of heroin use on Spanish society, especially for the female users of this substance. Heroin and its use have triggered a drug crisis in some Western societies [23], changing the relationship and view of psychotropic substances compared with the previous period.

A series of characteristics have been attributed to female heroin users that differ from the pattern of use by male users [1, 19]. Of these, we highlight the following:

- The start of heroin use in the first group of users was related to its use by their partner. In the following group of users, especially those born from the 1970s onward, the first use of heroin often took place among groups of male and female friends.
- The principal route of administration as this pattern of use spread was intravenous. For the first doses, women tend to behave cautiously, using routes other than intravenous injection, although as their use continues they then change the route of administration. The first times they use heroin, the women demonstrate certain cautious behaviors and previous familiarity with the substance. In other words, the perception of the risk and of putting oneself at risk is usually more

Table 14.4 Use of heroin (Last 12 months, DGPNsD)

AGES (15–64 years)	Males (%)	Females (%)
1995	0.8	0.3
1997	0.4	0.1
1999	0.2	0.0
2001	0.2	0.0
2003	0.2	0.1
2005	0.2	0.1
2007	0.1	0.0
2009	0.1	0.0
ESTUDES (14–18 years)		
1994	0.5	0.2
1996	0.6	0.2
1998	0.8	0.5
2000	0.7	0.1
2002	0.4	0.2
2004	0.8	0.1
2006	1.2	0.3
2008	1.1	0.4
2010	0.9	0.3

moderate than among men. This more cautious behavior is also reflected in the doses they administer.

- It has been recorded that the women tend to inject themselves after their partners. There seem to be two reasons behind this fact. On the one hand, women have more trouble finding their veins, taking longer to administer the drug than the men, who are faster and find it easier to inject as their veins are more protruding and visible. On the other hand, women tend to share and delegate the first turns to other people in their family setting, as happens with food, in addition to the power relations that exist within the couple's relationship, which influence the method of administration.
- Women tend to use drugs for the first time in a private or discreet setting, outside of the public sphere, given that the stigmatization already associated with heroin use is exacerbated for female users.
- Although we find some cases of coercion and intimidation concerning the taking of heroin among couples, the women make decisions about starting to use it. The subordinate and passive role assigned to women may be a way of justifying their inclusion in the use and in the rule-breaking behaviors associated with heroin.
- The significance of heroin use for many women is related to the rule-breaking, the conflict of gender roles and a rejection of the traditional roles assigned to women.
- Women tend to conceal their heroin use, given that their acknowledgement of it generates a higher level of social rejection than among men, calling into question a woman's worth as a colleague, mother, and wife.

We mentioned at the start that heroin use currently involves only a minority of the general population and the reasons and circumstances for its use may be different from those of the 1980s when this substance was more widespread and the social and economic conditions were very different. Nevertheless, the reasons for using an illegal substance with such a socially discredited image as heroin is related to rule-breaking, to what is prohibited, to pleasure, the evasion of personal problems and to peer group cohesion. Thus, women's reasons for taking this substance are no different to those of men, except in some isolated instances where it may have been motivated by a desire to lose weight.[3]

The decline in heroin use is linked to many factors, but of these we can highlight the pejorative images related to its use (overdose, deaths, crimes, marginalization, etc.), the AIDS epidemic in Europe and Western societies that was very much linked in the early years to the intravenous use of heroin; and above all the decline is linked with the emergence and popularization of other drugs that are deemed safer and that can be controlled.

14.2.4 Recreational Drug Use

The drugs that we look at in this section and that are usually associated with leisure activities are cocaine, ecstasy, and cannabis, which although they are not the only drugs found in recreational contexts, they are the principal substances used. We will cover the available epidemiological data for these substances, the reasons for their use, the way they are used, and the contexts in which they are used, focusing on women and comparing them with men.

14.2.4.1 Data on Use

According to the data we have available from various national and independent surveys, cannabis is the illegal psychotropic substance most frequently consumed in European and Western societies. Cannabis use generally generates higher percentages among men than women, although in some age groups the percentage differences are not so high. Thus, the ESTUDES surveys by the National Drug Strategy (PNsD) show a difference of approximately 5 % for male and female use of cannabis among school-goers. At the ages of 14 and 15 these percentage differences are practically even in both sexes. Thus, in the study by EDIS for the Women's Institute, we find a big difference in cannabis use among school goers (25.3 %) and other women (7 %). The user profile generated by this study relates to "young women, living in urban areas, with a good level of education, of all social classes, in work, with unconventional ideologies and religious beliefs" [16]. Among school-goers we can also add that there is a presence of young people from a low

[3] This reason appeared among younger groups of users who began using heroin in the 1990s, but we repeat again that this incidence involved a minority as there were other drugs with a better social image than heroin that could satisfy this motivation.

social class, who study and work at the same time and some of them have repeated years of academic study.

The average age for cannabis use among the female population is in the 15- to17-year-old age group, according to EDIS' work for the Women's Institute; around 18 years old in the home-based surveys; and 15 years for school-goers in the PNsD survey. These average starting ages are similar to those for men and boys.

As for cocaine, a high increase in use has occurred in recent years according to the results obtained in the different surveys carried out by the PNsD. It is the second most frequently used illegal psychotropic substance. The differences in percentage between the sexes for annual use, according to the various surveys carried out, are around 2 % less for women compared with men, for both school-goers and for the rest of the population. Also, the EDIS survey of the female population reveals a much higher annual prevalence among school-goers (6.1 %) than the PNsD survey in the same year (3 %).

The profile of cocaine users in the EDIS shows us that these are young women, aged between 14 and 34 years old, and from 17 years of age among school-goers; they are single women with a medium- and high-level of education, employed, students, and they are nonbelievers and agnostics. Among school-goers we also highlight those who work and study, who have repeated an academic year, live in the northern area along the Mediterranean coast, and they spend their leisure time going out with friends to bars, discos, and parties; drugs are being used in their peer groups [16].

The average age for cocaine use in the female population is around 19 years and among school-goers it is 16 [16]. This average starting age is higher in the home-based surveys of the PNsD, at between 20 and 21 years for women (similar to men) and around 15 years for school-goers (Table 14.5).

Finally, in the case of ecstasy and similar substances, the differences for annual prevalence by gender are similar to those for cocaine use. Women consume between 1 % and 2 % less than males. The data obtained in the EDIS survey with regard to women is also similar to the school-based and home-based surveys of the PNsD.

The user profile for ecstasy is similar to that for cocaine, among other reasons because both substances are mainly used in a recreational context. On the other hand, what stands out in the female group are that the users are aged between 14 and 24 years old and, among the school-goers, they are around 13–14 or 17–18 years old.

The average age for starting to use ecstasy is around 19 and 20 years among women, which is 1 year less than for males, in the home-based surveys; and around 15 years for both sexes in the school-based surveys.

Now that we have presented epidemiological data about male and female use that is most readily available, our questions turn to the reasons for the use, the contexts and forms of use among women, and the differences compared with men.

Table 14.5 Use of cannabis, cocaine, and ecstasy in the last 12 months

	Cannabis		Cocaine		Ecstasy	
	Males	Females	Males	Females	Males	Females
	Survey AGES (15–64 years)					
1995	10.7	4.4	2.7	1.0	1.9	0.7
1997	10.7	4.7	2.6	0.6	1.2	0.5
1999	9.6	4.3	2.3	0.8	1.2	0.5
2001	13.0	5.5	3.8	1.3	2.8	0.7
2003	16.2	6.3	4.1	1.2	2.0	0.8
2005	15.7	6.6	4.6	1.3	1.8	0.6
2007	13.6	6.6	4.4	1.5	1.6	0.5
2009	14.8	6.2	4.2	1.0	1.4	0.3
	Survey AGES (14–18 years)					
1994	21.0	15.3	2.3	1.2	4.2	2.2
1996	25.9	21.1	3.3	2.2	4.8	3.5
1998	28.2	23.5	5.4	3.6	2.9	2.1
2000	32.2	25.2	6.4	3.1	6.4	3.9
2002	36.2	29.8	7.5	5.1	4.7	3.8
2004	39.4	33.7	9.4	5.1	3.3	1.9
2006	31.6	28.2	5.2	3.1	3.3	1.6
2008	33.5	27.5	4.9	2.4	2.6	1.3
2010	28.2	24.7	3.3	1.8	2.2	1.2

14.2.4.2 Reasons and Circumstances for Use

The social and public participation of women, as well as their legal equality, has been increasing in Spain since the change to democracy. Although the Spanish Constitution of 1978 already established more possibilities for participation than under the previous regime, it took longer for social customs and norms to be assimilated and for profound changes to occur in the roles assigned to each gender. Thus, few women engaged in recreational drug use until the 1990s for various reasons [10].

First, the pattern of recreational drug use became more popular and widespread in the 1990s, even though it had been established in the previous decades. Recreational and leisure activities, especially night-time ones, have become an important concept for young people, in which young women are accepted and integrated, possibilities that their mothers and grandmothers could not have experienced.

Second, drug use for reasons related to pleasure, fun, and rule-breaking had existed in the male but not the female domain, and the latter was not tolerated until the 1990s. The changes in how leisure time was spent, sexual liberation, and the opening of social relations between both sexes, and the social tolerance toward some drugs compared with others have been changing over the last 10 years.

Third, some psychostimulants were substances traditionally prescribed in slimming programs and were also easy to access in the pharmacies during the decades of the dictatorship, as were amphetamines [20]. Cocaine and ecstasy are slimming substances and allow users to preserve a good physical image. Although this is not the principal reason for use, it is considered to be a good reason for maintaining its occasional use.

Fourth, the transition from positions of dependency on or subordination to men to more independent and autonomous situations has generated a conflict of roles among women on the one hand, owing to a lack of new female role models with which they may identify that are not based on the traditional roles of mother, wife, and carer or on male styles. On the other hand, the possibility of participating in all these spheres or environments from which women had been prohibited, has opened up a new space for conquest and equal rights. Certainly, leaving behind the seclusion of the home and domestic sphere to which they have been subject to then participate in all the social environments entails risks and benefits for women.

It has been suggested that women participate more frequently in the use of illegal drugs than in previous eras as a symbol of equality and liberation, but would it not be the opposite? In the historic times in which we live, do women still not have the same opportunities as men? Could this be related to a form of rebellion, nonconformism and a transgression of social roles that has yet to occur?

If we look at what has traditionally been valued in women, such as their behavior of self-control, security, and protection of others, all these related to their traditional roles, the use of psychotropic substances signifies a certain rebellion against these behaviors. Drug use offers an opportunity to satisfy curiosity, pleasure, seeking new sensations, fun, and integration into peer groups.

14.2.5 Problematic Uses of Psychotropic Substances

Approaching the problematic uses of legal and illegal psychotropic substances presents many methodological problems, especially if we want to obtain exhaustive data on them. Thus, we have some indirect indicators prepared by the PNsD in 1987, the SEIT (Government System of Information on Drug Addicts).[4] Perhaps the treatment indicator offers us the best coverage, although it is certain that not all the people who exhibit a dependency on drugs attend the care systems, as an undetermined percentage manage to recover naturally without professional support.

As we can see in Table 14.6, we present data on almost all the substances we have dealt with during the 7 years of this project. The demand for treatment for alcohol dependency is not recorded in SEIT, among other reasons because the drug dependency care programs have only recently incorporated this treatment, as other channels and mechanisms existed and continue to exist for this care, making it difficult for us to supply accurate data. It is also possible that the demand for treatment for psychotropic substance dependency is underestimated in this

[4] Government System of Information on Drug Addicts. There are three indirect indicators: treatment indicator, emergency indicator, and the indicator of mortality related to illegal drugs.

Table 14.6 Request for treatment per principal substance that motivated the request (Government System of Information on Drug Addicts, SEIT, 1996–2009; National Drug Strategy, PNsD)

	Heroin		Cocaine		Ecstasy		Cannabis		Psychotropic substances[a]	
	Males	Females	Males	Females	Males	Females	Males	Females	Males	Females
1996	84.5	15.5	86.0	14.0	80.5	19.5	88.8	11.2	54.7	45.3
1997	84.3	15.7	86.0	14.0	75.1	24.9	90.3	9.7	55.7	44.3
1998	84.4	15.6	86.7	13.3	80.5	19.5	88.9	11.1	57.7	42.3
1999	84.8	15.2	86.0	14.0	82.8	17.2	89.2	10.8	57.9	42.1
2000	84.3	15.7	87.5	12.5	83.1	16.9	90.1	9.9	60.6	39.4
2001	84.4	15.6	86.6	13.4	80.6	19.4	90.1	9.9	56.0	44.0
2002	84.0	16.0	87.2	12.8	80.8	19.2	89.2	10.8	60.9	39.1
2005	84.1	15.9	85.9	14.1	81.1	18.9	84.7	15.3	60.9	39.1
2009	84.8	15.2	85.8	14.2	87.4	12.6	86.3	13.7	60.9	39.1

As of 2002, the data have not been published annually

[a]In 1996 and 1997 the data refer to hypnotics and sedatives, and in 2002 to hypnotics and benzodiazepines

indicator. In all the substances we show, the principal clients of the treatment programs are male.

According to the above data, we find more women requesting treatment (according to the higher percentages of substances) for psychotropic drugs, ecstasy and similar, heroin, cocaine, and cannabis. The prevalence of psychotropic substances analyzed in the female group would be (in line with the higher percentages obtained) for psychotropic drugs, cannabis, cocaine, ecstasy, and heroin, a sequence that is different for men. As a general rule, requests for treatment in the first years are mainly for heroin addiction and later these are replaced by requests for treatment for cocaine abuse. Women account for no more than 20 % of the requests for care with regard to these substances. Why are fewer women demanding treatment for dependence on psychotropic substances?

Various hypotheses have been put forward concerning the low representation of women in the drug dependency care programs [19, 24]. Given that the prevalence of women in illegal drug use is much lower than that of men, their demand for treatment is logically lower as well. But it may also be the case that the pattern of use among women is very different to that of men and they do not require treatment, only a small section of women requiring professional help. As previously mentioned, female use may be more secretive, moderate, and sustained without generating problems, in other words, it leads less frequently to compulsive use. It may also be related to the roles they traditionally played of displaying greater self-control and security, so that once their behavior becomes compulsive, they have a greater capacity to stop taking drugs without professional care or treatment. In other words, they recover naturally from situations of dependency. In these latter aspects, the greater social exclusion and stigmatization of illegal drug use by women may inhibit their acquisition of a drug dependency, or their attendance for treatment. Another aspect that has also been mentioned with regard to women is that they leave the environments in which drugs are used earlier as they acquire responsibilities in the family before men [9]. But it has also been suggested that it is precisely because men constitute the majority in the treatment programs that women do not attend them, because of their male-centered orientation. They would not feel comfortable or find the services or care they require. There are currently very few programs that take women's needs into account and that have put together resources or strategies to cover them.

It is very likely that these hypotheses we are putting forward explain the lower representation of women, and a more in-depth investigation into gender and female drug use would be necessary to confirm them.

14.3 A Gender Approach in Drug Policies

Drug use is conditioned by the gender norms and the female and male role models that defined the social acceptance of drug use and related behaviors for each sex [25]. The traditional gender role models have influenced the adoption of certain types of drug use among women that were previously deemed to "belong to men."

This has been the case with alcohol and tobacco, and above all with illegal substances, associated with risk and rule-breaking. Also, the sexist stereotypes linked to the traditional female roles have contributed to the rise of other types of drug use that are "compatible" with female needs and problems, specifically the use of psychotropic drugs [26] and have "protected" women from tobacco and alcohol. Nevertheless, the "protective" function of the traditional gender roles is becoming less and less effective in the context of women's emancipation, which opens up interesting routes of inquiry around the adoption of certain types of drug use by women.

If we accept the analysis of policies to curb drug supplies, despite the long history of studies and publications about gender and development cooperation policies, few applications have been made under this approach to analyze the alternative development policies aimed at replacing the cultivation of plants prohibited by other agricultural products. Nor are there any exhaustive analyses of policies to control drug traffic that include a gender approach. The few studies that exist in this regard show that neither the public bodies nor the consumer rights agencies pay sufficient attention in their discourses to the differences in the patterns of use and sociocultural context between men and women [27].

Both the guidelines for drug use and the related gender roles vary according to the user's gender. In recent decades, surveys reveal an increase in the use of legally regulated substances such as tobacco, alcohol, and tranquillizers among women, or of socially accepted substances such as cannabis, while the use of prohibited drugs continues to be mainly masculine.

The core approach of the policies to curb drug demand in the European Union appears to focus on prohibited drugs. The EU Drugs Action Plan for 2009–2012 [28] translated the general aims and priorities of the EU Drugs Strategy (2005–2012) into specific actions, with indicators that measure progress. The first paragraph of the said Plan states that "illicit drugs are a major concern for the citizens of Europe, a major threat to the security and health of European society and a threat to living conditions worldwide " (EU Council 2008). But how are the risk and risk factors defined? How do you measure the damage caused by drug use? In Western culture, accounts of addictions focus mainly on the substance, the "drug," omitting other explanations such as relocation or the financial crisis, or cultural practices that induce the habit amongst many people in social contexts where the drug proliferates.

Insofar as the discourses about official drug policy define the risks that derive from using certain substances, in the collective imagination the "drug" becomes an element capable of transforming the users, removing any other desire or eroding the values of the people and the community. As in the social imagination, cultural values are incorporated into public policies in ways that do not always give rise to practical, ethical or fair policies.

Public policies are a central instrument in the organization of contemporary societies, to the point of categorizing people as "citizens," "delinquents," "ill persons," or "deviants," without those who are the object of such policies having any control over or being aware of the process for drafting them. Thus, drug use is managed using risk-based technologies that convert the users into delinquents or ill people.

For women, the construction of their image with regard to drugs is conditioned by gender roles; thus, a collective imagination is produced, which then circulates and takes shape, especially in public policies, about the significance or women and drugs, based on sex, gender, ethnic background, and class. The rights of women depend on the extent to which they fulfill their responsibilities as workers, consumers, and carers, buying their independence at the price of good behavior and social conformity. Thus, social stigma or the threat of withdrawing custody of their children becomes a disciplinary method of social regulation for effectively governing female drug users.

Conclusion

Social acceptance of drug use is not equal for male and female users, just as it is not equal for prohibited and legally regulated substances. Women are often affected to a greater extent by social criminalization (stigmatization) related to the prohibited substances and their compulsive use. This stigmatization and the fear of social sanction mean that many women do not admit to using prohibited substances and do not access the resources available for people with compulsive use disorders, making them invisible in the statistics and studies.

The vulnerability of women is exacerbated by their invisibility: few resources are allocated to cover the needs of female drug users; there is a shortage of staff trained on gender matters; treatments begin at a late stage; a growing number of women are imprisoned in men's prisons; few if any women hold responsible positions in drug user associations, etc. Thus, the invisibility that exacerbates their vulnerability results in complete exclusion in some cases. At the same time, the invisibility of female drug users is not only obvious when they are the object of policies, but also when they are the subject.

We can foresee that, as a gender approach is incorporated into the policy guidelines designed and issued by the various organizations dedicated to drafting drug policies in the European Union, and as these guidelines are effectively applied by the member States, we will be able to obtain clearer information about the problematic uses and the contexts in which drugs are used, about the treatment programs and the accessibility by all the people who need such programs, which also cover women's needs with their strategies and resources.

References

1. Meneses C. Mujer y heroína. Un estudio antropológico de la heroinomanía femenina. Tesis doctoral. Departamento de Antropología y Trabajo Social. Universidad de Granada; 2001.
2. Romo N. La mirada de género en el abordaje de los usos y abusos de drogas. Revista Española de Drogodependencias. 2010;3:269–72.
3. Reed BG. Drug misuse and dependency in women: the meaning and implications of being considered a special population or minority group. Int J Addict. 1985;20(1):13–62.

4. Meneses C. Invisibilidad y estigmatización del consumo de drogas en las mujeres, en García-Mina, Ana; Carrasco, Mª José, editors. Diferencias de género en el uso de las drogas. Madrid: Universidad P Comillas; 2006.
5. Camí J. 2000. Las sustancias: farmacología. In: Grup Igia y cols, editors. Contextos, Sujetos y Drogas: Manual sobre Drogodependencias. Madrid: Institut Municipal de Salut Pública-FAD; 2000, p. 159–85.
6. Kuntsche E, Rehm J, Gmel G. Characteristic of binge drinking in Europe. Soc Sci Med. 2004;59:113–27.
7. Wilsnack RW, Vogeltanz ND, Wilsnack SC, Harris TR. Gender differences in alcohol consumption and adverse drinking consequences: cross-cultural patterns. Addiction. 2000;95 (2):251–65.
8. Meneses C y Charro B. en prensa. Es necesaria una intervención diferencial de género en la prevención universal y selectiva del consumo de drogas en adolescentes. Revista de Psiquiatría y Salud Mental. http://dx.org/10.1016/j.rpsm.2013.01.003
9. Romo N. Cultura del baile y riesgo: la influencia del género en los nuevos consumos de drogas de síntesis. Granada. Tesis doctoral, Departamento de Antropología y Trabajo Social, Universidad de Granada; 2001.
10. Romo N. Técno y Baile. Mitos y realidades de las diferencias de género. Revista de Estudios de Juventud. 2004;64:111–6.
11. Keane H. Intoxication, harm and pleasure: an analysis of the Australian National Alcohol Strategy. Crit Public Health. 2009;19(2):135–42.
12. Romo N, Vega A, Meneses C, Gil E, Markez I, Póo M. Sobre el malestar y la prescripción: un estudio sobre los usos de psicofármacos por las mujeres. Revista Española de Drogodependencias. 2003;28(4):372–9.
13. Markez I, Póo M, Romo N, Meneses C, Gil E, Vega A. Mujeres y psicofármacos: la investigación en atención primaria. Revista de la Asociación Española de Neuropsiquiatría. 2004;XXIV(91):39–61.
14. Goudsmit E. ¡Todo es mental! Puntos de vista estereotípicos y la psicologización de las enfermedades de la mujer, en Wilkinson S y Kitznger C. Mujer y Salud. Una perspectiva feminista. Barcelona. Paidós; 1996.
15. Comas D. El uso de drogas en la Juventud. Madrid: Ministerio de Cultura. Instituto de la Juventud; 1985.
16. EDIS. Consumo de alcohol y otras drogas en el colectivo femenino. Madrid: Instituto de la Mujer; 2000.
17. Burin M. Mujeres al borde de un ataque de psicofármacos [en línea]. http://old.clarin.com/diario/2000/08/31/o-02901.htm
18. Levinton ND. El superyo femenino. Maristarán. 2002;14:13–22.
19. Meneses C. Mujeres y consumo de opiáceos. Una realidad específica. Trastor Adict. 2006;8 (4):261–75.
20. González DE. Consumo de Drogas en España. Madrid: Villalar; 1979.
21. Usó Arnal JC. Drogas y Cultura de Masas. (España 1855–1995). Tesis doctoral. Universidad Complutense de Madrid; 1995.
22. Meneses C. De la morfina a la heroína. El uso de drogas en la Juventud. Miscelánea Comillas. 2002;60(116):217–43.
23. Gamella J. Heroína en España (1977-1996). Claves de Razón Práctica. 1997;72:20–30.
24. Meneses C. Una atención específica para mujeres drogodependientes. Revista Proyecto. 2002;43:5–9.
25. Jiménez ML, Guzmán R. Género y usos de drogas: dimensiones de análisis e intersección con otros ejes de desigualdad. En: Diferencias invisibles: género, drogas y políticas públicas. Oñati Socio-Legal Series, vol. 2, no. 6; 2012.
26. Romo N, Gil E. Género y uso de drogas. De la ilegalidad a la legalidad para enfrentar el malestar. Trastor Adict. 2006;8(4):243–50.

27. Arana X, Markez I, Montañés V. Introducción al enfoque de género en las políticas europeas de drogas. En: Diferencias invisibles: género, drogas y políticas públicas. Oñati Socio-Legal Series, vol. 2, no. 6; 2012.
28. Consejo de la Unión Europea. 2008. Plan de Acción de la Unión Europea en materia de lucha contra la droga 2009-2012, Consejo de la Unión Europea, 2008/C 326/09, 20/12/2008.

Psychosis and Gender: Everything You Always Wanted to Know About Sex (and Gender) in Psychosis but Were Afraid to Ask

15

Maria Haarmans

Abstract

In Chap. 5 in "General Aspects," I argue for sex- and gender-based analysis (SGBA) to improve the science of psychosis research, describing how to conduct SGBA. I extend that argument in this chapter by reviewing what we currently know about sex and gender in psychosis, highlighting gaps in our knowledge and illustrating how SGBA might fill those gaps by clarifying research findings and/or enhancing methodology, ultimately increasing our understanding of the development, maintenance, and recovery of psychotic experiences, strengthening my argument from Chap. 5.

15.1 Introduction

> "If they get you to ask the wrong questions, they don't need to worry about your answers."
> Anonymous (cited in Hare-Mustin and Maracek, 1994, p. 531)

Unfortunately, the title of this chapter is misleading; as the reader shall see, there is actually very little we know about gender and much more we could understand about sex in terms of our knowledge of how they impact psychosis. As pointed out in Chap. 5, researchers in the psychosis field have been, for one reason or another, "afraid" or reluctant to ask questions about how the variables of gender and, to a lesser extent, sex influence psychosis risk, development, expression, and outcomes for the men and women so diagnosed. In Chap. 5 I argue for sex- and gender-based analysis (SGBA) in the psychosis field, underlining the neglect of incorporating the multivariables of sex and gender into psychosis research and describe SGBA and the relevant constructs. In this chapter, I review the literature, briefly outlining

M. Haarmans (✉)
Clinical Psychology, Institute of Psychology, Health and Society, University of Liverpool, Liverpool, UK
e-mail: maria.haarmans@liverpool.ac.uk

M. Sáenz-Herrero (ed.), *Psychopathology in Women*,
DOI 10.1007/978-3-319-05870-2_15

research that focuses on sex differences in the schizophrenia field in addition to the few studies that examine gender, pointing out how SGBA may have illuminated findings further.

15.1.1 Sex Differences

Much more research in the schizophrenia field has been devoted to sex differences than gender, although there are still many unanswered questions, particularly with regard to the underlying mechanisms of these differences [1]. For more extensive reviews on sex differences in schizophrenia see Abel et al. [2], Falkenburg and Tracy [3], Kulkarni and Gavrilidis [4], Leung and Chue [5], McGrath et al. [6], Riechler-Rössler and Hafner [7], and Seeman et al. [8].

15.2 Prevalence, Incidence, and Onset

Falkenburg and Tracy [3], in their recent review of sex differences, note the conflicting epidemiological findings regarding prevalence, incidence, and age of onset of schizophrenia. For example, some authors suggest that prevalence might be higher among men and others find no difference between the sexes [1, 3, 9–13]. Several authors attribute these inconsistencies to age limits of samples (women in older age groups are at a higher risk; thus, samples should include all ages) and diagnostic criteria used (e.g., the narrower the diagnostic criteria used, the more women are excluded from a diagnosis of schizophrenia [2, 14, 15]; when affective or atypical symptoms are included in the diagnostic systems, more women will be diagnosed [16]). However, Iacono and Beiser [9] report that they found incidence rates two to three times higher in men than in women, regardless of which diagnostic criteria were used. While incidence rates seem to be more consistent in the literature, with a recent meta-analysis by Aleman et al. [17] reporting a mean ratio of male-to-female incidence of 1.42, this is not reflected in the lack of sex differences in prevalence that has been demonstrated by major epidemiological reviews using various measures [6, 18] and a well-designed Finnish population study, one of the largest and most thorough, with a nationally representative sample of over 8,000 individuals [19]. Interestingly, Susser and Wanderling [20], using the ten-country World Health Organization (WHO) cohort, found almost double the annual incidence of nonaffective acute remitting psychosis per 10,000 people in women than men in developing countries and about ten-fold the incidence for both sexes compared with developed countries. Abel et al. [2] note that this finding is surprising considering these cases came from the original ten-country study that found no difference in incidence between developed and developing countries and a lower prevalence in developing countries. Some authors have also pointed to the doubly high mortality rates in men compared with women with schizophrenia diagnoses (especially from suicide) as an additional factor possibly related to the discrepant prevalence and incidence rates [2, 3, 17]. They suggest that because of this paradox, it is important to emphasize the uncertainty of values associated with sex differences in these domains [2].

Falkenburg and Tracy [3] draw attention to the fact that even with regard to age of onset, regarded as the most convincing sex difference, inconsistencies are revealed in the current literature. The authors report that most studies find an earlier age of onset of 3–4 years for male subjects regardless of such confounders as culture and better socio-occupational functioning in women. However, a study by Chang et al. [21] in Hong Kong in 2011 fails to find any difference. In one of the largest and most comprehensive epidemiological, population-based samples, the National "Low Prevalence" study from Australia, they also found no significant difference in age of onset and report that both marital status and familiarity confound the association between sex and age at onset [3]. In fact, they cite several studies that have not found sex differences in age at onset and even some that have reported earlier onset in women. For example, they cite Jablensky and Cole, who, in a re-analysis of the WHO ten-country study data, proposed that reported differences may be the result of confounding, particularly by marital status, which they suggest acts as a protective factor, delaying onset. However, interpreting marital status as a "protective" factor is questionable; Nasser and colleagues [22] argue the quality of the marital relationship is an important variable. For example, they draw attention to other studies that reveal an association of marital status with higher rates of mental illness and underline the impact of other psychosocial stressors such as poverty, homelessness, and victimization that women with psychotic illness are differentially exposed to regardless of marital status. Nonetheless, several researchers have suggested that men's higher admission rates may be related to differential gender role expectations such that there is more tolerance of women being unemployed with increased responsibilities for unpaid work such as the care of others and domestic duties such as housework [23, 24], and marriage may be a related factor in lower admission rates for these reasons. Conflicting findings with regard to the age at onset have also been attributed to differing definitions of "age of onset" (some definitions refer to age at admission, first treatment, first positive, or first noticeable signs of the disorder), younger age cutoffs, thus excluding late-onset women and including nonschizophrenic psychoses. Falkenburg and Tracy [3] point out that findings are more consistent regarding onset distribution over time, with admixture analyses demonstrating onset for both sexes as nonlinear and typically bimodal or trimodal for women, in whom onset peaks between age 25 and 30, with a smaller peak after 45 and some studies reporting a third after age 60 [3].

In a recent review and meta-analysis of the incidence rates over a 60-year period of schizophrenia and other psychosis in England, Kirkbride in 2012 found that the incidence of psychotic disorders varied strikingly by age, sex, migrant status/ethnicity, and place. The authors indicate that there was broad support for the most consistent findings of the sex differences in peak incidences for men and women in their twenties declining thereafter with a smaller second peak in women from midlife in addition to the elevated rates reported across several ethnic minority groups [25]. Interestingly, their review suggested raised rates for ethnic minority groups descendant from the Indian subcontinent in women only.

15.3 Phenomenology and Symptomatology

One of the most consistently reported findings of sex differences in symptomatology is that men experience more or worse "negative symptoms" and women more "positive symptoms," particularly auditory hallucinations and paranoia or persecutory delusions and affective symptoms [2, 5, 26–28]. Morgan and colleagues [28] report that women present with more depressive symptoms at entry and throughout illness progression. Other researchers have also reported that women with a schizophrenia diagnosis display higher levels of depression [7, 29], which may be why they are likely to be diagnosed as schizoaffective. According to Maric and colleagues in 2003, based on their findings from the NEMESIS general population study with a sample size of over 7,000 participants, men display more negative symptoms (this effect size increases when adjusted for depression) and women more positive symptoms, although when adjusting for depression, differences could be accounted for by overlap between positive symptoms and depression [27]. The investigators have suggested, as have other investigators [2, 30–32], that the higher levels of depression in women with psychosis may induce higher levels of positive symptoms. The investigators also suggest that this finding may help to explain the discrepant findings between studies with regard to sex differences in positive symptomatology. Interestingly, the researchers point out that these findings are consistent with earlier reports that affective symptomatology are not only more prevalent in women compared with men with schizophrenia, but also correlate more strongly with psychotic symptoms. Cotton in 2009 suggests that higher levels of depressive symptoms in women at service entry may be related to the greater prevalence of sexual abuse histories and mood disorder in women [33].

Maric and colleagues suggests that these findings might be interpreted using current psychological models of symptom formation, which emphasize the role of emotional processes in the cognitive biases that may lead to positive symptoms [27]. Here is an example of where SGBA has the potential for understanding these findings further by exploring the role of gender as well as sex.

Al-Issa [33], reviewing studies on gender and psychosis, states that delusions are more frequent in women than in men and cites Swanson, Bohmert, and Smith (1970), who report that the greatest sex differences in delusions occur between ages 40 and 50 when the incidence is twice as high in women as in men [34]. Similarly, Lucas et al. report from their sample of 206 female and 196 male hospitalized patients a significantly higher incidence of delusions in women than in men and more variation in terms of the content of delusions in women [35]. More recent studies also report an increased incidence of delusions, particularly persecutory delusions in women [2, 5, 28] and more severe paranoia in women [4] particularly in women with an older onset than in men with an older onset [2]. This is a very interesting finding in the light of Mirkowsky and Ross's research linking belief in external control with low socioeconomic status, Mexican heritage, and being female. They found that belief in external control interacts with low current socioeconomic status to produce mistrust, which in turn is the major factor directly associated with paranoia [36]. Women's declining social status with age as well as increased economic insecurity potentially could help explain the increased persecutory delusions that are reported in older women.

An interesting paradox in the findings by Danish investigators [16] is that men had more severe negative symptoms and a poorer social network, and women experienced more severe hallucinations; however, in spite of women's superior functioning in terms of education, employment, permanent relationships, and independent living they reported lower self-esteem than the men.

15.4 Course and Outcome/Recovery

Most studies suggest that socio-occupational functioning (including pre-morbid) and outcome is better in women, including in first-episode samples [1, 2, 4, 12, 16, 26, 37], but as pointed out previously, marital status is often used as a measure of this type of functioning without consideration of the quality of the marital relationship [22]. Some authors suggest that a better course and outcome for women is related to a later age at onset [2]; however, other researchers have found that this superior functioning is related to neither premorbid functioning nor age at onset [37].

Morgan and colleagues [28] report that women in their study had experienced a psychosocial stressor just prior to illness onset significantly more frequently than men, which consistent with the findings of McGlashan and Bardenstein [29]. This finding is also consistent with several clinical studies cited under the "Gender and Psychosis" section [39–45].

As Thorup [16] points out, the different course of the disorder for men and women needs more thorough investigation.

15.4.1 Gender

As noted previously, the role of gender has been severely neglected in the schizophrenia field, with the exception of a few interesting studies conducted from the 1950s to the early 1980s, and one as early as 1934. However, the majority of the papers that are reviewed in this section essentially compare sex differences and do not test gender constructs empirically. Thus, most could be included with those under the "Phenomenology/Symptomatology" section, but are discussed here as the authors consider gender in the explanation of their results. Another limitation with regard to these articles conducting SGBA is that much of the data is collected via chart reviews, case notes, or to a lesser extent structured interviews, and gender has not been defined clearly or explored in terms of individual life experiences, context, gender relations, intersections with other social categories such as "race" or class, or their impact on the development of psychotic experience with the exception of a few very interesting early studies that emphasize the significance of sociological factors in psychiatry [34, 35, 44–47]. However, it is interesting to note that the work reviewed here examines the content of psychotic phenomena and not merely form, particularly with regard to delusions. The reason for this earlier interest in gender and specifically delusional content may be related to the fact that psychodynamic models of mental illness including psychosis were more prevalent at that time and the role of psychiatrists included providing psychotherapy. In addition, there was a greater emphasis on the phenomenology of psychopathology, a tradition that continues to this day in Germany, with the aim of improving the accuracy of diagnosis [43]. It is also a period in history corresponding to the women's movement, where gender roles were beginning to be questioned and were beginning to change.

Included in this review are areas of inquiry where no SGBA has been conducted to date, but which would particularly benefit from such analyses in terms of increasing our understanding of the development and maintenance of psychotic experiences and have the potential to inform development of more responsive psychological interventions.

15.5 Gender Role/Identity and Psychosis

While there was much more interest in gender roles and gender identity and schizophrenia several decades ago [48, 49], Nasser and colleagues point out, most of the research focusing on gender identity specifically has methodological flaws and was conducted with hospitalized men [22]. Further, by and large, this earlier work was based on an outdated gender identity trait model, which later theorists have replaced with social constructionist models [50–54]. One of the leading theories among this earlier work, proposed by LaTorre [47] is the diathesis–gender–stress model of schizophrenia, which identifies gender identity or "gender role confusion" in which there is less identification with characteristics associated with normative gender roles. Although an intriguing model, the vulnerability–gender–stress model was based on an outdated theory. LaTorre in 1984 theorized that "faulty gender identity" results from dysfunctional family dynamics such as parental non-involvement or hostility and thus poor same-sex models leading to sex incongruent gender identity [47]. The underlying assumption of this work, as with much of the earlier work on gender and schizophrenia in general, is that the problem lies within the individual's "impairment" in their ability to incorporate "normal" gender role norms into one's personality or behavior, although LaTorre does suggest that, in the adolescent male, greater "gender identity uncertainty" is related to Western male role norms that emphasize aggression, thus explaining earlier onset in men. This latter idea is more consistent with the gender role strain paradigm.

Al-Issa [33] cites a number of studies that report that hospitalized men with a schizophrenia diagnosis tend to exhibit more passivity and withdrawal than non-psychotic men. Conversely, women are observed to be more active and domineering than their nonclinical counterparts. In addition, clinical observations on hospital wards and in psychotherapy according to several authors have reported that female patients are more sexual and aggressive than male patients. One could question, however, whether these observations are biased because of traditional gender role expectations so that women who do not fit the stereotyped gender roles are perceived and labeled as "more sexual and aggressive." Al-Issa suggests that selection factors may explain these purported sex differences in behavior such that "...overactive, aggressive females and underactive, withdrawn males are hospitalized more readily than those whose behaviour is socially acceptable" (1982, p. 159). He also questions whether institutionalization itself, is responsible for the sex differences observed in the behavior of hospitalized patients. He notes that the aggressive behavior of women appears to be situation-specific, for example, during staff interactions, but not, in the case of jointly admitted mothers and infants, in interactions of mothers with their infants. Interestingly, Al-Issa reports studies in which women who display "feminine" behavior such as "a feminine pattern of high anxiety" and "low ego strength" are rewarded by being more likely to be discharged from hospital than if they "...reveal a masculine pattern of low anxiety and high ego strength" (p. 160).

He proposes that cross-cultural studies reveal that conflicts associated with gender role ideals may be related to the development of schizophrenia in both men and women [33]. This idea is reminiscent of Pleck's [52] gender role strain paradigm described earlier. Al-Issa [33] suggests that these findings reflect gender role norms regarding sexual prescriptions and proscriptions for men and women in society, for example, greater restrictions on sexuality for women than for men. He cites Weinstein [55] who, in contrast to Western studies, found that sexual content is not very frequent in the delusions of native women in the Virgin Islands and attributed this finding to social expectations and his observation that biological sex does not determine social roles in this culture.

While current gender role theories, such as the gender role strain paradigm and the gender role conflict construct, attribute distress to the individual's perceived discrepancy between the actual self and the ideal self with regard to gender role norms, in addition to experiencing discrimination by others for violating gender role norms, these paradigms locate the problems not within the individual per se, but rather within the gender role norms themselves [50, 52, 56]. Further, a critical component of these constructs, as described earlier, are the harmful psychological consequences resulting when individuals do conform to gender role norms such as Pleck's subtype of "dysfunction strain" or the outcomes of gender role conflict [52, 53]. Nevertheless, some of the findings of this earlier research are thought-provoking, particularly those related to problems with body image, such as studies that found that hospitalized patients experience less sexual differentiation than control groups, as measured by various tests from projective tests such as the Draw-a-Person (DAP) test and the Sexual Differentiation Scale, which attempt to account for gradations of differentiation, to self-report scales such as the Body Parts Satisfaction test that measure satisfaction or dissatisfaction with body parts [33, 47, 49]. In the light of emerging research demonstrating clear links between childhood sexual abuse (CSA) and psychotic experiences, these findings are particularly interesting and possibly related to CSA; however, this was not investigated by any of the researchers. An additional limitation of this early work, as pointed out by Al-Issa [33] is the simplistic conceptualization of gender as a bipolar model as opposed to a multidimensional and multifaceted construct. He also criticizes this early work for its lack of recognition of the harmful psychological impacts of rigid gender typing and adopting stereotypical gender role norms that he theorizes could be related to the development of schizophrenia.

The only recent empirical study I could find that examines gender and psychosis was conducted by Sajatovic et al. [57] who examined "gender identity" with 49 men and 41 women diagnosed with schizophrenia or schizoaffective disorder and reported that both sexes endorsed traditionally male gender role statements on the Bem Sex Role Inventory (BSRI) to a lower extent than normative expectations for their respective sex. As mentioned in Chap. 5 in "General Aspects," the BSRI has been criticized as a rather crude measure of gender because it oversimplifies the constructs of masculinity and femininity [58, 59]. Some researchers suggest that the BSRI instead measures personality "traits," such as instrumentality versus expressiveness, which presumes that masculinity or femininity is located within the individual as opposed to being viewed as socially constructed and "...a component of a broader gender ideology that recommends the values, traits, and behaviors the members of a group believe a person should have as a man or woman (p. 131)." Nevertheless, the findings are interesting in the light of studies suggesting certain traits and behaviors reinforced as masculinity norms such as a sense of agency and assertiveness are associated with better mental health [58–60]. There is also a problem, however, with research relying on only one scale. Adopting the gender role strain paradigm is a more useful and comprehensive model because of its increased level of theoretical sophistication and sensitivity in that it captures the multidimensionality of the gender construct as well as accommodating the dynamism of gender and changing gender roles.

15.6 Gender and Psychosis Content/Symptom Expression

A limited number of studies in the schizophrenia field from various countries have examined sex differences in the content of delusional beliefs and even fewer of hallucinated voices, with investigators relying primarily on chart review, case report, and semi-structured interviews. Several of these authors explain results as being related to gender role socialization [39–43, 61–63]. However, we cannot be certain that the sampling methods such as those for psychosis criteria were sufficiently robust to avoid bias.

15.6.1 Delusions

15.6.1.1 Studies from the UK

Lucas et al. [35], predating the recent movement toward advocating individual formulation over diagnosis [64] based their research on the assumption that "...a patient's symptoms can often more reliably be identified and more meaningfully related to his *[sic]* social background than can a diagnosis" (p. 748), and examined the content of delusions of inpatients (196 men and 209 women) with a schizophrenia-spectrum disorder diagnosis in context. They based their assumption on previous research [45–47], which found psychotic symptom content to be related to environmental factors. The researchers aimed to investigate whether delusional content could be related in a meaningful way to sociocultural variables. In terms of sex differences, they report that significantly more women than men experienced delusions, and women had a much higher incidence of sexual delusions than men, which occurred more frequently in the married than in the single participants. In order to explore this finding further in terms of a possible influence of cultural gender roles, further analysis of content was conducted although the numbers were small. Prevalent among women, especially those who were single, were paranoid sexual ideas such as what the authors term "imposed intercourse," unusual terminology to say the least, a linguistic usage that perhaps reflects the very cultural gender role stereotypes and norms of the time that the researchers were attempting to examine, conveying the societal acceptability of sexual assault toward women. Women, again particularly those who were single, had a higher rate of delusions of being married, engaged, pregnant or having children. The authors report that the only sexual delusions more prevalent among men were masturbation among the single, and delusions of infidelity among the married. The authors explain these differences in terms of differential gender role norms, prohibitions, and prescriptions regarding sexuality:

> The content appears to reflect the more obvious sexual prohibitions and demands regarding the two sexes in our society—the greater social restrictions on intercourse, for example, in the single females as compared with the single males, the greater pressure on women to conform as regards marriage, and the more explicit condemnation of masturbation in men (p. 757).

Men had almost twice as many delusions of "inferiority," although this difference was not quite statistically significant. The authors defined "inferiority" as "having sinned, for example, or having committed a crime" and point out that many had a more "...depressive colouring...and included ideas of sin or crime, of poverty, and of unworthiness of some kind. Examples were beliefs of being a murderer, of being a thief, and of having blasphemed; such beliefs usually lacked the appropriate affect, or were associated with thought disorder" (p. 750). Interestingly, the authors point out that the trends are occurring in a small number of cases, but suggest that with larger sample sizes and more extensive analysis these differences will be more pronounced and may point to the influence of gender role norms for sexuality on "mental illness." Men had significantly more grandiose delusions of authority and power.

Walston et al. [65] examined sex differences in the content of persecutory delusions, basing their hypothesis that more women would identify familiar people as their persecutors and more men would identify strangers, on evolutionary psychology theory. The authors utilized discharge summaries (11 women and 13 men) as data for their study. They report that their hypothesis was confirmed although note the limitations in drawing any firm conclusions because of the small sample size and point to the cultural influence of gender socialization as possible explanatory factors in the sex differences in content. They recommend future replication with larger, more representative samples including cross-cultural studies and investigating sex differences in the nature of hostile threats. Interestingly, they report no between-sex differences in content and suggest this area for future prospective studies.

15.6.1.2 Studies from the United States

Sherman and Sherman [46], in one of the earliest studies in psychiatry detailing sociocultural variables, not only examined sex but also ethno-racial differences in psychosis content through examination of medical records of approximately 500 adult white and 400 adult black patients. One of the major differences in content was the finding that more men than women experience grandiose delusions. Interestingly, when examining ethnoracial differences, the authors report that while white women's delusional content consisted predominantly of paranoia compared with men, more black men experienced paranoia compared with black women. It must be emphasized that this study was carried out in 1934 where, as the authors note, men's participation in public life was far greater than women's. Therefore, the reverse finding with regard to paranoia being more prevalent among black men compared with black women may be due to black men's greater social participation than black women and thus greater exposure to victimization owing to discrimination and racism. The authors' explanation for grandiose delusions foreshadows the notion of normalization which views psychotic experiences on a continuum with ordinary experiences. In addition, the authors acknowledge the importance of the sociocultural context in shaping psychosis content:

> Grandiose delusions are probably among the most simple forms of escape from and compensation for, difficulties and frustrations which the individual is unable to overcome. In the ordinary daydreams of children and adults, and in their planning for the future, we see the mechanism of grandiose delusions, but it is under control. Grandiose delusions also give us insight into the ideals of the individual, and into the goals set by the cultural situation (p. 341).

They also report differences in the delusional content of American men, which emphasizes wealth; of foreign-born men which focuses on literary and of artistic talent; and of blacks where religious content is more predominant. The authors also looked at birthplace and found the highest rate of paranoid ideation among foreign-born whites. They also found that paranoid delusions were more prevalent among blacks from the more competitive northern regions and among individuals with little education, whereas grandiose delusions predominated among the college educated. Sherman and Sherman [46] also reported that hallucinations were more common among women than men and much more common among blacks than whites. However, the criteria for their broad diagnostic groups were not clearly defined.

Rudden et al. [43] compared the presentation of 44 men and 44 women, with delusions in addition to mania and depression according to DSM-III criteria, through examining delusion content, attendant symptomatology, and ease of diagnosis using patient charts. This study examined sex differences in phenomenology in order to understand sex differences in psychodynamic conflicts, and biological and sociocultural roles with the ultimate aim of improving diagnosis. The authors suggest that such empirical investigation of these differences is important because of the probability of sex biases in descriptions of clinical disorders, which are usually based on the observation of male patients. In their investigation, in terms of delusion content, they found sex differences only with regard to those related to sexual themes and/or erotomania. Erotomania refers to the persistent delusion of being loved from afar by another person [66]. The authors report that significantly more women had heterosexual erotic delusions and delusions of rape, impregnation or venereal disease, whereas significantly more men had homosexual erotic delusions, findings reported by several investigators [39, 63, 67–69]. The finding that more men reported delusions with homosexual themes and in particular, delusions centering on aggression by a male hostile figure, has been described by Rudden and colleagues [43] as a "male prototype of paranoid phenomenology," which the authors state "...has led to psychodynamic explanations that emphasize denied and projected homosexual impulses" (p. 1575). With psychodynamic theory not yet having gone out of favor, this interpretation may not be surprising; however, as mentioned previously, in the light of growing research demonstrating clear relationships between sexual abuse and psychosis (including sexual content of hallucinations/delusions predicting abuse histories), and the psychological impact of childhood sexual abuse on sexual identity and gender schemata (as discussed in Ch. 5) other interpretations may be equally valid. Other sex differences with regard to delusion content reported by the authors was that for women, more delusions centered around acquaintances, whereas men's delusions tended to be focused on strangers, a finding also repeated in other studies [39, 65, 70, 71]. The authors also reported that both sexes had many more male objects in their delusions than female and more men had delusions of reference.

The investigators also examined sex differences in precipitants finding that more of the women had interpersonal precipitants recorded in their charts, which included rape, extramarital affairs, and first sexual encounters, which may explain the predominance of delusions with sexual themes in the women although surprisingly this possibility is not suggested by the authors. One quarter of the women and only 13 % of the men had family-related precipitants (e.g., a quarrel with a spouse) recorded in their charts, a finding repeated in other studies [39]. The authors report that women also had significantly higher mean depression scores, significantly more diagnoses that are not well described discrete entities (e.g., atypical psychosis, schizoaffective disorder) and 3 women (and no men) received the diagnosis of atypical psychosis, using DSM-III criteria. The authors draw from sociological, ethological, and psychodynamic models to interpret their findings. For example, drawing on a sociological model, they explain the findings of sexual content differences, psychosocial precipitants for women, and male prevalence of the object of delusions with regard to gender role norms, male dominance, and less stigmatization of homosexuality for women than for men in Western society. They suggest that the predominance of sexual themes in women's delusions is related to self-worth and self-definition derived from roles as wives and mothers. Referring to psychodynamic and ethological frameworks, explanations offered for women's more prevalent sexual delusions include those related to a greater fear of loss of love than men. The authors also suggest that the fact that men are more physically aggressive and thus might be "a more ready symbol of threat or aggression" (p. 1577) helps to explain the greater prevalence of men as objects of persecutory delusions. As mentioned above, surprisingly the authors do not link the objective conditions of violence in these women's lives (i.e., 9.1 % of the women experienced precipitants such as rape and none of the men) to the prevalence of violent sexual delusions in the women (i.e., rape). Thus, for some of these women, male aggression may not be merely a "symbol," but in fact, an actual reality. The overwhelmingly high prevalence of violence against women and the impact of gender-based violence on mental health (WHO), should not be ignored as an important factor related to delusional expression, particularly when considering the recent research findings demonstrating strong links between childhood adversity and victimization and psychosis, as pointed out previously.

Here again we see how SGBA may have enhanced the methodology by taking life context into consideration in addition to incorporating a macro-level analysis of social structural factors such as women's increased risk for exposure to sexual violence.

15.6.1.3 Studies from India

Menon, Cornelio, and Saraswathy emphasize the prominence of socio-cultural roles, such as gender and occupational status in influencing sex differences in mental disorders. In a retrospective study, they examined all case records of patients over 18 years of age in a Government Mental Hospital in Madras, focusing on the documentation of delusions [63]. Of the 1,973 records examined from case notes over a period of 18 years registered during the year 1976, 1,219 were male and 754 female. Of the 214 records that documented delusions, 142 were male and 72 female. The majority of patients were diagnosed with schizophrenia, then affective disorders, and very few "puerperal and toxic" cases. Consistent with other studies, Menon and colleagues report that grandiose delusions regarding extraordinary wealth and power are more common among men than women. They also report the finding that women's delusions tend to be vague and "culture-bound," which they explain as possibly being related to a lack of education as the majority of women were illiterate, much less well educated than the men, and came from rural areas (p. 93). In their sample, significantly more men experienced what the authors termed "hypochondriacal" delusions such as "rotting or drying up of body parts" and more persecutory delusions than the women (p. 94). For women who were single, the authors report that there was a prevalence of what the authors describe as "persecutory delusions with erotic feelings," which may refer to erotomania, but no other details are provided (p. 94). Typically, more women than men were married and the majority of women in the sample were married. With regard to other demographic differences, the men were younger, more literate, and more frequently had outside employment.

Also in India, Kala and Wig [72], employing a sample of 200 (male $n = 107$; female $n = 93$) outpatients of a general hospital psychiatric clinic with a diagnosis of schizophrenia or "paranoid state," examined delusional content and frequency using the Present State Examination, adapting it according to the patient's linguistic and educational background. The majority of the sample ($n = 190$) had a diagnosis of schizophrenia. The main sex differences reported were that women were more likely to develop delusions of infidelity (i.e., taken to be present when the patient, on specific questioning, expressed a belief that one's spouse was having an extra-marital sexual affair, and when such a belief was of delusional quality and intensity), whereas men more often had grandiose delusions and delusions of thought reading. The authors interpret this finding as being related to gender relations and gender role norms in India, whereby women are granted lower social status than men and are expected to be submissive. They explain:

> In India, while extra-marital sex for males is considered just careless and irresponsible behavior, for females it is a grave moral transgression. It seems to be much easier for a woman to believe that her husband is having an affair than it is for a man to believe the same in respect of his wife (p.192).

They also examined differences according to age, urban vs rural, first vs last born, geographic mobility, family type, and SES. They point to social rank as also underlying their findings that delusions of persecution are higher in last-born individuals, whereas grandiose delusions are higher in first-borns. A similar pattern was reported with regard to SES, urban vs rural, and education, in which two distinct profiles emerged: one of wealthy, urban, educated, and male where grandiose delusions were more common, versus poor, rural, illiterate, and female, where persecutory and delusions of bodily control were more prevalent, a finding very similar to Suhail's study of men and women in Pakistan discussed below [73] and the previous study by Menon and colleagues in India [63].

15.6.1.4 Studies from Pakistan

In addition to analyzing sex and gender in delusional content, Suhail in 2003, using a structured interview, the Present State Examination, also examined social class, interviewing 48 men and 50 women with a schizophrenia diagnosis in Pakistan [73]. Two distinct profiles emerged: one rich and male with grandiose delusions being more prevalent; the other poor and female with persecutory delusions more common. Themes of grandiosity (e.g., being a star and having physical and psychic powers) were more prevalent among men and economically advantaged patients, whereas themes of black magic, fantasy lovers, persecution, and being controlled were more prevalent in the female and poor subgroup. Suhail interprets this finding as a manifestation of the helplessness perceived by women and the lower classes. Analysis of the content of religious delusions revealed that men have more delusions where they have a special relationship and communication with God. A greater number of patients of lower social class believed that someone was trying to harm, hurt or attack them, whereas patients of higher social class believed people were jealous of them and their possessions. Ideas of being controlled especially bodily movements and actions were more prevalent in the women and lower class subgroup than the male and higher social class group. Suhail suggests that:

> ...the development of such ideas in certain subgroups is no exception in a culture where women are granted a secondary social role and where large economic and social gaps exist

> between higher and lower social strata. Moreover, submissive behaviour is expected from both of [sic] groups (p. 198).

Suhail draws direct links between life experiences and delusional content, pointing out that the majority of erotomanic women had a low social status and were experiencing psychosocial stressors such as marital disputes, beliefs that their husbands were not interested in them, and suspicions that their husbands were having extra-marital affairs. It may be that erotomanic ideas reflect the sociocultural context for Pakistani women of a lower social class where infidelity and the possibility of separation is much more threatening as the women are not financially independent. The author also suggests that the excess of erotomanic ideas in women may reflect the suppression of any type of sexual activity of women (but not of men) in Pakistani society and could be viewed as a struggle between their own desires and the cultural gender proscriptions. Suhail reports that the finding that erotomanic ideas are seen more in women than in men is consistent with studies with patients in other countries, citing studies from the UK [35], Malaysia [74], and Saudi Arabia [75]. Sex differences were also found in the content of persecutory delusions where men more often perceived persecutors as friends, whereas for women, they were family members, a similar finding reported by other researchers as noted above [43, 70, 71]. The author also explains this difference by pointing to differences in gender role expectations of men and women in India such that "women have to keep themselves confined to family affairs while men are expected to venture outside to face challenges of a harsh world" (p. 198). This study is a good example for demonstrating the usefulness of SGBA as when the sample was analyzed as a whole, the delusion of persecution was most common followed by grandiose identity. However, when it was divided according to sex and social class the two subgroups emerged from the analysis.

15.6.1.5 Studies from Greece

From clinical practice as a psychiatrist in Greece, Kazamias [76] noted that his men patients expressed more grandiose delusions than his women patients. He investigated this impression more systematically through examination of the case notes of 50 patients (25 women and 25 men) and interviews of 43 (23 women and 20 men) of the 50 with diagnoses of paranoid schizophrenia and paranoid psychosis for confirmation of written accounts in the case records. He found that the investigation supported his initial impression and reported that in 14 of the men patients but only 1 of the women, grandiose delusions were evident. The author categorized delusions as grandiose if they were "concerned with the possession by the patient of exceptional or supernatural qualities or abilities" (p. 229). Content of delusions for the men involved the belief that they were great scientists, writers and/or thinkers with a great mission to carry out, great politicians or royalties, or God. The woman patient believed that she was Virgin Mary, Mother of God. For the majority of patients who experienced persecutory delusions, the persecutors were external to the family. There were no sex differences in this regard.

15.6.1.6 Studies from Australia

Allan and Hafner also explain their findings of sex differences in delusional content as being shaped by gender role norms [39]. In fact, they state: "In many respects the form and content of the delusions mirror with surprising accuracy aspects of prevailing sex-role stereotypes" (p. 48). They examined case notes of 30 women and 30 men with a DSM-III diagnosis of schizophrenic disorder and found that significantly more men reported grandiose delusions with sub-categories of social status, psychological strength, and sexual power. The authors note that the structure of grandiose delusions "...mirror aspects of the patients' social environment" (p. 48) with women's special powers conferred on them by others or exercised vicariously through association with powerful or famous men. Conversely, men were more often subjects (as opposed to objects as were the women in this sample) in their grandiose delusions and acquired their powers directly from being God or Jesus or having special skills or knowledge for the benefit of humankind. Another interesting difference was that the content of these grandiose delusions was nearly always positive for men, but for the minority of women who had grandiose delusions, their attributes nearly always described destructive effects such as floods, plagues, earthquakes or World War II. Furthermore, men were more likely to be the persecutors in women's delusions and, as reported in other studies, were more likely to be personally known by the women than the men. Significantly more women experienced delusions of jealousy, the majority concerning infidelity of a husband or partner. Again as with several other investigators cited previously, Allan and Hafner also report that in their sample the men had many more homosexual persecutory delusions than did the women. In addition to reporting sex differences in delusional content, Allan and Hafner, as with the previous cited study by Rudden et al. [43], additionally reported that the women in their sample were significantly more likely to have experienced severe or extreme psychosocial stress, which in about 80 % of cases was related to marital or family conflict [39]. In addition, the authors found that the level of functioning for women was significantly higher than for men in the year before admission, with 24 of the men scoring at the poor, very poor, or grossly disorganized level on Axis V of the DSM-III. While the above studies acknowledge that gender and social environment play a role in the expression of delusions, the authors do not directly link life experiences to these psychotic phenomena.

15.6.1.7 Studies from Germany

Musalek et al. [71] examined sex and age differences in delusional content by examining case records of 865 patients in Germany (authors do not report *n*-sizes for men and women) with varying diagnoses from schizophrenia spectrum disorders to bipolar and personality disorders. These authors emphasize the importance of life history and existential concerns, which are different for men and women. They hypothesize that these concerns correspond to differential developmental stages in the expression of delusions although they did not collect data on life history, psychosocial stressors or precipitants. Musalek and colleagues found that the delusion of love was noted almost exclusively in women (91.3 % of their sample), and not after the age of 50. They also report that the theme of persecution occurred significantly later in women than in men (age 41–50 for women; 21–30 for men) and was more predominant in women (62.5 % for women and 37.5 % for men). Interestingly, in this sample, the theme of jealousy was mostly found in men (69.2 % for men; 30.8 % for women) and peaked at age 41–50, with more than two-thirds developing the delusion after age 40 and only 8.6 % before age 30. This finding is in contrast to that of Allan and Hafner in Australia [39], Kala and Wig in India [72], and Gecici et al. in Turkey [68], who found that delusional jealousy was experienced predominantly by women in their samples.

15.6.1.8 Studies from Vienna

Gutiérrez-Lobos et al. [77] investigated links among age, sex, diagnoses with delusional content. Their sample consisted of 639 (men = 239, women = 400) first-admitted patients in Vienna from 1971 to 1974. Diagnoses, according to ICD-8, included: schizophrenia = 295; affective psychosis = 296; organic psychosis = 290–294; paranoid states 298, and other disorders = 297.

Similar to other studies reviewed here, women presented with more persecutory delusions than men and were older upon admission; men presented with significantly more delusions of grandiosity and unlike other studies with the exception of the previous study by Musalek and colleagues, with delusions of jealousy. They also reported that delusions were not specific to schizophrenia diagnoses in their sample, concluding that other symptomatology is required for a schizophrenia diagnosis [77].

15.6.1.9 Studies from Turkey

Gecici and colleagues, recognizing that the content of psychotic phenomena is likely to be influenced by social and cultural factors, point out that "...no culture is homogeneous and even within the same culture, there are different status classes, age and sex groups characterized by specific customs, social roles, and religious affiliations" (p. 204) and thus investigated differences in the content of delusions and hallucinations according to sex and geographic location within Turkey by examining case notes of 158 women and 215 men from Western and Central regions of Turkey, with a total of 346 experiencing delusions [68]. They reported that women experienced more delusions of poisoning and erotomania than male patients (21.5 % and 8.2 % respectively). Other sex differences in content reported were delusions of jealousy being more prevalent among women, objects of delusions tended to be family or neighbors in women, whereas they were strangers for men, consistent with previously reported studies. The authors explain this difference as related to gender role socialization, similar to Suhail's explanation of his findings in Pakistan cited previously, i.e. women are socialized to play the major role in child care domestic tasks limited to the home and conversely men are socialized to work in the public sphere. Delusions of physical/mental injury were more predominant among men and in the Western region of Turkey. Delusions with a religious theme were also more common in men and in Central Turkey. The content of these delusions concerned being controlled by the devil and were often treated by exorcism. Again similar with these findings, the authors report that grandiose delusions were more prevalent among men than women and among men from Central Turkey, which is more economically advantaged. Themes of these delusions consisted of being a star or important person and physical and psychic powers. Gecici and colleagues found no sex differences in hallucination themes. Demographic sex differences reported were women having less higher education than men, being more likely to be unemployed, having fewer hospitalizations than men (less than half) and more likely to be married.

All of the above studies reviewed here reporting on erotomanic content, found that the prevalence of delusions of erotomania were significantly higher in women than men [39, 43, 62, 63, 67–69, 71]. In fact, Kraepelin observed over a century ago that women exhibited more heterosexual delusions than men [78]. The incidence of erotomania is not known, but that of delusional disorder in general has been reported to be approximately 15 cases per 100,000 of the population per year, with a female:male ratio of 3:1 [79]. In a Japanese study by Yamada et al. of 4,144 first-time attendees at a psychiatric clinic, of the 1.2 % diagnosed with delusional disorder, women outnumbered men by a ratio of 3:1 [80]. Historically, the excess of erotomania in women was so marked that it was suggested that the condition occurred almost exclusively in women [79].

A limitation of the above studies reviewed is that the description of content is superficial (most studies do not describe specific individual content) and decontextualized (no explicit explanation of psychosocial history, narrative of individual life experiences or sociocultural context) with the exception of the study by Suhail in Pakistan [73], which examines social class and two other studies reporting on interpersonal precipitants [39, 43, 81] in their paper on childhood abuse and content of psychotic phenomena, recommend employing qualitative methodologies to generate this kind of data where open-ended questioning generates narrative accounts. Using qualitative methodology, Rhodes and Jakes found that delusional content for the 14 men and women in their sample (numbers for each sex are not reported) reflected fundamental life concerns and personal goals, though they did not examine sex differences per se [82]. The primary goal categories that the investigators report were expressed in the delusions of the participants in their sample: (1) Social: any goal related to social relationships was the most prominent (2) Competence: goals related to achievement and work as well as travel and hobbies (3) Experiential: goals to avoid physical or mental pain or suffering and the desire for the opposite of these (e.g., calm, relaxation, good feelings) (4) Material base: any goal related to acquiring money or accommodation, although the authors report that this was not often listed (5) Direction: refers to feeling directionless, but desiring a sense of direction or focus in life (6) Evaluation: refers to self-evaluations (or self-schema in terms of a cognitive psychological framework, although the authors do not define it as such) and self-evaluations in comparison to others In the paper, the authors report on only 4 of the 14 participants in their sample: 3 men and 1 woman. They analyze the content of participants' delusions in relation to participants' life experiences and context. While the authors do not compare findings by sex, it is noteworthy that the content of the three men relates to competence, status, and getting a job, whereas the delusional content of the female participant relates primarily to "loneliness" and attachment. However, the primary goal category that was identified in the delusional content in general was social. Rhodes and Jakes discuss the relevance of culture in influencing motivation and goals and also point to the cross-cultural variation of delusional content. As gender is a prominent component of culture, SGBA may have informed their findings further.

15.6.2 Hallucinations

Klaf obtained the records of 75 women with a diagnosis of paranoid schizophrenia comparing them with the records of 100 female nonpsychotic patients with diagnoses of personality disorders and psychophysiological disorders as a control group to investigate the Freudian hypothesis regarding the genesis of paranoid symptoms as a defense against unconscious homosexual wishes with women [62]. He reports that the hallucination and delusional content of the female paranoid group had prominent sexual content and religious preoccupations, but does not elaborate with further details except to indicate that the evidence did not support Freud's hypothesis as almost 84 % of the sexual content was "heterosexual." He also refuted Freud's hypothesis on the basis that the largest percentage of persecutors were male, which is similar to the studies reported below.

Alan and Hafner, similar to reports by other investigators, reported that both the men ($n = 30$) and women ($n = 30$) in their sample identified predominantly more male voices than female [39]. Interestingly, more women in their sample recognized the speaker. The researchers only reported on the content of the delusions of their sample (discussed above) and did not report on the content of hallucinations.

Nayani and David explored the phenomenology of hallucinated voices through semi-structured interviews with 100 patients, the majority of whom had a schizophrenia diagnosis (61 %) [83]. They found that all the patients were more likely to hear a male hallucinated voice than a female and when amalgamating data on age and sex, more likely to hear a middle-aged male voice, followed by a young adult male, and finally by a young adult female. The authors examined content verbatim and found that simple terms of abuse were the most prevalent, occurring in 60 % of the whole sample. They found a clear sex difference in such terms of vilification and abuse, often conveying contempt and anger where: "Female subjects described words of abuse conventionally directed at women (e.g., slut), and 32 male subjects similarly described 'male' insults such as those imputing homosexuality" (p. 182). The main findings regarding characteristics of hallucinated voices are that they are repetitive, emotive, context-driven, spatio-temporally organized, and highly personal.

The finding of the predominance of male hallucinated voices was also found in a qualitative study by Legg and Gilbert [70], who interviewed 10 women and 10 men examining the power and rank of hallucinated voices. They also found that the most common insult for men was sexual and that of being homosexual, whereas for females it was denigrating their appearance and being called "fat and ugly." They also reported that the men in their sample were never called "fat" and there was no homosexual insult for women. Similar to the study by Nayani and David, the content of the voices appears to reflect gender socialized norms [83]. Legg and Gilbert [70] conceptualize the types of derogations by the voices as "a direct social rank challenge designed to undermine confidence and maintain a subordinate position" (p. 523). They report that "... as the voices are experienced as demeaning and devaluing and indicating limitations on aspiration, they fit the dynamics of social rank theory" (p. 525). For both sexes the importance of sexuality, acceptability, and desirability (and their shaming) are highly represented in the voices. Although the authors do not interpret their findings as such, it could be noted that gender socialized prescriptions and proscriptions appear evident in the content for both sexes. Both men and women reported feeling more depressed and frightened when hearing insulting voices. Both male and female participants described feeling shame, degraded, alone and guilty.

The findings of this study alone implicate the significance of gender. However, it would be interesting to see if the study findings might have been more illuminating had the authors adopted SGBA and included gender in their research questions and analysis. In fact, this chapter's author is currently conducting such a study utilizing a mixed method approach.

15.7 Gender and Response to Psychotic Experiences

15.7.1 Interpersonal Relationships and the Social World

Birchwood and colleagues have conducted interesting research examining the relationship individuals experience with their voices, which for many who are distressed by their voices, is characterized by subordination and a sense of powerlessness [84, 85]. Birchwood and colleagues and others more recently [86] found that this subordination by voices parallels subordination by others in the social world. Birrell and Freyd [87] have pointed out that "...although oppression is often institutionalized at societal levels, it is necessarily enacted in the context of interpersonal relationships" (p. 52). Brown [88] also reiterates this perspective when describing feminist conceptualizations of power, which can also be conceptualized as internalized oppression:

> Bias, stereotype, and oppression all constitute social forces that create disempowerment; they can be enacted in the large context of society or culture, the smaller context of family and community and intra-psychically, internalized and felt as part of self (p. 31).

It is not surprising, then, that the experience of subordination by voices has been found to reflect the experience of subordination and marginalization in the social world and hence any attempts at enhancing understanding of both the subjective experience and the external environment would not be complete without an analysis of gender. A gender analysis, considering women's subordinate social status worldwide (WHO) [89] and a hegemonic masculinity that subordinates certain classes of men as well as women (e.g., men of color, sexual minorities), could potentially add to our understanding of the experience of subordination by voices specifically and to the experience and expression of psychotic phenomena in general.

Mary Boyle [90] criticizes the reluctance of the disciplines of psychology, psychiatry, and medicine to entertain the idea that:

> ...psychotic behaviours and experiences are *relational*, that they arise in social and interpersonal contexts that their form and content are given meaning by those contexts and that such behaviours are officially transformed to 'pathology' only through a relationship of unequal power. Context has been consistently marginalised or made secondary by traditional theory through, for example, the vulnerability-stress model which privileges an assumed inherent weakness or defect; through family research which insists on the family's influence only on the 'course of the illness' and through the claim that poverty or low social class are consequences and not antecedents of psychotic experiences (p. 317).

Boyle's argument for the centrality of context in understanding psychosis or other forms of psychological distress, which feminist scholars have long been making since they coined the slogan: "the personal is political," is consistent with Kaschak's work on how sociocultural phenomena are translated into personal experience [91]. The same might be said for psychotic experiences; in essence, they are a translation of sociocultural phenomena, which includes components of gender socialization. This perspective may help articulate, how Aschebrock's participants in 2005, in her qualitative exploration of women's experiences of delusions and hallucinations, "choose[s]" between "competing frames of reference" or "interpretive repertoires" (p. 121) when trying to make sense of and explain these phenomena. This process can also be elucidated by a cognitive psychological approach in which one's schemata or core beliefs about self, others/world, and future influence the appraisals one makes for various experiences. These schemata, or internal mental representations, are developed through life experience and shaped by culture, of which gender socialization is a critical component. Several of Aschebrock's participants explain their delusions/hallucinations as being related to trauma and "insecurity" or "low self-esteem" or self-schema. Although Aschebrock did not conduct a gender analysis per se, we can see how Bem's concept of gender schema could be relevant here.

The translation of sociocultural phenomena into personal experience provides another rationale for exploring subjectivity and utilizing qualitative methods in which participants are given voice to identify aspects of their lives and social and interpersonal contexts of which researchers may not have even conceived, let alone considered relevant. Furthermore, utilizing a qualitative method of analysis that incorporates grounded theory is consistent with Collins' definition of "interpretive theorizing," in which she suggests that the social can be found in the individual to expand the reach or scope of the developing theory. As observed previously, it is not surprising then, to find that social relationships are reflected not only in the content of an individual's hallucinated voices and "delusional" beliefs, but also in the relationship one has with their voices. Similarly, One would also expect gender relations and meanings to be reproduced in both the content and relationship one has with their voices.

Similarly, Jenkins [92], a medical anthropologist has argued that:

> ... (1) the subjective experience of persons with schizophrenia is forged at the nexus of culture and agency, desire and attachment, none of which are annulled by disease process; and (2) the study of schizophrenia casts a bright light on our understanding of culture and subjectivity more generally (p. 30).

Jenkins points out how earlier theorists in the 1920s, such as Edward Sapir and Harry Stack Sullivan, from the fields of anthropology and psychiatry respectively, have claimed that we can learn much about culture from the behavior of a person diagnosed with schizophrenia as well as from their subjective experience. In fact, it is how experience is interpreted that is shaped by culture. She explains: "Sapir's dynamic formulation of culture as created and recreated among persons in the process of social interaction paralleled Sullivan's (1953:10) conception of psychiatry as the study of interpersonal relations under any and all circumstances in which these relations exist" (p. 32)

15.7.2 Gender and Recovery

Sells et al. [93], in their review of qualitative research on recovery in schizophrenia, point out that: "Evidence suggests that recovery of an active and effective sense of self as a social agent may play a crucial role in improvement from schizophrenia" (p. 88). Schön, in a qualitative study, found that gender constructions and differential gender role expectations have a beneficial influence on recovery in women [24]. A total of 30 participants were interviewed dividing the sample equally between male and female informants. Many of the men in the sample have internalized masculine gender roles regarding the importance of independence, the prominence of work, and the ability to support themselves, leading to a greater discrepancy between gender role norms and their own ability to meet these norms or what could be termed gender role strain, which had a negative impact on the recovery process. Consistent with other studies, the women interviewed functioned better because of increased social support via a social network and differential gender role norms where there is more acceptance of dependency on family and society in comparison to men, in addition to lower expectations for women concerning work and studies. The male participants, on the other hand, were living a life quite different from that of other men in society, thus contributing to a sense of inadequacy and not feeling like a "normal man" (p. 563). Schön explains that in a Scandinavian context, for many men, work is still an integral part of their gender identity, it is for them: "what life is all about" (p. 563).

15.7.3 Summary

What seems quite clear from this review of the few studies that do examine content and sex differences in psychotic experiences is what Sherman and Sherman theorized as early as 1934; namely, that psychotic phenomena may be meaningfully related to sociocultural variables and in particular gender [46]. For example, this review has revealed that the pattern, formation, and content of delusions and hallucinations are shaped by various factors—such as age, sex, marital status, racial and cultural background, education, and social class. Many of the reported sex differences in hallucination and delusional content are related to sexuality and are more prevalent among women, which is not surprising in the light of the differential gender socialization of men and women with regard to control of one's sexuality [94], as well as recent research findings linking childhood sexual abuse and psychosis with women experiencing a greater incidence of sexual abuse according to the few studies examining sex differences in abuse [95, 96]. Furthermore, several studies have found that sexual content in hallucinations or delusions is related to a history of sexual abuse [81, 97, 98].

From the studies reviewed here, originating from several countries, the interaction of multiple factors with gender in shaping the phenomenology and expression of psychotic experiences is apparent. Consistent findings across countries, such as grandiose delusions being more prevalent among men and persecutory delusions among women could arguably be interpreted as possible evidence for underlying biological sex factors. However, in the light of cross-cultural studies demonstrating that gender role stereotypes are pan-cultural with differences mostly in terms of degree as opposed to kind [99, 100] together with social role theory [101], and empirical evidence of the universality of gender inequality and gender-based violence against women (WHO) [89], these findings could be interpreted as providing compelling evidence for the influence of environmental factors. In particular, the studies from Pakistan, Turkey [68], Greece [76], and India [63, 70], where gender inequality is more pronounced and women are poorer, less well educated, and more isolated in terms of being excluded from participation in the public domain than men, such lower social status, rank, social exclusion, and social deprivation is reflected in psychotic phenomena. These studies demonstrate how the lens of gender is ideal for examining the interaction of micro-level (individual/intrapsychic) and macro-level (social/structural) factors in the development, presentation, and experience of psychotic phenomena. Furthermore, they illustrate the significance of SGBA incorporating an intersectionality approach.

Conclusion

Sadly, this review has not been able to meet the title's promise of providing the reader with *everything* they have always wanted to know about sex and gender in psychosis. Rather, it has illustrated that we are very far indeed from knowing "everything" (although one could argue that this is the case for all scientific inquiry: see Popper, 1963/2004) about sex and gender in psychosis, but instead know very little at all, making the case for SGBA.

One of the main themes emerging in much of what has been reviewed in this chapter is the centrality of relations and context, both interpersonal and socio-cultural, from the intrapsychic to the institutional level, with regard to the development and expression of psychotic experiences and recovery for people diagnosed with schizophrenia. As Ratner and Sawatzky contend: "...Gender must be understood in context; gender is merely a mental representation that must acquire its content or meaning from context" (p. 82) [102]. Similarly, we could assert that psychotic phenomena must also be understood in context and derive their content or meaning from context. Thus, we can see how SGBA is not only ideal, but critical for examining the interaction of micro-level and macro-level factors mentioned above. Furthermore, SGBA may help to explain some of the many inconsistent findings with regard to sex differences and illuminate the underlying mechanisms, which heretofore have remained illusive.

Sex- and gender-based analysis examines the complex interactive contributions of biological, psychosocial, and cultural factors, avoiding the tendency of biological determinism to attribute unidirectional causation [103]. The analysis of multiple structural forms of oppression through SGBA would allow testing of hypotheses and measurement of how other social determinants such as ethnicity or class interact with gender and further explain the development, enactment, and experience of psychosis. Of course, SGBA will not help us know everything about sex and gender in psychosis, but at the very least, it has the potential to guide us in the direction of being able to discover more than we know now.

References

1. Mendrek A. Sex and gender differences in mental health research. In: Cohen S, Banister E, editors. What a difference sex and gender make: a gender, sex and health research casebook. Ottawa: Institute of Gender and Health of the Canadian Institutes of Health Research; 2012.
2. Abel KM, Drake R, Goldstein JM. Sex differences in schizophrenia. Int Rev Psychiatry. 2010;22(5):417–28.
3. Falkenburg J, Tracy DK. Sex and schizophrenia: a review of gender differences. Psychos Psychol Soc Integr Approaches 2012;6(1):1–9.
4. Kulkarni J, Gavrilidis E. Psychosis in women: gender differences in presentation, onset, course and outcome of schizophrenia. In: Women and health (pp. 1283–1291). 2nd ed.; 2013.
5. Leung A, Chue P. Sex differences in schizophrenia, a review of the literature. Acta Psychiatr Scand. 2000;101:3–38.
6. McGrath J, Saha S, Chant D, Welham J. Schizophrenia: a concise overview of incidence, prevalence, and mortality. Epidemiol Rev. 2008;30:67–76.
7. Riecher-Rössler A, Hafner H Gender aspects in schizophrenia: bridging the border between social and biological psychiatry. Acta Psychiatr Scand. 2000;102:58–62.
8. Seeman MV. Gender. In: Mueser KT, Jeste DV, editors. Clinical handbook of schizophrenia. New York: Guilford; 2008.
9. Iacono WG, Beiser M. Are males more likely than females to develop schizophrenia? Am J Psychiatry. 1992;I49:1070–4.
10. Iacono WG, Beiser M. Where are the women in first-episode studies of schizophrenia? Schizophr Bull. 1992;18:471–80.

11. McGrath JJ, Susser ES. New directions in the epidemiology of schizophrenia. Med J Aust. 2009;190(4):S7–9.
12. Thorup A, Waltoft BL, Pedersen CB, Mortense PB, Nordentoft M. Young males have a higher risk of developing schizophrenia: a Danish register study. Psychol Med. 2007;37:479–84.
13. Wahl OF, Hunter J. Are gender effects being neglected in schizophrenia research? Schizophr Bull. 1992;18(2):313–7.
14. Lewine RR. Sex: an imperfect marker of gender. Schizophr Bull. 1994;20(4):777–9.
15. Castle DJ, Wessley S, Murray RM. Sex and schizophrenia: effects of diagnostic stringency, and associations with premorbid variables. Br J Psychiatry. 1993;162:658–64.
16. Thorup A, Petersen L, Jeppesen P, Ohlenschlæger J, Christensen T, Krarup G, Jorgensen P, Nordentoft M. Gender differences in young adults with first-episode schizophrenia spectrum disorders at baseline in the Danish OPUS study. J Nerv Ment Dis. 1997;195:396–405.
17. Aleman A, Kahn RS, Selten JP. Sex differences in the risk of schizophrenia: evidence from meta-analysis. Arch Gen Psychiatry. 2003;60:565–71.
18. Saha S, Chant D, Welham J, McGrath J. A systematic review of the prevalence of schizophrenia. PLoS Med. 2005;2:e141.
19. Perala J, Suvisaari J, Saarni SI, Kuoppasalmi K, et al. Lifetime prevalence of psychotic and bipolar I disorders in a general population. Arch Gen Psychiatry. 2007;64(1):19–28.
20. Ezra Susser E, Wanderling J. Epidemiology of nonaffective acute remitting psychosis vs schizophrenia: sex and sociocultural setting. Arch Gen Psychiatry. 1994;51(4):294–301.
21. Chang WC, Tang JY, Hui CL, Chiu CP, Lam MM, Wong GH, Chung DW, Law CW, Tso S, Chan KP, Hung SF, Chen EY. Gender differences in patients presenting with first-episode psychosis in Hong Kong: a three-year follow up study. Aust N Z J Psychiatry. 2011;45:199–205.
22. Nasser EH, Walders N, Jenkins JH. The experience of schizophrenia: what's gender got to do with it? A critical review of the current status ofresearch on schizophrenia. Schizophr Bull. 2002;28(2):351–62.
23. Riecher-Rössler A, Pflüger M, Borgwardt S. Schizophrenia in women. In: Kohen D, editor. Oxford textbook of women and mental health. Oxford: Oxford University Press; 2010. p. 102–14.
24. Schön U. Recovery from severe mental illness, a gender perspective. Scand J Caring Sci. 2010;24:575–80.
25. Kirkbride JB, Errazuriz A, Croudace TJ, et al. Incidence of schizophrenia and other psychoses in England, 1950–2009: a systematic review and meta-analyses. PLoS ONE. 2012;7:e31660.
26. Andia AM, Zisook S, Heaton RK, Hesselink J, Jernigan T, Kuck J, et al. Gender differences in schizophrenia. J Nerv Ment Dis. 1995;183:522–8.
27. Maric N, Krabbendam L, Vollebergh W, de Graaf R, van Os J. Sex differences in symptoms of psychosis in a non-selected, general population sample. Schizophr Res. 2003;63(1–2):89–95.
28. Morgan V, Castle DJ, Jablensky AV. Do women express and experience psychosis differently from men? Aust N Z J Psychiatry. 2008;42:74–82.
29. McGlashan TH, Bardenstein KK. Gender differences in affective, schizoaffective, and schizophrenic disorders. A review. Schizophr Res 1990;3(3):159–72.
30. Verdoux H, van Os J, Maurice-Tison S, Gay B, Salamon R, Bourgeois M. Increased occurrence of depression in psychosis-prone subjects: a follow-up study in primary care settings. Compr Psychiatry. 1999;40:462–8.
31. Garety P, Kuipers E, Fowler D, et al. A cognitive model of the positive symptoms of psychosis. Psychol Med. 2001:31:189–95.
32. Van Os J, Verdoux H, Maurice Tison S, Gay B, Liraud F, Salamon R, Bourgeois M. Self-reported psychosis-like symptoms and the continuum of psychosis. Soc Psychiatry Psychiatr Epidemiol. 1999;34(9):459–63.

33. Al-Issa I. Gender and schizophrenia. In: Al-Issa I, editor. Gender and psychopathology. New York: Academic; 1982. p. 53–77.
34. Cotton S, Lambert M, Schimmelmann BG, Foley DL, Morley KI, McGorry PD, Conus P. Gender differences in premorbid, entry, treatment, and outcome characteristics in a treated epidemiological sample of 661 patients with first episode psychosis. Schizophr Res. 2009;114:17–24.
35. Lucas CJ, Sainsbury P, Collins JG. A social and clinical study of delusions in schizophrenia. J Ment Soc. 1962;108:747–58.
36. Mirowsky J, Ross CE. Paranoia and the structure of powerlessness. Am Sociol Rev. 1983;48:228–39.
37. Ochoa S, Usall J, Cobo J, Labad X, Kulkarni J. Gender differences in schizophrenia and first-episode psychosis: a comprehensive literature review. Schizophr Res Treatment. 2012;2012:1–9.
38. Grossman LS, Harrow M, Rosen C, Faull R, Strauss GP. Sex differences in schizophrenia and other psychotic disorders: a 20-year longitudinal study of psychosis and recovery. Compr Psychiatry. 2008;49(6):523–9.
39. Allan JA, Hafner JR. Sex differences in the phenomenology of schizophrenic disorder. Can J Psychiatr. 1989;34:46–8.
40. Hollander MH, Callahan AS. Erotomania and De Clerambault's Syndrome. Arch Gen Psychiatry. 1975;32:1574–6.
41. Modlin H. Psychodynamics and management of paranoid states in women. Arch Gen Psychiatry. 1963;8:262–8.
42. Raskin DE, Sullivan KE. Erotomania. Am J Psychiatry. 1974;131:1033–5.
43. Rudden M, Sweeney J, Frances A, Gilmore M. A comparison of delusional disorders in women and men. Am J Psychiatry. 1983;140(12):1575–8.
44. Benedict PK, Jacks I. Mental illness in primitive societies. Psychiatry. 1954;17:377–89.
45. Seeman MV. Schizophrenic men and women require different treatment programs. J Psychiatr Treat Eval. 1983;5:143–8.
46. Sherman M, Sherman IC. Psychotic symptoms and social backgrounds. In: Bentley M, Cowdry EV, editors. The problem of mental disorder: a study undertaken by the Committee on psychiatric investigations National research council. New York: McGraw-Hill; 1934. p. 339–45.
47. LaTorre RA. The psychological assessment of gender identity and gender role in schizophrenia. Schizophr Bull. 1976;2(2):266–85.
48. Yap PM. Mental diseases peculiar to certain cultures: a survey of comparative psychiatry. Br J Psychiatry. 1951;97:313–27.
49. Reed MR. The masculinity-femininity dimension in normal and psychotic subjects. J Abnorm Psychol. 1957;55(3):289–94.
50. Levant RF. Research in the psychology of men and masculinity using the gender role strain paradigm as a framework. Am Psychol. 2011;66(8):765–76.
51. O'Neil JM. Summarizing 25 years of research on men's gender role conflict using the gender role conflict scale—new research paradigms and clinical implications. [Review]. Couns Psychol. 2008;36(3):358–445.
52. Pleck JH. The myth of masculinity. Cambridge: MIT Press; 1981.
53. Pleck JH. The gender role strain paradigm: an update. In: Levant RF, Pollack WS, editors. A new psychology of men. New York: Basic Books; 1995.
54. Root MPP. Rethinking racial identity development: an ecological framework. In: Spickard P, Burroughs J, editors. We are a people: narrative in the construction and deconstruction of ethnic identity. Philadelphia, PA: Temple University Press; 2000.
55. Weinstein EA. Cultural aspects of delusion: a psychiatric study of the Virgin Islands. New York: The Free Press of Glencoe, Inc.; 1962.
56. Tolman DL, Impett EA, Tracy AJ, Michael A. Looking good, sounding good: femininity ideology and adolescent girls' mental health. Psychol Women Q. 2006;30(1):85–95.

57. Sajatovic M, Jenkins J, Strauss M, Butt Z, Carpenter E. Gender identity among men and women with schizophrenia. Psychiatr Serv. 2005;56(1):96–8.
58. Barrett AE, White HR. Trajectories of gender role orientations in adolescence and early adulthood: a prospective study of the mental health effects of masculinity and femininity. J Health Soc Behav. 2002;43:451–68.
59. Johnson JL, Greaves L, Repta R. Better science with sex and gender: a primer for health research. Vancouver: Women's Health Research Network; 2007. p. 557–64.
60. Whitely BE. Sex-role orientation and psychological wellbeing: two meta-analyses. Sex Roles. 1984;12:207–25.
61. Arieti S. An overview of schizophrenia from a predominately psychological approach. Am J Psychiatr. 1974;131:241–9.
62. Klaf FS. Female homosexuality and paranoid schizophrenia. Arch Gen Psychiatry. 1961;1:84–6.
63. Menon SM, Cornelio N, Saraswathy K. Delusions—a study in sex differences. Int J Soc Psychiatry. 1980;26:93–8.
64. Kinderman P, Read J, Moncrieff J, Bentall RP. Drop the language of disorder. Evid Based Ment Health. 2013;16:2–3.
65. Walston F, David AS, Charlton BG. Sex differences in the content of persecutory delusions: a reflection of hostile threats in the ancestral environment? Evol Human Behav. 1998;19:257–60.
66. Segal JH. Erotomania revisited: from Kraepelin to DSM-III-R. Am J Psychiatry. 1989;146 (10):1261–6.
67. Galdos P, van Os J. Gender, psychopathology, and development: From puberty to early adulthood. Schizophr Res. 1995;14:105–12.
68. Gecici O, et al. Phenomenology of delusions and hallucinations in patients with schizophrenia. Bull Clin Psychopharmacol. 2010;20:204–12.
69. Klaf FS, Davis CA. Homosexuality and paranoid schizophrenia: a survey of 150 cases and controls. Am J Psychiatr. 1960;116:1070–5.
70. Legg L, Gilbert P. A pilot study of gender of voice and gender of voice hearer in psychotic voice hearers. Psychol Psychother. 2006;79:517–27.
71. Musalek M, Berner P, Katschnig H. Delusional theme, sex and age. Psychopathology. 1989;22(5):260–7.
72. Kala AK, Wig NN. Delusion across cultures. Int J Soc Psychiatry. 1982;28(3):185–93.
73. Suhail K. Phenomenology of delusions in Pakistani patients: effect of gender and social class. Psychopathology. 2003;36(4):195–9.
74. Azhar MZ, Verma SL, Hakim HR. Phenomenological differences of delusions between schizophrenic patients of two cultures of Malaysia. Singapore Med J. 1995;36:273–5.
75. El-Assra A. Erotomania in a Saudi woman. Br J Psychiatry. 1989;155:553–5.
76. Kazamias NG. Sex difference in the incidence of grandiose delusions in paranoid patients in Greece. Int J Soc Psychiatry. 1970;16(3):228–31.
77. Gutiérrez-Lobos B, Schmid-Siegel B, Bankier B, Walter H. Delusions in first-admitted patients: gender, themes and diagnoses. Psychopathology. 2001;34:1–7.
78. Goldstein JM. The impact of gender on understanding the epidemiology of schizophrenia. In: Seeman MV, editor. Gender and Psychopathology. Washington, DC: American Psychiatric Press, Inc.; 1995.
79. Kelly BD. Erotomania: epidemiology and management. CNS Drugs. 2005;19(8):657–69.
80. Yamada N, Nakajima S, Noguchi T. Age at onset of delusional disorder is dependent on the delusional theme. Acta Psychiatr Scand. 1998;97:122–4.
81. Reiff M, Castille DM, Muenzenmaier K, Link B. Childhood Abuse and the content of adult psychotic symptoms. Psychol Trauma. 2012;4:356–69.
82. Rhodes JE, Jakes S. Correspondence between delusions and personal goals: A qualitative analysis. Br J Med Psychol. 2000;73:211–25.

83. Nayani TH, David AS. The auditory hallucination: a phenomenological survey. Psychol Med. 1996;26(01):177–89.
84. Birchwood M, Gilbert P, Gilbert J, Trower P, Meaden A, Hay J, Miles JNV. Interpersonal and role-related schema influence the relationship with the dominant 'voice' in schizophrenia: a comparison of three models. Psychol Med. 2004;34(08):1571–80.
85. Birchwood M, Meaden A, Trower P, Gilbert J, Plainstow J. The power and omnipotence of voices and significant others. Psychol Med. 2000;30(2):337–44.
86. Hayward M, Berry K, Ashton A. Applying interpersonal theories to the understanding of and therapy for auditory hallucinations: a review of the literature and directions for further research. Clin Psychol Rev. 2011;31(8):1313–23.
87. Birrell PJ, Freyd JJ. Betrayal trauma: relational models of harm and healing. J Trauma Pract. 2006;5(1):49–63.
88. Brown LS. Feminist therapy Washington, DC: American Psychological Association; 2009.
89. World Health Organization. Gender in mental health research report. 2004. Geneva: Author. Available at: http://whqlibdoc.who.int/publications/2004/9241592532.pdf?ua=1. Accessed 29/03/2011.
90. Boyle M. Schizophrenia: a scientific delusion? 2nd ed. London: Routledge; 2002.
91. Kaschak E. Engendered lives. New York: Basic Books; 1992.
92. Jenkins JH. Schizophrenia as a paradigm case for understanding fundamental human processes. Cambr Stud Med Anthropol. 2004;11:29–61.
93. Sells DJ, Staynor DL, Davidson L. Recovering the self in schizophrenia: an integrative review of qualitative studies. Psychiatry Q. 2004;75(1):87–97.
94. Leaper C. The social construction and socialization of gender during development. In: Miller PH, Kofsky-Scholmick E, editors. Toward a feminist developmental psychology. Florence, KY: Taylor & Francis/Routledge; 2000. p. 127–52.
95. Bebbington PE, Jonas S, Kuipers E, King M, Cooper C, Brugha T, Meltzer H, McManus S, Jenkins R. Sexual abuse and psychosis: data from an English National survey. Br J Psychiatry. 2011;199:29–37.
96. Fisher H, Morgan C, Dazzan P, Craig T, Morgan K, Hutchinson G, Jones PB, Doody GA, Pariente C, McGuffin P, Murray RM, Leff J, Fearon P. Gender differences in the association between childhood abuse and psychosis. Br J Psychiatry. 2009;194:319–25.
97. Beck JC, van der Kolk B. Reports of childhood incest and current behavior of chronically hospitalized psychotic women. Am J Psychiatr. 1987;144:1474–6.
98. Hardy A, Fowler D, Freeman D, Smith B, Steel C, Evans J, et al. Trauma and hallucinatory experience in psychosis. J Nerv Ment Dis. 2005;193:501–7.
99. Rudman LA, Glick P. The social psychology of gender: how power and intimacy shape gender relations. New York: The Guilford Press; 2008.
100. Williams JE, Satterwhite RC, Best DL. Pancultural gender stereotypes revisited: the five factor, Health Organization. (Undated) Gender and women's mental health; 1999
101. Eagly AH, Wood W. The origins of sex differences in human behaviour: evolved dispositions versus social roles. American Psychologist. 1999;54(6):408–23.
102. Ratner PA, Sawatzky RG. Approaches to the measurement of gender. In: Oliffe JL, Greaves L, editors. Designing and conducting gender, sex, and health research. Los Angeles: Sage; 2012. p. 65–84.
103. Read J, Bentall RP, Fosse R. Time to abandon the bio-bio-bio model of psychosis: exploring the epigenetic and psychological mechanisms by which adverse life events lead to psychotic symptoms. Epidemiol Psychiatr Soc. 2009;18(4):299–310.

16 Psychopathology, Art, and Gender

María del Río Diéguez and Belén Sanz-Aránguez Ávila

Abstract

The intention of this chapter is to show how the artistic medium brings an experiential framework into play. This framework facilitates the integration of sensorial, affective, cognitive, and relational elements, wherein it is possible to address some of the difficulties derived from the patriarchal structure inherent to Western societies.

Many of the creative processes developed within the framework of the therapeutic device we are proposing, which have proven to be key in initiating significant individual subjectivity, must be observed from a gender perspective to be understood, and addressed from that "network of beliefs, personality traits, attitudes, values, behaviours and activities that differentiate men from women." We take these processes, insofar as they are discursive inscriptions allowing formulas to be reframed with regard to power, control, and regulation which, a priori, seem to be unshakeable, as the axes of our presentation.

16.1 Introduction

The intent of this chapter is to show how the artistic medium brings an experiential framework into play. This framework facilitates the integration of sensorial, affective, cognitive, and relational elements, wherein it is possible to address some of the difficulties derived from the patriarchal structure inherent to Western societies.

M. del Río Diéguez (✉)
Autónoma University of Madrid, Madrid, Spain
e-mail: maria.delrio@uam.es

B. Sanz-Aránguez Ávila
University Hospital Puerta de Hierro Majadahonda, Madrid, Spain
e-mail: belenosanz@terra.com

M. Sáenz-Herrero (ed.), *Psychopathology in Women*,
DOI 10.1007/978-3-319-05870-2_16

Many of the creative processes developed within the framework of the therapeutic device we are proposing, which have proven to be key in initiating significant individual subjectivity, must be observed from a gender perspective to be understood, and addressed from that "network of beliefs, personality traits, attitudes, values, behaviours and activities that differentiate men from women" [1]. We take these processes, insofar as they are discursive inscriptions allowing formulas regarding power, control, and regulation to be reframed, which, a priori, seem to be unshakeable, as the axes of our presentation.

We show these processes through several clinical examples; however, before doing so, we must pause and consider a few aspects.

16.2 Artistic Languages

Because of their liberalizing condition and illogical nature, artistic languages are excellent pathways to developing personal, singular interpersonal, flexible, and capacitating resources; they bring one to unusual levels of conscience, unlike those in which meaning tends to be given to problems, and they promote the development of individual subjectivity based on positions of self-determination, freedom, and spontaneity.

The artistic medium is symbolically and factually engraved in that which is real, both as a language and as an action. It interposes a world without defined borders or a previous shape between the being and the world, allowing one to integrate territories of a different nature, even when they have no margins in common. A place where the creative act is possible, the event by means of which a subject's Imaginary goes out to find what the world has to offer them and from there constructs a figure, a symbol, a cultural artifact that links these two realities, which, up until then, flowed separately: a *bridge*. It enables a pathway that connects two differentiated yet interdependent experiential spaces, turning their discontinuity into continuity, making it possible to go from shore to shore without any loss in demarcation, limit, shape, or content.

The text of art is not a linear discourse, but rather a maze of dialogues between thought and material, the inside and the out, memory and time, the body and space, and impulse and action. Preparing oneself for artistic creation requires a singular, differentiated operation: setting aside, at least for a moment, one's prejudices, and listening to one's own discursive practices. Putting a pen to a blank page is not the same as holding a brush.

Custom, history, and habit bequeath us with a perspective of the human being that leads us to think of its nature in terms of all or nothing and implies the existence of pairs of unquestionable realities defined by opposition: man/woman, ill/healthy, or psyche/body. However, as occurs when we contemplate a work by Escher, it is impossible to pay attention to only one of the figurative orders shown to us by the piece without needing to renounce its contemplation. The complexity brought to the ensemble by the duality in composition is not resolved by exclusion; on the contrary, only one capable of regarding the work in its ensemble as nondual, but

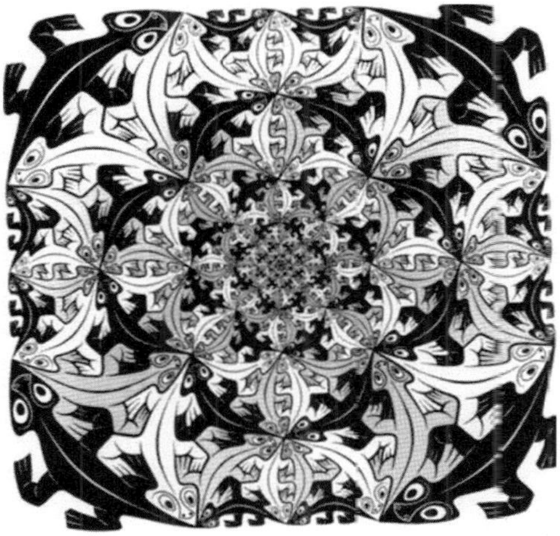

Fig. 16.1 Author: Maurits Cornelis Escher

rather integrated, can understand it in its simplicity and apprehend its endless movement and the wonder of its self-engendering (Fig. 16.1).

The pretense of depriving psychopathology of its contextual dimension means renouncing the reality that is the person. The body of psychopathology cannot be an ordered ensemble of neurons, hormones, structures, and substances. No such body exists if a physical, relational, social, and theoretical context to refer it to does not exist. The body is also a representation, a formula based on language. It is also an experiential ensemble, or ideological concept.

Merleau Ponty wrote: "Corporal space can be distinguished from exterior space and envelop its parts instead of unfolding them, because this space is the darkness in the room necessary for clarity of the spectacle, the depths of somnolence or the reserve of vague potency over which the gesture and its objective stand out, the non-being zone before which precise beings, figures and points may appear" [2].

We must be capable of paying attention to the body, not as a surface to be demarcated, but rather a place that is theoretical, political, affective, aesthetic, sensory, relational, etc., and also takes into account that, in this sense the limitations imposed on thought by logical discourse are not dismissible.

16.3 Experience and Language

In addressing mental illness with psychotherapy, "words" and logical thought have taken precedence as preferred methods. This implies that a person is capable of using them. In other words, that the person is disposed to construct and be constructed based on logical thought, and equipped with language that allows them "to tell and be told based on words."

However, with some pathologies or with determined aspects related to them, experiences take place that are far from capable of being constructed as structured thoughts and they cannot be approached with verbal language. On occasions, these experiences are disassociated from cognition and affect, and remain in psychic space as flashbacks that are only accessible on a sensory level.

Within this context, we ask ourselves about the viability of a expressive–communicational process that is not ruled by cognition, implying what some authors refer to as bottom-to-top processing [3], allowing access to "important regulating, sensorial-motor, holistic, autobiographic, stress-reducing functions, based on images inherent to non-verbal processing modalities" (Siegel in the prologue to Ogden) [3]. This is a process that implies cognitive and affective levels, but also physiological, sensorial, motor, social, and cultural levels.

Human beings, just like the other living beings, possess memory linked to the species and another memory related to their own existence as individuals. Both of them are essential for their biological survival, but for psychological survival, they need another memory, interlinked with their relational, cultural, and transcendent dimension. Thanks to the latter, it is possible for them to make experience something lived, to transpose affect, knowledge, discourses, and the unconscious within that which is sensory, generating spaces and relationships that give meaning to their everyday life. In essence, the work of an artist consists of transforming feelings into something visible, making an ensemble of inscriptions on the outside: strokes, movements, volumes, etc., that allow them to link their memory to the memory of the world in an explicit and long-lasting fashion.

One might say that all artistic products imply symbolization, but also implicated therein is movement, the footprint of that movement, the memory over which it passes and the memory proposed within as a new representational configuration. This movement, understood as an exteriorization process, thanks to which that which is sensitive being spatially and temporally dimensioned, transforms the thought that it represents, thereby affecting perception in and of itself. As such, all artistic production alludes to subjective production interdependent on the context and the subject carrying it out, configuring it as an artistic object. In this sense, it includes at least a social–political (inter-subjective) dimension, another cognitive–affective (intra-subjective) dimension, and a poetic–transcendental (artistic) dimension.

16.4 Gender, Art, and Health

As far as the gender perspective is concerned, we could ask ourselves if it is possible to speak of a differential artistic production in relation to gender, or if a correlational component derived from the different subjective meanings of the artistic experience in relation to this variable exist. One might also consider (mental) health in relation to art and gender, as both things are social constructions modulating the perception–interpretation–representation continuum and operate thereupon qualitatively, according to whether one is man or woman, artist or not. Last, one might argue as to a therapeutic method that works based on the interaction between different mental positions, the models and ideals socially maintained and constructed regarding femininity and masculinity, and the artistic products and processes that are produced according to them.

The construction of what we call identity includes an identification process in which, at minimum, biological, cultural and biographical elements, and the social structure are involved. For healthy development, the baby must be within a setting they can handle, and to this end, it needs someone else capable of sustaining, protecting, providing, and feeding their experience. This mediating function must exist, beyond whoever holds it, so that they, in turn, may develop it.

When gender roles (masculine/feminine) are articulated around rigid social models that counter masculine omnipotence with feminine abnegation, parental figures assume differentiated forms that are expressed through relations and attitudes such as power/submission, activity/passivity, strength/suffering, and control/guilt. As a consequence, the caretaking functions are divided, and they become vertebrae in the masculine–defense–strength–external/feminine–sustain–sensitivity–internal duo.

The internalization of a complete caretaker figure is mandatory for a subject's development, regardless of whether they are biologically a man or woman. When this figure breaks or proves to be insufficient, it promotes a gender construction based solely on the biological factor, constituted as a stereotype, leading to over-identification/rejection of social bonds. However, and additionally, it becomes a vulnerability factor that may be at the base (at the origin) of, or modulate, different psychopathological alterations that are either conflictive or structurally deficient in nature.

On occasion, the intolerable nature of a thought, affection or sensation is not considered in relation to another one that is better or more credible; rather, it is the fact in and of itself of being unable to self-sustain when faced with it that is intolerable. When this *sufficiently good* maternal function fails, as Winnicott so magisterially presents, it may be that it is impossible for an individual to be in the world without warning themselves, no longer of a lack, but as a result of an empty space.

"Spaces cannot be reduced to the concepts of I-think as conscience, the instruments with which nature draws on the landscape of subjectivity. As such, they must be experienced outside of time, outside of history, because they are outside of the interior of conscience." [4]

16.5 Clinical Examples

16.5.1 Lola

Reality may be taken as a maze of relations (as well as an ensemble of correspondences) in which the body and language form part of the same system that gives the subject meaning, as they are called upon to be activated in each new situation in which the subject finds themselves. Both body and language share something we might call an updating vector that operates in two senses: in conservation and in transformation. There is something in the corporal element that remains and something that is moved by experience and transformed by it, and the same thing occurs with language (especially nonverbal). In this fashion, every experience is engraved in a subject's mental framework, mobilizing their structure, ascribing it to the body and language in order to bequeath it with subjectivity.

Language and body embrace the experience of living and give it meaning. Habit is the base upon which different experiences are outlined, the condition for the development of new experiences, which puts the instant when it becomes real into play, and in which it is possible to play or create, to imagine something different, and to prepare for change. "One must be capable of imagining something different than what there is in order to be capable of wanting; and one must want something different than what there is in order to be capable of imagining" [5]. In this sense, art facilitates a certain "resonance" between the body and language, thanks to which the capacity for self-regulation is increased, and the capacity to create changes along with it.

The factual condition of artistic products induces one to collate, evaluate, realize, detect problems, try solutions, make adjustments, etc. Experiencing an achievement, even when not absolute, provided by artistic work hearkens to the very capacity to modulate, facing every situation from the emotion, sensation, and thought it produces.

"In *poiesis*, everything is radically different. The nature of what could be is attributed to that which is presented in the creation or production. It is always the result of doing, of *facere* (*fictio*). More than resembling existence, it is a revelation of its conditions of possibility." [6]

Lola is a 63-year-old woman who has suffered a brain stroke affecting the left side of her body. Her motor capacity appears to have recuperated, but she says she has lost her freedom. Her husband, recently retired, has taken charge of the situation and controls all of her movements, preventing her from doing anything that would imply decision-making or change.

At the beginning of the session, she appears uneasy, constantly looking every which way, and when she is asked to close her eyes to remember, for example, a landscape, she is incapable of doing so. She sits on the edge of the chair, which is too high for her, because she says she needs to have her feet on the floor, and she keeps her arms on the armrests. Her body language is ambiguous; she appears to be anchored to the chair and about to take off running all at once.

She has always lived under a man's protection; first her father, and then her husband. She has never needed anything that had to do with taking care of herself. Since she married, she has dedicated her life to her family. Her day-to-day always consisted of the house and children: she got up, prepared breakfasts, took care of her family, and once they had all left, she got ready and went to the market. There, she met up with other women with whom she chatted and drank coffee. Then she went home and took care of domestic tasks, meals, and once again, taking care of her children and husband.

Now her husband does the grocery shopping for her. He says that she cannot take care of everything and that it is better for her to rest. Lola does not understand what is happening; she feels guilty and ungrateful for his care, and explains a feeling of intense sadness and malaise that she feels as an after effect of the stroke.

After considering different materials, we worked with play dough, which interested her because she said it allows her to exercise her hands, especially the left one. From this point, we focused especially on the connection between the imagination and the manual realization of what was imagined, proposing experiences to her that allow her to effortlessly experience this connection. We worked with very basic shapes: a ball (that she called a bouncy ball), a ball with a hole (a washing-up bowl), and a solid cylinder (worm).

It is easy to observe her great difficulty in imagining, and especially in separating herself from the literality where she finds herself, and in thinking of some change; with each new suggestion, her breathing becomes ragged and she begins looking at her fingers with greater unease (perhaps anxiety), so we suggest that she tells us something that she likes. After a moment of uncertainty, she tells us that she likes flowers. When we show our curiosity regarding which ones she appears indecisive, and finally says, "roses." We ask her to think about a rose, and then go one step further. "Once you have the image in your head, don't you think you could make a rose out of play dough?" we affirm. Her response is immediate and unequivocal: both her words and her body say no, she cannot, that is impossible.

Then we ask her if she can make a stem. She looks at us, surprised, and affirms, "Yes, of course!" and makes a thin cylinder from green play dough. Then we ask her what the rose is like, what it is made of. She says it has petals, and we ask her if she can make one. She is still surprised, and makes one. We ask her how many it has, and she says she doesn't know. We ask her if it has two, and she says no, there are more, so she continues making them. When she has several, she makes something that she says is the centre of the flower. Then we suggest that she make the flower. She places the petals around the center, and from there, she adjusts sizes, the number, and position. Then she sticks the flower on the stem and adds leaves.

Her face has totally changed, and she looks at the flower she has made, half-surprised and half in admiration. We comment that it is perhaps not exactly as she had imagined, and we ask her what she thinks of it. She says that she likes it and then adds that life is that way: sometimes, one thinks about how things will be and then they don't turn out that way, but, oh well.

Working with art allows one to bring what they are feeling to the body, and then manage it through materials. Finishing implies a "retreat," but it is also conserving that which has been achieved. It is difficult for Lola to spurn her flower, but more than anything, she will not allow it to be spurned by others; she will protect it from critical voices that undervalue it or try to invalidate it. It is also a way for one to become aware of responsibility with regard to oneself and one's life, making it possible to receive and welcome what arises from it.

In this fashion, a receptive, and not reactive, position is facilitated; it allows one to work with processes and not with results, with personal rhythms, considering subjectivity as a founding element in creative value.

16.5.2 Julia

"... being or feeling like a man, woman, or however one wishes to live gender, is a substantially corporal experience, a lived experience made real, situated in determined historical, social and changing coordinates. In other words, a process produced through basically corporal actions: ways of feeling, walking, talking, moving, dressing, adorning, touching, feeling emotion. . .in continuous interaction with others, actions that are modified in time and in space." [7]

Gender differentiation is the fruit of a group of practices that are socially legitimized, infiltrated without familiar gender models, referring to a group of differentiated beliefs, values, and attitudes, inscribed within a system that includes roles and conducts of domination/submission. Within this system, that which is feminine is constructed, affectively and cognitively, as per a masculine exterior that holds strength and control, in opposition to that which is masculine, and must be repressed, including the capacity for self-determination, negotiation, and leadership.

The emplacement of that which is feminine within the borders of private space implies, in turn, an emplacement within the public space, with everything that this implies in terms of power, control, and regulation. Space is presented as a guarantee of gender identity, in the sense that certain psychological characters such as maternal instinct, empathy, commitment to others, generosity, noncompetition, etc., cannot be developed within normative practices inherent to that other public/masculine nature.

Julián and Marisa's first child was a daughter. The father's wish to have a boy crashed against the reality of the birth, and perhaps to reinstate order, he called the new-born Juliana.

The expectations Julián had placed on that son–daughter, Marisa's affective ambivalence, the birth of a sickly sister who required all their attention and care, and finally, the arrival of the boy, complicated Juliana's childhood. She spent her first four years trying to find her own way to be in the world.

A few years ago, and as a continuation of the therapeutic process she had begun for learning purposes, Juliana began another one with artistic means as the preferred method.

She had never shown any psychiatric symptomology of note, but a constant element in her life was a certain feeling of malaise, which she never quite managed to figure out, and she related it to her difficulty in developing true bonds of trust. She was a successful woman, both socially and professionally; she had a partner with great qualities, and she had recently become a mother. She had decided to become a mother at the moment when she desired to do so, and she had prepared everything to enjoy what motherhood implied.

The biological situation of motherhood coincided with her decision to begin the process that led her to legally change her name. One of the issues worked on the most during her previous therapy had led her to the conclusion that being named Juliana had significantly conditioned her life, especially insofar as her appropriation of her feminine condition was concerned. Surely for this reason, during her adolescence, she had decided to go by the name of Julia. Currently, practically all of those around her, except for her original family, knew her by that name.

However, both things, maternity and changing her name, were in actuality more difficult that she had supposed, and this led to a notable increase in the underlying malaise that began causing moments of great anxiety, a feeling of uselessness, lack of meaning, and even existential emptiness.

The image of a woman (Fig. 16.2) *she found in a newspaper in one of the first sessions, and to which she returned on several occasions, proved to be a key element in developing what might be called a "genderization" based on the body, appropriating from that feminine image what she could not integrate when she was a child, and it allowed her to sustain herself beyond her biology, biography, and the paternal desire for a son. To this end, it was necessary for the image to no longer be the center of her thought and to become the nucleus of a creative action.*

The huge emotional destabilization that the image produced in her had led Julia to work with it several times, always from a perspective of rationally searching for answers, but verbal language did not achieve the goal of freeing her from the abyss she saw interposed between herself and the image. Finally, the discourse found new materials and structure to put into play, and the image became the matrix for an identity fabric that was generated based on those three places, interlacing memories, desires, and present realities.

The discovery of repetition as the compositional base to generate new meanings was the first step. It took place coincidentally, based on carrying out artwork with canvas, which began as an exercise in color with small adjacent squares. They were added to session-by-session over the course of a month, making a multi-color space that, as it formally grew, contributed sensory content. She called it Blanket. *The blanket as a protective, sheltering, and caring element, but also as a hiding, clandestine element, sheltered the intensity of some of the contents, which, in the*

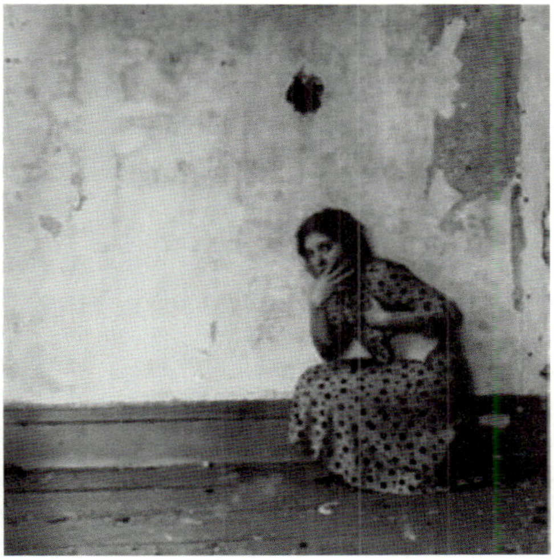

Fig. 16.2 Author: Francesca Woodman

form of sensations, affective remnants or automatic defensive thoughts, brought the square along with it. In parallel fashion, Julia recuperated a hobby she had previously entertained, and in her free time, she began to crochet squares which, once joined together, made way for a real blanket. Making this blanket was extended over the course of the entire posterior process, like a parallel activity, giving continuity to global process.

This pictorial artwork made clear the enormous transforming potential that the action in and of itself held in relation to the affective mobilization/performance. Upon finishing it, Julia was interested in some pieces of cardboard from leftover boxes in the studio and began to work with them, using them as the base, but also as plastic material. In this fashion, the material had a twofold quality: as a base, it was containing and permanent, rigid enough to hold up the rest of the elements being placed on top of it, and as flexible and versatile material, it adapted and was able to function under various regimes. One could cut, fold, wrinkle, soften, wrap, pulverize it, etc. Additionally, glue as a cohesive element gave the ensemble strength, in such a way that the more elements were added, the stronger and more consistent it became, and the more hardy and resistant the artwork became.

The cardboard base acted as the foundation for the composition, all the while functioning as a producer of new materials and plastic qualities. The cut-out image of the woman was pasted to the surface, and work was begun on the background as if it were a material field; the cardboard was scratched, scored, and separated into layers revealing different reliefs and textures. Julia saved the ripped leftovers, and when she had enough, she mixed them with glue and made a paste that, in turn, acted as a new material. With it, she covered part of the surface, and taking advantage of its plasticity, she shaped volumes, made incisions, defined rigidity, etc.

As the blanket had covered sensory–affective memories that could hardly be verbalized, this new work with cardboard took on a new, unlimited capacity in the affective realm, also giving way to a labor of unloading. Aspects regarding vulnerability, the need for protection and care, containing, receptiveness, and playing, were connected to others such as rage, aggressiveness, and control. In this fashion, the background figure ensemble became a battlefield where the figure, who never directly participated, was modified through the constant, profound transformations taking place in the background.

The artwork took on a huge level of complexity, both from a formal and a thematic point of view. Its bi-dimensional condition appeared to be questioned by the diversity of superimposed cardboard planes and paste, the mono-color brought about by the fact that the image, made of photocopies in black and white, was squelched by the cardboard, whose textures and mixture with the glue created different nuances: shadows, a shine, tones, etc. Each one of these qualities was experientially put into play, and only on occasion was some verbal correlate derived; the material condition of the text with which she was working implied the emergence of emotional movements congruent with the intervention, which interlaced with others of a more reflective, perhaps projective, origin. There was great emotional mobilization in the form of frustration, rage, fear, expectation, curiosity, disgust, shame, feeling of achievement, empathy, love, care, etc., which interacted with the evocations, projections, and reflections that the image as such provoked.

Once this artwork was finished, Julia began making a great number of photocopies of the image of the woman, which she used as vertebrae elements for new cardboard compositions. The elements that appeared gave her the opportunity to develop a set of artworks whose central axis was her own femininity. In this sense, within the framework of the vital tensions sustained by the creation process, it was also possible to integrate them: action/passivity, strength/fragility, freedom/subjugation, transgression/abidance, certainty/uncertainty, expansion/drawing inward, etc.

Pieces of mirror, ropes, spring, nails, fabrics, silk paper, wool, feathers, stones, and many other real elements were conjugated with visual elements, such as tunnels, nets, high heels, peepholes, doors, windows, rain, wings, etc. and were composed in different orders as a ship, a house or a body.

Each creation process constitutes in and of itself a spontaneously generated experience that includes the human being in their totality and in action.

In this sense, it is linked to that which is corporal, and from this point, to the very body of the artwork itself, to its factuality, which appears not only as the support for language, but as a part constituting language. The artwork body operates as the signifier, and also as the significance and signification agent, capable of expressing itself through a rhetoric based on relations with other scopes of knowledge and the flow of experience: memory, cognition, setting, and emotion—all come together therein to form an ensemble with meaning. The relation between this ensemble is finally corporal and is in the nature of the language, on its edges, at its limits, and each one of us has developed different ways of founding and giving shape to these relations.

16.5.3 Elena

"Fear is a passive state. The goal I set for myself is to go from being a passive to an active element, to take control, to move from passivity to implication," as Louise Bougeois expressed [8].

The condition of motherhood as a building block of feminine nature is upheld by an ensemble of beliefs, inherent to patriarchal organizations, which implies a system of power relations from whence, in many cases, it is difficult to extract oneself. The woman–mother identification is articulated by a series of "natural" capacities that often prove to be unavoidable for women: love, bonding, empathy, sacrifice, etc., and they imply commitment, not only to sons and daughters, but also to that which is human in its broadest meaning: family, community, culture, health, education, etc.

This form of subjectivity implies a woman *being* dedicated to being a *being* for others which, when this is made impossible, may prove to be excessive for the psyche. The need to be accepted, wanted, and even indispensable for the other being, goes hand-in-hand with the fear of being alone, of invisibility, and in the last instance, of the condition of not existing; not being wanted is also not being seen or recognized as singular, as valuable; being dispensable or substitutable. Even when motherhood as such does not come about, generalization of the role of the mother regarding other relationships is superimposed on a way of being in the world that takes values such as collaboration, solidarity or surrender as nuclear units for construction as a valid subject. In this fashion, the question, "Who am I?" is inseparably formulated with "Who am I for the other one?," announcing the important component of affective dependency thereby implied.

The mandate to attend to the other being's necessities implies total deployment from the body, insofar as their own consistency is concerned: sexuality, pregnancy, birth, and breastfeeding, as well as the external space it articulates: the home. A body conceived for the other, that has suffering, sacrifice, and pain as founding elements of subjectivity, a body–home that presents itself as the main legitimizing element of the being, in such a way that renouncing it also implies renouncing one's own space wherein they are deployed as a subject.

Elena is a 40-year-old woman. In her psychiatric file, three suicide attempts and an imprecise diagnosis stand out: post-traumatic stress disorder, eating disorder, melancholic depression, attachment disorder, general anxiety disorder, toxic addiction, and finally, borderline personality disorder.

She was born into a conservative, religious family, with a high socioeconomic level; she was the first girl out of a total of 8 children, including her twin brother, José.

She says that she was happy during her childhood, and especially that she was never bored. Her brothers and sisters were always driving forces in her life, especially after the death of her mother owing to childbirth complications when she was 7 years old. She says she is passionate about children, that she understands them well, unlike adults. She does not have children, but she has several godchildren whom she adores. She considers motherhood for herself to be impossible, and that her body and head would resist pregnancy, since both of them are only apt for death.

She explains that when her mother (a woman with strong religious convictions, who put the divine command to procreate before recommendations of those who warned her as to the danger of new pregnancies) died, and with a father who only spent time with his sons and daughters to judge their progress, she assumed the role of caretaker and rose up as an affective point of reference for the rest of the family.

Five years later, her father married again. The new wife could not have children and joined the family nucleus as an indisputable maternal figure, leaving the position Elena had filled until then worthless. At the time, she was 12 years old. In addition to the initial powerlessness, rage, and bitterness, she first felt guilt and then transgression as a singular way of being.

She began interpreting her mother's death as an abandonment, thinking that her mother knew the risks she was running with each new child, and that even so, she continued getting pregnant until death. This brought with it unacceptable feelings and thoughts that first filled Elena with rage, and then with guilt. Then she idealized her mother, taking her as a model of what she said she could never be: perfection, sweetness, balance, happiness, and safety. She compared her mother with her father's new wife and felt that the latter's mere presence was already a betrayal of her mother's memory. Finally, Elena wished to follow in her mother's footsteps and become, like her, an exceptional woman, dedicated to others, in social action and in religion.

At 17, she was molested by an acquaintance of the family. She says that her father did not want to believe her, alleging her lack of attractiveness, so she never received support. She remembers that moment as a brutal blow to her condition as a woman that, in addition to being discarded from her role as caretaker/mother for her brothers and sisters, she received definitive nonrecognition of her feminine values: motherhood and sexuality. Along with the impunity to which she felt men had both physically and psychologically subjected her, this shattered her already precarious mental structure. She began to radicalize control of her body, to distance herself from the family home, and to increase her activity as a student and religious leader. She drastically reduced her food intake, she dedicated herself to camp activities and social projects, and began university studies. In a parallel fashion, she began feeling an ever-increasing feeling of emptiness and guilt that she tried to neutralize with constant self-punishments, including bodily self-harm. At 20 years of age, given her clear physical and emotional deterioration, and after a suicide attempt, she was admitted to a psychiatric institution.

She attributes the two fundamental, vital consequences that those years brought to the collapse of the bonding model offered by the mother and the impossibility of any bond with the father: rejection of religion and homosexuality. Upon leaving the institution, she began to dress as a man, she joined a high-competition sports team, and was filled with intense anti-system political passion.

Her personal achievements at that time did not manage to make her feel sufficiently valued. Additionally, the rhythm she had with her father progressively moved her away from the recognition she increasingly intensely desired. She says that all of that wasted energy ended up throwing her toward a position of insufferable impotence and guilt, which was paradoxically experienced as dependency. The impossibility of obtaining control and authority over herself, along with feeling empty, as if there were an abyss under her feet, led her to a second suicide attempt that had serious physical consequences.

Thanks to a family inheritance, she purchased a house and decided to live alone. She had some income, and a disability pension that permitted her to manage expenses without many problems. Little by little, she recuperated some of her previous activities, all the while becoming aware of her many limitations. She also picked up some of her more radical positions regarding religion, sexuality, and politics again. She began to look for more and more experiences of extreme pleasure that led her to a period of great promiscuity, toxic consumption, and risky behaviors, which, in turn, brought large doses of guilt and increased feelings of emptiness. After another suicide attempt, she was once again admitted. At this point, and as a complementary method to her treatment (pharmacological and psychotherapeutic), she began a therapeutic approach focused on languages and artistic processes.

Elena had been a brilliant philosophy student; her capacity for reflection and criticism was notable, and she tirelessly searched for explanations and reasoning. On occasions, however, logical thought could not explain or give meaning to a large part of what was happening to her. When this occurred, the only escape route she could find was her body: controlling it, exhibiting it, inflicting self-harm, disguising herself, inebriating herself, purging herself, binging, and practicing extreme sex. Plastic surgery allowed her, more than anything else, to experience and integrate beauty–ugliness, creation–destruction, malaise–pleasure, and control–chance pairs. From that point, it was possible for her to undertake a self-construction process that allowed her to manage the ambivalence of her desires/ impulses, especially in relation to her father and everything he stood for.

Sensory, cenesthetic, and poetic work opened up a new pathway for her. We suggested beginning with some techniques used by surrealists. She liked the history of art and was aware of many of its movements, so we thought this could act as a bridge between that which is intellectual, to which she was accustomed, and the proposal we were making. Additionally, surrealism has a large dose of transgression, rebellion, and insubordination. Techniques such as dripping, collage, frottage, and stamping allowed us to introduce playing and chance as discursive elements, that initially prevented a great part of the possibility of control, but opened a wide range of valid solutions that could be managed later on; more than anything else, it allowed her to give meaning to the process and the different moments undergone by the artwork as it evolved.

Here, the body was fundamental (Fig. 16.3). *The techniques required concentration and patience if one desired to obtain a result even slightly similar to that which was being sought: regulating the amount of water on the painting for dripping, tones, and fillers for stamping, the pressure used to transpose color from one surface to another and the selection of images and materials for collages.*

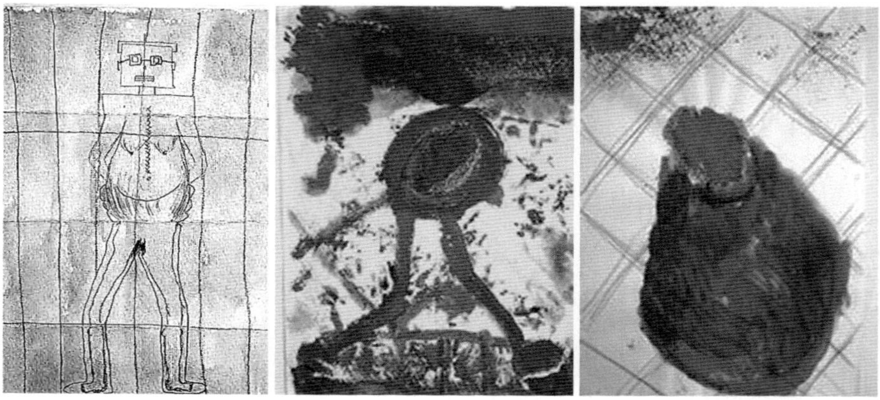

Fig. 16.3 Body

All of this forced the body to be currently present, it pushed it take the reins and forced the mind to be available to the body: planning the steps, careful execution, paying attention, evaluating, and correcting. It required appropriate and flexible handling of materials rather than exhaustive control, which in turn, was not possible. Once this pathway was available to her, she began working with freedom, enjoying the ludic moment created by the activity and creating different mental content that came into play.

The experience of her split femininity, which derived in a construction of herself that she was unable to sustain as a man, either, along with her current state as "a broken body," began to come together in a reparative artistic action, wherein everything that was significant to her was incorporated: food, crafting, personal hygiene, pharmaceuticals, a brush, empty refreshment cans, candles, rice cakes, wrappers and fruit peelings, scrap wood, medication bubble-packs, etc. Everything was useful as a way to connect to her body, to reality, and to her affection that the therapeutic device offered to her. Constructions were organized from the interior, around a base structure that became increasingly solid, in which elements from different places, of different colors, materials, lightness, etc., were involved (Fig. 16.4).

She began alternating tri-dimensional compositions, which offered her a more physical space, with other bi-dimensional ones, which allowed her wordplay later on, and bit by bit, verbal language was able to regain meaning. She was also able to selectively use techniques, according to the mental state she was in, both to reinforce it and to change it: she sought relaxation, unloading, playing, bonding, explaining herself, avoiding, etc. Little by little, she developed a set of artworks arranged as if they were a text to be decoded; some took on meaning according to others, as she organized them chronologically, thematically or technically.

Her last composition was a collage (Fig. 16.5). *She made it on the floor and as a summary of all of the work carried out. From many magazines, she extracted words*

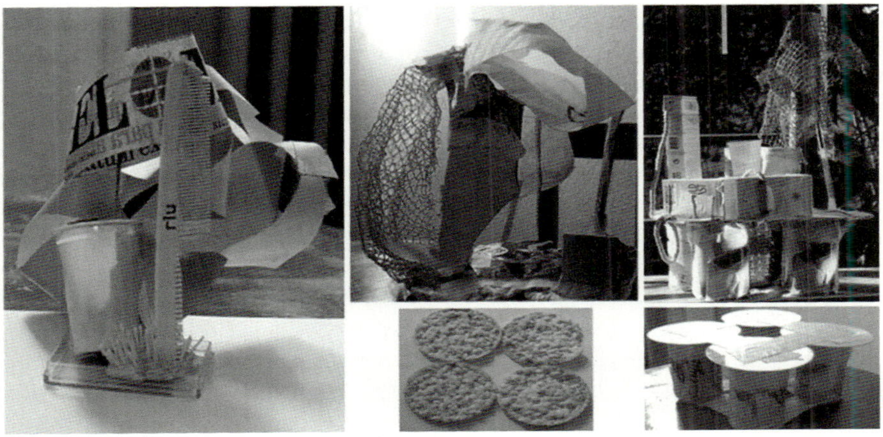

Fig. 16.4 Constructions

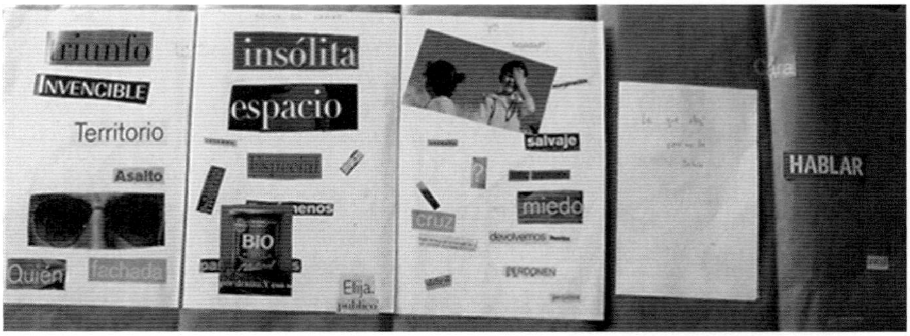

Fig. 16.5 Collage

and images, one-by-one, that had somehow had an impact on her. Then she put them onto three sheets of paper. She says that each one of them represents a different type of person: the first two are people she hates and that she once was, and the third is what she is. She says that the images help her to clarify words. Once the three compositions are made, she warns that she still has words left to use. She rejects two of them: "virtues" (theological virtues, she says), and "stars," and throws them into the rubbish bin. Then she makes a fourth pile that refers to the favorable aspects that she recognizes in herself.

She takes a large piece of paper and puts the three sheets on it, directly gluing the last ones to it. She warns that she still has some left. When she picks them up again, she looks at them and looks at the therapist, half-surprised, half-happy. She laughs. "I'm also all the ones that are left," she says. Then she folds a paper in half and glues them inside. On the outside, she writes: "What I chose, but didn't know."

What she wrote afterward, she said, was a declaration of intent.

"Triumph, the invincible ones, those who believe they have a right to an inviolable territory, those who assault that which is private, that which is personal and belongs to another...Who? ALL of them are a façade. They hide behind imaginary glasses. They believe that they can bully. I HATE them.

"Those who are unlikely, those who believe themselves to be special (not because they are unique, but because they believe themselves to be above the rest), those who, when they need personal space, invade the space of another, those who believe they are made of iron, the champions, distant and therefore exclusive, may they select an AUDIENCE, may they feed off of the latest, the most organic, but may they leave me in peace, may they stray from my path.

"Fatalists, the marginalized, those who have at times been wild, those of us who feel fear, those who shun (vomit) eagerness, those of us who are a burden to the rest, but more than anything, to oneself, those of us who see life as difficult, those of us who believe we have an equivocal life, those who they almost always say must be forgiven, those we harm...they, them, me, we have no place in this life other than the path of death. We do not know how to see or hear; we turn our back on life.

"I like personal relationships, those that collaborate so the heart speaks and talks, those who have a family, but I do not see them at first sight.

I would like to be able to speak to life face-to-face, to live in that which is real, even for just a few instants; not everything need be forever."

The construction of a gender identity, just like the rest of one's aspects, takes place within a dialectic relationship with one's setting: relational, social, experiential, linguistic, geographical, etc. In opposition to all domination practices, by principle, there is a being that resists, that struggles to maintain its singularity. However, the possibility that this singularity emerges as something primary, and not reactive, does not depend on the quantity or quality of reasoning we may carry out in this respect, but on the fact that a potentially appropriate medium for the development of personal resources allowing to do so exists, or has existed.

Offering spaces for free creation, putting nonverbal areas of experience into play within a sufficiently sustaining therapeutic device, is fundamental to developing resources and strategies that facilitate the handling of uncertainty, fear, frustration, and rage so that all of this may be integrated into one experience of achievement on all levels: cognitive, affective, sensory, motor, and relational. Only in this fashion will transformation be viable: creating something new for the person that shows that they are a capable, free, and autonomous individual.

References

1. Burin M, Meler I. Varones. Género y subjetividad masculina (Men. Gender and masculine subjectivity). Paidós: Buenos Aires; 2000.
2. Merleau-Ponty M. Fenomenología de la percepción (Phenomonelogy of perception). Barcelona: Editorial Altaya; 1999.
3. Ogden P. The healing power of the emotion. In: Fosha D, Siegel DJ, Solomon MF, editors. Affective neuroscience, development and clinical practice. Los Angeles: UCLA School of Medicine; 2009.
4. Pardo JL. Sobre los espacios pintar, escribir, pensar. Barcelona: Del Serbal; 1991.
5. Castoriadis C. El psicoanálisis, proyecto y elucidación (Psychoanalysis, project and elucidation). Buenos Aires: Nueva Visión; 1992.
6. Trias E. Ciudad sobre ciudad. Arte, religión y ética en el cambio de milenio (City over city. Art, religión and ethics at the change of the millennium). Barcelona: Ediciones Destino; 2001.
7. Esteban Galarza ML. Etnografýa, itinerarios corporales y cambio social: apuntes teóricos y metodológicos (Ethnography, corporal itineraries and social change; theoretical and methodological notes). In: Elixabete Imaz Martýñez M, Coordinator. La materialidad de la identidad (The materiality of identity). Trans. Revista Transcultural de Música. 2008;(12):135–58.
8. Bourgeois L. Destrucción del padre/reconstrucción del padre. Madrid: Síntesis; 2002.

Part III

Psychopathology Related to Hormonal Aspects

Adolescent Depression

17

Emma Noval-Aldaco, María Ruiz-Torres, Jose López-Gil,
and Beatriz Payá-González

Abstract

Mood disorders are one of the most commonly experienced mental disorders during childhood and adolescence. Before adolescence, depression rates are similar in boys and girls, but from puberty, the incidence of depression in women increases in a ratio of 2:1 compared with men, a tendency that remains during adulthood. Some authors speculate that this phenomenon originates from the hormonal changes that occur at this stage of development and their effects on neurobiological level. Currently, a multifactorial etiological model in which several risk factors interact and enhance reciprocally is already accepted. Considering that adolescence is a key period in the acquisition of autonomy and the formation of personal identity, sociocultural pressure becomes particularly important. In this sense, the familiar and social context, which is closer to the adolescent, is crucial for the transmission of cultural values and stereotypes. In this chapter, differences between male and female subjects in diverse aspects of the clinical manifestations of depressive disorders, as well as biological, cognitive, and social factors that attempt to explain gender differences in adolescent depression, are reviewed. Finally, it is necessary to take into account that the role and gender stereotypes internalized by patients and health professionals can influence both the way in which depressive disorders manifest and the clinical attention provided.

E. Noval-Aldaco • M. Ruiz-Torres • J. López-Gil • B. Payá-González (✉)
Department of Psychiatry, Valdecilla University Hospital, Santander, Spain
e-mail: bpaya@humv.es

M. Sáenz-Herrero (ed.), *Psychopathology in Women*,
DOI 10.1007/978-3-319-05870-2_17

17.1 Introduction

The first descriptions of depressive disorders in children and adolescents were carried out in the seventeenth century. These early theories underestimated the importance of the disorder, hypothesizing that psychological mechanisms involved in the vulnerability to depression were not present in children and adolescents.

It was in 1975, after a meeting conducted by the National Institute of Mental Health to discuss the diagnosis of depression in children, that the existence of this disorder in the pediatric population was widely accepted. From this moment onward, the existence of this disorder was recognized in children and adolescents and new lines of investigation and theoretical models of pathogenesis were developed.

Epidemiological studies estimate prevalence rates of depression in children of around 2 % [1, 2], increasing in adolescents up to 5 % [3]. By sex, the prevalence of depressive disorders in childhood is similar for boys and girls. However, in adolescence there is a significant increase in the female prevalence, up to a ratio of 2:1 [4–6]. It has been speculated that this phenomenon originates from the hormonal changes that occur at this stage of development and the effects on a neurobiological level. Nevertheless, the sole attribution of these differences to assumed biological variables would be a simplistic approach and would not explain other changes in prevalence observed among different ethnicities and cultures.

It points to the consideration of other types of variables more related to culture and/or society values in the genesis of adolescent depressive disorders. Currently, a multifactorial etiological model, in which several risk factors interact and enhance reciprocally, has already been accepted. Considering that adolescence is a key period in the acquisition of autonomy and the formation of personal identity, sociocultural pressure becomes particularly important. In this sense, the familial and social context, which is closer to the adolescent, is crucial for the transmission of cultural values and stereotypes [7, 8].

We think that the higher prevalence of depression observed in women after adolescence may have some particularly influential variables such as those linked to gender social stereotypes.

In this chapter, differences between males and females in clinical manifestations of depressive disorders, as well as sex divergences in biological, cognitive, and emotional variables that may predispose to a greater vulnerability to depression, are reviewed. Furthermore, the role of sociocultural factors, highlighting those intrinsically linked to gender and their involvement in the variability found in depression prevalence between sexes, are discussed [9].

17.2 Epidemiology

Mood disorders are one of the most common mental disorders in childhood and adolescence with estimated prevalence rates for major depressive disorder between 0.4 % and 2.5 % in children and between 7 % and 9.8 % in adolescents [10–12].

For dysthymia, the prevalence rates are between 0.6 % in children and between 1.6 % and 8 % in adolescents [13, 14].

Although the prevalence of depressive disorders in childhood is similar in both sexes, in adolescence there is a significant increase in the female prevalence [4–6].

The female predominance of depressive disorders has been observed in different countries and cultures as well as across multiple generations [12].

Different authors propose that the difference observed between men and women in adolescence is due to a decrease in depressive disorders in boys that is greater than a real increase in girls. This suggests that women's reactivity to life events does not change along the course of development; meanwhile, in boys this does happen [15, 16].

Naninck et al. [17] propose that this phenomenon might be related to a greater tendency of women to seek help for psychological problems while men show a greater tendency to cope with sadness or depressive symptoms in other ways, such as by increasing toxic consumption.

A variety of factors, including hormonal changes, coping styles, and socialization experiences have been hypothesized to be causes of gender differences.

However, these assumptions are not totally able to explain the existence of gender differences in the incidence of depressive disorders.

17.3 Clinical Characteristics in Children and Adolescent Depression

From the third version of the *Diagnostic and Statistical Manual of Mental Disorders* (APA, 1980), diagnostic criteria for depression in pediatric and adolescent populations are the same as those given to adults, with special consideration of the possible occurrence of an irritable mood instead of a low one, and the failure to make expected weight gain by age instead of weight loss or gain.

Clinical expression of depression changes depending on the stage of development. During childhood physiological and motor manifestations are predominant, while cognitive manifestations will become more important over the years. Nissen [18] describes different symptoms depending on the age. At pre-school ages, depressive symptoms usually appear in the form of rejection of playing, psychomotor agitation and hyperactivity, shyness, tantrums, encopresis, sleeplessness, eating disorders, and other somatic symptoms. At school age, the most common manifestations include irritability, insecurity, learning difficulties, shyness, enuresis, encopresis, nail biting, night terrors, temper tantrums, and somatic symptoms. At puberty and adolescence, rumination, suicidal ideation, feelings of inferiority and oppression, changes in appetite and sleep, and rebellious behaviors prevail.

Regarding sex differences, some authors have suggested that women are more likely than men to suffer somatic symptoms. Other studies have shown that women tend to exhibit greater fatigue, more frequent changes in appetite, weight, and sleep [19].

Other cognitive symptoms, such as increased crying, feelings of failure and guilt, and low self-esteem, are more frequent in women than in men [20–25]. Men with depression used to report anhedonia, diurnal variation of mood, loss of energy, social withdrawal, and occupational impairment [20, 21, 24].

17.4 Explanatory Hypotheses of Gender Differences

17.4.1 Biological Factors

The significant increase in the number of depressive disorders in adolescence has generated many hypotheses on its biological basis, stressing the importance of sexual hormones, as well as brain or genetic factors.

17.4.1.1 Hormones

The neuroendocrine system plays an important role in the physical changes that begin in adolescence. The hypothalamus stimulates the pituitary gland, which releases hormones that trigger physical changes on several aspects such as body growth, cell metabolism, and the development of the sexual characters.

Implication of sexual steroids (androgens) in brain sexual differentiation was also supported by Phoenix in a paper published in 1959 [26]. Phoenix's paper put forward the concept that prenatal exposure to testosterone masculinized the behavior of genetic female guinea pigs. Specifically, authors proposed that testosterone acted on the central nervous tissues in which patterns of sexual behavior are organized. Later, the same authors went on to demonstrate similar effects in nonhuman rhesus monkeys [27] by showing that play behavior by female monkeys prenatally treated with testosterone was masculinized as well.

These behaviors include both sexual and social behaviors, all of which are also influenced by social experience. Phoenix argued that there are different periods of maximal susceptibility to the organizing actions of androgens. In the prenatal period two neural circuits get differentiated by sex, involving an organizational effect, which would activate subsequently again in adolescence owing to sex steroids, leading to different behavior patterns according to sex.

The Phoenix's organizational–activational hypothesis has received much empirical support. Later studies with animals [28] replicated the finding that the androgens' organizational effects are not limited to the early stages of infant development, but that they can also occur during adolescence, when brain plasticity still exists.

Other studies with adolescent rodents have also proven the role of sexual steroids in modifying other neuronal and brain neurotransmission systems [17, 29] with a secondary influence in mood or behavior [30].

Along these lines, Martel et al. [31] suggest a theory that considers that sexual hormones would activate negative affects by influencing the neurotransmitter systems of serotonin and related neural structures, such as the amygdala and the hypothalamic–pituitary–adrenal circuit (HPA axis).

Human studies have also related both the increase [32] and the decrease [33] in estrogen levels to a greater incidence of depression and negative mood in adolescents [34].

It has been argued that, rather than the level of estrogens, it is their fluctuation that is the most influential variable in the development of depressive symptoms [35].

Positive associations have been also observed between testosterone levels and proactive and reactive aggression [36], which may explain the greater frequency of men in exhibiting externalizing symptoms compared with women, in whom internalizing symptoms are predominant.

Even though some of these findings cannot be extrapolated to the human species since they have been conducted in animals, they point to the role of sexual hormones in gender differences of prevalence founded in depression.

17.4.1.2 Hypothalamic–Pituitary–Adrenal Axis

There are indications that the higher risk of depression in adolescent women could be related to a stronger, genetically conditioned sensitivity to stressful life events, which has opened up new lines of research focused on possible gender differences in stress regulation patterns.

Much of the research carried out in this field has been focused around the hypothalamic–pituitary–adrenal (HPA) axis, since it is a critical part of the neuro-endocrine system, which regulates a large number of physiological processes such as controlling stress reactions.

It is known that physiological reactions to stress are deeply influenced by the increase in gonadal hormone levels that occurs during adolescence [37]. The impact that the gonadal hormones have on brain receptors could explain differences in stress regulation patterns by sex [38].

Studies in humans and animals suggest that the HPA axis is more sensitive to female sexual hormones [39], showing that the fluctuation in steroid levels might be the main factor implicated in stress sensitivity in women [40].

Since the most consistent neuroendocrine alteration found in depressive disorders is the dysregulation of the HPA axis [41] and since depressive disorders are more prevalent amongst women, it has been theorized that girls are more prone to depression as a result of a dysregulation of the HPA axis [42].

The HPA axes of men and women react in different ways depending on the nature of the stress factor. Whereas men secrete more cortisol as a response to target achievements, women do so as response to social rejection situations, which suggests that psychosocial stressors have a deeper impact on girls [43].

Research suggests that the HPA axis responds differently in men and women to stressful situations and that there seems to be a link between the HPA axis function and a higher level of sensitivity to stress-related depressive disorders in female teenagers [44].

17.4.1.3 Differences at Brain Level

Research with imaging brain techniques has showed both structural and functional brain differences between males and females.

Discrepancies by sex have been described in both size and brain structure [17]. In addition, there are specific changes in the neuronal network at puberty, which determines male–female differences in cognition, emotion, and motivation [45]. These structural differences have been considered a critical factor, which may predispose to a higher female vulnerability to depression [17].

Regarding brain function, there is evidence that female sexual hormones may regulate brain neurotransmitters such as the serotonergic system, which is involved in depression [46].

Oxytocin [47–49] is a hormone that also works as a neurotransmitter that plays an important role in the development of attachment behaviors in animals by facilitating birth delivery and breastfeeding of newborns, as well as the development of maternal cares [47]. The biological hormonal changes occurring at adolescence have been linked with an increase in the attachment behaviors among female teenagers, driven by a rise in oxytocin level. From an evolutionist point of view, the development of affective attachment to the newborns contributes to the species survival.

Still, from an evolutionist viewpoint, we observe that women have played the role of caretakers, being more involved in child upbringing and more sensitive to their needs, while men have played a more instrumental role. In this respect, depressive behaviors have been linked to mechanisms of search for security and danger aversion [50]. Therefore, vulnerability to external stress factors may be an adaptive tool in women, especially those with dependent children [44]. It is important to highlight that mechanisms that were adaptive in the past may no longer be so at the current time [51]; however, the impact of the new social roles of women on their biological predisposition to greater attachment behaviors is unknown, since these actual social roles are not in line with the biological findings above.

17.4.1.4 Genetics

Descriptive studies suggest that having a parent suffering from depressive disorder is one of the main risk factors in child depression [52]. Goodman and Gotlib [53] suggest four mechanisms by which depressed parents transmit depression to their children: inheritability, dysfunctional neuroregulatory mechanisms, learning dysfunctional coping styles, and more exposure to stress factors.

Research shows the importance of genetic factors in the appearance of depression [54], finding higher rates of this disorder amongst the relatives of a depressed person [55]. The influence of genetic factors is also confirmed by a higher correlation in monozygotic than in dizygotic twins, and by research on adoption that shows a higher correlation in biological than in adoptive parents [56]. Nevertheless, there is no evidence of differences in genetic vulnerability between males and females.

17.4.2 Cognitive Factors

Hankin and Abramson [57] have developed a theory based on cognitive vulnerability to explain gender differences in depressive disorders. According to the general model of cognitive vulnerability to depression [58, 59], people with a tendency toward negative interpretations of life events are more likely to develop depressive symptoms. This model has considerable empirical support in predicting the development of depression in adults [60, 61], as well as in children and adolescents [57, 62–64].

From this general model, the authors develop a cognitive vulnerability-based theory within a transactional model of stress. The starting point, according to the general theory, would be related to a vulnerability that causes the person to experience higher levels of negative affect. This cognitive bias is characterized, according to the authors, by a ruminative response style [65], dysfunctional attitudes [58], and a negative attributional style [59]. This cognitive processing style would be initiated upon the occurrence of negative life events leading to an increase in the initial levels of negative affect and the emergence of depressive symptoms.

Regarding to cognitive predisposition, a ruminative response style has been defined by Nolen-Hoeksema [66] as a way of responding to negative life events characterized by excessive focus on negative emotions, their causes and consequences. Research has found that this style of response results in increased severity of depressive symptoms, supports their maintenance over time, and is associated with an increased likelihood of developing other psychopathological disorders. The results of the studies have confirmed a greater tendency in women to ruminate, in both adolescents [67–69] and adults [70–73]. Moreover, several studies have found that girls score higher than boys in neuroticism [74, 75], a variable that has been linked to higher levels of negative affect [76].

17.4.3 Sociocultural Factors

The familial and social background of the child, and later of the adolescent, is the main vehicle for transmitting socio-cultural values and beliefs in which people build their identity.

Although socio-cultural stereotypes are not the same in all families and social contexts, they usually tend to vary according to the sex of the person. This leads, as a general rule, to differences in the education and socialization patterns of children according to the attitudes and behaviors that are considered appropriate for each gender [77]. These gender differences begin early in childhood, when parents choose different clothing or toys for the children, and continue throughout childhood development through an education based on values and attitudes that are considered appropriate for members of their biological sex [78].

Through a social learning model, based on behavior modeling and reinforcement, children and adolescents build personality traits of their own internalized sex as either male (rationality, competitiveness, and assertiveness) or female (warmth, care, and sensitivity). Girls are educated in a role of caretakers in which relational aspects acquire more importance than other individual aspects of their personality. In contrast, men are educated toward developing individual coping skills.

Hill and Lynch [79] suggest the hypothesis of "gender intensification." According to this theory differences between men and women become accentuated in adolescence because of the social pressure to fulfill established gender roles. At this developmental stage in which adolescents also initiate partner relationships, the predominant social gender values, which usually maintains a male supremacy over female and motherhood as an essential condition of women, may lead to the establishment of unequal relations that favors gender violence and other manifestations of inequality between women and men that lead to emotional discomfort.

In this way, sociocultural pressure predisposes adolescent girls to become exposed to higher stress levels and more negative life events than men, which may explain the dramatic increase in the rates of depression among women in this development period. In fact, several studies have shown that women experience more depressogenic and a greater number of negative life events than men, such as violence or sexual abuse [57].

Since women are under greater pressure to reach physical attractiveness, the physical changes of puberty lead to higher rates of dissatisfaction in women's body image [80–84]. This has also been associated with lower levels of self-esteem and increased depressive symptoms [81, 83].

In conclusion, there is evidence that the socio-emotional adjustment at the adolescent stage is highly mediated by gender issues. Educational attitudes in the family related to social gender stereotypes are a key factor in the construction of adolescent identity and in their level of emotional comfort.

17.5 Discussion

A female predominance in the prevalence of depression becomes evident in the transition from childhood to adolescence. This points to the role of biological factors, especially hormonal ones.

Nonetheless, as in other mental disorders, a strong interrelation between biological and environmental factors seems to underlie the etiological basis of adolescent depression. There's current evidence of the influence of cultural stereotypes as strong modulators of the emotional experience that men or women have in the presence of certain life events.

The gender, as a global concept, determines that a single life event may simultaneously act as a risk factor or as a protective factor for depression; it may also predispose to a greater or lesser degree of vulnerability to suffering traumatic life experiences.

Men and women have adopted different social roles over the years, resulting in different cognitive styles, with a predominance of interpersonal sensibility in women. As a result of this, and given that adolescence is a time when interpersonal stressors increase, it becomes another risk factor that increases the vulnerability of women to depression.

The effect that gender social stereotypes has on the vulnerability to suffering from a depressive disorder provokes the need to design and develop new intervention strategies aimed at enhancing cognitive styles to promote the strengthening of abilities that are scantly stimulated in the social environment. These include the identification and verbalization of feelings in men, and the reinforcement of assertiveness in women.

The modification of cognitive styles and attitudes in a key period that is involved in the formation of personal identity, such as adolescence, may be relevant to neutralizing the negative influence of some of the sociocultural stereotypes.

This is an important field for prevention and intervention programs in adolescent depression, which should also involve families as well as the educational sphere, since they are the main channels for the transmission of sociocultural values during childhood.

Gender will also exert an influence on the symptomatic manifestation of the disease, enhancing and/or inhibiting the expression of certain depressive symptoms. Thus, the incorporation of the gender dimension into clinical assessment broadens the phenomenological understanding of depression.

Finally, the diagnostic bias that may result from the social gender stereotypes internalized by the professionals who work with adolescents should be emphasized. Since social gender stereotypes can change the vision we have of our patients and their problems, we must consider the weight that our own gender values have when making our usual diagnostic and therapeutic decisions.

References

1. Méndez J, Olivares J, Ros CM. Características clínicas y tratamiento de la depresión en la infancia y adolescencia. In: Caballo VE, Simón MA, editors. Manual de psicología clínica infantil y del adolescente. Madrid: Pirámide; 2001. p. 139–85.
2. Egger HL, Angold A. Common emotional and behavioral disorders in preschool children: presentation, nosology, and epidemiology. J Child Psychol Psychiatry. 2006;47:313–37.
3. Lewinson PM, Rohde P, Seeley JR. Major depressive disorder in older adolescents: prevalence, risk factors, and clinical implications. Clin Psychol Rev. 1998;18(7):765–94.
4. Thapar A, Collishaw S, Pine DS, Thapar AK. Depression in adolescence. Lancet. 2012;379: 1056–67.
5. Fleming J, Offord DR. Epidemiology of childhood depressive disorders: a critical review. J Am Acad Child Adolesc Psychiatry. 1990;29:571–80.
6. Lewinsohn PM, Clarke GN. Major depression in community adolescents: age at onset, episode duration, and time to recurrence. J Am Acad Child Adolesc Psychiatry. 1994;33:809–18.
7. Kessler RC, McGonagle KA, Zhao S, et al. Lifetime and 12-month prevalence of DSM-III-R psychiatric disorders in the United States. Results from the National Comorbidity Survey. Arch Gen Psychiatry. 1994;51:8–19.
8. Richardson LP, Katzenellenbogen R. Childhood and adolescent depression: the role of primary care providers in diagnosis and treatment. Curr Probl Pediatr Adolesc Health Care. 2005;35(1): 6–24.

9. Le HN, Boyd RC. Prevention of major depression: early detection and early intervention in the general population. Clin Neuropsychiatry. 2006;3(1):6–22.
10. Zahn-Waxler C, Shirtcliff EA, Marceau K. Disorders of childhood and adolescence: gender and psychopathology. Annu Rev Clin Psychol. 2008;4:275–303.
11. Kessler RC, Avenevoli S, Ries-Merikangas K. Mood disorders in children and adolescents: an epidemiologic perspective. Biol Psychiatry. 2001;49:1002–14.
12. Lewinsohn PM, Essau CA. Depression in adolescents. In: Gotlib IH, Hammen CL, editors. Handbook of depression. New York: Guilford; 2002. p. 541–59.
13. Rao U, Chen LA. Characteristics, correlates, and outcomes of childhood and adolescent depressive disorders. Dialogues Clin Neurosci. 2009;11(1):45–62.
14. Birmaher B, Ryan ND, Williamson DE, Brent DA, Kaufman J, Dahl RE, et al. Childhood and adolescent depression: a review of the past 10 years, Part I. J Am Acad Child Adolesc Psychiatry. 1996;35:1427–40.
15. Birmaher B, Ryan ND, Williamson DE, Brent DA. Childhood and adolescent depression: a review of the past 10 years, Part II. J Am Acad Child Adolesc Psychiatry. 1996;35:1575–83.
16. Bouma E, Ormel J, Verhulst FC, Oldehinkel AJ. Stressful life events and depressive problems in early adolescent boys and girls: the influence of parental depression, temperament and family environment. J Affect Disord. 2008;105:185–93.
17. Naninck EFG, Lucassen PJ, Bakker J. Sex differences in adolescent depression: do sex hormones determine vulnerability? J Neuroendocrinol. 2011;23:383–92.
18. Nissen G. Depressive syndromes in childhood and adolescence. Symptomatology, etiology and prognosis. Monogr Gesamtgeb Psychiatr Psychiatry Ser. 1971;4:1–174.
19. Uebelacker LA, Strong D, Weinstock LM, Miller IW. Use of item response theory to understand differential Functioning of DSM IV major depression symptoms by race, ethnicity and gender. Psychol Med. 2009;39:591–601.
20. Baron P, Joly E. Sex-differences in the expression of depression in adolescents. Sex Roles. 1988;1988(18):1–7.
21. Bennett DS, Ambrosini PJ, Kudes D, Metz C, Rabinovich H. Gender differences in adolescent depression: do symptoms differ for boys and girls? J Affect Disord. 2005;89:35–44.
22. Carter JD, Joyce PR, Mulder RT, Luty SE, McKenzie J. Gender differences in the presentation of depressed outpatients: a comparison of descriptive variables. J Affect Disord. 2000;61: 59–67.
23. Angst J, Dobler-Mikola A. Do the diagnostic criteria determine the sex ratio in depression? J Affect Disord. 1984;7:189–98.
24. Vredenburg K, Krames L, Flett GL. Sex-differences in the clinical expression of depression. Sex Roles. 1986;14:37–49.
25. Wilhelm K, Roy K, Mitchell P, Brownhill S, Parker G. Gender differences in depression risk and coping factors in a clinical sample. Acta Psychiatr Scand. 2002;106:45–53.
26. Phoenix CH, Goy RW, Gerall AA, Young WC. Organizing action of prenatally administered testosterone propionate on the tissues mediating mating behavior in the female guinea pig. Endocrinology. 1959;65:369–82.
27. Thornton J, Zehr JL, Loose MD. Effects of prenatal androgens on rhesus monkeys: a model system to explore the organizational hypothesis in primates. Horm Behav. 2009;55(5):633–45.
28. Lenroot RK, Giedd JN. Sex differences in the adolescent brain. Brain Cogn. 2010;72:46–55.
29. Steiner M, Dunn E, Born L. Hormones and mood: from menarche to menopause and beyond. J Affect Disord. 2003;74:67–83.
30. Rubinow DR, Schmidt PJ, Roca CA. Estrogen-serotonin interactions: implications for affective regulation. Biol Psychiatry. 1998;44:839–50.
31. Martel MM, Klump K, Nigg JT, Breedlove SM, Sisk CL. Potential hormonal mechanisms of attention-deficit/hyperactivity disorder and major depressive disorder: a new perspective. Horm Behav. 2009;55(4):465–79.
32. Angold A, Costello EJ, Erkanli A, Worthman CM. Pubertal changes in hormone levels and depression in girls. Psychol Med. 1999;29:1043–53.

33. Buchanan CM, Eccles JS, Becker JB. Are adolescents the victims of raging hormones: evidence for activational effects of hormones on moods and behaviour at adolescence. Psychol Bull. 1992;11:62–107.
34. Warren MP, Brooks-Gunn J. Mood and behavior at adolescence: evidence for hormonal factors. J Clin Endocrinol Metab. 1989;69:77–83.
35. Freeman EW, Sammel MD, Lin H, Nelson DB. Associations of hormones and menopausal status with depressed mood in women with no history of depression. Arch Gen Psychiatry. 2006;63:375–82.
36. Van Bokhoven I, van Goozen SH, van Engeland H, Schaal B, Arseneault L, Séguin JR, Assaad JM, Nagin DS, Vitaro F, Tremblay RE. Salivary testosterone and aggression, delinquency, and social dominance in a population-based longitudinal study of adolescent males. Horm Behav. 2006;50(1):118–25.
37. McCormick CM, Mathews IZ. HPA function in adolescence: role of sex hormones in its regulation and the enduring consequences of exposure to stressors. Pharmacol Biochem Behav. 2007;86:220–3.
38. Levine JE. Stressing the importance of sex. Endocrinology. 2002;143:4502–4.
39. Bangasser DA, Curtis A, Reyes BAS, Bethea TT, Parastatidis I, Ischiropoloulos H, et al. Sex differences in corticotrophin-releasing factor receptor signaling and trafficking: potential role in female vulnerability to stress-related psychopathology. Mol Psychiatry. 2010;15:896–904.
40. Young E, Korszun A. Sex, trauma, stress hormones and depression. Mol Psychiatry. 2010;15: 23–8.
41. Carroll BJ, Curtis GC, Mendels J. Neuroendocrine regulation in depression I. Limbic system-adrenocortical dysfunction. Arch Gen Psychiatry. 1976;33:1039–44.
42. Weiss EL, Longhurst JG, Mature CM. Childhood sexual abuse as a risk factor for depression in women: psychosocial and neurobiological correlates. Am J Psychiatry. 1999;156:816–28.
43. Stroud LR, Salovey P, Epel ES. Sex differences in stress responses: social rejection versus achievement stress. Biol Psychiatry. 2002;52:318–27.
44. Oldehinkel AJ, Bouma MC. Sensitivity to the depressogenic effect of stress and HPA-axis reactivity in adolescence: a review of gender differences. Neurosci Biobehav Rev. 2011;35: 1757–70.
45. Giedd JN, Clasen LS, Lenroot T, Greenstein D, Wallace GL, Ordaz S, Molloy EA, Blumenthal JD, Tossel JW, Stayer C, Samango-Sprouse CA, Shen D, Davatzikos C, Merke D, Chrousos GP. Puberty-related influences on brain development. Mol Cell Endocrinol. 2006;254–255:154–62.
46. Andrade TG, Nakamuta JS, Avanzi V, Graeff FG. Anxiolytic effect of estradiol in the median raphe nucleus mediated by 5-HT1A receptors. Behav Brain Res. 2005;163(1):18–25.
47. Insel TR. A neurobiological basis of social attachment. Am J Psychiatry. 1997;154:726–35.
48. Amico JA, Crowley RS, Insel TR, Thomas A, O'Keefe JA. Effect of gonadal steroids upon hypothalamic oxytocin expression. Adv Exp Med Biol. 1995;395:23–35.
49. Cyranowski JM, Frank E, Young E, Shear MK. Adolescent onset of the gender difference in lifetime rates of major depression. Arch Gen Psychiatry. 2000;57:21–7.
50. Nettle D. Evolutionary origins of depression: a review and reformulation. J Affect Disord. 2004;81:91–102.
51. Uher R. The role of genetic variation in the causation of mental illness: an evolution-informed framework. Mol Psychiatry. 2009;14:1072–82.
52. Wickramaratne PJ, Weissman MM. Onset of psychopathology in offspring by developmental phase and parental depression. J Am Acad Child Adolesc Psychiatry. 1998;37:933–42.
53. Goodman SH, Gotlib IH. Risk for psychopathology in the children of depressed mothers: a developmental model for understanding mechanisms of transmission. Psychol Rev. 1999;106: 458–90.
54. Moldin SO, Reich T, Rice JP. Current perspectives on the genetics of unipolar depression. Behav Genet. 1991;21:211–42.

55. Harrington RC, Fudge H, Rutter M, Bredenkamp D, Groothues C, Pridham J. Child and adult depression: a test of continuities with data from a family study. Br J Psychiatry. 1993; 162:627–33.
56. Kendler KS, Gardner CO, Prescott CA. Clinical characteristics of mayor depression that predict risk of depression in relatives. Arch Gen Psychiatry. 1999;56:322–7.
57. Hankin BL, Abramson LY. Development of gender differences in depression: an elaborated cognitive vulnerability-transactional stress theory. Psychol Bull. 2001;127(6):773–96.
58. Beck AT. Cognitive models of depression. J Cogn Psychother. 1987;1:5–37.
59. Abramson LY, Metalsky GI, Alloy LB. Hopelessness depression: a theory-based subtype of depression. Psychol Rev. 1989;96:358–72.
60. Abramson LY, Alloy LB, Hogan ME, Whitehouse WG, Donovan P, Rose DT, Panzarella C, Raniere D. Cognitive vulnerability to depression: theory and evidence. J Cogn Psychother. 1999;13:5–20.
61. Ingram RE, Miranda J, Segal ZV. Cognitive vulnerability to depression. New York: Guilford; 1998.
62. Nolen-Hoeksema S, Girgus JS, Seligman MEP. Predictors and consequences of childhood depressive symptoms: a 5-year longitudinal study. J Abnorm Psychol. 1992;101:405–22.
63. Panak WF, Garber J. Role of aggression, rejection, and attributions in the prediction of depression in children. Dev Psychopathol. 1992;4:145–65.
64. Robinson NS, Garber J, Hilsman R. Cognitions and stress: direct and moderating effects on depressive versus externalizing symptoms during the junior high transition. J Abnorm Psychol. 1995;104:453–63.
65. Nolen-Hoeksema S. Sex differences in depression and explanatory style in children. J Youth Adolesc. 1991;20:233–45.
66. Nolen-Hoeksema S. Responses to depression and their effects on the duration of depressive episodes. J Abnorm Psychol. 1991;100:569–82.
67. Broderick PC. Early adolescent gender differences in the use of ruminative and distracting coping strategies. J Early Adolesc. 1998;18:173–91.
68. Hart IB, Thompson JM. Gender role characteristics and depressive symptomatology among adolescents. J Early Adolesc. 1996;16:407–26.
69. Schwartz JAJ, Koenig LJ. Response styles and negative affect among adolescents. Cogn Ther Res. 1996;20:13–36.
70. Butler LD, Nolen-Hoeksema S. Gender differences in responses to depressed mood in a college sample. Sex Roles. 1994;30:331–46.
71. Nolen-Hoeksema S, Morrow J. Effects of rumination and distraction on naturally-occurring depressed mood. Cogn Emot. 1993;7:561–70.
72. Nolen-Hoeksema S, Larson J, Grayson C. Explaining the gender differences in depressive symptoms. J Pers Soc Psychol. 1999;77:1061–72.
73. Nolen-Hoeksema S, Parker LE, Larson J. Ruminative coping with depressed mood following loss. J Pers Soc Psychol. 1994;67:92–104.
74. Del Barrio V, Moreno-Rosset C, López RM, Olmedo M. Anxiety, depression and personality structure. Personal Individ Differ. 1997;23:327–35.
75. Goodyer IM, Ashby L, Altham P, Vize C, Cooper PJ. Temperament and major depression in 11 to 16 years old. J Child Psychol Psychiatry. 1993;34:1409–23.
76. Clark LA, Watson D. Tripartite model of anxiety and depression: psychometric evidence and taxonomic implications. J Abnorm Psychol. 1991;100:316–36.
77. Bussey K, Bandura A. Social cognitive theory of gender development and functioning. In: Eagly AH, Beall A, Sternberg R, editors. The psychology of gender. New York: Guilford; 2004. p. 92–119.
78. Deaux K, Lewis LL. Structure of gender stereotypes: interrelationships among components and gender label. J Pers Soc Psychol. 1984;46:991–1004.
79. Hill J, Lynch M. The intensification of gender-related role expectations during early adolescence. In: Brooks-Gun J, Petersen A, editors. Female puberty. New York: Plenum; 1983.

80. Harter S. The construction of the self: a developmental perspective. New York: Guilford; 1999.
81. Kostanski M, Gullone E. Adolescent body image dissatisfaction: relationships with self-esteem, anxiety, and depression controlling for body mass. J Child Psychol Psychiatry. 1998;39:255–62.
82. Paxton SJ, Wertheim EH, Gibbons K, Szmukler GI, Hillier L, Petrovich JL. Body image satisfaction, dieting beliefs, and weight loss behaviours in adolescent girls and boys. J Youth Adolesc. 1991;20:361–79.
83. Rierdan J, Koff E, Stubbs ML. A longitudinal analysis of body image as a predictor of the onset and persistence of adolescent girls' depression. J Early Adolesc. 1989;9:454–66.
84. Wertheim EH, Paxton SJ, Maude D, Szmukler GI, Gibbons K, Hillier L. Psychosocial predictors of weight loss behaviours and binge eating in adolescent girls and boys. Int J Eat Disord. 1992;12:151–60.

Premenstrual Experience Premenstrual Syndrome and Dysphoric Disorder

18

Miriam Santamaría and Irantzu Lago

Abstract

Premenstrual syndrome (PMS) is considered as a health problem that affects millions of women of reproductive age and, in some cases, may be severe enough to be considered a premenstrual dysphoric disorder (PMDD). Both PMS and PMDD are composed of affective, behavioral, and physical symptoms. Risk factors identified that predispose to PMS/PMDD are age between 25 and 35 years, a psychiatric history, a family history of PMDD, unhealthy living habits, and stressful life events. In addition, a comorbidity of PMDD with various psychiatric disorders such as major depression and anxiety disorders has been established. Although the etiology is unknown, it is considered that PMDD is of a multifactorial nature and is likely to develop because of the interactions among genes, biological variables (the neurotransmitters and gonadal hormones), and environmental influences. The first-line treatment for PMDD is pharmacological with selective serotonin reuptake inhibitors. From a medical point of view there is some evidence of the efficacy of nonpharmacological treatments such as relaxation, aerobic, and cognitive behavioral therapy, which are used mostly in mild cases.

The major criticisms made to the conceptualization of PMDD as a clinical syndrome focus on pathologizing women's biology and its consequent medicalization, which perpetuated misconceptions related to menses. Medicine would be opened up to other fields such as anthropology, sociology, and gender studies with qualitative studies to look for context and meaning to women's

M. Santamaría • I. Lago (✉)
Clinical Psychologists Residents, Alava University Hospital, Vitoria 01004, Spain
e-mail: MIRIAN.SANTAMARIACRESPO@osakidetza.net; IRANTZU.LAGOSANTIAGO@osakidetza.net

M. Sáenz-Herrero (ed.), *Psychopathology in Women*,
DOI 10.1007/978-3-319-05870-2_18

suffering. It has been suggested that it might be more appropriate to introduce the concept of premenstrual or perimenstrual experience instead of PMDD.

18.1 Introduction

Throughout their reproductive age women experience a number of physiological and endocrinological changes associated with ovulation. It is estimated that between 75 and 80 % have experienced some premenstrual symptoms as a result of the hormonal changes that occur during the normal menstrual cycle. The recurrent pattern of emotional, behavioral, and physical symptoms that occur during the last week of the luteal phase and reverse during the first days of menses is called premenstrual syndrome (PMS). These symptoms do not normally affect women's daily life; thus, they are not clinically relevant and do not require a specific treatment [1].

PMS symptoms that are very severe and produce a decrease in functional impairment are defined as premenstrual dysphoric disorder (PMDD). The symptoms, as in the case of PMS, usually start 5–7 days before menses, although in some women they may appear even 12 or 14 days before, reaching the peak of greatest intensity during the 2 days before the start of menses [2] and disappearing in the first few days after. Unlike PMS, which includes mostly somatic symptoms such as breast tenderness and bloating [3], the most common symptoms in PMDD are affective and include affective lability, irritability, depressed mood, and anxiety.

Currently, the relationship between PMS and PMDD is unclear, although most clinicians consider that there is a continuum between these premenstrual problems; PMDD constitutes the more severe stage [4]. PMS/PMDD have been traditionally considered minor health problems affecting only a subset of women during the luteal phase without a significant continuing impact on daily life. However, as pointed out by Stoddard et al. [5], "women have between 400 and 500 menstrual cycles over their reproductive years, and since premenstrual distress symptoms peak during the 4–7 days prior to menses, consistently symptomatic women may spend from 4 to 10 years of their lives in a state of compromised physical functioning and/or psychological well-being"; thus, it could constitute a major health problem for women.

However, despite the disruption that PMS/PMDD can have to women's quality of life, the World Health Organization (WHO) 2001 report on mental health, listing as many as 2,000 disability rates for about 90 disorders, did not even mention PMS/PMDD [6]. This could reflect the fact that many professionals were still unaware of the implications arising from premenstrual experience. But it also makes us question whether we are faced with a major health problem, as they are trying to ascertain, or it is just a physiological state including hormonal, emotional, and physical changes that are not pathological per se. In our opinion it is closer to the latter assumption. The moon cycle changes every month and it has been related to mental health problems without empirical success. Menstrual cycles could be included in the same way.

18.2 History

Despite the physical and psychological changes associated with the menstrual cycle having been recognized and described for thousands of years, it was not until the twentieth century that the concept of PMDD emerged as a clinical disorder.

Hippocrates in the fifth century BC observed that in the days prior to menses mood swings occurred in women, and Galen in the second century AD associated premenstrual hysterical reactions to a toxic uterine fluid, which was eliminated through menstruation. In general, the Hippocrates considered that the most likely cause of any disease in women was the retention of menses. Such retention could result in headaches, fever, hot flashes, etc., and in extreme cases, even loss of reason. This is reported in the Hippocratic treatise "On the diseases of virgins," which tells how in some virgins, retained blood can move through the body causing in the first place a heart dysfunction and in severe states of the disease, stupor, delirium, and madness:

> "Women go crazy as a result of the acute inflammation, as a result of the putrefaction, they feel the desire to kill; as a result of the darkness that builds inside them, they feel terrors and fears, as a result of pressure on the heart they desire choking; because of the spoiling of their blood, their spirit, agitated and distressed, is perverted. In addition, the patient says terrible things. (The visions) command them to jump and throw themselves to wells or strangle themselves as if it was the better and was something useful..." [7]

The problems did not occur only because of the retention of menstrual blood. In some Hippocratic texts the idea remains that an excessive of loss of menstrual blood could also cause a number of complications, such as heat loss, lethargy, fever, anorexia, anxiety, weight loss, general weakness, sterility, and in extreme cases, increased sex drive.

Therefore, according to the Hippocratic perspective, menses is viewed as somewhat therapeutic, as a mechanism that protects women from disease but, at the same time, is its primary cause. The Aristotelics, however, suggested that menses was a weakness, with no therapeutic purpose, whose function was restricted to procreation.

Although the connotations of menses for these classical philosophers are opposed, in both cases women are at constant risk of being damaged by their own nature. This produces a negative view of women as a being sick, weak, and inferior to men by nature, a view that continued over the following centuries and even holds today. This is related to the excessive medicalization of a normal process in women from our point of view.

The first to use menses as a scientific basis to explain some of the female behavior was the American neurologist Robert Frank. In 1931 he published a descriptive study conducted with 15 women who relate recurring physical, emotional, and behavioral symptoms during the luteal phase, which disappeared at the beginning of menses. He called this set of symptoms "premenstrual tension syndrome."

Frank proposed the existence of three groups of women based on the gravity of the symptoms:

- A first group in which are included those women with mild symptoms, such as fatigue, considered to be within normal limits.
- Another group of women diagnosed with other clinical conditions who suffer variations in them during the premenstrual phase.
- Finally, a group with "premenstrual tension," considered a severe emotional disorder with irritability, tension, emotional instability, and reckless behavior [8].

In 1953, Green and Dalton [9] suggest that the emotional tension was just a symptom of the many that compound this state and they replace the term "premenstrual tension" with "premenstrual syndrome." In her book *The Premenstrual Syndrome*, Katerina Dalton reported that "the premenstrual syndrome is the most common endocrine disturbance, frequently meeting in general medical practice, due to the impact of cyclical changes and their effects on the patient and the family circle. It infiltrates in many medical specialties, so that the issue should be of great interest to psychiatrists, endocrinologists, gynecologists, medical officers of the industry and the prison system." Dalton identifies an imbalance between estrogen and progesterone during the luteal phase as the cause of the syndrome, proposing a treatment with progesterone during the premenstrual period, treatment of questionable reliability that acquired great popularity in the 1980s [10].

Finally, in 1987, the Diagnostic and Statistical Manual of Mental Disorders III (DSM-III) included PMDD in the research criteria under the name of "late luteal phase dysphoric disorder, LLPDD." After that, the DSM-IV-TR (text revision) criteria categorized it in Appendix B "Criterion Sets and Axes Provided for Further Study" with its current name. The new DSM-5 considers that there is enough empirical evidence to consider PMDD as a new diagnostic category (see below: "Diagnosis").

18.2.1 Criticism of the Concept and Diagnosis of Premenstrual Syndrome

Some authors such as Chrisler and Caplan [11] criticize "menstrual tension" being used to justify the exclusion of women from the labor market and certain positions of power. This idea is also developed by Shopie Laws in her critique of Dalton's work. Laws, without denying the premenstrual experience, considers it a normal experience and opposes its inclusion within a syndrome or disease. She also wondered why these experiences were not described clearly as diseases until the twentieth century and suggests that there may be a double benefit in its creation: on the one hand, it serves to maintain and reinforce the patriarchal society model and on the other, it is profitable for the pharmaceutical industry, as the medicalization of premenstrual experience has increased their market [10, 12].

In terms of the social impact, PMS was gradually becoming embedded in western culture. This was exposed during a murder trial carried out in the UK in which PMS was the defense for the two accused. It was accepted as mitigation to reduce the sentence and the degree of responsibility. Chrisler and Caplan [11] report that one of the lawyers described his client as a typical case of *Dr. Jekyll and Mr. Hyde* (Robert Louis Stevenson, 1886), because without the progesterone treatment the hidden animal that was living inside her had appeared. This type of judgment is also obvious in Mary Shelley's novel *Frankenstein* (1818), an allegory of the situation of women in the Victorian era, independently of whether it was in the pre-, intra- or postmenstrual period and they have been used to justify the situation of legal inferiority of women: they really could feel (like Frankenstein's monster), but are considered "apart." Indeed, the references about the "monstrous nature" of women has been reported and supported during history many times.

After these events, a committee of psychiatrists in the United States called the premenstrual syndrome the "late luteal phase dysphoric disorder," incorporating it into the DSM-III-R. Despite criticism from the feminist community and many members of the American Psychiatric Association it was permanently defined as a psychiatric disorder. Their main criticism is similar to the criticism made previously of the other terms. They propose that it reflects a destructive vision of women's biology, making them psychiatrically ill through the pathologizing of their natural cycles and their consequent medicalization [13, 14]. Caplan [15] states: "The problem with PMDD is not the women who report that they have premenstrual emotional problems; the problem is with the diagnosis of PMDD itself" (p. 62).

Other critics suggest that the association of premenstrual changes with the diagnosis might affect the way we understand the emotions, in principal gender-neutral [16]. We question whether there are emotional pathological changes per se, or whether they are socially built. Nowadays, there is no evidence that mood changes resulting from hormonal changes are more severe in women than in men [17]. Despite this, an equivalent diagnosis for men has not been proposed, and in this way, the PMDD may be perpetuating a gender bias. Even more mood changes related to hormonal changes could be physiological in women. They also warn of the possibility of perpetuating myths and stereotypes about women's "raging hormones" [18], although the diagnosis does not imply that all menstruating women have a disorder and it represents only a small proportion of the female population.

Finally, some authors suggest that the changes occurring during the premenstrual period might be socially learned and propose a social constructivist understanding view. That is, young women may be influenced by cultural and mostly negative beliefs about menses and this could provoke the psychological and physical symptoms [19]. However, the social learning theory of PMDD is problematic because it is not clear what results measure, if learning, a genetic vulnerability to developing symptoms or both.

18.3 Prevalence

It is estimated that over 75 % of women of reproductive age have experienced symptoms in the premenstrual period [20]. But feeling or experiencing some kind of physiological changes would not be necessary pathological per se. According to the DSM-5, 12-month prevalence of premenstrual dysphoria is between 1.8 % and 5.8 % of menstruating women [21]. The PMS incidence rates vary considerably because, to date, there has been no clear definition of the syndrome and rigorous diagnostic criteria that allow an accurate differentiation of the PMDD have not been developed.

One of the first epidemiological studies of PMDD made following the DSM criteria was conducted by Wittchen et al. in 2002 with 1,000 German women, obtaining a prevalence of 5.8 % [22]. Similar data have been found in other community samples. The prevalence estimated in British women was 6 % [23], while in Canada 5 % of women had PMDD [24].

In a study by Dueñas Diez [25], which estimated the prevalence in Spain of PMS and PMDD, it was found that 91.1 % of women showed isolated PMDD symptoms (PMS), 8.9 % moderate/severe PMS, and only 1.5 % met Steiner's criteria for PMDD. Dueñas reported that these lower percentages for moderate/severe PMS and PMDD could be explained by the notion that Steiner's criteria are more restrictive than those used in other studies.

18.4 Clinical Symptomatology

The main feature of the clinical representation of the PMS/PMDD is the recurring expression of symptoms during the late luteal phase of the menstrual cycle (approximately over 4 days) that ends in the first or second day after the onset of menses [26]. For most women, the symptoms are consistent between cycles and last an average of 6 days per month [27].

The literature has ascribed to PMS/PMDD over 150 symptoms. However, the number of symptoms that patients usually present are much more limited [28]. Most referrals show the following symptoms:

- Physical: swelling; breast tenderness; aches; headache; bloating/weight.
- Behavioral: sleep disturbances; appetite changes; poor concentration; decreased interest; social withdrawal.
- Mood: irritability; mood swings, anxiety/tension; depression; feeling out of control [29].

Some studies suggest that women with PMDD, especially those with more severe symptoms, are at an increased risk of suicidal ideation [30]. Therefore, it is considered an important area in the evaluation of severe PMDD. When it occurs along with symptoms of depression or other mood symptoms they should be referred to a specialist.

Regarding the evolution, symptoms can start at any time from the onset of menarche and are usually maintained throughout the woman's reproductive life if they are not specifically treated [31]. This is, at least, questionable. It has been observed that some women experience more severe symptoms during the late reproductive years [23] and this condition has been associated with an increased risk of developing affective disorders during the transition to menopause [32]. PMS/PMDD resolve completely after menopause, and temporarily during pregnancy or during any menstrual cycle interruption [23, 32, 33].

Finally, no specific abnormalities were found in physical examinations of women with PMS/PMDD, nor were there any specific biochemical abnormalities in laboratory tests [34, 35].

18.4.1 Negative Impact of PMDD Symptoms in Functional Impairment

One of the criteria required by the current classifications for the diagnosis of PMDD is that symptoms must be severe enough to cause a significant deterioration in the quality of life, interfering with work, interpersonal relations, and/or social activities. In fact, the negative impact that this disorder has on the quality of life of women could be compared with that of other affective disorders, including major depression [6]. Most women with PMDD diagnosis report a significant alteration in social adjusting, an increase in interpersonal difficulties and perceive a decrease in quality of life [6, 36–38]. In a study conducted with women from the USA, UK, and France 30 % of women reported serious interference in family life, 17 % interference in social life, and 14 % at work [36]. The question that follows is how other important variables become key influences: social inequality, glass ceiling, gender roles, and domestic violence, having lower salaries in the same jobs within the labor market are all important factors.

The economic burden generated by PMDD has revealed both directly, through the use of health resources, and indirectly, causing a drop in productivity and increasing absenteeism, the latter being much more significant than the former. Borenstein et al. associated in relation to direct costs an annual increase per patient in a year of $59 and an increase of $4,333 in relation to the indirect ones [39]. In women with PMS the number of days off work (measured as 2 days or more of absence in a month) was significantly higher than those without PMS (2.5 vs 1.3 days respectively). Regarding productivity, women with PMS are more likely to have a "high productivity loss" (5 days or more per month with a 50 % drop in productivity) during one menstrual cycle compared with asymptomatic patients (7.2 days vs 4.2 days) [40].

18.5 Diagnosis

The evolution of the diagnostic criteria for PMS and PMDD has been controversial history and has created confusion with regard to what symptoms constitute the disorder. Several diagnostic criteria for PMS and PMDD have been published by many groups including the WHO, the American College of Obstetrics and Gynecology (ACOG), the Royal College of Obstetricians and Gynecologists (RCOG), the International Society for Premenstrual Disorders (ISPMD), and the American Psychiatric Association (DSM-5).

The ICD-10 diagnosis requires only one symptom of a list to make the diagnosis and does not require a reduction in functional impairment; thus, over-diagnosis with these criteria is quite frequent. By contrast, the ACOG, which published its criteria in 2000 combining the National Institute of Mental Health (NIMH) and the University of California criteria, contemplated a significant decrease in functionality as being compulsory for diagnosis [41]. In general, there is an agreement that the ACOG criteria describe adequately the PMS while the DSM criteria describe the most severe form of the syndrome, PMDD [26].

18.5.1 Premenstrual Syndrome

The ACOG defines PMS as the presence of at least one affective or somatic symptom during the luteal phase of the menstrual cycle. To make a diagnosis using these criteria a 30 % increase in reported symptoms during the 6 days preceding menses should be calculated compared with symptoms experienced during the 5–10 days after menses. This pattern of symptoms should be documented in a diary register for 2–3 cycles. Furthermore, the severity of the change should result in functional impairment. The change must be clinically meaningful and not just a mathematical representation [41].

18.5.2 Premenstrual Dysphoric Disorder

Premenstrual dysphoric disorder is a clinical entity that was included in DSM-III in 1987 under the name "late luteal phase dysphoric disorder, LLPDD" in the research criteria. DSM-IV-TR criteria categorized it in Appendix B "Criterion Sets and Axes Provided for Further Study." However, the DSM-5 considers that there is enough empirical evidence to consider PMDD a proper diagnostic category.

The DSM-5 criteria for PMDD do not differ much from those proposed by the DSM-IV-TR. For diagnostic purposes, five or more symptoms must be presented during the week before menses and settle a few days after the start of it. Prospective information is required for physical and behavioral symptoms (using a diary) for at least two cycles. These criteria also specify that the PMDD can overcome other psychiatric disorders, but it must not be confused with the exacerbation of the characteristic symptoms of these disorders. Finally, the symptoms must interfere

Table 18.1 DSM-5 diagnostic criteria

A. In the majority of menstrual cycles, at least five symptoms must be present in the final week before the onset of menses, start to improve within a few days after the onset of menses, and become minimal or absent in the week postmenses
B. One (or more) of the following symptoms must be present:
1. Marked affective lability (e.g., mood swings; feeling suddenly sad or tearful or increased sensitivity to rejection)
2. Marked irritability or anger or increased interpersonal conflicts
3. Marked depressed mood, feelings of hopelessness, or self-deprecating thoughts
4. Marked anxiety, tension, feelings of being "keyed up" or "on edge"
C. One (or more) of the following symptoms must additionally be present, to reach a total of five symptoms when combined with symptoms from criterion B above
1. Decreased interest in usual activities (e.g., work, school, friends, hobbies)
2. Subjective sense of difficulty in concentration
3. Lethargy, easy fatigability, or marked lack of energy
4. Marked change in appetite, overeating, or specific food cravings
5. Hypersomnia or insomnia
6. A sense of being overwhelmed or out of control
7. Physical symptoms such as breast tenderness or swelling, joint or muscle pain, a sensation of "bloating," or weight gain
B. The symptoms are associated with clinically significant distress or interference with work, school, usual social activities or relationships with others (e.g., avoidance of social activities, decreased productivity and efficiency at work, school, or home)
C. The disturbance is not merely an exacerbation of the symptoms of another disorder, such as major depressive disorder, panic disorder, persistent depressive disorder (dysthymic), or a personality disorder (although it may co-occur with any of these disorders)
D. Criterion A should be confirmed by prospective daily ratings during at least two symptomatic cycles. (The diagnosis may be made provisionally prior to this confirmation)
E. The symptoms are not attributable to the physiological effects of a substance (e.g., a drug of abuse, a medication, or other treatment) or another medical condition (e.g., hyperthyroidism)

with daily activity or be causes of stress and therefore, be significant clinically (Table 18.1) [42].

18.5.3 Diagnosis in Women Without Menstruation

The diagnosis of the premenstrual syndrome is more complex but still possible in women with ovulation in the absence of menses. These women experience the typical symptoms of PMS/PMDD, but cannot use menses as a benchmark for the evaluation of the symptoms. This causality can occur in:

- Women who have undergone a hysterectomy (with ovarian conservation) or an endometrial ablation. In these cases 35–40 % develop amenorrhea.

– Women using a levonorgestrel intrauterine device (for contraception or heavy menstrual bleeding). After 6 months women develop amenorrhea, but ovulation can persist in approximately 75 % of the patients.

18.6 Comorbidity

In spite of the growing amount of literature on PMDD, there are not many studies that evaluate its comorbidity with other disorders. The higher rates of comorbidity have been established with mood and anxiety disorders. More research is necessary to clarify this issue, and it is necessary to include the sociocultural construct of gender that has been denied.

Women with PMDD have an incidence of psychiatric disorders such as major depression, seasonal affective disorder, postpartum depression, and anxiety disorders during their lifetime of 50–70 % [43]. Dysthymia, major depressive disorder (MDD), panic disorder (PD), and generalized anxiety disorder (GAD) are Axis I disorders with higher comorbidity or exacerbation premenstrually.

Studies that evaluate the PMDD prospectively suggest comorbidity between no seasonal depression and PMDD of 12–25 %, major depression is reported in 2–12 % of samples, and seasonal affective disorder occurs in 38–46 % of women [44]. Furthermore, it appears that women with PMS suffer more frequently postpartum depression [20]. Anxiety disorders in general are comorbid with PMDD in 11–38 % of the women. Comorbidity between various anxiety disorders and prospectively estimated PMDD is 25 % in panic disorder, 19–23 % in social phobia, and 11–13 % in obsessive compulsive disorder (OCD). In the generalized anxiety disorder (GAD), studies report more variation (4–38 %) [44].

Some of these medical conditions that may be exacerbated in the premenstrual period are: migraines, asthma, seizure disorders, irritable bowel syndrome, diabetes, chronic fatigue symptom, allergies, and autoimmune disorders. Although the mechanisms underlying these conditions are not known, the differential diagnosis is simple because the main symptoms of these disorders are not typical of PMDD [45].

18.7 Etiology

Although the etiology of PMDD is as yet unknown, there is a consensus on its complex and multifactorial nature. The etiology involves biological, psychological, environmental, and social variables. The biological hypotheses are those that have attracted more research, emphasizing the implication in the pathogenesis of certain central neurotransmitters and ovarian steroids. It looks obvious, from our point of view, that medical research has neglected the sociocultural aspects in the construct of this syndrome in our culture, and it is necessary to further research in these fields to be able to understand it.

18.7.1 Female Sex Hormones

Since PMDD only affects women of reproductive age, it is supposed that female sex hormones play a causal role in the disorder. However, studies comparing the levels of progesterone, estradiol, follicle-stimulating hormone, luteinizing hormone (LH), prolactin, cortisol, testosterone, and dihydrotestosterone in women with and without premenstrual symptoms found similar levels [34, 35].

The deficits of progesterone, metabolites (some of which have anxiolytic properties), and its receptors have been proposed as possible mediators of PMS/PMDD. However, as already noted, progesterone concentrations are normal in women with PMS. Furthermore, although the results of the studies are contradictory, it seems that concentrations of progesterone metabolites happen to be similar in women with PMS to those in control women [46].

Since women with PMS have normal levels of estrogen and progesterone, it is postulated that they may have a greater vulnerability to normal hormonal changes that occur during the menstrual cycle, suggesting that gonadal hormones might be necessary but not sufficient to explain the etiology of the disorder.

The basis of this vulnerability could be in the interaction that occurs with other neurohormonal systems, including the renin–angiotensin–aldosterone system and the CRH, as well as neurotransmitters of the central nervous system, particularly the gamma-aminobutyric acid (GABA) and serotonergic systems [47, 48], as discussed below.

18.7.2 Neurotransmitter Systems

Animal studies provide evidence that the cyclical fluctuations of estrogen and progesterone in blood changes produce changes in the opioid [49], GABA [50], and serotonin systems [6].

18.7.2.1 Beta-Endorphins

The role of endogenous opioid activity in the late luteal phase was one of the first hypotheses for the pathogenesis of PMDD. Specifically, the significant decrease in opioid levels may contribute to the emergence of irritability, an increment in appetite, and a lower ability to control impulses, aggression, and anxiety [51]. Nevertheless, more research is needed to corroborate this hypothesis.

18.7.2.2 Serotonin

The serotonergic system has emerged as the most likely cause of PMDD and PMS, as most research has been carried out in this field. One of the pioneers was Wirst [52], who showed that the levels of free tryptophan (an amino acid precursor of serotonin) showed changes during the menstrual cycle that correlated with plasma concentrations of estrogens. There is wide evidence in the literature suggesting that PMDD is caused by a deregulation in the serotonergic system in response to fluctuations of gonadal female hormones during the menstrual cycle. In fact, it has been shown that during the lutein phase, women with PMS have lower plasma levels of serotonin reuptake and fewer minor recognition sites for this neurotransmitter [53].

Several findings support this hypothesis. For example, the administration of L-tryptophan is more effective than placebo in treating premenstrual symptoms, including mood swings, dysphoria, irritability, and tension [52]. Also, it has been reported that flenfluramine, which increases the release of serotonin and decreases its reuptake, produces a significant improvement in PMS symptoms [54]. Besides, selective serotonin reuptake inhibitors (SSRIs) are the most effective drugs for the treatment of PMDD. In fact, the administration of metergoline (a serotonin antagonist) in women treated with fluoxetine produces a recurrence of symptoms [55].

All these findings justify the efficacy of SSRIs for the treatment of PMDD. However, the fact that there are women who do not respond to these antidepressants, suggests that serotonin might not be the only causal variable involved in PMDD [56].

18.7.2.3 GABA

The GABA system has also been studied, though not as widely as the serotonin system in the pathogenesis of PMDD. Several studies have shown low levels of GABA in patients with mood disorders, including PMDD [57]. This decrease in GABA activity could explain the appearance of some of the premenstrual symptoms such as the depressed mood, irritability, tension, and anxiety [6].

In spite of this, the data obtained on the levels of progesterone and its metabolites in symptomatic and asymptomatic women are contradictory [58, 59]. Some works suggest that the differences in women with PMDD and asymptomatic women might not be associated with the levels of allopregnanolone; the differences are due to their sensitivity to this metabolite. This metabolite response to stress in asymptomatic women may be inadequate owing to a reduction in the sensitivity of the GABA-A receptor [60].

18.7.3 Vitamins and Minerals

Attempts to determine if there are vitamin deficiencies in women with premenstrual symptoms have not been successful. It has also been suggested that women with PMS might have lower levels of intracellular magnesium during the menstrual cycle [61, 62]. However, as in the case of vitamin B, the results are inconsistent.

18.7.4 Central Nervous System

The development of neuroimaging techniques has opened up a new stage in the study of biological alterations in mental disorders. Through functional neuroimaging techniques, specifically SPECT, fluctuations of glutamate in the medial prefrontal cortex have been discovered during the menstrual cycle in women with

PMDD as well as in asymptomatic women. Thus, there are lower levels during the luteal phase compared with the follicular phase. These variations in the levels of glutamate are probably due in part to hormonal changes that occur during the menstrual cycle, as mentioned previously, as women with PMDD are more sensitive to these changes produced during the menstrual cycle [63].

On the other hand, magnetic resonance studies revealed that during the premenstrual phase, the gray matter volume is relatively larger in the right anterior hippocampus and, at the same time, is relatively reduced in the right region of the right dorsal basal ganglia [64].

The autonomic nervous system has also been extensively studied in the premenstrual syndrome. Classic studies demonstrated that parasympathetic nervous system activity in women with PMDD was smaller in the luteal phase than in the follicular phase. Recently, Matsumoto et al. have managed to establish a relationship between the decline in autonomic nervous system activity and PMS. This group conducted a study with a sample of 62 women divided into three groups: controls (who manifest few or no symptoms), a group with PMS, and a PMDD group. Heart rate variability and hormone levels in the follicular and luteal phase were recorded, in addition to administering behavioral, physical, and emotional questionnaires to record the different symptoms. Results indicate that there were no changes in the autonomic nervous system activity in the control group, whereas the group of women with PMS showed a significant decrease during the luteal phase that is more marked in women with PMDD [65, 66].

Regarding electrophysiological abnormalities, women with PMS have a lower incidence of delta activity and a higher incidence and amplitude of theta waves during electroencephalographic studies [67].

18.7.5 Psychosocial Factors

The psychosocial model considers that PMDD is a syndrome influenced by Western culture where most women have negative believes about menses. In this culture, menses has been related to affective symptoms and has always had negative connotations (see "History" below). For this reason, they suggest that women have ended up interpreting negatively normal physiological changes that occur during the menstrual cycle [68].

The role that psychosocial factors play in the etiology of PMDD has been very poorly investigated. There are some studies that mention attributional and coping styles playing a central role in the PMS [69]. For example, Blake [70], who developed a cognitive therapy for the treatment of PMDD, suggests that premenstrual symptoms might be caused by negative attributions that women give the symptoms. They perceive a loss of control and use an emotion-focused coping style that leads them to feelings of anger and depression and increases negative thoughts in relation to symptoms.

18.8 Risk Factors

The following are factors that have been associated with an increased risk of PMDD.

18.8.1 Age

Although this disorder can appear at any time from the onset of menarche until the end of the reproductive cycle, research shows that the risk is higher in young women aged 25 to 35 years. This is exemplified by a study conducted with a sample of women aged 18–44 years old that found that the older age group (35–44 years) was the least likely to experience premenstrual symptoms (4.5 %) compared with the groups aged 18–24 (8.7 %) and 25–34 years (10.4 %) [71].

Most of the women seeking treatment for PMDD are in the first half of the fourth decade of life, but recognized the appearance of the symptoms in their teenage years. This suggests that the symptoms tend to become more severe over time until they eventually disappear with the menopause [72]. Although over time the belief that women with irregular menstrual cycles have a higher incidence of PMS/PMDD has been maintained, the fact is that recent studies have found no such difference [73].

18.8.2 Past or Current Psychiatric Disorders

Women with a history of mood disorders, anxiety disorders, personality disorder, and substance abuse disorder have a higher incidence of severe premenstrual symptoms [74]. Specifically, PMDD is usually associated with a history of depression [23] and anxiety disorders [75] (see "Comorbidity" above).

On the other hand, some studies show that during the premenstrual period, certain psychiatric symptoms can be exacerbated such as obsessive–compulsive behavior, increased alcohol consumption, and a higher rate of suicide or schizophrenic symptoms [76]. This is why in the DSM, one of the diagnostic criteria for PMDD is that symptoms cannot be mere exacerbations of another disorder.

18.8.3 Family History of PMS

Numerous studies have explored the role that genetic factors play in the predisposition in PMS and PMDD. Women whose mothers suffer from premenstrual symptoms are at a higher risk of developing PMS than women whose mothers are not affected.

Twin studies also point in this direction. Kendler et al. [78], with a sample of 1,000 twins, found a level of agreement of 56 % in monozygotics. It was estimated in another Australian study population (454 monozygotic and 266 dizygotic) that genetic factors accounted for 44 % of the total variance [77, 78].

18.8.4 Genetic Variations of Estrogen Receptor ESR1

Recent studies have found an association between PMDD and polymorphisms in the *ESR1* gene [79, 80]. This is promising for several reasons. First, the ESR1 plays an important role in the physiological activation, whose dysfunction could occur on the basis of the somatic, cognitive, and affective symptoms [81]. Second, the ESR1 is a hormone receptor that could be relevant in the development of PMDD [46]. Finally, allelic variations in the ESR1 could explain the abnormal sensitivity experienced by women with this disorder to normal fluctuations in estrogen and progesterone during the menstrual cycle [82].

18.8.5 Healthy Behaviors

Smoking has been associated with an increased incidence of PMDD [83]. Women smokers are 2.1 times more likely to suffer from premenstrual symptoms than nonsmokers. Furthermore, this risk is much higher for women who started smoking during adolescence [84].

Body mass index (BMI) has also been associated with PMS, with a three times higher risk in women with a BMI greater than or equal to 30 [85, 86].

18.8.6 Educational Level and Work Situation

Cohen et al. [23] found an association between PMDD and lower educational level. Also, they reported that women who do not work outside the home were less likely to have the disorder [23]. Krantz and Ostergren's results [83] suggested that, in addition to the symptomatology increment observed in unemployed women, those who are exposed to a high level of job strain suffered it too. Despite these data, Potter et al. [85], with a sample of 2,863 French women, did not find associations among the educational level, employment status, and PMDD.

To sum up, studies have not found consistent associations between sociodemographic variables and PMDD. Because of the diverse results, the role of sociodemographic variables as risk factors for PMDD is as yet unknown.

18.8.7 Stressful Events

It appears that women diagnosed with PMDD experience more stressful events than asymptomatic women, and they are also more vulnerable to daily stress [60, 87]. Traumatic events, including sexual and psychological abuse, have been considered risk factors for developing PMDD. A longitudinal study with a 4-year follow-up in a sample of 1,488 women diagnosed with PMDD revealed that traumatic events greatly increase the chances of developing PMDD. The other predictor found was an elevated daily hassles score [88].

18.9 Treatment

The therapeutic options available for the treatment of PMS and PMDD can be classified into nondrug interventions and pharmacological approaches.

18.9.1 Nondrug Interventions

The ACOG recommends changes in daily life as the first choice of treatment for PMS [41]. However, the pharmacological treatment, with SSRIs or oral contraceptives, is most frequently used. The ACOG recommendations are often ignored owing to the absence of information about the effectiveness of behavioral interventions to produce long-term changes in lifestyle and are typically reserved for mild cases of PMS. The results observed in this type of treatment occur over a longer period of time than in the pharmacological intervention. Nondrug interventions that have shown some evidence of effectiveness, or at least have a consensus supporting their use, are described below.

18.9.1.1 Aerobic Exercise and Relaxation

There is some evidence to indicate the effectiveness of aerobic exercise [89, 90] and relaxation [91] as a treatment for PMS/PMDD. Correlational studies show a positive correlation between the maintenance of aerobic exercise and the increments in quality of life (QOL) reports [92, 93]. However, it has not yet been verified whether the improvement is superior to that with placebo.

18.9.1.2 Cognitive Behavioral Therapy

Although there is some evidence for its effectiveness for PMS/PMDD [94, 95] a recent meta-analytic study undertaken by Kathleen et al. [96] shows that such evidence is still scarce and highlights the need to develop more studies in order to evaluate its effectiveness.

Regarding the practical application, one of the most important limitations of cognitive behavioral treatment for PMS/PMDD is that it requires months to produce improvements. Since the therapeutic recommendation is to proceed with another treatment if symptoms do not improve in 2–4 cycles, its application is very limited.

18.9.1.3 Others

Caffeine, sugar, and alcohol are associated with an increase in the symptoms associated with PMS [97]. However, dietary interventions, such as reducing sugar intake and eating small but frequent meals, have little scientific evidence to support their effectiveness. Some vitamins such as B6, calcium, and magnesium have been studied as therapeutic agents for premenstrual syndrome, but there is no evidence to indicate that their effect is superior to that of placebo [62, 98–103].

18.9.2 Pharmacological Approaches

Pharmacological agents with proven efficacy for the treatment of PMS or PMDD include: SSRIs, anxiolytics, GnRH agonists, and combined oral contraceptives.

18.9.2.1 SSRIs

Selective serotonin reuptake inhibitors (fluoxetine, sertraline, paroxetine, and venlafaxine) have been proven to have a safety profile [104] and have been effective in the treatment of PMDD in clinical trials [105] as well as in systematic reviews [106, 107]. SSRIs can be administered daily or specifically during the luteal phase. Many women prefer this treatment mode [32]. Intermittent therapy starts on the 14th day of the cycle and continues until the onset of menses. It can be maintained for some days longer if the symptoms persist during menses. This modality of treatment has the advantage of being cheaper and has fewer side effects. While individual trials suggest the efficacy of this approach [102–104], a meta-analysis of 29 studies reported that intermittent dosing was less effective than continuous therapy [32].

The rates of success of the SSRIs are high; 60–70 % of the patients respond positively. Women who do not respond can benefit from the administration of a second SSRI or daily therapy [105].

Generally, side effects are well tolerated by patients. Nausea is a common symptom and decreases after the first few days of treatment, not to return, even in the intermittent treatment modality [106]. Sexual effects (decreased libido and anorgasmia) persist throughout the treatment period, but not during periods without it [107]. The discontinuation of symptoms that may occur if the treatment ceases abruptly do not occur in the intermittent modality, indicating that 2 weeks are insufficient to provoke them [104].

Other antidepressants that inhibit serotonin reuptake (but are not SSRIs) and have proven somewhat effective for PMDD include clomipramine (administered throughout the menstrual cycle or only during the luteal phase) [108, 109], nefazodone [110], and venlafaxine [111], a drug that selectively inhibits the reuptake of serotonin and norepinephrine.

18.9.2.2 Anxiolytics

Anxiolytics that have been evaluated for the treatment of premenstrual syndrome include alprazolam and buspirone. The therapeutic recommendation is to add alprazolam to treatment with SSRIs at low doses (0.25 mg three or four times a day) when treatment with SSRIs has been ineffective or has not reduced all symptoms [104, 112–114]. It is considered a second treatment option because there is a risk of addictive use.

18.9.2.3 Combined Oral Contraceptives

The treatment with oral contraceptives (OC) for PMDD, despite being widespread in clinical practice, is not supported by strong empirical evidence. Placebo-controlled trials are limited, and the first results are negative [115, 116]. However, it seems that OC treatment with fewer hormone-free days could be more effective [117]; the reduction in the number of hormone-free days results in fewer symptoms [118].

The use of the OC drospirenone plus ethinyl estradiol is promising [119–121]. This treatment modality reduces the symptoms of PMDD, including the reduction in work productivity and the impairment in social relationships, at least in short-term studies [120]. The studies also support the efficacy of drospirenone with only four hormone-free days [3, 122].

18.9.2.4 Hormone Treatment

If the treatment with SSRIs or oral contraceptives has not been effective or is not well tolerated, GnRH agonist with estrogen–progestin add-back therapy is recommended. The goal of hormone therapy is to suppress the hypothalamus–gonadal cyclicity that triggers the symptoms. It is important to take into account that GnRG agonists administered alone produce hypoestrogenism (hot flashes and loss of bone mineral density). Studies report the effectiveness of the maintained administration of leuprolide when low doses of estrogens and progestin are continuously added [123–125]. This combined treatment modality prevents the loss of bone density [126, 127].

18.9.2.5 Surgery

Surgery is reserved for refractory cases with severe and very disabling symptoms. Three observational studies found that bilateral oophorectomy, usually along with hysterectomy, is effective for these patients [128–130]. However, further research is necessary in this area.

18.10 Criticism of the Concept of PMS/PMDD

18.10.1 The Premenstrual Experience as a Social Construction

The premenstrual experience has not always been considered a disease. In fact, as we mentioned above, it was not until the twentieth century that professionals started talking about PMS and PMDD. The anthropological model considers that culture is responsible for determining which groups of signs and symptoms are recognized as a disease in a particular population; thus, similar experiences would be described as a disease in some cultures but not in others. Illnesses that are specific to a culture have been denominated "folk illnesses" [131]. In the case of the PMS/PMDD, it has been affirmed that it actually is a syndrome that has been influenced by Western culture, in which most women have negative beliefs about menses, as it is systematically associated with affective and physical symptoms. For this reason, women have ended up making a negative interpretation about normal changes that occur during the menstrual cycle [68].

To determine whether PMS/PMDD is a social construction it would be necessary to prove that women of other countries, in addition to Europeans or Americans, have premenstrual experiences. However, conducting such cross-cultural studies encounters several problems. First, the main scales used in the assessment of premenstrual symptoms are not adapted to different cultures. Second, we cannot forget the great influence that English-speaking cultures have on other countries. In fact, studies with samples of developing countries show that the women with more Western influences are the ones who report more psychological and emotional symptoms when describing their premenstrual experiences [132]. Finally, it seems that these cultural studies can promote new health politics that can create negative concepts related to health. Therefore, women can be influenced by this type of politics, developing negative perceptions about some feminine phenomena. This has been shown in a study conducted in Thailand by Chirawatkul and Maderson [133] about the menopause, so it would also have happened with PMS/PMDD.

18.10.2 The Premenstrual Experience from a Socio-Historical Point of View

Throughout history, the female body has been systematically associated with negative conceptions including the idea of femininity as being something sick and dirty. This vision could be involved in both the birth and the development of the SPM and other phenomena such hysteria in the nineteenth century or the menopause in this century [134].

The search for the influence of the reproductive system in female behavior responds to a reproductivist vision of health and the female body in which women's behavior is explained only through its reproductive potential. In this way, women are constantly at the mercy of their reproductive system. While before, the main influence came from the uterus, as in the case of hysteria, it has lately been focused on the hormones, as in the case of PMS/PMDD and the menopause [135]. This idea has been maintained until the present day, when, instead of abandoning it, it has emerged more strongly because of the attention given to it by medical professionals and the media [10].

The appearance during the twentieth century of the terms of PMS/PMDD has been proposed as something beneficial. On the one hand, women, because PMS is a clinical entity, could receive health care, an idea supported by Dr. Dalton. PMS would be considered a real problem that requires active intervention by the healthcare system. However, on the other hand, it could be used to reinforce and maintain the patriarchal model. If women are treated medically because of their own biology, they would respond again to the female stereotype of women as mild, placid, and undemanding [12]. At the same time, for some women it could represent an attractive explanation to justify their oppression and their relative lack of success compared with men. This means that women can attribute their subordination and oppression to something identifiable and potentially curable, rather than attributing it to gender power relations [136]. Finally, the concept is clearly of benefit to the pharmaceutical industry, as the medicalization of premenstrual experiences has increased their market [10, 12].

18.10.3 Alternative Proposal

García Porta [10] suggests that it might be more appropriate to talk about the premenstrual or perimenstrual experience rather than PMS. This does not deny the experience itself, although it would exclude it as an expression that defines a pathological state [11, 137].

The role that reproductive health education can play in changing the social construction made for the PMS/PMDD has been emphasized. Apart from that, if biomedicine was opened up to social disciplines such anthropology, sociology, history and gender studies, and their qualitative methodology, the context and meaning of many of these phenomena could be clarified. Only through an approach like this could women be active agents who try to make sense of their own experiences [10].

Conclusions

- The main aim of this chapter is to consider the premenstrual experience as a phenomenon that involves biological, psychological, social, and anthropological aspects.
- PMDD includes mood, somatic, and behavioral symptoms, which cause functional impairment. PMDD is considered to be the severe form of PMS.
- While mild premenstrual symptoms are very common in women of reproductive age, PMDD is much less common, with a prevalence in Western countries of around 5–6 %.
- To diagnose PMDD it is necessary to present five or more symptoms during the week before menses that finish a few days after onset. Information regarding the physical and behavioral symptoms is collected prospectively using diaries of symptoms for at least two cycles. Symptoms must interfere with daily activity or cause stress and therefore be significant clinically.
- The most common comorbid disorders associated with PMDD are mood disorders such as depression and anxiety disorders. Frequently, symptoms of other medical illnesses can be exacerbated during the luteal phase.
- Although the etiology of PMDD is unknown, the literature showed abnormalities in central nervous system neurotransmitters, also influenced by ovarian steroids, as the serotonergic system and the neurotransmitters are

more frequently implicated in the onset of the clinical syndrome. However, to consider only one etiological factor would be a mistake, given the multi-faceted and biopsychosocial nature of PMDD. It might be more appropriate to talk about the influence of genetic vulnerability and biological variables (neurotransmitters and gonadal hormones) in interaction with environmental factors as being the cause of PMDD.

- Certain factors have been identified that may predispose to the disorder, such as a history of psychiatric disorders (especially major depression), stressful events of everyday life, past traumatic events, and an unhealthy lifestyle (obesity, smoking, etc.). Regarding sociodemographic factors, although PMDD is usually associated with a lower educational level and unemployment the results of different studies are inconsistent.
- The first-line treatment for PMDD is treatment with SSRIs and the second anxiolytics, combined oral contraceptives, and finally GnRH agonist add-back estrogen–progestin therapy. Surgery is reserved for very severe refractory cases. Nonpharmacological treatments are recommended in milder cases. There is some evidence of the effectiveness of relaxation, aerobic exercise, and CBT.
- Critics of the diagnosis focus on the disapproving of the pathologizing of women's biology and consequent medicalization. Negative stereotypes about menses have been maintained throughout centuries, limiting women's lives.
- The psychosocial model considers PMS/PMDD to be a syndrome developed in Western culture, where most women already have negative beliefs about menses.
- Some authors remind us of the historical and negative conceptions with regard to the female body plus a reproductivist vision as the causes of many women's behavior that have had a determinate influence on the consideration of women's experiences as diseases. In our opinion, it is important to rethink and talk about the premenstrual experience rather than syndrome.

References

1. Pearlstein T, Yonkers KA, Fayyad R, Gillespie JA. Pretreatment pattern of symptom expression in premenstrual dysphoric disorder. J Affect Disord. 2005;85(3):275–82.
2. Bocchino S. Salud Mental de la Mujer. Boletín Sociedad de Psiquiatría del Uruguay. 2005: 3–10.
3. Steiner M, Born L. Psychiatric aspects of the menstrual cycle. In: Kornstein S, Clayton A, editors. Women's mental health. A comprehensive textbook. 1st ed. New York: The Guilford Press; 2002. p. 48–69.
4. Schechter D. Estrogen, progesterone, and mood. J Gend Specif Med. 1999;2(1):29–36.
5. Stoddard JL, Dent CW, Shames L, Bernstein L. Eur J Appl Physiol. 2007;99:27–37.
6. World Health Organization. Mental health: new understanding, new hope. Geneva Halbreich; 2001.
7. Jensvold MF, Dan CE. Psychological aspects of women's health care: the interface between psychiatry and obstetrics and gynecology. Washington, DC: American Psychiatric Publishing; 2001.

8. Richardson J. The premenstrual syndrome: a brief history. Soc Sci Med. 1995;6(41):761–7.
9. Dalton K. El Síndrome Premenstrual. México: Proteo; 1967.
10. García Porta M. Síndrome premenstrual: Aproximación crítica. AIBR Revista de Antropología Iberoamericana. 2006 [cited 2013 Jun 25]; 1(1):80–102. Available from: http://www.aibr.org/antropologia/01v01/articulos/010105.pdf
11. Chrisler JC, Caplan P. The strange case of Dr. Jekyll and Ms. Hyde: how PMS became a cultural phenomenon and a psychiatric disorder. Annu Rev Sex Res. 2002;13:274–306.
12. Laws S. Issues of blood: the politics of menstruation. London: Palgrave Macmillan; 1990.
13. Caplan PJ, McCurdy-Myers J, Gans M. Should premenstrual syndrome be called a psychiatric abnormality? Fem Psychol. 1992;2:27–44.
14. Offman A, Kleinplatz PJ. Does PMDD belong in the DSM? Challenging the medicalizaton of women's bodies. Can J Hum Sex. 2004;13:17–28.
15. Caplan P. The debate about PMDD and Sarafem: suggestions for therapists. Women Ther. 2004;27:55–67.
16. Nash HC, Chrisler JC. Is a little (psychiatric) knowledge a dangerous thing? Psychol Women Q. 1997;21:315–22.
17. Fausto-Sterling A. Myths of gender: biological theories about women and men. New York: Basic Books; 1985.
18. Gallant SJ, Hamilton JA. On a premenstrual psychiatric diagnosis: what's in a name? Prof Psychol Res Pr. 1988;19:271–8.
19. Anson O. Exploring the bio-psycho-social approach to premenstrual experience. Soc Sci Med. 1999;49(1):67–80.
20. Grady-Weliky TA. Clinical practice. Premenstrual dysphoric disorder. N Engl J Med. 2003; 348:433–8.
21. American Psychiatric Association. Diagnostic and statistical manual of mental disorders-V. 5th ed. Washington, DC: American Psychiatric Association; 2013.
22. Wittchen HU, Becker E, Lieb R, et al. Prevalence, incidence and stability of premenstrual dysphoric disorder in the community. Psychol Med. 2002;32:119–32.
23. Cohen LS, Soares CN, Otto MW, et al. Prevalence and predictors of premenstrual dysphoric disorder (PMDD) in older premenopausal women. The Harvard study of moods and cycles. J Affect Disord. 2002;70:125.
24. Steiner M, Macdougall M, Brown E. The premenstrual symptoms screening tool (PSST) for clinicians. Arch Womens Ment Health. 2003;6(3):203–9.
25. Dueñas JL, Lete I, Bermejo R, Arbat A, Pérez-Campos E, Martínez Salmeán J, Serrano I, Doval JL, Coll C. Prevalence of premenstrual syndrome and premenstrual dysphoric disorder in a representative cohort of Spanish women of fertile age. Eur J Obstet Gynecol Reprod Biol. 2011;156(1):72–7. doi:10.1016/ejogrb.2010.12.013.
26. O'Brien PM, Bäckström T, Brown C, et al. Towards a consensus on diagnostic criteria, measurement and trial design of the premenstrual disorders: the ISPMD Montreal consensus. Arch Womens Ment Health. 2011;14:13–21.
27. Yonkers KA, O'Brien PM, Eriksson E. Premenstrual syndrome. Lancet. 2008;371(9619): 1200–10.
28. Freeman EW, Halberstadt SM, Rickels K, et al. Core symptoms that discriminate premenstrual syndrome. J Womens Health (Larchmt). 2011;20(1):29–35.
29. Freeman EW. Premenstrual syndrome and premenstrual dysphoric disorder: definitions and diagnosis. Psychoneuroendocrinology. 2003;3:25–37.
30. Pilver CE, Libby DJ, Hoff RA. Premenstrual dysphoric disorder as a correlate of suicidal ideation, plans, and attempts among a nationally representative sample. Soc Psychiatry Psychiatr Epidemiol. 2013;48(3):437–46.
31. Rapkin AJ, Winer SA. Premenstrual syndrome and premenstrual dysphoric disorder: quality of life and burden of illness. Expert Rev Pharmacoecon Outcomes Res. 2009;9(2):157–70.
32. Freeman EW, Sammel MD, Rinaudo PJ, Sheng L. Premenstrual syndrome as a predictor of menopausal symptoms. Obstet Gynecol. 2004;103(5 Pt 1):960–6.

33. Di Giulio G, Reissing ED. Premenstrual dysphoric disorder: prevalence, diagnostic considerations, and controversies. J Psychosom Obstet Gynaecol. 2006;27(4):201–10.
34. Andersch B, Abrahamsson L, Wendestam C, et al. Hormone profile in premenstrual tension: effects of bromocriptine and diuretics. Clin Endocrinol (Oxf). 1979;11:657.
35. Taylor JW. Plasma progesterone, oestradiol 17 beta and premenstrual symptoms. Acta Psychiatr Scand. 1979;60:76.
36. Hylan TR, Sundell K, Judge R. The impact of premenstrual symptomology on functioning and treatment-seeking behaviour: experience from the United States, United Kingdom and France. J Womens Health Gend Based Med. 1999;8:1043–52.
37. Kuan AJ, Carter DM, Ott FJ. Distress levels in patients with premenstrual dysphoric disorder. Can J Psychiatry. 2002;47:888–9.
38. Campbell EM, Peterkin D, O'Grady K, Sanson-Fisher R. Premenstrual symptoms in general practice patients: prevalence and treatment. J Reprod Med. 1997;42:637–46.
39. Borenstein J, Chiou C, Dean B, Wong J, Wade S. Estimating direct and indirect costs of premenstrual syndrome. J Occup Environ Med. 2005;47(1):26–33.
40. Dean B, Borenstein J. A prospective assessment investigating the relationship between work productivity and impairment with premenstrual syndrome. J Occup Environ Med. 2004; 46(7):649–56.
41. ACOG. ACOG practice bulletin: premenstrual syndrome. Int J Gynecol Obstet. 2000;73: 183–91.
42. Epperson CN, Steiner M, Hartlage SA, et al. Premenstrual dysphoric disorder: evidence for a new category for DSM-5. Am J Psychiatry. 2012;169:465.
43. Endicott J. The menstrual cycle and mood disorders. J Affect Disord. 1993;29(2–3):193–200.
44. Kim DR, Gyulai L, Freeman EW, Morrison MF, Baldassano C, Dube' B. Premenstrual dysphoric disorder and psychiatric co-morbidity. Arch Womens Ment Health. 2004;7:37–47.
45. Pearlstein T, Steiner M. Premenstrual dysphoric disorder: burden of illness and treatment update. J Psychiatry Neurosci. 2008;33:291–301.
46. Schmidt PJ, Nieman LK, Danaceau MA, Adams LF, Rubinow DR. Differential behavioral effects of gonadal steroids in women with and in those without premenstrual syndrome. N Engl J Med. 1998;338:209–16.
47. Chrousos GP, Torpy DJ, Gold PW. Interactions between the hypothalamic-pituitary-adrenal axis and the female reproductive system: clinical implications. Ann Intern Med. 1998;129(3): 229–40.
48. Wardlaw SL, Thoron L, Frantz AG. Effects of sex steroids on brain beta-endorphin. Brain Res. 1982;245:327.
49. Majewska MD, Harrison NL, Schwartz RD, et al. Steroid hormone metabolites are barbiturate-like modulators of the GABA receptor. Science. 1986;232:1004.
50. Bethea CL. Regulation of progestin receptors in raphe neurons of steroid-treated monkeys. Neuroendocrinology. 1994;60:50.
51. Chuong CJ, Hsi BP, Gibbons WE. Periovulatory beta-endorphin levels in premenstrual syndrome. Obstet Gynecol. 1994;83:755.
52. Yonkers KA. The association between premenstrual dysphoric disorder and other mood disorders. J Clin Psychiatry. 1997;58 Suppl 15:19–25.
53. Wirst-Justice et al. Citado en Jensvold MF. Nonpregnant reproductive age women. In: Psychopharmacology and women. Washington, DC: American Psychiatric Press; 1996. p. 139–69.
54. Roca CA, Schmidt PJ, Smith MJ, et al. Effects of metergoline on symptoms in women with premenstrual dysphoric disorder. Am J Psychiatry. 2002;159:1876.
55. Steinberg S, Annable L, Young SN, Liyanage N. A placebo controlled clinical trial of L-tryptophan in premenstrual dysphoria. Biol Psychiatry. 1999;45:313–20.
56. Brzezinski AA, Wurtman JJ, Wurtman RJ, Gleason R, Greenfield J, Nader T. d-Fenfluramine suppresses the increased calorie and carbohydrate intakes and improves mood of women with premenstrual depression. Obstet Gynecol. 1990;76:296–301.

57. Indusekhar R, Bose Usman S. Psychological aspects of premenstrual Síndrome. Best Pract Res Clin Obstet Gynaecol. 2007;2(Pt 21):207–20.
58. Schmidt PJ, Purdy RH, Moore Jr PH, et al. Circulating levels of anxiolytic steroids in the luteal phase in women with premenstrual syndrome and in control subjects. J Clin Endocrinol Metab. 1994;79:1256.
59. Rapkin AJ, Morgan M, Goldman L, et al. Progesterone metabolite allopregnanolone in women with premenstrual syndrome. Obstet Gynecol. 1997;90:709.
60. Girdler SS, Klatzkin R. Neurosteroids in the context of stress: implications for depressive disorders. Pharmacol Ther. 2007;116:125–39.
61. Sherwood RA, Rocks BF, Stewart A, Saxton RS. Magnesium and the premenstrual syndrome. Ann Clin Biochem. 1986;23(Pt 6):667.
62. Facchinetti F, Borella P, Fioroni L, et al. Reduction of monocyte's magnesium in patients affected by premenstrual syndrome. J Psychosom Obstet Gynaecol. 1990;11:221.
63. Batra NA, Seres-Mailo J, Hanstock C, et al. Proton magnetic resonance spectroscopy measurement of brain glutamate levels in premenstrual dysphoric disorder. Biol Psychiatry. 2008;63:1178–84.
64. Protopopescu X, Butler T, Pan H, et al. Hippocampal structural changes across the menstrual cycle. Hippocampus. 2008;18:985–8.
65. Kondo M, Hirano T, Okamura Y. Changes in autonomic nerve function during the normal menstrual cycle measured by the coefficient of variation of R-R intervals. Nippon Sanka Fujinka Gakkai Zasshi. 1989;41:513–8.
66. Matsumoto T, Ushiroyama T, Morimura M, et al. Autonomic nervous system activity in the late luteal phase of eumenorrheic women with premenstrual symptomatology. J Psychosom Obstet Gynaecol. 2006;27:131–9.
67. Baker FC, Kahan TL, Trinder J, Colrain IM. Sleep quality and the sleep electroencephalogram in women with severe premenstrual syndrome. Sleep. 2007;30:1283–91.
68. Chrisler JC, Johnston-Robledo I. Raging hormones? Feminist perspectives on premenstrual syndrome and postpartum depression. In: Ballou M, Brown LS, editors. Rethinking mental health and disorder: feminist perspectives. New York: Guilford Press; 2002. p. 174–97.
69. Sigmon ST, et al. The role of anxiety level, coping styles and cycle phase in menstrual distress. J Anxiety Disord. 2004;18:177–91.
70. Blake F. Cognitive therapy for premenstrual syndrome. Cogn Behav Pract. 1995;2:167–85.
71. Deuster PA, Adera T, South-Paul J. Biological, social, and behavioral factors associated with premenstrual syndrome. Arch Fam Med. 1999;8:122–8.
72. Ramcharan S, Love EJ, Fick GH, Goldfien A. The epidemiology of premenstrual symptoms in a population-based sample of 2650 urban women: attributable risk and risk factors. J Clin Epidemiol. 1995;45:377–92.
73. Perarnau MP, et al. Síntomas, Síndrome y Trastorno Disfórico Premenstrual en una muestra de mujeres universitarias. Fundamentos en Humanidades. 2010;2(Pt11):195–209.
74. Bocchino S. Salud Mental de la Mujer. Boletín Sociedad de Psiquiatría del Uruguay. 2004;68(1):78–89.
75. American Psychiatric Association. Diagnostic and statistical manual of mental disorders-IV-TR. Barcelona: Masson; 2002.
76. Perez-Lopez FR, et al. Premenstrual syndrome and premenstrual dysphoric disorder: symptoms and cluster influences. Open Psychiatr J. 2009;3:39–49.
77. Kendler KS, Karkowski LM, Corey LA, Neale MC. Longitudinal population-based twin study of retrospectively reported premenstrual symptoms and lifetime major depression. Am J Psychiatry. 1998;155:1234.
78. Treloar SA, Heath AC, Martin NG. Genetic and environmental influences on premenstrual symptoms in an Australian twin sample. Psychol Med. 2002;32:25.
79. Miller A, Vo H, Huo L, et al. Estrogen receptor alpha (ESR-1) associations with psychological traits in women with PMDD and controls. J Psychiatr Res. 2010;44:788.

80. Huo L, Straub RE, Roca C, et al. Risk for premenstrual dysphoric disorder is associated with genetic variation in ESR1, the estrogen receptor alpha gene. Biol Psychiatry. 2007;62 925.
81. Garey J, Goodwillie A, Frohlich J, Morgan M, Gustafsson JA, Smithies O, et al. Genetic contributions to generalized arousal of brain and behavior. Proc Natl Acad Sci USA. 2003; 100:11019–22.
82. Rubinow DR, Schmidt PJ, Roca CA. Review estrogen-serotonin interactions: implications for affective regulation. Biol Psychiatry. 1998;44(9):839–50.
83. Krantz G, Ostergren PO. Common symptoms in middle aged women: their relation to employment status, psychosocial work conditions and social support in a Swedish setting. J Epidemiol Community Health. 2000;54(3):192–9.
84. Bertone-Johnson ER, Hankinson SE, et al. Cigarette smoking and the development of premenstrual syndrome. Am J Epidemiol. 2008;168(8):938–45.
85. Potter J, Bouyer J, et al. Premenstrual syndrome prevalence and fluctuation over time: results from a French population-based survey. J Womens Health (Larchmt). 2009;18(1):31–9.
86. Masho SW, Adera T, South-Paul J. Obesity as a risk factor for premenstrual syndrome. J Psychosom Obstet Gynaecol. 2005;26:33–9.
87. Woods NF, Lentz M, Mitchell ES, Heitkemper M, Shaver J. PMS after 40: persistence of a stress-related symptom pattern. Res Nurs Health. 1997;20:319–40.
88. Perkonigg A, Yonkers KA, Pfister H, et al. Risk factors for premenstrual dysphoric disorder in a community sample of young women: the role of traumatic events and posttraumatic stress disorder. J Clin Psychiatry. 2004;65:1314.
89. Steege JF, Blumenthal JA. The effects of aerobic exercise on premenstrual symptoms in middle-aged women: a preliminary study. J Psychosom Res. 1993;37(2):127–33.
90. Aganoff JA, Boyle GJ. Aerobic exercise, mood states and menstrual cycle symptoms. J Psychosom Res. 1994;38:183.
91. Goodale IL, Domar AD, Benson H. Alleviation of premenstrual syndrome symptoms with the relaxation response. Obstet Gynecol. 1990;75:649.
92. Lustyk MKB, Widman L, Paschane A, Ecker E. Women Health. 2004;39:35–44.
93. Lustyk MKB, Widman L, Paschane A, Olson KC. Behav Med. 2004;30:124–31.
94. Christensen AP, Oei TP. The efficacy of cognitive behaviour therapy in treating premenstrual dysphoric changes. J Affect Disord 1995;33(1):57–63.
95. Hunter MS, Ussher JM, Browne S, et al. A randomized comparison of psychological (cognitive behavioural therapy), medical (fluoxetine) and combined treatment for women with premenstrual dysphoric disorder. J Psychosom Obstet Gynaecol. 2002;23(3):193–9.
96. Kathleen B, Wislow G, Shelley S, Shaunie L. Cognitive-behavioral therapy for premenstrual syndrome and premenstrual dysphopic disorder: a systematic review. Arch Women Ment Health. 2009;12:85–96.
97. Portella AT, Haaga DA, Rohan KJ. The association between seasonal and premenstrual symptoms is continuous and is not fully accounted for by depressive symptoms. J Nerv Ment Dis. 2006;194:833–7.
98. Dalgleish T, Rosen K, Marks M. Rhythm and blues: the theory and treatment of seasonal affective disorder. Br J Clin Psychol. 1996;35:163–82.
99. Parry BL, Newton RP. Chronobiological basis of female-specific mood disorders. Neuropsychopharmacology. 2001;25(5 Suppl):102–8.
100. Krasnik C, Montori VM, Guyatt GH, Heels-Ansdell D, Busse JW. The effect of bright light therapy on depression associated with premenstrual dysphoric disorder. Am J Obstet Gynecol. 2005;193:658–61.
101. Lam RW, Carter D, Misri S, Kuan AJ, Yatham LN, Zis AP. A controlled study of light therapy in women with late luteal phase dysphoric disorder. Psychiatry Res. 1999;86:185–92.
102. Parry BL, Berga SL, Mostofi N, Sependa PA, Kripke DF, Gillin JC. Morning versus evening bright light treatment of late luteal phase dysphoric disorder. Am J Psychiatry. 1989;146:1215–7.

103. Rossignol AM, Bonnlander H. Caffeine-containing beverages, total fluid consumption, and premenstrual syndrome. Am J Public Health. 1990;80:1106–10.
104. Stewart A. Vitamin B6 in the treatment of the premenstrual syndrome–review. Br J Obstet Gynaecol. 1991;98:329.
105. Thys-Jacobs S, Starkey P, Bernstein D, Tian J. Calcium carbonate and the premenstrual syndrome: effects on premenstrual and menstrual symptoms. Premenstrual Syndrome Study Group. Am J Obstet Gynecol. 1998;179:444.
106. Walker AF, De Souza MC, Vickers MF, et al. Magnesium supplementation alleviates premenstrual symptoms of fluid retention. J Womens Health. 1998;7:1157.
107. London RS, Murphy L, Kitlowski KE, Reynolds MA. Efficacy of alpha-tocopherol in the treatment of the premenstrual syndrome. J Reprod Med. 1987;32:400.
108. Wyatt KM, Dimmock PW, Jones PW, Shaughn O'Brien PM. Efficacy of vitamin B-6 in the treatment of premenstrual syndrome: systematic review. BMJ. 1999;318:1375.
109. Brown J, O'Brien PM, Marjoribanks J, Wyatt K. Selective serotonin reuptake inhibitors for premenstrual syndrome. Cochrane Database Syst Rev. 2009; (2):CD001396.
110. Shah NR, Jones JB, Aperi J, et al. Selective serotonin reuptake inhibitors for premenstrual syndrome and premenstrual dysphoric disorder: a meta-analysis. Obstet Gynecol. 2008;111:1175.
111. Wikander I, Sundblad C, Andersch B, et al. Citalopram in premenstrual dysphoria: is intermittent treatment during luteal phases more effective than continuous medication throughout the menstrual cycle? J Clin Psychopharmacol. 1998;18:390.
112. Sundblad C, Hedberg MA, Eriksson E. Clomipramine administered during the luteal phase reduces the symptoms of premenstrual syndrome: a placebo-controlled trial. Neuropsychopharmacology. 1993;9:133.
113. Halbreich U, Bergeron R, Yonkers KA, et al. Efficacy of intermittent, luteal phase sertraline treatment of premenstrual dysphoric disorder. Obstet Gynecol. 2002;100(6):1219–29.
114. Landen M, Nissbrandt H, Allgulander C, Sorvik K, Ysander C, Eriksson E. Placebo-controlled trial comparing intermittent and continuous paroxetine in premenstrual dysphoric disorder. Neuropsychopharmacology. 2007;32:153–61.
115. Sundblad C, Wikander I, Andersch B, Eriksson E. A naturalistic study of paroxetine in premenstrual syndrome: efficacy and side effects during ten cycles of treatment. Eur Neuropsychopharmacol. 1997;7:201–6.
116. Yonkers K, Holthausen G, Poschman K, Howell H. Symptom-onset treatment for women with premenstrual dysphoric disorder. J Clin Psychopharmacol. 2006;26:198–202.
117. Sundblad C, Modigh K, Andersch B, Eriksson E. Clomipramine effectively reduces premenstrual irritability and dysphoria: a placebo-controlled trial. Acta Psychiatr Scand. 1992;85:39.
118. Freeman EW, Rickels K, Sondheimer SJ, et al. Nefazodone in the treatment of premenstrual syndrome: a preliminary study. J Clin Psychopharmacol. 1994;14:180.
119. Freeman EW, Rickels K, Yonkers KA, et al. Venlafaxine in the treatment of premenstrual dysphoric disorder. Obstet Gynecol. 2001;98:737.
120. Smith S, Rinehart JS, Ruddock VE, Schiff I. Treatment of premenstrual syndrome with alprazolam: results of a double-blind, placebo-controlled, randomized crossover clinical trial. Obstet Gynecol. 1987;70:37.
121. Harrison WM, Endicott J, Nee J. Treatment of premenstrual dysphoria with alprazolam. A controlled study. Arch Gen Psychiatry. 1990;47:270.
122. Berger CP, Presser B. Alprazolam in the treatment of two subsamples of patients with late luteal phase dysphoric disorder: a double-blind, placebo-controlled crossover study. Obstet Gynecol. 1994;84:379.
123. Bancroft J, Rennie D. The impact of oral contraceptives on the experience of perimenstrual mood, clumsiness, food craving and other symptoms. J Psychosom Res. 1993;37:195–202.
124. Graham CA, Sherwin BB. A prospective treatment study of premenstrual symptoms using a triphasic oral contraceptive. J Psychosom Res. 1992;36:257–66.

125. Sulak P, Scow R, Preece C, Riggs M, Kuehl T. Hormone withdrawal symptoms in oral contraceptive users. Obstet Gynecol. 2000;95:261–6.
126. Sulak P, Kuehl T, Ortiz M, Schull B. Acceptance of altering the standard 21-day/7-day oral contraceptive regimen to delay menses and reduce hormone withdrawal symptoms. Am J Obstet Gynecol. 2002;186:1142–9.
127. Freeman EW. Evaluation of a unique oral contraceptive (Yasmin) in the management of premenstrual dysphoric disorder. Eur J Contracept Reprod Health Care. 2002;7 Suppl 3:27–34.
128. Lopez L, Kaptein A, Helmerhorst F. Oral contraceptives containing drospirenone for premenstrual syndrome. Cochrane Database Syst Rev. 2008;(1):CD006586.
129. Rapkin AJ, Winer SA. Drospirenone: a novel progestin. Exp Opin Pharmacother. 2007;8:989–99.
130. Yonkers K, Brown C, Pearlstein T, Foegh M, Sampson-Landers C, Rapkin A. Efficacy of a new low-dose oral contraceptive with drospirenone in premenstrual dysphoric disorder. Obstet Gynecol. 2005;106:492–501.
131. Simon RC, Hughes CC. The culture bound syndromes: folk illness of psychiatric and anthropological interest. Dordrecht: Reidel; 1985.
132. McMaster J, et al. Menstrual and premenstrual experiences of women in a developing country. Health Care Women Int. 1997;18:533–41.
133. Chirawatkul S, Manderson L. Perceptions of menopause in northeast Thailand: contested meaning and practice. Soc Sci Med. 1994;39(11):1545–54.
134. Martin E. The woman in the body. A cultural analysis of reproduction. Boston: Beacon; 1987.
135. Esteban, Ma Luz. Re-producción del cuerpo femenino. Discursos y prácticas acerca de la salud. Donostia: Tercera Prensa-Hirugarren Prentsa S.L. 2001
136. Nicolson P. The menstrual cycle, science and femininity: assumptions underlying menstrual cycle research. Soc Sci Med. 1995;41(6):779–84.
137. Rodin M. The social construction of premenstrual syndrome. Soc Sci Med. 1992;35 (1):49–56.

Pregnancy Depression from a Gender Perspective

19

Izargi Lacunza and Mónica Martinez-Cengotitabengoa

Abstract

There is a significant number of pregnant women who eventually have some kind of psychiatric symptoms during pregnancy. This is a period that involves significant biological, psychological, and social changes. In this chapter, we review this issue in its entirety, examining in detail how gender roles and social models of maternity/paternity may contribute to the development of gestational depression in women. We also review the different treatments used. Finally, we include a section focusing on the father figure from the same perspective and emotional disorders that he could also have in this process.

19.1 Introduction

The World Health Organization has estimated that depression is one of the most significant causes of illness worldwide that affect women of childbearing age [1] (a message from the Director General. http://www.who.int/whr/2001/dg_message/en/index.html, 2001). Nowadays, both gynecologists and obstetricians accept depression as one of the most frequent illnesses during pregnancy and puerperium [2]. It confirms that the gestational process is not always, and by definition, a "happy process."

Traditionally, pregnancy has always been related to an emotional welfare state, satisfaction, and being in the prime of one's life. Almost up to the 1990s, it was known that, on the one hand, mentally ill women could get pregnant and, on the other hand, puerperal women, as a general rule, were slightly more vulnerable psychologically speaking. But without a doubt, the dominant concept was the one

I. Lacunza (✉) • M. Martinez-Cengotitabengoa
Alava University Hospital, Vitoria, Spain
e-mail: IZARGI.LACUNZAARETA@osakidetza.net; monica.martinezcengotitabengoa@osakidetza.net

M. Sáenz-Herrero (ed.), *Psychopathology in Women*,
DOI 10.1007/978-3-319-05870-2_19

that stated that an expectant mother would not suffer from any specific mental disturbances [3]. Gisela B. Oppenheim, a London psychiatrist, was the person who, in 1985, in a chapter talking about psychological disorders during pregnancy, gave voice for the first time to all those women who had refuted the prevailing myth up to then [4].

Today, it is well known that pregnancy is a period in which great metabolic changes occur, hormonal as well as immunological, both considerably noticeable by women and potentially influential for her from the very beginning of gestation. But far beyond such biological involvement, gestation brings about, from a psychosocial point of view, an important change in the lives of women [5].

Although the physiological process is universally similar for all women (no matter her culture, race, or social status, the biological event is always the same), the psychosocial experience we are talking about can vary enormously, in view of the fact that pregnancy and maternity can be conceptualized and represented in many diverse ways by women [6]. To that experience contributes first the woman as an individual, as an individual human being in the world, with her personality and her background [7]; but beyond that culture, education, the current social ideal regarding pregnancy, the maternal models shared around her, as well as the established social standards of what is supposed to be a mother and what is supposed to be a father also have an influence.

19.2 Maternity, Gender, and Society

To talk about psychopathology and gender with regard to pregnancy, we believe it is important and necessary to open a window to social and cultural facts, to the reading of the expression of maternity, and to reach the process in our occidental world.

In her characteristic book *The Second Sex* [8], Simone de Beauvoir launched the idea of placing maternity in a privileged position into the reflection raised of the question "What is woman?" Historically, the maternal function has set up the identity core we know as "femininity."

Being a mother, far beyond a role, is a function or a position; it shows up as a figure full of meanings, sometimes opposite to each other, but deeply rooted. Maternity is defined in our society as a substantial part of being a woman, a vital dimension that frequently emerges as the dominant one [9].

It is obvious that maternity does not only have a unique sense, but it includes several definitions: it is sometimes drawn up as an instinct to seek fulfillment inside women. Other times, it is reproduction, the unique and biological process of generating a human being. It is drawn up, too, as one of the strongest representations of Western culture, being even stronger in the case of Catholic tradition, where the figure of the Virgin Mary, a virgin and mother at the same time, has had absolute prominence in the "feminine" concept definition [10].

To consider maternity is, consequently, examining a clutter of symbols and models of femininity that overcome the field of procreation. This is why it also implies litigation with strong gender stereotypes that rely on supposed evidence of the biological—the generic conferring of the expectant capacity—as the last model of the construction of the concept woman [9]. All in all, maternity is a cultural construction in which very strong and deeply rooted representations that form a great part of what we understand by "feminine" are included.

Talking about maternity leads us first to talk about our body, a place where the primary difference in sexual organs and their specific function in reproduction lays. It is all about sexual dimorphism, the axis of the difference. The female body, biologically speaking, owns the capacity of reproduction and of generating new life, that is something evident and natural. However, the dominant patriarchal system has contributed significantly during its whole history to "naturalize" the characteristics socially assigned to each sex, transforming crude biological sex into gender. Inequality was made out of the difference [11].

This way, during decades of western history, and in mostly all cultures, women have been assigned the assumption of a prominence, vital in the creation of new human beings: in their socialization, upbringing and care. The feminine role, focused on maternity, has been defined by attributes linked to sensitivity, affection as well as delicacy features and mainly to the special interest in children and family care. Something so forged in our minds that the assumption that claims that all women like boys and girls prevails in our culture. To express the opposite is probably branded as something abnormal, something "surprising and strange."

So, in short, it has not been easy to demarcate the feminine from maternal, something that has not happened with men, who have been defined mainly by other attributes and not for that of being a father [12]. In fact, today is the day in which in spite of the socio-cultural changes, maternity is still being understood, in general terms, as something inherent in the feminine condition and there are still dozens of beliefs revolving around the fact that a woman is only fulfilled if she is mother [13].

It is a fact that the topics regarding maternal function of women that have been passed on to date, push and condition women enormously, up to the point when most of them get to idealize it and assume an overriding need to have a baby [13]. Those who do not at least consider it at some time. It is without a doubt, a link in the feminine subjectivity.

In this context, the idealization of pregnancy comes together too, knowing it as the process to reach full personal development (up to then incomplete). In this way, a process has been drawn: the gestation process as something satisfying, idyllic, a full welfare state. An idea: "If you are pregnant, you will be happy."

We can identify this even in images used in publicity and in images of publications destined for future mothers, in which the expectant mother is shown in a calm introspective way, dressed in tulles, gauzes, and pastel colors, typical of baby clothing. The pregnant women seem to be sober, balanced, patiently waiting, and connected with her inside [9]. It is pregnancy's idealization. These are still sociocultural carriers, and are the ones we should get rid of.

Another important aspect widely defined in psycho-social literature, is that the transition to maternity means, in the case of women, the most obvious and clear inclusion in the social legal age; in other words, "The shifting to a symbolic adult social age" [14].

In a study conducted by Lasén [15] it was observed that in the case of women, maternity, knowing it is an irreversible process, breaks with the dynamism typical of youth, indefinition, encouraging them to enter an adulthood in which the expected role the woman would still be the same as the traditional feminine model of children and family care.

According to this study, in the case of men, even if the transition to maturity is seen as something unavoidable, it is conceived in a blurred way. In the few cases in which paternity is mentioned, unlike with maternity, it is not appearing as a clear milestone in the discourse, but just another element of that whole called maturity. Becoming a father is not, in this case, the transition to adulthood itself, but an effect or consequence of being into it. Therefore, gestation is not only the creation of a new son or daughter, but also the transformation of a woman into a mother, and the gestation of a mother is a complex social process.

It is true that, in the last few years, the perception that women and society have of maternity has been evolving, and today it is a field that is in a full process of change, in which important aspects for equality between men and women are dealt with. In fact, currently, a great number of women who become mothers cannot be considered passive and submissive compared with the social models and structures they have been exposed to; instead, they should be considered social beings who display tactics from inside their own private and social circumstances, which, at the same time, leads to change what was thought to be so strongly stipulated.

In the last decades, women have conquered a greater social space; far beyond the limited domestic environment, she has been gaining new definitions and new bases in her subjective identity. That is why maternity is more and more one base amongst others, not just the only one. But this socio-cultural change has brought new realities for women that do not always seem to be easy: the antagonism between maternity demand and labor demand appears during pregnancy itself [16]. For many women it is difficult to handle that passive situation in which pregnancy subjugates them and the split from the professional field and labor environment, mainly when the work constitutes an important part of their personal identity and their vital satisfaction. A great number of women affirm having qualms with regard to announcing their pregnancy in the company they work for. Many women admit to fearing the consequences of sick leave in their development as workers. They can return to work after maternity leave and they should be offered their old job back, but this is something that does not always happen. This is discrimination. There are quite a lot of women who accept this guilty feeling, coming from the strange sensation of unfulfillment and breach with the company [9]. It is important to remember that only women are the ones forced into that precise planning, whereas their partners are still in the same working situation, where their coming paternity will almost never lead them to situations such as confrontation, negotiations or hiding, which are common in women. It is fully accepted that equality between men and women is a legal principle universally recognized. But it is something undeniable too that despite all the progress gained in all women's situations, real equality does not exist at all. This is something relevant to living through a pregnancy and anticipating the idea of creating a family [17].

At this point is where the new feminine role emerges, and here is where feelings of guilt can appear, all of them bound to the difficulties in answering the consecrated legend of maternity and bound also to uniting satisfyingly vital antagonistic spaces, but both interesting for women. Becoming aware that the proper offer to the others is always to the detriment of one's interests, necessities, and wishes can cause great feelings of frustration that necessarily influence the mood of the person [18].

All in all, the relationship between maternity and work is, from before the birth, one of the sources of stress that could bring a slight dose of angst to a woman's life.

A recent field study [9] demonstrates that even if it is clear that nowadays maternity is not considered as the only possible social destiny for women, it is quite striking (or maybe it is not as much) that this option is still being imagined by future mothers as a clear producer of disadvantages at other levels, not being able to reach and break the clichés and the traditional assignment.

19.3 Other Psychosocial Components

As a part of the experience that women obtain from pregnancy, the corporeality derived from the physiological process gains, without a doubt, a special prominence. In fact, the first difference between maternity and paternity is that the former happens inside the body whereas the latter is a process alien to it [9].

The transition to maternity goes always with a temporary physical transformation that is outwardly perceptible and socially loaded with meaning. In the same way, the concern about one's image and for one's body's attractiveness becomes a critical aspect during this period. Physical transformations and substantial changes in weight occur in all senses.

As an obvious feature of this process, we relate pregnancy to a weight gain and to a size increase in the body of the expectant woman, which engenders greater discomfort, tiredness, decreased mobility, and even increased clumsiness. This might be accepted, in general terms, as a cost linked to proper maternity; something women must go through inevitably. Nevertheless, and even if the idea of having a son or a daughter compensates for these costs, psychologically, these costs could be greater.

We recall at this point the strong aesthetic canons that have been established for women in our culture: the imposition of an impeccable body image and the demand by which women see themselves compelled to show and exhibit a body in accordance in order to be valued. Women, and not the men (but more and more often) are demanded a great deal in physical terms; upto a point that nowadays, there is an important internalization of these models even inside women against them.

Pregnancy invades, suddenly and inevitably (we talk about natural gestation processes), the self- control of women with regard to her body. Any body change remains out of control and self-regulation. That is when a strong psychiatric conflict occurs; the confrontation between what is socially stipulated by the sexual category and the "physical reproductive disagreement," also defined by their sexual organ. The dread of gaining weight and not being able to return to the weight previous to pregnancy is one of the incessant complaints and dreads during this stage [9]. Such is the case that we consider that at this point conflicts, intolerances, frustrations, and strong ambivalences could arise that might affect women's mental health.

On the other hand, our body gains the power to become the opening to the social world of maternity. The body gives "visibility" to maternity. Intimacy loses space and the woman opens herself up to public life, to an external view that will go on later on: others know with certainty that she is pregnant. From this point on, the others begin to "maternize" that person, with her behavior and attitude, rebuilding a whole host of stereotypes, models, and values about what it is to be an expectant woman (a future mother) and what it should be [9].

Maybe we should not reflect at this point about what it is required and awaited from a pregnant woman. In fact, what it is required is nothing but full dedication to one's son or daughter from the very first moment of their conception. Dedication means care, protection against everything, even against herself. The future baby becomes the individual of the first importance inside her own individual being.

This means in practice, a social censorship for maternal behavior that implies any kind of influence (large or small) on the health and welfare of the fetus she carries inside her belly. It implies interjections and criticisms when they act in a form that is socially considered inadequate for a pregnant woman. This behavior includes the following: drinking alcohol, smoking, practicing intense physical activities or eating in an irresponsibly way. It implies that people around her feel to be within their rights to give their opinion and judge (even with a mere glance) the other person just for her condition of being pregnant. Together with this, we are not supporting the idea of legitimizing such acts (true as it is, they fact that these behaviors could harm the fetus' development is empirically checked); what we want instead is to remark on the de-individuation that the woman undergoes during this period, the vigilance and external judgment to which she has to submit, without taking into account (as a general norm) either her capacity to decide, or her circumstances.

Conceiving a new creature requests lots of changes and lots of sacrifices. Stop consuming certain types of food and beverages, restricting sports activities, withdrawing from social life. Women (and not men) are obliged to assume during the 9 months of gestation what for them are significant privations and repressions under the banner of the fact that "a mother has to sacrifice everything for her son or daughter." This is not assigned to the father in such complete terms at all. Women sees her place in a position of "not complaining," in a place in which only acceptance and dedication fit in, once again. As an alternative: to be criticized, to be judged, and almost with complete certainty, to feel guilty for "not being a good mother," even before she is a mother.

For the reasons mentioned above, it is impossible to think of all the things related to the social and cultural process of becoming a mother (with the generic constructions we find in it), which contains heavy emotional baggage. There may be someone who develops it, adapting to it, but there will be someone who does not, leading to variations (minor, moderate or even serious) in the emotional state during the moment of preparation for maternity: pregnancy.

19.4 Depression During Pregnancy

The existence of the "melancholy of pregnancy" was first mentioned in 1840 [19]. However, it was not until the late twentieth century when, in a very gradual way, studies on the subject started to be published. In those studies, it is confirmed that pregnant women compared with nonpregnant women had higher percentages of mental disorders [20]. It was also observed that these women had, mostly, a previous psychiatric history. These data led us to suspect the presence of a specific pathology associated with the gestational process itself.

It is estimated that one out of ten pregnant women presents features that predispose to depression. These numbers may even be higher depending on other variables such as the cultural and socioeconomic status. A recent review has suggested that depressive symptoms affect 18.4 % of pregnant women, 12.7 % of them having an episode of major depression [21]. Regarding the course, longitudinal studies have found an almost linear decrease in the symptoms after pregnancy until the third month postpartum [22]. It is generally known as one of the most significant clinical problems in pregnant women [2].

Despite the epidemiological data, studies focused on maternal depression are limited, especially those about depression during the prenatal period [23].

For starters, we must think about the place of the psychology of "pregnant women" (and consequently psychopathology) in the scientific literature, which has been very limited as we have already revealed above. Many authors have noted longstanding scientific negligence concerning pregnancy and mental health (compared with other subjects). It is an obvious reflection of the dominant androcentric bias in the development of health sciences in particular, and the development of Western thought in general. In fact, this issue has been totally invisible for many years and "pregnancy" and its emotional implications have not awakened interest until recently.

In the last decade, there has been a greater need for understanding maternal depression (owing to the evidence of negative consequences in both the mother and the fetus). It has led to an increase in the number of studies conducted in this area. Nevertheless, they have paid more attention to the postpartum maternal depression, forgetting the uniqueness of the pathology associated with gestation. This inattention is observed in the media as well as in the scientific literature [24].

It is striking that most current psychiatric treatment has few specifications about mood and maternity disorders up to the postpartum period, minimizing or even completely forgetting the pregnancy period and its emotional disturbances.

19.5 Clinical Symptomatology

The new revision of the *Diagnostic and Statistical Manual of Mental Disorders* (DSM-5, 2013) refers to the entity of "peripartum depression" as a nonspecific mood disorder including in it all the depressive symptoms associated with the gestational process, both pre- and post-partum [25].

The clinical characteristics of depression during the postpartum period are essentially similar to those observed in depressive episodes that occur at other times of life [3]. However, the correct detection of depressive symptoms relevant for the diagnosis is complex in these cases.

First, because pregnancy involves multiple symptoms such as fatigue, emotional lability, sleep disturbances, and appetite variations, which can be present during this period of time without clinical implications, that is, they can be symptoms directly derived from physiological processes underlying the gestational process. Similarly, pregnant women can also have medical conditions such as anemia, gestational diabetes, and thyroid dysfunction, which are often associated with depressive symptoms [3].

For many years, targeting the medical interventions in the maternal–fetal physical well-being in addition to attributing maternal complaints (such as fatigue, changes in appetite and weight) to the physical and hormonal changes of pregnancy have been able to mask depression symptoms, probably contributing to an infrared diagnosis of depression during pregnancy [26].

It was not until the twenty-first century that a study conducted by Kelly et al. [27] confirmed for the first time the existence of a significant difference between the physical complaints of nondepressed pregnant women and pregnant women who were eventually diagnosed with depression.

Therefore, the detection of major and minor affective disorders during pregnancy requires a thorough clinical examination of all the symptoms, but perhaps showing a special interest in the psychological components such as anhedonia, feelings of guilt, hopelessness, and suicidal ideation, considered highly relevant differential elements for the diagnosis [3].

Although suicide rates during pregnancy are low, there has been an increment in the number of young women who commit suicide [28]. The risk increases in these cases: women with psychiatric diagnosis or prior hospitalizations, in case of perinatal death and during puerperium [29]. In a review by Lindahl et al., they found that approximately 14 % of pregnant women have suicidal ideation [30]. In the same study, it was concluded that social support, contact with health professionals, and concern for the fetus significantly reduced the risk as well as the probability of self-harming.

It is important to mention also that the comorbidity between anxiety symptoms and depression is frequently cited during pregnancy [31–34]. A nonlinear pattern is detected in clinical anxiety, the first and third trimesters being identified as the high-risk periods [35].

Data suggest that the first trimester is a period of increased psychological vulnerability specifically for first-time mothers because of the awareness of the pregnancy status and the impact and reactions to the first symptoms. Regarding the third trimester, it appears to be higher levels of stress associated with fear of childbirth and the imminent arrival of the baby. In this case, the stress level is higher for multiparous couples [36].

Finally, it is important to point out the existence in the clinical practice of several tests that assess this pathology. The most commonly used scale is the EPDS [37], validated during pregnancy in different contexts [38]. Mothers have to choose one among four statements, taking into account how they felt during the previous week. Recommended cut-off values are 11/12 for pre-natal depression and 9/10 for postpartum depression [39]. The PRIME-MD (Patient Health Questionnaire) is also used as a validated psychometric instrument for obstetrics–gynecology patients as another option for assessing mood [40].

19.6 Etiology and Risk Factors

As has been said previously, the gestational period is a time of great vulnerability for women. After reviewing the scientific literature gathered up to now, we find that some etiological factors have been mentioned more frequently: hormonal changes, neuroendocrine modifications, and psychosocial adjustments. In the medical bibliography (neither in the psychiatric nor even in the gynecological–obstetric one) we have not found, to date, pieces of work that revise this pathology from a clear gender point of view. That is why right after we gathered the findings in this review, we tackled the ideas and references of the social and gender analysis previously carried out.

Health science, out of sheer spite, has maximized the biological part of the diseases. The changes in the feminine hormones (estrogen and progesterone) that happen throughout a woman's life, during adolescence, their menstrual cycle, pregnancy, puerperium, and menopause, have been commonly identified as mainly responsible for the discrepancy between the rates of depression in men and women [41].

Estrogen is believed to have an effect on the neurotransmitters, including serotonin, which is directly associated with mood modulation and anxiety [42, 43]. Women also show differences in the thyroidal function and in the cortisol levels as well as in the adrenocorticotropic hormone (ACTH), both part of the hypothalamus–pituitary–adrenal axis, which is responsible for modulating the mood in response to environmental stress. These differences have been demonstrated to have the potential to increase the susceptibility to suffering a depressive disorder [41, 43, 44].

However, the direct implication of psychosocial factors as an etiological component of the expected depression is widely accepted in the scientific community.

In a recent wide reaching review [45] it was found that stress, the severe emotional alterations prior to gestation, the absence of social support, a complicated couple relationship, and domestic violence are predictors of higher relevance in the depressive symptomatology during pregnancy.

Regarding the first factor, it seems that the presence of stressful vital events (psychologically significant, such as a divorce or a death) during the previous year to the gestational period increases the risk of developing a depressive mood during such a period [45]. The lack of social support that is perceived plays an important role as a hastening element of the depressive disorder in this setting. Several studies confirm the idea saying that the perceived support (not the actual support) received from the familial environment can help the mother [45–47]. The satisfaction with the family seemed to be, in general, a protective factor [45, 48, 49].

Regarding the perceived support, it is of vital importance to observe the role of the father as a protective factor for maternal prenatal depression. In a recent study [50] it has been proved that paternal implication during the 9 months of pregnancy has a direct impact upon the results of gestation itself and the infants. When the fathers get involved during the pregnancy, the negative symptoms in women's health diminish. This remains in line with the three-dimensional theory that Lamb [51] proposes as the definition of a new paternal role (accessibility, commitment, responsibility): the involved father, beyond being a simply financial supporter, and without caring about his status association, becomes an emotional as well as a physical support for the pregnant woman [50].

However, in that study, despite the participants understanding the importance of these kinds of paternal behaviors regarding the maternal and fetal welfare, lots of barriers were identified that would block an optimal implication. Factor such as individual, familial, community and social (mainly fundamental principles and values) played a vital role excluding and reducing the father's implication during pregnancy in many cases. Here, the evidence to keep affirming the burden that social and cultural stereotypes still have when a father is about to involve himself, more or less, during the pregnancy of his future son/daughter. Thus, the security that in the cases in which he is capable of accepting other nontraditional roles, the welfare of the partner, future son/daughter, and family in general, is ensured with certainty.

It has also been observed that people with a low educational level and with employment problems or people who are into a long-term situation of low incomes (many times related to the lacking school attendance, but not always) are at a higher risk of developing depressive symptoms during pregnancy [47, 48]. Considering the social inequalities (in terms of power, educational possibilities, employment conditions) also results in a high degree of global poverty in women. This is an important risk factor.

As for other familial characteristics, we must add that in contrast to what it is used to happening in postpartum depression, the probability of antenatal depressive symptoms is lower in primiparous women [52]. Multiparous women, thus, show a higher risk of antenatal depression (taking care of another child increases the burden and stress, even more so when the woman is the one who takes on the largest amount of those cares and responsibilities).

19.7 Unplanned Pregnancy

An unwanted or unplanned pregnancy can become a great risk factor for the development of severe emotional disorders at this stage [45]. It was already found in a previous study [53] that psychiatric symptomatology measured in women with an accidental pregnancy during the SCL-90 questionnaire was much higher than in women who had planned their pregnancy.

If maternity and paternity are complex and complicated by themselves when the individuals want the baby, it gets even more complicated when they occur unexpectedly. Once it is there, however, there are differences. It seems that it may have been unplanned, but it is accepted with excitement; instead, it could be rejected and live with unhappiness. In the second case, the impact on the mental health of women will be higher.

The amount of studies dealing specifically with this point is large, and they demonstrate that women do not always want to have children, and when they already have one or two, especially, lots of women do not want to have any more.

Chodorow talks about the maternal ambivalence in one of his studies [54]. Like the fact of having offspring, or the same as not having it, can be freely chosen or pathologically inspired, involved in conflicts or relatively conflict-free. For example, a woman can decide to continue with gestation with a free desire to do so or she could feel to be under the responsibility of assuming the consequences of having reached that point and accept it with "morality." Do men feel and suffer from these very cultural products? Are men aware of this same introjected moral pressure? A man who gives priority to other interests over the decision of paternity is believed to be an independent man; when this is done by a woman, we talk about "selfishness" [55]. Has the scientific community considered this when it thinks and talks about pregnancy and about what it refers to as depressive symptoms?

It is important to remark on how the rate of women who do not want to have children in the Western world has doubled in these last 20 years [56]. Also, it has been confirmed that the more education and power they have in their societies, the less children they have.

It is important to take into consideration this last piece of information. As mentioned before, the scarce school attendance and the low socio-economical level appear to be factors related to depression during pregnancy. On the other hand, women with more educational and economic resources seem to decide to have fewer children. We could hypothesize then, that higher culturalization and development permit women to forge more complex subjective identities (defined by more pillars than just the only and exclusive one of maternity), more sovereignty and more personal autonomy, gaining distance from the traditional destiny that was previously established for women. Just like that, the fact that the socio-economic status may coincide with the underdevelopment (higher patriarchal hierarchies, more deeply rooted gender stereotypes) explains the fact of these women to be subdued, to a greater extent (familial pressure, morality, submission before the partner) to accept the maternal role without wanting it truly (what has been established as a clear risk of suffering from prenatal depression).

19.8 Abortion

We introduce at this point a review about miscarriage and abortion and its implications for psychopathology.

Miscarriage implicates a difficult grief process. This is one of the loneliest losses a woman may suffer. Mothers are the most aware of the existence of their babies because they carry them in their wombs. The mother (also the father, but with greater distance) suffers it as the death of a child with whom she had a strong emotional bond. Considering this conditions and the gestational time when the loss occurs its vital, since the more evolved the pregnancy, the higher would be the emotional impact and the post-abortion trauma.

Of all the feelings of grief resulting from the death of a baby, Fonnegra highlights three that are almost always present, no matter the case: anger, guilt, and sadness, accompanied by an incapacitating sense of failure [57]. It is probable that they can even feel shame for not being able to maintain a pregnancy without difficulties [58]. These feelings have also been associated with an increased risk of psychopathology during subsequent pregnancies [59].

On the contrary, having infertility or in vitro fertilization antecedents can convert being finally pregnant into a very positive experience for these women and their partners. According to Kozinszky et al. [60], these can be protective factors that reduce the prevalence of mood disorders before birth.

Regarding the abortion, it is important to analyze the reasons that led to this decision as different emotions will emerge from different reasons. The abortion is in almost universal terms an aggression to the woman's body and psyche. It must be avoided as far as possible, without forgetting that it can be less aggressive than continuing with pregnancy if the woman wants to terminate it [61]. The legislation on abortion is very diverse depending on the country and its government: it can be a right or a punishable offense. In spite of the different points of view, the reality is that abortion has always been controlled by a set of laws (decided mostly by men) that make women a mere instrument of gestation and not human beings with rights. The right of the fetus has been prioritized against the right of women to decide. Even today, there are countries where the decriminalization of abortion is limited to a number of conditions. Governments are the ones who determine what a women "can" or "cannot" do with their corporality. They speak and decide for them, depriving them, in this way, of the most basic sovereignty, their most intimate territory: their body [61].

After this social labeling in which women are denied, the unwanted pregnancies probably have a serious negative impact on the female psyche with a clear risk of damaging their mental health.

On the other hand, it is also important to say that despite the voluntary nature of the process, the interruption of a pregnancy also involves strong emotional consequences for women who will experience ambivalence, sadness, relief, and also some degree of guilt as a result of the moral learned.

19.9 Gender Violence

Gender violence during pregnancy is a problem that exists in all societies of the world, regardless of class, race, age or religion [62] (although the forms of appearance may be very different).

Worldwide figures report that 2 out of 10 women are assaulted physically, psychologically or sexually during pregnancy [63–65]. Besides, in social groups with less cultural development, in which stereotypical gender roles are present, conceptualization of women as a possession, an idiosyncratic patriarchal model and associations of masculinity with strength and authority, the prevalence of mistreatment during pregnancy is much higher [66, 67].

A direct and significant association between gender violence and mood disorders during pregnancy has recently been demonstrated [68]. However, despite the consequences for both the mother and fetus, this topic remains under-researched in the field of mental health. Female victims of abuse or mistreatment suffer much higher levels of gestational depression. Thus, the development of this pathology is also mediated by social beliefs that have placed men in a role of superiority and women, in contrast, in a role of inferiority and submission.

19.10 Reflections

Lots of expectant women mention a state of anxiety, fear, and preoccupation as being something common. Together with fantasies, hopes, and illusions assigned to pregnancy, it also brings together a bunch of dreads, musings, and fears for both the mother and the father. The possibility of problems in the fetus' health, the excitement upon the moment of birth, and the possibility of having a miscarriage are in general those that are mentioned most frequently. Regarding birth, even if regular narrations talk about fear of pain, of death, and risks to the fetus during birth, the presence of a "fear of lack of control" has also been confirmed [9]. "Fear of lack of control", or in other words, "demand for regulation, self-control and care conduct", has been attributed to women's lives. We can perceive it in how women face what it has to do with diet control, physical exercise control, sexual control, and control in general of any kind of public conduct that seeks the adaptation to what is right [69]. In this sense, fear of giving birth alludes to the interiorized mechanism of regulating ourselves and behaving just as we are expected to behave. An unease in not knowing if they will be able to control their behavior at the moment of birth, the fear of acting hastily, of not being able to make the grade, of attracting attention and in short, of losing proper decency. All these experiences can amplify the level of "maternal anxiety" inherent in pregnancy.

To finish, just recall at this point how confrontations with other destinies and possible frustrations in many women in current Western society can affect the significant levels of psychological unease. After all, any new self-fulfillment constitutes in the most Eriksonian sense [70] an "identity crisis" and a grief regarding everything left behind; even more so when it comes to entering adulthood and anticipating a social model, with which a woman can feel unidentified [15].

Few clinical relevance studies with an appropriate methodology about the direct effects of depression on pregnancy have been published. Again, empirical articles have focused on the effects of postpartum depression without considering gestational depression [24]. Depression, given its biopsychopathological nature, can affect (even at subclinical levels) both mother and fetus, in the short and long term [71]. Having gestational depression may lead mothers to neglect their basic care, presenting in these cases higher rates of self-medication, poor diet, and use of alcohol, tobacco, and other drugs. The damaging effects of these behaviors to fetal growth and placental function are well known [72, 73]. These women usually tend to reduce obstetric visits and/or fail to follow prenatal counseling, all of which can harm the fetus and also the mother [74, 75].

First studies on the subject estimated that these pregnancies often finish prematurely and often have major obstetric complications (miscarriages, fetal malformations, low birth weight, preeclampsia, preterm birth, fetal growth restriction, and hyperemesis gravidarum) [76]. However, one recent piece of research concludes that the current evidence does not allow the effect of depression during pregnancy to be supported or disproved [77].

On the other hand, other studies have shown the relationship between some psychological variables (such as stress, depression, low self-esteem, and anxiety) and longer births [78].

It is also known that untreated depression can predispose to the development of psychosis and to suicide ideation [42]. In addition, the presence of depression during pregnancy increases the risk of postpartum depression [79]. The 30 % of women with prenatal depression still had it after giving birth.

Finally, it has been suggested that depressed mothers cannot be capable of establishing a secure attachment bond with their children and this can have negative consequences for them in the long term [80].

19.11 Treatment

The main goal in the treatment of prenatal depression is in almost all cases the maintenance or improvement of the mental health of women, minimizing the risks to the fetus and future baby.

19.11.1 Pharmacological Treatment

In this section we will review the available information on antidepressant treatment and its impact on pregnancy, trying to provide clinical recommendations for the management of patients, but we started saying in advance that the information on the matter is sometimes scarce and often contradictory. Given that untreated depression during pregnancy is associated with increased mortality and morbidity

Table 19.1 Most common risks from untreated depression during pregnancy

Risks	Possible consequences
Intensification of depressive symptoms	Poor self-care Inappropriate prenatal care Substance abuse Suicide Postpartum depression
Problems in pregnancy and during delivery	Abortion Preeclampsia Preterm delivery Cesarean and instrumental delivery Minor head circumference Low birth weight Perinatal complications Neonatal intensive care Disturbances of the hypothalamic–pituitary–adrenal
Long-term effects for the child	Poor postnatal care High cortisol levels Poor adaptation to stress Stunting Delayed psychomotor development Behavioral and cognitive problems

both the newborn and the mother [81], it is important to use the most optimal strategy for addressing this disease. To take the decision of starting pharmacological treatment, first of all it is necessary to weigh up the potential harm of untreated disease, compared with the adverse effects of exposure to drugs. Table 19.1 sets out the risks of untreated depression during pregnancy [82].

The exclusion of pregnant women from clinical trials, makes the information available to us regarding the use of drug therapies in pregnancy low, while the only information we have is through observational studies, which logically include numerous confounding factors [83]; thus, it would require rigorous randomized controlled treatment trials (RCTs) to assess whether antidepressant drugs are efficacious in pregnant women, whether any antidepressant are harmful to the fetus, and whether untreated depression is harmful itself.

In the aforementioned meta-analysis by Ross [81] the authors find small associations between exposure to pharmacological treatment for depression in pregnancy and pregnancy outcomes, and conclude that the differences between groups are small; thus, it is important to consider the clinical importance of the decision to treat or not treat maternal depression versus low risk of exposure.

19.11.1.1 Antidepressants

Most women of childbearing age who are treated with antidepressants receive selective serotonin reuptake inhibitors (SSRIs) or serotonin–norepinephrine reuptake inhibitors (SNRIs), and considering the high percentage of unplanned pregnancies, it is expected that in many cases, when the woman detects pregnancy, the fetus has had weeks of exposure to the drug [84].

The most recent reviews and guidelines on the use of antidepressants in pregnancy recommend the use of SSRIs and SNRIs versus classic monoamine oxidase inhibitors (MAOIs) and tricyclic antidepressants (TCAs) for their better safety profiles and lower risk to the fetus.

Selective Serotonin Reuptake Inhibitors

Both SSRIs and SNRIs cross the placental barrier and are detected in umbilical cord blood and amniotic fluid. In the early years after the marketing of fluoxetine in 1987, studies found no relationship between the use of SSRIs and the occurrence of congenital malformation. But it was not until 2005, following the publication of a report by GlaxoSmithKline, which suggested an increase of 1.5 times the risk of cardiac malformations in fetuses exposed to paroxetine (primarily ventricular septal defects) [85].

Based on these studies, the FDA (US Food and Drug Administration) issued a notice recommending avoiding the use of paroxetine during pregnancy and changing its classification category from teratogen risk class C to class D [86]. In the following years numerous epidemiological studies were published relating both positively and negatively to the use of paroxetine with the occurrence of these malformations. A meta-analysis published in 2010, suggested a slightly increased risk of heart defects with exposure to paroxetine during the first trimester of pregnancy, with an OR of 1.46 (CI 1.17–1.82) [87]. Still, there are authors who claim that women who suffer from anxiety and depression during pregnancy are more likely to be screened by echocardiography tests, relative to healthy pregnant women; thus, there is a greater probability of detection of cardiac malformations [88]. Furthermore, these women are more likely to take their children to the emergency services, so there is also a higher probability of the detection of malformations. Most of the malformations seen tend to resolve spontaneously during childhood, so that if we examine children not exposed to paroxetine, after resolution of the malformation, there is another confounding factor. It may even be possible that depression itself causes externally detected fetal risks.

All these potential confounders have been confirmed by a recent population-based study in Denmark in which the authors conclude that exposure to SSRIs during pregnancy was not significantly associated with cardiac malformations reported so far, and blamed the previous findings for the biases described above [89].

On the other hand an association between the use of SSRIs and persistent pulmonary hypertension in the newborn has been reported. A recent meta-analysis concludes that although the risk cannot be determined, it is very small, less than 1 %, and if a pregnant woman needs pharmacological treatment this low risk does not support its discontinuation or lowering the dose of her antidepressant [90].

Another meta-analysis recently published reaches similar conclusions to those described, adding that other SSRIs widely used such as sertraline and citalopram are not associated with an increased risk of fetal malformations [91]. The review concludes that the only recommendation to keep in mind is that you should avoid as far as possible fluoxetine and paroxetine in the first trimester of pregnancy or among those women planning to become pregnant. The added risk is very low with both medications and the risk of untreated illness should always be assessed.

Serotonin–Norepinephrine Reuptake Inhibitors

In relation to SNRI there are fewer data and perhaps the most studied drug during pregnancy has been duloxetine. Duloxetine is approved in many countries for the treatment of major depressive disorder, general anxiety disorder, diabetic peripheral neuropathic pain, and fibromyalgia. Since it has been marketed, millions of women have received duloxetine, with many of them of childbearing age. Duloxetine crosses the placenta and passes into breast milk [92]. In a preliminary work published in 2012, the authors recorded the pregnancy outcomes of 208 pregnant women taking duloxetine. It was found that malformation rates were similar to those of pregnant women treated with other antidepressants and women who were taking no medication ($p = 0.991$); thus, although the sample size is not enough to detect rare malformations, the study results suggest that duloxetine does not appear to increase the baseline risk of major malformations [93].

More recently, a record-linkage study carried out by Lilly Company concludes that there is a slightly higher, but not significant proportion of abnormal pregnancy outcomes in those women taking duloxetine during pregnancy, but probably because of a bias toward reporting abnormal versus normal outcomes. There is also a higher prevalence of risk factors for abnormal pregnancy outcomes, including smoking and alcohol use, in depressed women than in the general population [94]. Indeed, in this study, more women with abnormal pregnancy outcomes had a history of using concomitant medications with positive evidence of human fetal risk (benzodiazepines, nonsteroidal anti-inflammatory drugs, anticonvulsants, and angiotensin-converting enzyme inhibitors). In summary, the frequency of abnormal outcomes reported in duloxetine pregnancy cases is generally consistent with the rates in the general population.

The limited information available in the literature about mirtazapine use during pregnancy suggests that there is no evidence that this drug increases the risk of major fetal malformations [95]. In general, mirtazapine is more likely to cause weight gain or increased appetite; thus, these effects will be appropriate in depressed women with severe loss of weight or appetite. Mirtazapine is sometimes used in combination with SSRI drugs for treatment of major depression or panic disorders including symptoms of severe nausea, insomnia, and decreased appetite [96].

There are few studies regarding the use of venlafaxine during pregnancy. Perhaps the study that includes a larger sample is that carried out by Polen et al. [97], which analyzed a cohort of women exposed to venlafaxine from the month before conception and at least during the first 3 months of pregnancy. The study finds that perinatal exposure to venlafaxine may be related to certain birth defects, principally anencephaly, cleft palate, gastroschisis, and some heart defects; however, the study has the limitation of a small sample size of exposed pregnant women. In a previous study, comparing exposure to venlafaxine with SSRIs they found no increased risk of birth defects overall or for cardiovascular defects in particular, but the study included only a small number of women [98]. Further studies are needed to confirm these results.

Bupropion

Overall, 10–20 % of pregnant women smoke, which is a great public health problem. Smoking cessation drugs such as nicotine replacement therapy (NRT), varenicline, and bupropion are effective for pregnant women [99], but, to date, they have not been recommended as a first option, because their efficacy and safety have not been yet established. In the meta-analysis carried out by Myung et al., assessing NRT and bupropion, only one of the included studies used bupropion [100]; thus, further studies are warranted to explore this issue. Moreover, there is insufficient evidence to determine whether or not NRT is effective and safe when used for smoking cessation in pregnancy [99]. In a more recent review article from the Cochrane Database, Hajek et al., six studies using bupropion in pregnant women trying to quit tobacco consumption were included and they found no significant effect (RR 1.15, 95 % CI 0.98–1.35) [101].

Besides failing to show efficacy in smoking cessation, use of bupropion in the first trimester of pregnancy has been associated with an increased incidence of cardiac malformations [102].

In short, if we have a pregnant woman smoking, she should try to give up the habit through psychological techniques and if pharmacological interventions are needed, it seems more appropriate to use NRT.

Norepinephrine Reuptake Inhibitors

We have found practically no published information about the use of reboxetine during pregnancy.

Agomelatine

Owing to the good tolerability and low incidence of side effects with agomelatine, we assume that this drug could be an alternative to consider in the treatment of perinatal depression, but in fact there is still no evidence for this.

Tricyclic Antidepressants

Two case–control studies have been published that did not find an increased risk of major congenital malformations or developmental delay after the use of TCAs during pregnancy. However, a study using a birth registry that included 395 infants exposed to TCAs found an increased risk of preterm birth, low birth weight, respiratory distress, hypoglycemia, low Apgar score, and convulsions [103]. For these reasons, the myth that MAOIs are safer antidepressants during pregnancy has been dismissed [104].

Table 19.2 Teratogen risk according to categorization by the FDA

Chemical name	FDA classification
Amitriptilyne	C
Bupropion	C
Citalopram	C
Clomipramine	C
Doxepin	C
Duloxetine	C
Escitalopram	C
Fluoxetine	C
Fluvoxamine	C
Imipramine	D
Maprotiline	B
Mirtazapine	C
Paroxetine	D
Sertraline	C
Trazodone	C
Trimipramine	C
Venlafaxine	C

B: Reproduction studies in animals indicate no risk to the fetus, but there are no controlled studies in pregnant women; or reproductive studies with animals have shown adverse effects (other than a decrease in fertility) that are not confirmed in controlled studies in pregnant women in the first trimester (and there is no obvious risk in later trimesters)
C: Studies in animals have revealed adverse effects on the fetus (teratogenic in the embryo or other), but no controlled studies in women; or there are no studies available neither in women nor in animals. Drugs should be given if the potential benefit justifies the potential risk to the fetus
D: There is positive evidence of human fetal risk, but it is accepted for use in pregnant women despite the risk (e.g., if the drug is needed for a life-threatening situation or for a serious disease for which drugs can not be prescribed more safely or they are ineffective)

Monoamine Oxidase Inhibitors

It is not suitable to use MAOIs during pregnancy because of the risk of hypertensive crisis, requirement for dietary restrictions, etc.

An increased risk of malformations after the use of tranylcypromine in a small sample of patients has also been described. For other MAOIs information is scarce or non-existent.

Teratogenicity of Antidepressant Drugs

According to the FDA classification we present in Table 19.2 the teratogenic risk of commonly used antidepressants.

19.11.1.2 Electroconvulsive Therapy

Despite a demonstrated efficacy, ECT still remains a controversial treatment in psychiatry, even more during the pregnancy, when associated risk may be higher [105]. Nonetheless, ECT plays a role in the more severe cases of depression during pregnancy. Mainly during the beginning of pregnancy ECT is indicated when there is a poor nutritional intake, a high risk of suicide, a high level of tormenting thoughts, a history of poor response to drug treatment or a history of a good response to ECT. The most common reason to use ECT during the third trimester used to be in a patient who has not responded to other treatments. These reasons and the potential teratogenic effects of drugs increase the attractiveness of ECT use in depressed pregnant women, both unipolar and bipolar depression or mixed states.

Electroconvulsive therapy is safe throughout the pregnancy, although it must be carried out in a hospital to manage any possible emergencies. Several early reviews reported no increase in the risk of labor complications after the use of ECT [106]. The Collaborative Perinatal Project did not find an excess of malformations in newborns with the use of ECT and drug use during the procedure [107].

Summarizing, ECT may be a safe treatment during the first trimester of pregnancy. In the second and third trimesters, ECT is recommended when medications do not control the illness or when a history of a good response to ECT exists from a previous episode.

19.11.1.3 Clinical Approach to Major Depression During Pregnancy

A first step would be to treat all women of childbearing age and pregnant or if it were to be. When we think about treating a woman of childbearing age with major depression, the treatment will be administered over a long period of time; thus, we should question the patient about her plans for future pregnancy, to take them into account from the beginning.

Treatment options should include the depressive history of the patient. Therefore, patients in treatment without symptoms during the last year, and no severe history of depressive episodes could be candidates for stopping medication (obviously in a gradual manner) some months before getting pregnant. They should be monitored often to detect or prevent a relapse. Women with suicidal behavior or severe episodes would not leave treatment.

If depression occurs during pregnancy, its intensity will determine the treatment. If depression is mild we could try nonpharmacological treatments such us psychotherapy. But, if even if it is mild, if the depression presents with insomnia or suicidal risk, then pharmacological treatment will be indicated.

In order to choose an antidepressant, the previous history of drug response in this patient must be taken into account, and whether breast-feeding is included in her plans. Those most frequently used are the SSRIs, specifically fluoxetine, because it is the drug for which there is more evidence of use. However, fluoxetine is not the drug of choice if the mother is going to undertake breastfeeding. In this case, sertraline has a favorable profile in pregnancy and is safe during breastfeeding. Citalopram has been more frequently studied during pregnancy than sertraline, but it crosses the BBB in a more extensive way, and is therefore considered as a second option, or a first option if there is a history of a good response to citalopram.

Tricyclic antidepressants are also a safe option, but owing to their side effects they are considered as a second-line alternative, in case of a nonresponse to the aforementioned medications.

Electroconvulsive therapy is a safe and effective alternative, and according to the APA [108], it can be used in the primary treatment of depression during the first 3 months of pregnancy. Because ECT can promote uterine contractions proper coordination with obstetrics is essential.

19.11.2 Psychotherapy Interventions

Despite the recent evidence pointing toward the relevance of the exposed issue, the literature on the effectiveness of psychotherapy interventions for antenatal depression is still limited. On the one hand, cognitive behavioral therapy has been validated for depression, but without specificities for pregnant women. On the other hand, it has been shown that the interpersonal psychotherapy facilitates the reduction of depressive symptoms in these women [109], probably because of the emphasis given by this model to changing roles, the transition among state, and the acquisition of new skills throughout life.

A recent study [110] carried out an experiment with women (some pregnant and others in their postpartum period), trying to give them space to express their thoughts and feelings about motherhood. Expectations, moods, and feelings about their daily lives were explored. Likewise, the opportunity was offered to build a vision of pregnancy in which they included their own needs. These authors allowed women to claim their life, maternity, and health goals. The results confirmed that the intervention improved the mood of the participants in all cases, especially the pregnant women.

19.12 Fatherhood and Pregnancy

Traditionally, especially in patriarchal societies, it has been believed that the father's role during pregnancy, childbirth, and early childhood is less important than woman's, because the emphasis falls on the mother–child binomial [111]. Directly or indirectly, men have been excluded from sexual and reproductive health for a long time and, in particular, from pregnancy and birth [112]. Their role has been limited to protection and providing help [113]. Although today it still is common in health systems and social circles for the woman to place the father in a secondary role, in industrialized societies this attitude is changing and fathers have begun to be increasingly involved in these processes. The maternity/paternity project is almost always a consensus decision made by both members of the couple. The active involvement of men in the reproductive aspects of their partners fosters a much needed change in gender conceptions.

Fatherhood is also a fundamental part of men's identity. Studies of social roles described how fatherhood can be the point at which they achieve maturity by acquiring a "public identity" as a representative of a family group. It operates as a structuring element of duty in their life cycle [114]. However, the practice of fatherhood is presented as a right or a free choice not as an imposition in the case of maternity [115].

Man lives the gestation process from another perspective. Although involved in their partner's pregnancy, they sometimes have difficulties in imagining the future baby as a real human being. Many men can feel confused and ambivalent about what is expected of them during pregnancy. Despite being on a conscious level very happy, it is frequent that they feel anxiety and fear of the future. Common concerns involving what it is to be a father have been reported, how they have to behave, and whether they could provide for their child and family [111]. The demands of responsibility, protection, and control defined in their role, can confront the father with their self-perceived capacity to occupy that "socially relevant" place. In addition, data suggest that first-time fathers show higher levels of anxiety and depression between the fourth and eighth month compared with men with previous experience [116].

At the end of pregnancy most of the attention is directed to the pregnant woman and after birth to the baby. Relatives look after the mother, while nobody shows an explicit concern for the father [111]; how many times do people ask for him? How many people are interested in his preparation for parenthood? It might be necessary to think about how they will experience it, and how, from a "less important" position, they may have felt during the 9 months in which the arrival of a son/daughter is expected.

19.13 Fatherhood Depression During Pregnancy

Recently, owing to the sociocultural changes in the conceptualization of paternity, fathers have been included in the studies on pregnancy and depression. The results suggest that fathers with depressive tendencies suffer more symptoms of depression and anxiety during pregnancy than parents without those traits. It was also noted that these symptoms do not differ from the symptoms of depression and anxiety during pregnancy identified in depressed mothers [117]. However, the rates of parental depression tended to be lower than those for the mothers, which means that perhaps as the result of hormonal influences together with the cultural factors already described in this chapter, women become depressed more than men during pregnancy. With regard to men, the higher peak of distress seems to be around the second term of pregnancy (18 %) and decreases steadily after birth [118].

Another study found an interaction between depressive symptoms in the father and those in the mother [119]. It was observed that the presence in the father of depressive symptoms directly affects the mental health of the mother, increasing her risk of depression. Therefore, identifying and treating fathers who suffer from depression in the prenatal period must be a priority to increase their psychological well-being and to prevent the negative influence that they may have on the mood of the prenatal mother and the unborn child [120].

The active participation in the gestational process has a favorable impact on the construction of fatherhood and generates a healthy emotional environment for him and his partner [112]. The WHO conducted in 2007 [121] a compilation of several group interventions made with fathers in the field of health, which were specifically aimed at preventing gender inequality. These group experiments tried to train men in sexual and reproductive health, as well as transform the role of men in relation to paternity.

Finally, we will talk about the Couvade syndrome. Currently, this term is used in psychiatry to describe psychosomatic manifestations in men during their partner's pregnancy or during the postpartum period. Sometimes, they have common pregnancy symptoms such as weight gain, morning nausea, fatigue, and mood disturbances. They reproduce the expected symptoms of a pregnant woman. Not many studies make reference to this syndrome, but a wide range in prevalence (13–97 %) has been described. Therefore, it may be more useful to think that almost all parents manifest any of the symptoms, but not the syndrome per se, which would imply that we are faced with a dimensional phenomenon [111]. Although no one knows for sure what its causes are, different theories have been proposed: some authors suggest that the father envies the protagonist role of the woman during pregnancy; others propose that an identification with the mother occurs in an emphatic way and others consider that the anxiety of the father is the origin of these unusual symptoms [111].

In any case, this phenomenology is interesting from the point of view of this chapter. The need to understand these events leads us beyond the purely biological aspects (which is what has been used to justify the psychopathological disturbances of women), reinforcing the idea that pregnancy, for both for man and woman, is much more than the process of creating a new life.

19.14 Conclusion

Pregnancy, apart from being a physiological process, means breaking into the place that is given to the mother and the father: a new individual, family, and social reality.

Despite the cultural changes in the last decades, even today, the attributions associated with each sex in the conception of maternity and paternity, are still alive in the social mind. However, the psychiatric epistemology forgets how men, and especially how contemporary women, face and manage those representations that have been incorporated and the effects they can have on their mental health.

Despite the evidence, the reality is that health policies give the biological issues the main point of the different situations and maternal attitudes during pregnancy. Research and knowledge of mental health assumes that social elements such as violence, poverty, and lack of support are risk factors for psychopathology in pregnant women. However, there are no treatment and prevention interventions focused on these social elements.

We should consider the emotional connotations of what it means to be a mother and father in the societies with a strong patriarchal legacy. This situation could include in the clinical practice different issues (previously neglected) in the understanding of gestational mental health.

References

1. World Health Organization (WHO). A message from the Director General. 2001. Available from: http://www.who.int/whr/2001/dg_message/en/index.html
2. Hendrick V, Altshuler L. Management of major depression during pregnancy. Am J Psychiatry. 2002;159:1667–73.
3. Enrique JM. Depresión en el embarazo y el puerperio. Rev chil neuro-psiquiatr. 2010;48(4): 269–78.
4. Oppenheim G. Psychological disorders in pregnancy. In: Priest R, editor. Psychological disorders in obstetrics and gynaecology. London: Butterworths; 1985.
5. Smith RP, editor. Netter: Obstetricia, Ginecología y Salud de la Mujer. 1st ed. Barcelona: Masson; 2006.
6. Enrique JM. Depresión postparto: aspectos antropológicos y transculturales. Psykhe. 1996;5(2):149–57.
7. Cloninger S. Cattell y los cinco grandes: Teorías analítico-factoriales de los rasgos. In: Cloninger S, editor. Teorías de la personalidad. México: Pearson Education; 2003. p. 227–74.
8. De Beauvoir S. El segundo sexo. Buenos Aires: Siglo XXI; 1999
9. Imaz E. Convertirse en madre. Etnografía del tiempo de gestación. Madrid: Col Feminismos, Ediciones Cátedra; 2010.
10. Warner M. Tú sola entre las mujeres. El mito y el culto de al virgen María. Madrid: Taurus; 1991.
11. Martínez Benlloch, I. Actualización de conceptos en perspectiva de género y salud. Programa de Formación de Formadores/as en Perspectiva de Género el Salud, establecido mediante Convenio entre el Ministerio de Sanidad y Consumo (Observatorio de la Salud de la Mujer) y la Universidad Complutense de Madrid (Grupo de Investigación Estilos Psicológicos, Género y Salud. Madrid; Noviembre de 2005.
12. Arvelo Arregui L. Maternidad, paternidad y género. Red de Revistas científicas de América Latina, Caribe, España y Portugal. Otras Miradas Dic. 2004;4(2):92–8.
13. Muruaga S. La depresión Postparto una forma de Depresión de Género. "La boletina". 2009 nº XXIX. Revista publicada por Mujeres para la salud. Atención especializada a mujeres AMS. Available from: http://www.mujeresparalasalud.org/spip.php?article43
14. Langevin A. Pour une nouvelle réflexion sur les âges de la vie. In: Langevin A, editor. Ces maternités que l'on dit tardives. París: Robert Laffont; 1982.
15. Lasén, A. Le devenir fémenin des temporalités juvéniles. In : Langevin A, Coord. Temporalités du social. Cahiers du Genre; 1999. 24, p. 99–114.
16. Malenfant R. Concilier travail et maternité: un sens, des pratiques, des effets. In: Francine D, Christine C, editors. Espaces et temps de maternité. Montreal: Les ëditions du Remue-Ménage; 2002.
17. Gisbert M. Mujer y sociedad: Evolución de la mujer en la sociedad y mundo laboral del siglo XX. Realidad actual de al mujer en España. La igualdad. Mujer y trabajo en el siglo XXI: estudios y prevención de riesgos laborales. Universidad Internacional Menéndez Pelayo: Santander; Junio 2007.
18. Martínez Benlloch I, Bonilla A. Sistema sexo/género, identidades y construcción de la subjetividad. Valencia: Universitat de València; 2000.

19. Brockington I. Motherhood and mental health. Oxford: Oxford University Press; 1996.
20. Bibring GL, Dwyer TF, Huntington DS, Valenstein AF. A study of the psychological processes in pregnancy and of the earliest mother-child relationship. Psychoanal Study Child. 1961;16: 9–27.
21. Gavin NI, Gaynes BN, Lohr KN, Meltzer-Brody S, Gartlehner G, Swinson T. Perinatal depression: a systematic review of prevalence and incidence. Obstet Gynecol. 2005;106(5 Pt 1): 1071–83.
22. Figuerido B, Conde A. Anxiety and depression symptoms in women and men from early pregnancy to 3-months postpartum: parity differences and effects. J Affect Disord. 2011;132: 146–57.
23. Misri S, Kendrick K. Treatment of perinatal mood and anxiety disorders: a review. Can J Psychiatry. 2007;52:489–98.
24. Davalos DB, Yadon CA, Tregellas HC. Untreated prenatal maternal depression and the potential risks to offspring: a review. Arch Womens Ment Health. 2012;15:1–14.
25. American Psychiatric Association. Diagnostic and statistical manual of mental disorders. 5th ed. Arlington, VA: American Psychiatric Publishing; 2013.
26. Depression in pregnancy [Internet] 2002 [Cited 2005 Jan]. University of Michigan Health Sciences. Available from: http://www.med.umich.edu/depression/pregnancy.htm
27. Kelly RH, Russo J, Katon W. Somatic complaints among pregnant women cared for in obstetrics: normal pregnancy or depressive and anxiety symptom amplification revisited. Gen Hosp Psychiatry. 2001;23:107–13.
28. Levey LC, Newport DJ, Stowe ZN. Suicidal ideation in pregnancy. In: Poster presentation at American Psychiatric Association. New York: Emory University; 2004 May
29. Grigoriadis S, Vonder Porten EH, Mamisashvili L, Tomlinson G, Dennis CL, Koren G, Steiner M, Mousmanis P, Cheung A, Radford K, Martinovic J, Ross LE. The impact of maternal depression during pregnancy on perinatal outcomes: a systematic review and meta-analysis. J Clin Psychiatry. 2013;74(4):e321–41.
30. Lindhal V, Pearson JL, Colpe L. Prevalence of suicidality during pregnancy and the postpartum. Arch Womens Ment Health. 2005;8:77–87.
31. Field T, Diego M, Hernandez-Reif M, Schanberg S, Kuhn C, Yando R, Bendell D. Pregnancy anxiety and comorbid depression and anger: effects on the fetus and neonate. Depress Anxiety. 2003;17:140–51.
32. Matthey S. Using the Edinburgh postnatal depression scale to screen for anxiety disorders. Depress Anxiety. 2007;26:1–6.
33. Littleton HL, Breitkopf CR, Berenson AB. Correlates of anxiety symptoms during pregnancy and association with perinatal outcomes: a meta-analysis. Am J Obstet Gynecol. 2007;196: 424–32.
34. Austin MP, Tully L, Parker G. Examining the relationship between antenatal anxiety and postnatal depression. J Affect Disord. 2007;101:169–74.
35. Lee AM, Chong CSY, Chiu HW, Lam SK, Fong DYT. Prevalence, course, and risk factors for antenatal anxiety and depression. Obstet Gynecol. 2007;110:1102–12.
36. Teixeira C, Figueiredo B, Conde A, Pacheco A, Costa R. Anxiety and depression during pregnancy in women and men. J Affect Disord. 2009;119(1–3):142–8.
37. Buist A, Condon J, Brooks J, Speelman C, Milgrom J, Hayes B, Ellwood D, Barnett B, Kowalenko N, Matthey S, Austin MP, Bilszta J. Acceptability of routine screening for perinatal depression. J Affect Disord. 2006;93(1–3):233–7.
38. Gibson J, McKenzie-McHarg K, Shakespeare J, Price J, Gray R. A systematic review of studies validating the Edinburgh postnatal depression scale in antepartum and postpartum women. Acta Psychiatr Scand. 2009;119(5):350–64.
39. Mattheyy S, Henshaw C, Elliott S, Barnett B. Variability in use of cut-off scores and formats on the Edinburgh postnatal depression scale: implications for clinical and research practice. Arch Womens Ment Health. 2006;9:309–15.

40. Spitzer RL, Williams JB, Kroenke K, Hornyak R, McMurray J. Validity and utility of the PRIME-MD patient health questionnaire in assessment of 3000 obstetric-gynecologic patients: the PRIME-MD patient health questionnaire obstetrics-gynecology study. Am J Obstet Gynecol. 2000;183:759.
41. Miller LJ. Psychiatric disorders during pregnancy. In: Stewart DE, Stotland NL, editors. Psychological aspects of women's mental health. Washington, DC: American Psychiatric Press; 1993.
42. Kornstein SG, Clayton AH, editors. Women's mental health: a comprehensive textbook. New York: The Guilford Press; 2002.
43. Frank E, Novick D, Masalehdan A. Women and depression. In: National alliance for the mentally illness [Internet]. 2003 [Cited February 2005]. Available from: http://www.nami.org/Content/ContentGroups/Helpline1/Depression_in_Women.htm
44. Muramaki J. Gender and depression: explaining the different rates of depression between men and women. Perspect Psychol. 2002;5:27–34.
45. Lancaster CA, Gold KJ, Flynn HA, Yoo H, Marcus SM, Davis MM. Risk factors for depressive symptoms during pregnancy: a systematic review. Am J Obstet Gynecol. 2010; 202:5–14.
46. Pajulo M, Savonlahti E, Sourander A, Helenius H, Piha J. Antenatal depression, substance dependency and social support. J Affect Disord. 2001;65:9–17.
47. Melville JL, Gavin A, Guo Y, Fan MY, Katon WJ. Depressive disorders during pregnancy: prevalence and risk factors in a large urban sample. Obstet Gynecol. 2010;116:1064–70.
48. Goyal D, Gay C, Lee KA. How much does low socioeconomic status increase the risk of prenatal and postpartum depressive symptoms in first- time mothers? Womens Health. 2010; 20:96–104.
49. Evans J, Heron J, Francomb H, Oke S, Golding J. Cohort study of depressed mood during pregnancy and after childbirth. Br Med J. 2001;323:257–60.
50. Alio AP, Lewis CA, Scarborough K, Harris K, Fiscella K. A community perspective on the role of fathers during pregnancy: a qualitative study. BMC Pregnancy Childbirth. 2013;13: 60.
51. Lamb ME, Tamis-Le M, Catherine S. The role of the father: an introduction, chap. 1. In: Lamb ME, editor. The role of the father in child development. 4th ed. Hoboken, NJ: Wiley; 2004. p. 1–31.
52. Hayes BA, Muller R, Bradley BS. Perinatal depression: a randomized controlled trial of an antenatal education intervention for primiparas. Birth. 2001;28(1):28–35.
53. Bao L. Mental health of women with accidental pregnancy. Chin Ment Health J. 2001;97(6): 988–93.
54. Chodorow NJ. "Too late". Ambivalence about Motherhood, choice, and time. In: Brown SF, comp. What do mothers want? Developmental perspectives, clinical challenges. Hillsdale: The Analytic Press; 2005.
55. Imaz E. Condicionantes sociológicas de la fecundidad: pareja, maternidad y paternidad en el contexto de al sociedad asca contemporánea. In: Arregi B, editor. Reproduciendo la vida, manteniendo la familia. Una reflexión sobre la fecundidad y la familia desde Euskadi. Leioa: Editorial de la Unversidad del País Vasco; 2005.
56. Rosen A. Facts and fantasies about infertility. In: Brown SF, comp. What do mothers want? Developmental perspectives, clinical challenges. Hillsdale: The Analytic Press; 2005.
57. Fonnegra I. De cara a la muerte. Cómo afrontar las penas, el dolor y la muerte para vivir plenamente. Andrés Bello: México; 2001.
58. Gutiérrez Romero M, Gómez Castillo B, León Guzmán MI. Consecuencias psicopatológicas del aborto espontáneo. Revista de la Universidad Autónoma del Estado de Mexico. 2011;4:48–55.
59. Gong X, Hao J, Fangbiao Tao F, Zhang J, Wang H, Xu R. Pregnancy loss and anxiety and depression during subsequent pregnancies: data from the C-ABC study. Eur J Obstet Gynecol Reprod Biol. 2013;166(1):30–6.

60. Kozinszky Z, Orvos H, Katona M, Zoboki T, Pai A, Kovács L. Perinatal outcome of induced and spontaneous pregnancies of primiparous women aged 35 or over. Int J Gynecol Obstet. 2002;76(1):23–6.
61. Sau V. Diccionario Ideológico Feminista. Icaria. 1990;1:11–6.
62. Mac Millan HL, Wathen CN, Jamieson E, Boyle M, McNutt L-A, Worster A, Lent MD, Webb M. Approaches to screening for intimate partner violence in health care settings: a randomized trial. JAMA 2006; 296(5):530–6. Available from: http://jama.ama-assn.org/cgi/content/full/296/5/530
63. Moraes CL, Reichenheim ME. Domestic violence during pregnancy in Rio de Janeiro, Brazil. Int J Gynaecol Obstet. 2002;79(3):269–77.
64. Rachana C, Suraiya K, Hisham AS, Abdulaziz AM, Hai A. Prevalence and complications of physical violence during pregnancy. Eur J Obstet Gynecol Reprod Biol. 2002;103(1):26–9.
65. Calderon SH, Gilbert P, Jackson R, Kohn MA, Gerbert B. Cueing prenatal providers effects on discussions of intimate partner violence. Am J Prev Med. 2008;34(2):134–7.
66. Suárez L, Menkes C. La violencia familiar ejercida en contra de los adolescentes mexicanos. Rev Saúde Pública. 2006; 40(4):611–9. Available from: http://www.scielo.br/pdf/rsp/v40n4/ao-5005.pdf
67. Vladislavovna S, Pámanes-González V, Billings D, et al. Violencia de pareja en mujeres embarazadas en la Ciudad de México. Rev Saúde Pública 2007; 41(4):582–90. Available from: http://www.scielo.br/pdf/rsp/v41n4/5821.pdf
68. Lau Y, Chan KS. Influence of intimate partner violence during pregnancy and early postpartum depressive symptoms on breastfeeding among Chinese women in Hong Kong. J Midwifery Womens Health. 2007;52(2):e15–20.
69. Esteban ML. El cuidado de la imagen en los procesos vitales. Creatividad y miedo al descontrol. In: Kobie. Bizkaiko Foru Aldundia. 1997–1998; 8:27–54.
70. Erikson E. Identidad, Juventud y Crisis. Buenos Aires: Editorial Paidós; 1968.
71. Dudas RB, Csatordai S, Devosa I, Annamaría T, Bálint A, Barabás K, Pál A, Kozinszky Z. Obstetric and psychosocial risk factors for depressive symptoms during pregnancy. Psychiatry Res. 2012;200(2):323–8.
72. Kahn RS, Certain L, Whitaker RC. A re-examination of smoking before, during, and after pregnancy. Am J Public Health. 2002;92(11):1801–8.
73. Zhu S, Valbo A. Depression and smoking in pregnancy. Addict Behav. 2002;27:649–58.
74. Bonari L, Bennett H, Einarson A, Koren G. Risks of untreated depression during pregnancy. Can Fam Physician. 2004;50(1):37–9.
75. Kim HG, Mandell M, Cranall C, Kuskowski MA, Dieperink B, Buchberger RL. Antenatal psychiatric illness and adequacy of prenatal care in ethnically diverse inner-city obstetric population. Arch Womens Ment Health. 2006;9:103–7.
76. Chung TKH, Lau K, Yip ASK, Chiu HFK, Lee DTS. Antepartum depressive symptomatology is associated with adverse obstetric and neonatal outcomes. Psychosom Med. 2001;63(5):830–4.
77. Yonkers K, Wisner K, Stewart D, Oberlander T, Dell D, Stotland N, Ramin S, Chaudron L, Lockwood C. The management of depression during pregnancy: A report from the American Psychiatric Association and the American College of Obstetricians and Gynecologists. Obstet Gynecol. 2009;114(3):703–13.
78. Neggers Y, Goldenberg R, Cliver S, Hauth J. The relationship between psychosocial profile, health practices, and pregnancy outcomes. Acta Obstet Gynecol Scand. 2006;85(3):277–85.
79. Robertson E, Grace S, Wallington T, Stewart DE. Antenatal risk factors for postpartum depression: a synthesis of recent literature. Gen Hosp Psychiatry. 2004;26(4):289–95.
80. Nylen K, Moran T, Franklin C, O' Hara M. Maternal depression: a review of relevant treatment approaches for mothers and infants. Infant Ment Health J. 2006;27(4):327–43.
81. Ross LE, Grigoriadis S, Mamisashvili L, Vonderporten EH, Roerecke M, Rehm J, Dennis CL, Koren G, Steiner M, Mousmanis P, Cheung A. Selected pregnancy and delivery

outcomes after exposure to antidepressant medication: a systematic review and meta-analysis. JAMA Psychiatry. 2013;70:436–43.
82. Medrano J, Zardoya M, Pacheco L. Uso de psicofármacos en el embarazo y la lactancia Euromedice ed.; 2009. ISBN: 978-84-96727-57-1
83. Howland RH. Antidepressant medication and pregnancy: time for randomized controlled trials. J Psychosoc Nurs Ment Health Serv. 2013;51:11–4.
84. Koren G, Nordeng HM. Selective serotonin reuptake inhibitors and malformations: case closed? Semin Fetal Neonatal Med. 2013;18:19–22.
85. GlaxoSmithKline. Epidemiology study: paroxetine in the first trimester and the prevalence of congenital malformation. http://ctr.gsk.co.uk/summary/paroxetine/studylist.asp. 2013.
86. US Food and Drug Administration. FDA public health advisory: Paroxetine. http://www.fda.gov/cder/drug7advisory/paroxetine200512.htm. 2013.
87. Wurst KE, Poole C, Ephross SA, Olshan AF. First trimester paroxetine use and the prevalence of congenital, specifically cardiac, defects: a meta-analysis of epidemiological studies. Birth Defects Res A Clin Mol Teratol. 2010;88:159–70.
88. Bar-Oz B, Einarson T, Einarson A, Boskovic R, O'Brien L, Malm H, Berard A, Koren G. Paroxetine and congenital malformations: meta-analysis and consideration of potential confounding factors. Clin Ther. 2007;29:918–26.
89. Jiménez-Solem E, Andersen JT, Petersen M, Broedbaek K, Jensen JK, Afzal S, Gislason GH, Torp-Pedersen C, Poulsen HE. Exposure to selective serotonin reuptake inhibitors and the risk of congenital malformations: a nationwide cohort study. BMJ Open. 2012;2(3):e001148.
90. 't Jong GW, Einarson T, Koren G, Einarson A. Antidepressant use in pregnancy and persistent pulmonary hypertension of the newborn (PPHN): a systematic review. Reprod Toxicol. 2012;34:293–7.
91. Myles N, Newall H, Ward H, Large M. Systematic meta-analysis of individual selective serotonin reuptake inhibitor medications and congenital malformations. Aust N Z J Psychiatry. 2013;47:1002–12.
92. Boyce PM, Hackett LP, Ilett KF. Duloxetine transfer across the placenta during pregnancy and into milk during lactation. Arch Womens Ment Health. 2011;14:169–72.
93. Einarson A, Smart K, Vial T, av-Citrin O, Yates L, Stephens S, Pistelli A, Kennedy D, Taylor T, Panchaud A, Malm H, Koren G, Einarson TR. Rates of major malformations in infants following exposure to duloxetine during pregnancy: a preliminary report. J Clin Psychiatry. 2012;73:1471.
94. Hoog SL, Cheng Y, Elpers J, Dowsett SA. Duloxetine and pregnancy outcomes: safety surveillance findings. Int J Med Sci. 2013;10:413–9.
95. Gentile S. Drug treatment for mood disorders in pregnancy. Curr Opin Psychiatry. 2011;24:34–40.
96. Uguz F. Low-dose mirtazapine in treatment of major depression developed following severe nausea and vomiting during pregnancy: two cases. Gen Hosp Psychiatry. 2013;10:S0163–8343.
97. Olen KN, Rasmussen SA, Riehle-Colarusso T, Reefhuis J. Association between reported venlafaxine use in early pregnancy and birth defects, national birth defects prevention study, 1997–2007. Birth Defects Res A Clin Mol Teratol. 2013;97:28–35.
98. Oberlander TF, Warburton W, Misri S, Riggs W, Aghajanian J, Hertzman C. Major congenital malformations following prenatal exposure to serotonin reuptake inhibitors and benzodiazepines using population-based health data. Birth Defects Res B Dev Reprod Toxicol. 2008;83:68–76.
99. Coleman T, Chamberlain C, Davey MA, Cooper SE, Leonardi-Bee J. Pharmacological interventions for promoting smoking cessation during pregnancy. Cochrane Database Syst Rev. 2012;9:CD010078.
100. Myung SK, Ju W, Jung HS, Park CH, Oh SW, Seo H, Kim H. Efficacy and safety of pharmacotherapy for smoking cessation among pregnant smokers: a meta-analysis. BJOG. 2012;119:1029–39.

101. Hajek P, Stead LF, West R, Jarvis M, Hartmann-Boyce J, Lancaster T. Relapse prevention interventions for smoking cessation. Cochrane Database Syst Rev. 2013;20:8.
102. Thyagarajan V, Robin Clifford C, Wurst KE, Ephross SA, Seeger JD. Bupropion therapy in pregnancy and the occurrence of cardiovascular malformations in infants. Pharmacoepidemiol Drug Saf. 2012;21:1240–2.
103. Patel BN, Beste J. Antidepressant use during pregnancy. Am Fam Physician. 2011;83:1211–5.
104. Pariante CM, Seneviratne G, Howard L. Should we stop using tricyclic antidepressants in pregnancy? Psychol Med. 2011;41:15–7.
105. Saatcioglu O, Tomruk NB. The use of electroconvulsive therapy in pregnancy: a review. Isr J Psychiatry Relat Sci. 2011;48:6–11.
106. Abrams R. Electroconvulsive therapy. 4th ed. New York: Oxford University; 2002.
107. Walker R, Swartz CM. Electroconvulsive therapy during high-risk pregnancy. Gen Hosp Psychiatry. 1994;16:348–53.
108. APA: American Psychiatric Association, Committee on Electroconvulsive Therapy. The practice of electroconvulsive therapy, recommendations for treatment, training, and privileging: a task force report of the American Psychiatric Association; 2001.
109. Spinelli M, Endicott J. Controlled clinical trial of interpersonal psychotherapy versus parenting education program for depressed pregnant women. Am J Psychiatry. 2003;160:555–62.
110. Chavez-Courtois M, Hernandez-Maldonado A, Arce Zacarías E., Bolaños-Delfin I, González Pacheco I, Lartigue Becerra T. Experiencia grupal de mujeres embarazadas y en etapa postparto, y su relación con la depresión y algunos factores sociales. Perinatol Reprod Hum 2008; 22:270–8. Available from: http://www.medshool.uccsf.edu/latino/manuals.aspx
111. Maldonado-Durán M, Lecanne Elier F. El padre en la etapa perinatal. Perinatol Reprod Hum. 2008;22:145–54.
112. García D, Díaz Z. Anthropological and gender perspective in the analysis of care provided to pregnancy, delivery and puerperium. Revista Cubana de Salud Pública. 2010;36(4):330–6.
113. Figueroa JG. Algunos elementos para interpretar la presencia de los varones en los procesos de salud reproductiva. Cad Sáude Pub. 1998;1(14):87–96.
114. Olavarria J. Y todos querían ser (buenos) padres. Varones de Santiago de Chile en conflicto. Santiago: Lom Ediciones; 2001.
115. Montes-Muñoz MJ. Las culturas del nacimiento. Representaciones y prácticas de las mujeres gestantes, comadronas y médicos. PhD Thesis, Universitat Rovira i Virgili, Tarragona; 2007.
116. Ferkeitch SL, Mercer RT. Predictor of role competence for experienced and inexperienced fathers. Nurs Res. 1995;44:89–95.
117. Field T, Diego M, Dieter J, Hernandez-Reif M, Schanberg S, Kuhn C, Yando R, Bendell D. Prenatal depression effects on the fetus and the newborn. Infant Behav Dev. 2004;27:216–29.
118. Condon JT, Boyce P, Corkindale CJ. The First-Time Fathers Study: a prospective study of the mental health and wellbeing of men during the transition to parenthood. Aust N Z J Psychiatry. 2004;38(1–2):56–64.
119. Field T, Diego M, Hernández-Reif M, Figueiredo B, Deeds O, Contogeorgos J, Ascencio A. Prenatal paternal depression. Infant Behav Dev. 2006;29(4):579–83.
120. Buist A, Morse CA, Durkin S. Men's adjustment to fatherhood: implications for obstetric health care. J Obstet Gynecol Neonatal Nurs. 2003;32(2):172–80.
121. Barker G, Ricardo C, Nascimento M. Cómo hacer participar a los hombres y los niños en la lucha contra la inequidad de género en el ámbito de la salud: Algunos datos probatorios obtenidos de los programas de intervención. OMS; 2007. Available from: http://www.who.int/gender/documents/Men-SPAN.pdf

Postnatal Depression

20

Amaia Ugarte and Miryam Fernández

Abstract

Postnatal depression is the most common psychopathological disorder during the postnatal period. It is a mood and anxiety disorder and affects around 15 % of mothers. It involves the development of a major depressive episode whose onset can occur during pregnancy or within 4 weeks of giving birth, and depressive symptoms must be present for at least 2 weeks, but in clinical practice it is considered that it can also have an onset from pregnancy to 3–6 months postpartum, although it is more common during the postpartum period.

There are still many cases of postnatal depression that are not detected in clinical practice; in spite of that, it has deleterious consequences for the mother and for the baby and can delay the physical, social, and cognitive development of the baby.

Social, psychological, and biological factors can contribute to the development of postnatal depression. It is important to educate both professionals and mothers about the risk factors for early detection to prevent depression from developing.

The treatment of depressed women in the postpartum period may be different according to the characteristics of every clinical case; psychotherapy or pharmacotherapy may be used alone or in combination. The therapy may be beneficial for the symptoms and drug treatment is a good option in cases where postpartum depression is considered moderate or severe and in which therapy was not effective.

A. Ugarte (✉) • M. Fernández
Department of Psychiatry, Alava University Hospital, Vitoria, Spain
e-mail: AMAIA.UGARTEUGARTE@osakidetza.net

M. Sáenz-Herrero (ed.), *Psychopathology in Women*,
DOI 10.1007/978-3-319-05870-2_20

20.1 Introduction

Even though women have the same prevalence of psychiatric disorders as men in most countries, there are differences in the psychiatric diagnosis made by sex. Epidemiological studies show rates of depressive and anxiety disorders twice as high in women compared with men. Biology explains some differences in the diagnosis, but mental illnesses are influenced by both biological and psychosocial factors.

The rates of depressive disorders increase in women during maternity. Throughout the whole postpartum period the risk of suffering them is particularly high considering that the mother suffers stressful and important changes physically and also in her surroundings, for example, during the breastfeeding period and transformation in the couple relationship and in the familial structure [1]. Postnatal depression (PND) creates negative outcomes in the mother, her partner, and in the newborn; thus, early detection and treatment nowadays must be a priority for public health.

20.2 Depressive Disorders in the Perinatal Period

Gestational depression and PND are the most common psychopathological disorders during pregnancy and the postnatal period they are mood and anxiety disorders. There are different forms of depression, from minor and temporary episodes of sadness to more severe and persistent forms.

On the one hand is gestational depression that is suffered by 14–23 % of the pregnant women [2], of whom 3 to 5 % are such severe cases that if they do not receive any treatment they can get worse after delivery [3]. For women with a history of major depression the risk of relapse during pregnancy is high, especially if pharmacological treatment has ceased [4].

Postpartum dysphoria occurs in about 50 % of births [5]. It is a transitory mild condition that remits naturally and usually does not require treatment. It appears in the first hours after childbirth and can last a few weeks, but if it lasts more than 2 weeks, and if there is a history of recurrent depressive episodes, it requires an evaluation to rule out the development of a more severe mood disorder.

Postpartum depression, which we focus on in this chapter, affects around 15 % of mothers and can appear in the first few weeks and even for up to a year after childbirth. Medical, psychological, and pharmacological intervention is required so as not to affect the ability of the mother to care for her child.

Postpartum psychosis is a severe disease with an incidence of 0.1–0.2 % [6] that may appear in the first weeks after birth and has an abrupt start and evolves quickly. The characteristic symptoms are depressed or exalted mood, behavioral maladjustment, emotional lability, delusions, and hallucinations. Medical, psychological, and pharmacological interventions are important to avoid it evolving into a major psychiatric disorder.

20.3 Symptoms and Prevalence

In 2013 The American Psychiatric Association changed the name of this condition to peripartum depression in the *Diagnostic and Statistical Manual of Mental Disorders*, fifth edition (DSM-5). This involves the development of a major depressive episode whose onset can occur during pregnancy or within 4 weeks of giving birth [7] and, as in other major depressive episodes, depressive symptoms must be present for at least 2 weeks. However, in clinical practice it is considered that postpartum depression can also occur from pregnancy to 3–6 months postpartum [8, 9], although it is more common in the postpartum period.

The clinical symptomatology is characterized by sadness, anhedonia, tearfulness, fatigue, and anxiety. Also, eating and sleep disorders, loss of energy, and feelings of guilt commonly associated with the care of bringing up a child may appear. These symptoms are also observed in the ordinary postpartum period, which makes diagnosis more difficult. Therefore, it is recommended to explore for more specific symptoms such as impaired concentration, thoughts of death or self- or hetero-aggressiveness toward the newborn. Postnatal depression must be carefully distinguished from both normal and other postpartum psychiatric disorders common in this period, among which postpartum dysphoria and puerperal psychosis deserve social attention.

Each year PND occurs in between 15 and 20 % of all women of childbearing age, resulting in approximately 600,000–800,000 cases annually, and is one of the most common postpartum complications [10]. However, the prevalence is highly variable; some studies found rates from 0 to almost 60 % [11] and the rates vary between countries and within them [12].

20.4 Screening

Postnatal depression can be effectively treated and prevented [13], but there are still many cases continuing undetected in clinical practice [14]. Several tools for detecting depression exist, but few studies have evaluated their use in the postpartum period. The most commonly used in the scientific literature has been the Edinburgh Postnatal Depression Scale (EPDS) [15], a 10-item self-report scale to detect depressive symptoms in women who have just given birth that takes into account the severity of symptoms present during the previous 7 days. It has been translated into several languages and has been used both in clinical practice and in epidemiological studies [16, 17]. It has demonstrated its validity and reliability in several studies and has been recommended as a screening tool indicating the possible presence of depression in women after birth [18], but not as a diagnostic tool. The diagnosis of PND is made by detailed exploration of signs and symptoms in the context of the clinical interview as the Post-Partum Depression (PPD) must be distinguished both from normal puerperium and from other common psychiatric disorders in this period such as postpartum psychosis and postpartum dysphoria.

20.5 Etiology and Risk Factors

Social, psychological, and biological factors can contribute to the development of PND. However, most of the existing literature is focused on the social and psychological causes rather than on the biological ones.

20.6 Biological Factors

During pregnancy and postpartum, women experience hormonal changes, which are aimed at preparing the organism for both childbirth and the breastfeeding period. These changes affect the hormones and the neurotransmitters. Despite the fact that they are necessary to ensure the health of the women during this period, occasionally these alterations provoke deterioration in women's mental health after childbirth.

The concentration in plasma of hormones such as estrogens, progesterone, testosterone, cortisol, and corticotrophin-releasing hormone increases during the 40 weeks of pregnancy, decreasing drastically during childbirth [19, 20]. Several research works indicate that those hormonal changes can cause depression in a subgroup of vulnerable women. However, the origin of this sensitivity has not yet been clarified [21].

Alkistis Skalkidu [22] describes the biological changes associated with the development of postpartum depression, including elements such as the gonadal steroids, the hypothalamic–pituitary–adrenal (HPA) axis, the serotonergic neurotransmitter system, the thyroid system, inflammatory markers, and genetic risk factors.

20.6.1 Gonadal Steroids

Since progesterone and estradiol decrease rapidly after childbirth, their possible implications in the development of the PND have been studied often. In addition, low levels of estrogens have been associated with a reduction in a woman's well-being, and with the onset of depression after childbirth.

In more than 60 % of the cases of women with PND antecedents the low production of endogenous hormones has been linked to the emergence of depressive symptoms [23]. Some research works also corroborate that high-level estradiol treatments improve PND [24, 25]. On the other hand, there are studies that question the hypothesis of hypoestrogenism, as some evidence shows that women suffering deep depression sometimes have higher estradiol serum concentrations than mothers affected by PND in the early postpartum period [26].

As far as progesterone is concerned, in most of the cases it has been associated with postpartum dysphoria [27, 28]. However, in PND the evidence is not strong enough. Some research states that the decrease in progesterone levels coincides with the highest peak of the depressive symptoms in the early postpartum period.

Other studies, on the contrary, show no change [29], or even an increase in the progesterone [30].

Finally, Lawrie et al. [31] carried out a randomized, double-blinded, placebo-controlled clinical trial that demonstrated that the administration of progestogen in the early postpartum increases the risk of PND.

20.6.2 Hypothalamic–Pituitary–Adrenal Axis

The hormonal secretion system works in interrelationship with both the nervous and the immune system. External agents also affect it. During depression there are alterations in the operation of the HPA axis [32]. These three glands, namely, the hypothalamus, the pituitary, and the adrenal glands, operate in a synchronized way thanks to a feedback system. In specific types of depression this self-regulation system does not work. As a consequence the level of hormone production is higher than normal.

The alterations in the HPA axis observed in deep depression and during pregnancy and childbirth are similar to those mentioned above. In this way, the concentration of cortisol increases both in plasma and in urine [21].

A different origin and evolution of depression during pregnancy and in the PND have been pointed out. Thus, normally in the PND, the HPA axis reduces its activity [33], while in the depression suffered during pregnancy there is hyperactivity. Some studies demonstrate how women with PND have a reduced response capacity of the HPA axis compared with the controls [34, 35].

20.6.3 Other Factors in the Etiopathogenesis of PND

The activation of the inflammatory response system can be involved in the pathophysiology of PND [36]. This hypothesis states that external stressors, such as psychosocial factors, and internal stressors, such as organic inflammatory conditions that occur during the postpartum period, can trigger depression through the inflammatory processes [37, 38].

Oxytocin has been linked with childbirth and the breastfeeding period [39], suggesting that it has a positive effect on the mood [40]. The role of oxytocin in the mother–child attachment and social–cognitive processes has been highlighted [41]. These studies are addressed at searching for biomarkers, which, associated with the behavior of mothers affected by depression, could condition the development of the child.

A subgroup of the PND is founded in thyroid dysfunction. Up to 7 % of new mothers experience alterations in the thyroid system during and after childbirth compared with 3–4 % of the general population [42]. In addition, there is evidence that links thyroid dysfunction during pregnancy to depression in the first year after childbirth [43]. Therefore, the evaluation of the thyroid performance in the early period after childbirth is important in order to monitor effectively the women at risk.

The serotonergic system plays a fundamental role in mood disorders and in PND treatment. The use of selective serotonin reuptake inhibitors (SSRIs) has been shown not only to be effective in PND, but also to be well tolerated by the mothers. However, this treatment has not been demonstrated to be well above any other treatments [44].

Epigenetics, genetics, and stress–environment interaction, including the interactions in the early development of their own mother, are factors that have an influence on the propensity for developing PND [45]. Long-term monitoring of the children whose mothers suffered PND shows that they have a tendency to be depressed that is four times higher than the rest of the population [46]. This fact suggests an intergenerational transference that increases the propensity for depression and PND in the descendants. Apparently, multiple genes play an important role in this vulnerability, but not many studies have researched this subject [47, 48].

20.7 Psychosocial Factors

All women are prone to developing depression following childbirth; however, women who have certain risk factors are at a significantly increased risk of experiencing the illness. Many investigators have already described various risk factors with differing views on their importance. In this sense, Robertson et al. described different categories of risk factors.

20.7.1 Strong to Moderate Risk Factors

Depression or anxiety during pregnancy: Experiencing depressed mood or anxiety during pregnancy was a significant predictor of postpartum depression [49–52] and higher levels of anxiety during pregnancy predict the level of postpartum depressive symptomatology.

Past history of psychiatric illness: Having previously experienced depressive symptoms at any time, not just related to childbirth [49–51, 53] leads to a significantly increased risk of postpartum depression.

Life events: Strong–moderate relationship between experiencing a life event and developing postpartum depression was found in a study [49].

Social support: Receiving social support through friends and relatives during stressful times is thought to be a protective factor against developing depression [54] and several earlier studies have evaluated the role of social support in reducing postpartum depression.

20.7.2 Moderate Risk Factors

Psychological factors: Maternal personality characteristics including neuroticism and cognitive attributional style have been measured as risk factors for postpartum depression [49, 55].

Marital relationship: Studies have reported an increased risk of postpartum depression in women who experienced marital problems during pregnancy [49, 50, 56].

20.7.3 Minor Risk Factors

Obstetric factors: Obstetric factors including pregnancy-related complications have been examined as potential risk factors for postpartum depression [49, 53, 57, 58].

Socioeconomic status: Socioeconomic deprivation indicators such as unemployment, low income, and low education have been cited as risk factors in mental health disorders, and in depression in particular [59–61].

20.8 Effects of Illness

Postpartum depression has not only deleterious consequences for the mother but also for the baby and can delay the physical, social, and cognitive development of the baby. Therefore, it is very important to prevent this disease at the centers of women's care using a multidisciplinary approach.

The interaction disturbances of depressed mothers and their infants appear to be universal, across different cultures and socioeconomic status groups. All mothers have in common that they show less sensitivity to and responsibility for the infants [62].

Maternal depression can have a negative impact in different areas of the infants, a range of cognitive functions [63], and verbal abilities [64], as well as children's abilities to regulate their own emotions and behaviors [65]. Parenting can often be influenced by the effects of maternal depression; this may be caused by depressed mothers exhibiting decreased sensitivity in interactions with children, and the lack of contingency in response to the actions of child [66, 67].

Maternal depression is not the only factor that affects children's development; contextual risks can also have a negative impact on children's cognitive functioning, including executive functions such as attention [68], inhibitory control [69], IQ [70], and language development [71].

The possible impact of risks in the context of children's cognitive functioning may be higher in parents with a lower educational level and fewer resources to encourage them cognitively [72].

The interpersonal stress of depressed mothers can negatively affect the well-being of adolescents [73, 74] and children [75], considering that early in the life course, the mother constitutes the primary social environment for the child [76].

It is important to highlight the importance that the immediate social environment has for the baby and his/her experiences; the effect of both maternal depression and contextual risks on the children may be considerable [73].However, postpartum depression also has important consequences for the mother. At this important moment of her life, she is supposed to meet certain expectations, and discomfort caused by not being able to do so is added to the discomfort of depression.

20.9 Effects on the Mother

Depression after childbirth affects the woman's feelings about herself and her interpersonal relationships. It is remarkable in the mother–baby relationship, the couple relationship, and relationships with older children and the wider family are influenced by the depression of the mother. It is important to note that women with postnatal depression are at an increased risk of future depressive episodes. In the postnatal period, an additional challenge for the mother is coping with depression at a time when there is a strong societal expectation that motherhood is joyful and rewarding [77, 78]. Thus, we must not forget that social expectations about motherhood can increase women's reluctance to disclose negative feelings.

20.10 Effects of Depression on the Child

There are many factors that contribute to the healthy development of the child, but development can also be disrupted by many factors. Early relationships are central in promoting healthy social and emotional child development [79]. Having a depressed mother has an impact on the cognitive development of the children, including language development and intelligence. All this varies with the child's gender, different social factors, and the timing and course of the mother's depression [80, 81]. It is obvious to think that the mother's ability to regulate her baby's state plays an important role in helping children develop strategies for managing their feelings and emotions [82, 83]. Some studies showed that mothers with postnatal depression display more negative behaviors toward their babies and that their babies are less positive than those of nondepressed mothers [82, 84].

20.11 Treatment

Nowadays, the idea that postpartum depression is similar to nonpuerperal depression has changed. Until recently, this idea was supported by most investigators and clinicians, but at present and because of the results of some studies that showed that sex steroids have pronounced effects on the central nervous system, including the areas responsible for mood and cognition, this idea has changed [85]. Furthermore, the observation that women become depressed at twice the rate of men and are particularly vulnerable at times of hormonal fluctuation suggests that depression occurring at such times may be, in part, hormonally driven. Because of this association, several investigators have examined the role of estrogen in the treatment and prophylaxis of postpartum depression [25, 86].

In the meantime, the treatment of postpartum depression is based on that of nonpuerperal depression [87–89]. Psychotherapy or pharmacotherapy may be used alone or in combination. Because no modality has been shown to be superior to any other, some authors argue that the choice of therapy, pharmacological and/or psychotherapeutic, for mild to moderate postpartum depression, may be left to the patient [87].

20.12 Psychotherapy

Puerperal women may benefit from psychotherapy, as it focuses on the patient's interpersonal relationships and changing roles [90]. Although pharmacological treatment is also an option, because of the relative paucity of information about the safety of antidepressant use during breastfeeding, many women may choose a nonpharmacological treatment to avoid exposing the baby to psychotropic medication. Marriage counseling is warranted when marital conflicts are distressing and perhaps contribute to depression in women.

20.13 Antidepressant Therapy

Antidepressant treatment may be a suitable medication for any woman with postpartum depression, but especially in cases of persistent depression, or in women who have difficulties caring for themselves or who even have thoughts of harming themselves or the baby, antidepressant treatment has to be the therapy of choice after a comprehensive assessment of the case.

Besides antidepressants, a woman with postpartum depression may benefit from treatment with benzodiazepines to treat the anxiety and agitation that accompany depression. However, the use of antidepressants at this stage of life is something to be controlled, and many of the mothers take the option to breastfeed. In different reviews we have seen that the blood concentration of tricyclic and SSRI antidepressants have been below the detection limit of the laboratory [91]. However, the evidence shows that although well tolerated in the plasma of some babies, detectable levels of antidepressants were found, since these metabolites pass to the baby through breast milk [87, 92–96]. Thus, it is especially important to determine the duration of antidepressant treatment in lactating women [97].

20.14 Discussion

In the last few years this disorder has been considered a public health problem. The World Health Organization/United Nations Population Fund (WHO-UNFPA) [98] has identified maternal mental health as fundamental in achieving the Millennium Development Goals and the Marcé Society for Perinatal Mental Health [99] proposes a debate on the need for a universal psychosocial assessment and detection of depression in perinatal women in the field of primary health care.

Postnatal depression must be carefully distinguished from both normal and other postpartum psychiatric disorders common in this period, among which are dysphoria and postpartum psychosis. For this reason, it is important to have good screening tools to detect the possible presence of these symptoms in order to assess the severity and make a differential diagnosis.

The duration of postpartum depression is not equal in all cases. In some cases it is resolved within a few months of initiation; others, however, are extended in duration [56]. For many women, childbirth is the stress factor that has led them to trigger a series of recurrent depressive episodes that may become chronic. After an episode of postpartum depression the risk of recurrence is 25 %, i.e., they are likely to have more depressive episodes throughout their life, besides being more likely to have them in the postpartum period [56, 58, 100, 101].

It is important to educate about the risk factors for both healthcare professionals who have contact with the mother during pregnancy and the mother, as detecting these early can prevent her from developing depression. Practitioners have to be aware and education about the issue is of vital importance, for mothers not to confuse depression symptoms with pregnancy process symptoms.

Although the theory of hormonal changes in delivery is based on the influence of endocrine factors on the development of PND, there are contradictory findings in the literature so it is essential to continue researching new hypotheses about how the different causes such as psychosocial aspects and gender issues referred to in the previous chapter make some women more vulnerable to developing the disease.

Women in more vulnerable groups to which we must pay special attention include women with conflictive relationships, those who have suffered stressful life events, women of a lower socioeconomic level, as these women are, along with those with a lack of social support at a higher risk of developing postpartum depression.

Treatment of depressed women in the postpartum period may be different according to the characteristics of the case. In general, therapy may be beneficial for the symptoms, both individual and group therapy. Drug treatment is also a good option, especially in cases where postpartum depression is considered moderate or severe, where there are suicidal thoughts, or where it actually affected functionality in women in whom therapy was not effective. The use of tricyclic antidepressants and SSRIs are not contraindicated during lactation, but in cases that thrive and choose breastfeeding for the baby, taking antidepressants must be done with exhaustive control so that this does not affect the child, because the benefits of taking an antidepressant are probably greater than the risk of psychotropic exposure of the child.

References

1. Burt VK, Stein K. Epidemiology of depression throughout the female life cycle. J Clin Psychiatry. 2002;63 Suppl 7:9–15.
2. Gaynes BN, Gavin N, Meltzer-Brody S, Lohr KN, Swinson T, Gartlehner G, et al. Perinatal depression: prevalence, screening accuracy, and screening outcomes. Evid Rep Technol Assess (Summ) 2005;(119):1–8.
3. MacArthur. Initiative on depression and primary care. Patient health questionnaire (PHQ-9). http://depressionprimarycare.org/clinicians/toolkits/materials/forms/phq9; 2010 April 10.
4. Bonari L, Pinto N, Ahn E, Einarson A, Steiner M, Koren G. Perinatal risks of untreated depression during pregnancy. Can J Psychiatry. 2004;49(11):726–35.
5. Kendell RE, McGuire RJ, Connor Y, Cox JL. Mood changes in the first three weeks after childbirth. J Affect Disord. 1981;3(4):317–26.
6. Sit D, Rothschild AJ, Wisner KL. A review of postpartum psychosis. J Womens Health (Larchmt). 2006;15(4):352–68.
7. American Psychiatric Association. Diagnostic and statistical manual of mental disorders. 5th ed; 2013.
8. Wisner KL, Parry BL, Piontek CM. Clinical practice. Postpartum depression. N Engl J Med. 2002;347(3):194–9.
9. Not author listed. The management of postnatal depression. Drug Ther Bull 2000;38(5):33–7.
10. Gavin NI, Gaynes BN, Lohr KN, Meltzer-Brody S, Gartlehner G, Swinson T. Perinatal depression: a systematic review of prevalence and incidence. Obstet Gynecol. 2005;106 (5 Pt 1):1071–83.
11. Halbreich U, Karkun S. Cross-cultural and social diversity of prevalence of postpartum depression and depressive symptoms. J Affect Disord. 2006;91(2–3):97–111.
12. Affonso DD, De AK, Horowitz JA, Mayberry LJ. An international study exploring levels of postpartum depressive symptomatology. J Psychosom Res. 2000;49(3):207–16.
13. Brugha TS, Morrell CJ, Slade P, Walters SJ. Universal prevention of depression in women postnatally: cluster randomized trial evidence in primary care. Psychol Med. 2011;41 (4):739–48.
14. Dennis CL. Preventing and treating postnatal depression. BMJ. 2009;338:a2975.
15. Cox JL, Holden JM, Sagovsky R. Detection of postnatal depression. Development of the 10-item Edinburgh Postnatal Depression Scale. Br J Psychiatry. 1987;150:782–6.
16. Buist AE, Barnett BE, Milgrom J, Pope S, Condon JT, Ellwood DA, et al. To screen or not to screen—that is the question in perinatal depression. Med J Aust. 2002;177(Suppl):S101–5.
17. Lanes A, Kuk JL, Tamim H. Prevalence and characteristics of postpartum depression symptomatology among Canadian women: a cross-sectional study. BMC Public Health. 2011;11:302.
18. Georgiopoulos AM, Bryan TL, Wollan P, Yawn BP. Routine screening for postpartum depression. J Fam Pract. 2001;50(2):117–22.
19. Dorr HG, Heller A, Versmold HT, Sippell WG, Herrmann M, Bidlingmaier F, et al. Longitudinal study of progestins, mineralocorticoids, and glucocorticoids throughout human pregnancy. J Clin Endocrinol Metab. 1989;68(5):863–8.
20. Stalla GK, Bost H, Stalla J, Kaliebe T, Dorr HG, Pfeiffer D, et al. Human corticotropin-releasing hormone during pregnancy. Gynecol Endocrinol. 1989;3(1):1–10.
21. Bloch M, Daly RC, Rubinow DR. Endocrine factors in the etiology of postpartum depression. Compr Psychiatry. 2003;44(3):234–46.

22. Skalkidou A, Hellgren C, Comasco E, Sylven S, Sundstrom PI. Biological aspects of postpartum depression. Womens Health (Lond Engl). 2012;8(6):659–72.
23. Bloch M, Schmidt PJ, Danaceau M, Murphy J, Nieman L, Rubinow DR. Effects of gonadal steroids in women with a history of postpartum depression. Am J Psychiatry. 2000;157 (6):924–30.
24. Ahokas A, Kaukoranta J, Wahlbeck K, Aito M. Estrogen deficiency in severe postpartum depression: successful treatment with sublingual physiologic 17beta-estradiol: a preliminary study. J Clin Psychiatry. 2001;62(5):332–6.
25. Gregoire AJ, Kumar R, Everitt B, Henderson AF, Studd JW. Transdermal oestrogen for treatment of severe postnatal depression. Lancet. 1996;347(9006):930–3.
26. Klier CM, Muzik M, Dervic K, Mossaheb N, Benesch T, Ulm B, et al. The role of estrogen and progesterone in depression after birth. J Psychiatr Res. 2007;41(3–4):273–9.
27. Harris B, Lovett L, Newcombe RG, Read GF, Walker R, Riad-Fahmy D. Maternity blues and major endocrine changes: Cardiff puerperal mood and hormone study II. BMJ. 1994;308 (6934):949–53.
28. Nappi RE, Petraglia F, Luisi S, Polatti F, Farina C, Genazzani AR. Serum allopregnanolone in women with postpartum "blues". Obstet Gynecol. 2001;97(1):77–80.
29. Harris B, Lovett L, Smith J, Read G, Walker R, Newcombe R. Cardiff puerperal mood and hormone study. III. Postnatal depression at 5 to 6 weeks postpartum, and its hormonal correlates across the peripartum period. Br J Psychiatry. 1996;168(6):739–44.
30. Bou-Saleh MT, Ghubash R, Karim L, Krymski M, Bhai I. Hormonal aspects of postpartum depression. Psychoneuroendocrinology. 1998;23(5):465–75.
31. Lawrie TA, Hofmeyr GJ, De JM, Berk M, Paiker J, Viljoen E. A double-blind randomised placebo controlled trial of postnatal norethisterone enanthate: the effect on postnatal depression and serum hormones. Br J Obstet Gynaecol. 1998;105(10):1082–90.
32. Chrousos GP, Gold PW. The concepts of stress and stress system disorders. Overview of physical and behavioral homeostasis. JAMA. 1992;267(9):1244–52.
33. Kammerer M, Taylor A, Glover V. The HPA axis and perinatal depression: a hypothesis. Arch Womens Ment Health. 2006;9(4):187–96.
34. Jolley SN, Elmore S, Barnard KE, Carr DB. Dysregulation of the hypothalamic-pituitary-adrenal axis in postpartum depression. Biol Res Nurs. 2007;8(3):210–22.
35. Taylor A, Glover V, Marks M, Kammerer M. Diurnal pattern of cortisol output in postnatal depression. Psychoneuroendocrinology. 2009;34(8):1184–8.
36. Corwin EJ, Pajer K. The psychoneuroimmunology of postpartum depression. J Womens Health (Larchmt). 2008;17(9):1529–34.
37. Maes M, Yirmyia R, Noraberg J, Brene S, Hibbeln J, Perini G, et al. The inflammatory and neurodegenerative (I&ND) hypothesis of depression: leads for future research and new drug developments in depression. Metab Brain Dis. 2009;24(1):27–53.
38. Raison CL, Capuron L, Miller AH. Cytokines sing the blues: inflammation and the pathogenesis of depression. Trends Immunol. 2006;27(1):24–31.
39. Pter-Levy Y, Feldman M, Vakart A, Ebstein RP, Feldman R. Impact of maternal depression across the first 6 years of life on the child's mental health, social engagement, and empathy: the moderating role of oxytocin. Am J Psychiatry. 2013;170(10):1161–8.
40. Viero C, Shibuya I, Kitamura N, Verkhratsky A, Fujihara H, Katoh A, et al. Review: oxytocin: Crossing the bridge between basic science and pharmacotherapy. CNS Neurosci Ther. 2010;16(5):e138–56.
41. Feldman R. Oxytocin and social affiliation in humans. Horm Behav. 2012;61(3):380–91.
42. Basraon S, Costantine MM. Mood disorders in pregnant women with thyroid dysfunction. Clin Obstet Gynecol. 2011;54(3):506–14.
43. Kuijpens JL, Vader HL, Drexhage HA, Wiersinga WM, van Son MJ, Pop VJ. Thyroid peroxidase antibodies during gestation are a marker for subsequent depression postpartum. Eur J Endocrinol. 2001;145(5):579–84.

44. De CF, Perelli F, Armando M, Vicari S. Selective serotonin reuptake inhibitors (SSRIs) for post-partum depression (PPD): a systematic review of randomized clinical trials. J Affect Disord. 2014;152–154:39–44.
45. Anderson G, Maes M. Postpartum depression: psychoneuroimmunological underpinnings and treatment. Neuropsychiatr Dis Treat. 2013;9:277–87.
46. Pawlby S, Hay DF, Sharp D, Waters CS, O'Keane V. Antenatal depression predicts depression in adolescent offspring: prospective longitudinal community-based study. J Affect Disord. 2009;113(3):236–43.
47. Mehta D, Quast C, Fasching PA, Seifert A, Voigt F, Beckmann MW, et al. The 5-HTTLPR polymorphism modulates the influence on environmental stressors on peripartum depression symptoms. J Affect Disord. 2012;136(3):1192–7.
48. Mitchell C, Notterman D, Brooks-Gunn J, Hobcraft J, Garfinkel I, Jaeger K, et al. Role of mother's genes and environment in postpartum depression. Proc Natl Acad Sci USA. 2011;108(20):8189–93.
49. O'Hara MW, Swain AM. Rates and risk of postpartum depression—a meta-analysis. Int Rev Psychiatry. 1996;8:37–54.
50. Beck CT. Predictors of postpartum depression: an update. Nurs Res. 2001;50(5):275–85.
51. Josefsson A, Angelsioo L, Berg G, Ekstrom CM, Gunnervik C, Nordin C, et al. Obstetric, somatic, and demographic risk factors for postpartum depressive symptoms. Obstet Gynecol. 2002;99(2):223–8.
52. Neter E, Collins NL, Lobel M, Dunkel-Schetter C. Psychosocial predictors of postpartum depressed mood in socioeconomically disadvantaged women. Womens Health. 1995;1 (1):51–75.
53. Johnstone SJ, Boyce PM, Hickey AR, Morris-Yatees AD, Harris MG. Obstetric risk factors for postnatal depression in urban and rural community samples. Aust N Z J Psychiatry. 2001;35(1):69–74.
54. Brugha TS, Sharp HM, Cooper SA, Weisender C, Britto D, Shinkwin R, et al. The Leicester 500 Project. Social support and the development of postnatal depressive symptoms, a prospective cohort survey. Psychol Med. 1998;28(1):63–79.
55. Lee DT, Yip AS, Leung TY, Chung TK. Identifying women at risk of postnatal depression: prospective longitudinal study. Hong Kong Med J. 2000;6(4):349–54.
56. Kumar R, Robson KM. A prospective study of emotional disorders in childbearing women. Br J Psychiatry. 1984;144:35–47.
57. Nielsen FD, Videbech P, Hedegaard M, Dalby SJ, Secher NJ. Postpartum depression: identification of women at risk. BJOG. 2000;107(10):1210–7.
58. Warner R, Appleby L, Whitton A, Faragher B. Demographic and obstetric risk factors for postnatal psychiatric morbidity. Br J Psychiatry. 1996;168(5):607–11.
59. Bartley M. Unemployment and ill health: understanding the relationship. J Epidemiol Community Health. 1994;48:333–7.
60. Patel V, Araya R, de Lima M, Ludermir A, Todd C. Women, poverty and common mental disorders in four restructuring societies. Soc Sci Med. 1999;49(11):1461–71.
61. World Health Organization. The World Health Report 2001: determinants of mental and behavioural disorders. Web Site World Health Organization 2001.
62. Field T. Postpartum depression effects on early interactions, parenting, and safety practices a review. Infant Behav Dev. 2010;33(1):1–6.
63. Hughes C, Roman G, Hart MJ, Ensor R. Does maternal depression predict young children's executive function?—a 4-year longitudinal study. J Child Psychol Psychiatry. 2013;54 (2):169–77.
64. Barker ED, Jaffee SR, Uher R, Maughan B. The contribution of prenatal and postnatal maternal anxiety and depression to child maladjustment. Depress Anxiety. 2011;28(8):696–702.

65. Feldman R, Eidelman AI. Biological and environmental initial conditions shape the trajectories of cognitive and social-emotional development across the first years of life. Dev Sci. 2009;12(1):194–200.
66. Cox AD, Puckering C, Pound A, Mills M. The impact of maternal depression in young children. J Child Psychol Psychiatry. 1987;28(6):917–28.
67. Hay DF, Pawlby S, Sharp D, Asten P, Mills A, Kumar R. Intellectual problems shown by 11-year-old children whose mothers had postnatal depression. J Child Psychol Psychiatry. 2001;42(7):871–89.
68. Rueda MR, Posner MI, Rothbart MK. The development of executive attention: contributions to the emergence of self-regulation. Dev Neuropsychol. 2005;28(2):573–94.
69. Farah MJ, Shera DM, Savage JH, Betancourt L, Giannetta JM, Brodsky NL, et al. Childhood poverty: specific associations with neurocognitive development. Brain Res. 2006;1110 (1):166–74.
70. Duncan GJ, Brooks-Gunn J. Family poverty, welfare reform, and child development. Child Dev. 2000;71(1):188–96.
71. Noble KG, McCandliss BD, Farah MJ. Socioeconomic gradients predict individual differences in neurocognitive abilities. Dev Sci. 2007;10(4):464–80.
72. Conger RD, Donnellan MB. An interactionist perspective on the socioeconomic context of human development. Annu Rev Psychol. 2007;58:175–99.
73. Garber J, Cole DA. Intergenerational transmission of depression: a launch and grow model of change across adolescence. Dev Psychopathol. 2010;22(4):819–30.
74. Hammen C, Shih JH, Brennan PA. Intergenerational transmission of depression: test of an interpersonal stress model in a community sample. J Consult Clin Psychol. 2004;72(3):511–22.
75. Barker ED. The duration and timing of maternal depression as a moderator of the relationship between dependent interpersonal stress, contextual risk and early child dysregulation. Psychol Med. 2013;43(8):1587–96.
76. Murray L, Kempton C, Woolgar M, Hooper R. Depressed mothers' speech to their infants and its relation to infant gender and cognitive development. J Child Psychol Psychiatry. 1993;34(7):1083–101.
77. Hall PL, Wittkowski A. An exploration of negative thoughts as a normal phenomenon after childbirth. J Midwifery Womens Health. 2006;51(5):321–30.
78. Petch J, Halford WK. Psycho-education to enhance couples' transition to parenthood. Clin Psychol Rev. 2008;28(7):1125–37.
79. Thompson RA. Early sociopersonality development. In: Damon WE, editor. Handbook of child psychology, Social, emotional and personality development, vol. 3. 5th ed. New York: Wiley; 1998. p. 25–104.
80. Grace SL, Evindar A, Stewart DE. The effect of postpartum depression on child cognitive development and behavior: a review and critical analysis of the literature. Arch Womens Ment Health. 2003;6(4):263–74.
81. Hay DF, Pawlby S, Angold A, Harold GT, Sharp D. Pathways to violence in the children of mothers who were depressed postpartum. Dev Psychol. 2003;39(6):1083–94.
82. Hay DF. Postpartum depression and cognitive development. In: Cooper P, Murray L, editors. Postpartum depression and child development. New York: Guilford; 1997. p. 85–110.
83. Tronick E, Reck C. Infants of depressed mothers. Harv Rev Psychiatry. 2009;17(2):147–56.
84. Murray L, Cooper P. Effects of postnatal depression on infant development. Arch Dis Child. 1997;77(2):99–101.
85. Boyce P, Stubbs J, Todd A. The Edinburgh Postnatal Depression Scale: validation for an Australian sample. Aust N Z J Psychiatry. 1993;27(3):472–6.
86. Sichel DA, Cohen LS, Robertson LM, Ruttenberg A, Rosenbaum JF. Prophylactic estrogen in recurrent postpartum affective disorder. Biol Psychiatry. 1995;38(12):814–8.

87. Appleby L, Warner R, Whitton A, Faragher B. A controlled study of fluoxetine and cognitive-behavioural counselling in the treatment of postnatal depression. BMJ. 1997;314(7085):932–6.
88. Stowe ZNCJLJNC, Casarella J, Landry J, Nemeroff CB. Sertraline in the treatment of women with postpartum major depression. Depression. 1995;3:49–55.
89. Epperson CN, McDougle CJ, Ward-O'Brien D, Price LH. A controlled study of sertraline versus placebo in the treatment of postpartum depression: preliminary findings. Soc Neurosci. 1996;22:179. Ref Type: Abstract.
90. Stuart SOM, O'Hara MW. Treatment of postpartum depression with interpersonal psychotherapy [Letter]. Arch Gen Psychiatry. 1995;52:75–6.
91. Wisner KL, Perel JM, Findling RL. Antidepressant treatment during breast-feeding. Am J Psychiatry. 1996;153(9):1132–7.
92. Epperson CN, Anderson GM, McDougle CJ. Sertraline and breast-feeding. N Engl J Med. 1997;336(16):1189–90.
93. Lester BM, Cucca J, Andreozzi L, Flanagan P, Oh W. Possible association between fluoxetine hydrochloride and colic in an infant. J Am Acad Child Adolesc Psychiatry. 1993;32(6):1253–5.
94. Spigset O, Carleborg L, Norstrom A, Sandlund M. Paroxetine level in breast milk. J Clin Psychiatry. 1996;57(1):39.
95. Wisner KL, Perel JM, Findling RL, Hinnes RL. Nortriptyline and its hydroxymetabolites in breastfeeding mothers and newborns. Psychopharmacol Bull. 1997;33(2):249–51.
96. Wright S, Dawling S, Ashford JJ. Excretion of fluvoxamine in breast milk. Br J Clin Pharmacol. 1991;31(2):209.
97. American Academy of Pediatrics Work Group on Breastfeeding. Breastfeeding and the use of human milk. Pediatrics. 1997;100:1035–9.
98. WHO-UNFPA. The Millennium Development Goals Report 2012. https://www.unfpa.org/public/publications/pid/6090; 2013
99. Marcé International Society. http://www.marcesociety.com/About-Marce.aspx; 2013. Ref Type: Internet Communication.
100. Nott PN. Extent, timing and persistence of emotional disorders following childbirth. Br J Psychiatry. 1987;151:523–7.
101. Philipps LH, O'Hara MW. Prospective study of postpartum depression: 4 1/2-year follow-up of women and children. J Abnorm Psychol. 1991;100(2):151–5.

21 Puerperal Psychosis

Jaime del Corral Serrano

Abstract

The period of time after childbirth is, by far, the time of life of the woman in which the incidence of psychosis is the highest. Numerous cultural, psychological, and biological stressors converge around motherhood. Clinical aspects of the various forms of puerperal psychosis, and a specific and well-defined clinical picture (the "classical puerperal psychosis" described in the ancient texts), are addressed. The emergence of this disease has important prognostic implications. The absence of standardized classification criteria for puerperal psychosis has meant that, in many studies, it has been considered almost exclusively as one of the major psychiatric syndromes, such as bipolar disorder. At present, a biological paradigm in explaining these disorders seems to prevail, although numerous scientific data support the idea that this disorder should be considered from a complex and dimensional perspective.

21.1 Introduction

Postpartum psychosis is defined as psychosis commencing within 3 months of delivery. It is a severe and potentially dangerous clinical picture for the mother and baby. As discussed below, consideration of postpartum psychosis as a separate "entity" has been debated since interest in the disease reemerged in the nineteenth century.

In recent years, research has been conducted to support the existence of a specific type of psychosis associated with the postpartum period [1–3], and there have also been other studies that argue that it belongs to other forms of psychosis [4–6].

J. del Corral Serrano (✉)
Clínica Nuestra Señora de la Paz, Madrid, Spain
e-mail: jaicorser@gmail.com

M. Sáenz-Herrero (ed.), *Psychopathology in Women*,
DOI 10.1007/978-3-319-05870-2_21

Postpartum psychosis can be defined as any form of psychosis that happens after childbirth, or as a modality, characteristic of the postpartum period and with specific psychopathology. Many classical texts provide descriptions of puerperal psychosis with a number of characteristic symptoms, which have been reproduced in the current studies on the disease. To bring clarity, we hereafter refer to puerperal (or postpartum) psychosis as any form of psychosis after birth, and we use "classical psychosis" to refer to the specific mode of psychosis after delivery.

Postpartum psychosis is caused by the confluence of a number of stressors. These factors include strong biological and psychosocial influences.

This chapter aims to outline some of the possible causes of puerperal psychosis (and thus, the causes of psychosis in general). Psychopathology, epidemiology, and evolutionary aspects of the disorder also are addressed. In addition, we explore, in a summarized form, the conceptual dialectic of the disorder.

21.2 Conceptual History

The first references linked to postpartum psychosis can be found in ancient literature. Hippocrates described an entity called *phrenitis*, associated with the postpartum period, as a disturbance of thought, mood, and action, accompanied by physical changes such as fever (and equivalent to delirium), and separated from conventional madness (*mania*) in which fever is absent [7]. Soranus of Ephesus also described a febrile clinical picture accompanied by acute mental illness [8]. Many of the earliest descriptions of puerperal psychosis described the clinical symptoms of delirium, with (especially infectious) a probably physical cause. There are also writings on confusional psychosis episodes with no fever, approaching the future concept of puerperal psychosis. The doctrines of Hippocrates remained in place from the fourth century BC until the 19th century.

In the nineteenth century, two main lines of thought on puerperal psychosis that extend to the present were configured. Although some previous references exist, the first accurate descriptions of the disorder appear in the work of Esquirol [9], who observed a high incidence of psychosis in the immediate postpartum and in the breastfeeding period. The most famous pupil of Esquirol, Marce, concluded that, in fact, the post-birth period increased the incidence of various forms of psychosis, and described a puerperal syndrome characterized by the diversity of psychotic symptoms and confusion.

Conversely, other authors considered that the low specificity of symptoms suggests that puerperal psychosis does not meet the criteria to be considered a nosological category, and that the clinical picture "reveals" preexisting psychiatric tare. This vision, inserted into the line of "mental degeneration" of Morel, was defended by Magnan (1877) and Toulouse (1893), among others [10]. In the twentieth century, both lines of thought were maintained. The first, Anglo-Saxon and inspired by Kraepelin, holds that postpartum pathology existed previously, and is triggered by stress factors that appear in this period. The second, supported by French authors (such as Henry Ey), but also by the Anglo-Saxons (Kendell and

Hamilton), holds that there is a postpartum psychotic pathology. Hamilton is probably the best defender of the existence of postpartum psychosis as a disease entity in which the perplexity and symptomatic variability are the core aspects [1].

In many European countries the existence of a postpartum syndrome has been recognized for years. It was thought to be psychogenic or reactive and that it occurred in women with dysfunctional personality traits. The term "amentia" (considered practically synonymous with puerperal psychosis) refers to confusion and/or perplexity, and comes from the German-language literature. For decades, the "classic" puerperal psychosis has been considered one of the types of Bonhoeffer [11] acute exogenous reaction.

Throughout the twentieth century, a neo-Kraepelinian classification scheme, under which there are two basic disease entities in psychosis, manic-depressive psychosis and schizophrenia, was imposed. Moreover, the "classic" puerperal psychosis appears with much lower incidence than other forms of psychosis, which are also favored by stress factors and physical alterations. Thus, many studies on puerperal psychosis [12, 13] conclude that it does not exist as such, and that puerperal psychosis is most classifiable as an affective disorder [14]. Another feature that has been attributed to puerperal psychosis, which explains its absence in modern classifications, is the lack of specific symptoms. This fact, coupled with the presence of symptoms that overlap with other diagnostic categories makes it difficult to individualize. As discussed below, some recent studies suggest the existence of a number of typical symptoms, which coincide with the observations made in the nineteenth century.

ICD-10 employs the category of mental and behavioral disorders associated with the puerperium (F53), but warns that:

> The inclusion of this category should not be taken to imply that, given adequate information, a significant proportion of cases of postpartum mental illness cannot be classified in other categories. Most experts in this field are of the opinion that a clinical picture of puerperal psychosis is so rarely (if ever) reliably distinguishable from affective disorder or schizophrenia that a special category is not justified.

In the DSM-IV, the specification of postpartum onset (within 4 weeks) was included. It can be applied to manic or depressive episodes, within a major depressive disorder, bipolar I disorder, bipolar II disorder, or brief psychotic disorder. Therefore, the international classifications do not record a specific set of symptoms for postpartum psychosis, but allow the use of the term [15, 16].

McGorry and Connell, two Australian authors, have reviewed the scientific literature on puerperal psychosis. According to their research, studies clearly show vulnerability to puerperal episodes, and indicate a higher risk for affective and cycloid psychoses [17]. References to cycloid psychosis are common in work on puerperal psychosis, because there are many symptoms of the two diseases that overlap.

A current Dutch author we quote in this paper repeatedly, Klompenhouwer, defends the existence of "classic psychosis" as an entity [18]. He defines the disease as a confusional psychosis that develops in healthy women during a period of

2 weeks after delivery. The author makes a detailed study of puerperal psychosis based on the Research Diagnostic Criteria (RDC). The study concludes that there is a characteristic syndrome. Later, we will describe the symptoms and the evolution of this classic "psychosis," based primarily on the work of Klompenhouwer, Hamilton, Ey, and Esquirol.

In summary, during the nineteenth century, numerous writings about psychotic syndromes associated with the postpartum period reappeared. Some of them describe a picture of confusional characteristics and mood fluctuations that was categorized as a specific disease, while others tend to view puerperal psychosis as a manifestation of great psychiatric syndromes. The imposition of a consensual truth from classification models DSM and ICD have imposed the second option to the detriment of the first. At present, some authors provide evidence for the existence of a definite form of puerperal psychosis. It remains to be established whether this set of symptoms should be considered a disease in itself or a variant of other puerperal disorders.

21.3 Symptomatology

Postpartum conditions of physical and psychological stress cause an increase in all forms of psychosis. Studies of psychotic episodes associated with postpartum agree that there is a predominance of affective symptomatology. In many cases, it is stated that most of the episodes are classifiable in a bipolar spectrum [5, 19] and in other studies they are labeled as functional psychosis or schizoaffective disorders [18].

Those works that defend the existence of a specific disorder (the "classical" puerperal psychosis), define the following symptoms [20–22].

1. Fast onset, usually from 2 to 10 days after birth, with a decreasing incidence over time. The onset occurs with no previous symptoms, sometimes beginning with confusion and rapidly evolving to the full syndrome.
2. A fluctuating confusional state with variable intensity, in which the level of consciousness ranges from simple obnubilation to a state of severe stupor. Henry Ey described it as "a confused-oniric state with a tone of anxiety" [10]. Most papers agree on the high incidence of this symptom in relation to its presence in other forms of psychosis (manic-depressive psychosis or schizophrenic psychosis). The degree of confusion and perplexity usually fluctuates. After remission of the episode, amnesia for periods of confusion is a common fact.
3. Depersonalization and derealization. These are less specific symptoms of the disorder, and are present in most puerperal psychiatric disorders, both psychotic and nonpsychotic. These states of anxiety often induce a poor mother–child bond that generates intense feelings of guilt in the mother.
4. Dreamlike states of variable depth, independent of the degree of confusion. Thus, very rich dream experiences with little disorientation can appear, and

vice versa. The great complexity and polymorphism of these states are characteristic of puerperal psychosis.

5. Affective disturbances with melancholic, mixed or manic forms, often emerge after the dream phase. They constitute one of the most characteristic symptoms of the disorder, and the alternating mood is particularly frequent. The mood swings establish links with bipolar and cycloid psychosis.
6. Misrecognitions. Characteristically, the parent or husband is involved. They constitute one of the major symptoms of the disorder.
7. Hallucinations. The auditory and visual hallucinations are common in the "classical" puerperal psychosis, but also in schizophrenic and schizoaffective psychosis, and very rare in purely affective psychosis. They include verbal and non-verbal hallucinations (crying, screaming.). The presence of hallucinations is one of the main clues to differentiating the "classical" puerperal psychosis from bipolar psychosis.
8. Delusions. Delusional content related to motherhood, although not uncommon, appears more frequently in other forms of psychosis. The presence of thematic delusions has been interpreted as an argument in favor of psychogenic etiology in these patients. However, modern studies do not show a clear predominance of this delusional theme. It has been noted that persecutory and erotomanic delusions are also characteristic. A pathognomonic pattern of delirium has not been found.
9. Psychomotor symptoms. Agitation and retardation are the most common features. Stupor is less frequent.
10. Changeability of symptoms in the course of the illness, called the "kaleidoscopic picture" by Klompenhouwer. This alternation of altered level of consciousness, psychotic symptoms, and mood swings is one of the defining characteristics of "classical" puerperal psychosis.
11. Remissions and relapses. Often, after several days of symptoms, an apparent complete remission, and a few days later, a new outbreak occurs. These recurrences should be considered carefully, as the symptom-free periods can lead to a premature meeting between mother and child that may involve a significant risk for both.
12. Symptoms are infrequent after the 3rd week.

In a study of recurrences in patients who met the criteria for "classical" puerperal psychosis, 95 % had symptoms in the first 3 weeks. 95 % also presented confusional symptomatology. Other symptoms such as changes in the presented symptoms (kaleidoscopic image; 70 %), depersonalization (70 %), and, to a lesser degree, assault (60 %) were also observed [17].

There are specific symptoms of "classic" puerperal psychosis and nonspecific symptoms. Certain properties considered by ancient authors as characteristic of this disease, such as thematic delusions or mood changes, occur in other psychotic disorders. However, some characteristics do exist that can be conceptualized as indicators of "classic" psychosis. They are:

- Confusional symptoms
- Depersonalization
- Misrecognitions
- The "kaleidoscopic course"

It is worth mentioning another variety of psychosis that appears to be related to postpartum psychosis: psychosis associated with menstruation. The menstrual cycle, especially the fourth quarter, in which a dramatic reduction in the levels of sex hormones occurs, in an attenuated form mimics the hormonal milieu that occurs postpartum. As in puerperal psychosis, we found descriptions referring to it from the nineteenth century [23]. Over two centuries there have been observations on cases of psychosis with a cyclic evolution depending on the phase of the menstrual cycle. Although there are celebrated works about this subject (see Krafft-Ebing) [24], menstrual psychosis has not attained the status of a clinical entity. In a recent article, Brockington [25] reviews the literature on the subject and proposes a new classification, adapted to the work of Krafft-Ebing and Jolly [26]. These psychoses are considered to be presentations of bipolar disorder. He describes a picture characterized by:

- Acute onset, in a context of normality and no previous psychiatric history
- Short duration, with a full recovery
- Psychotic symptoms: confusion, stupor, mutism, delusions, hallucinations, or mania
- Cyclic course, with a monthly rate that coincides with the menstrual cycle

It is important to specify that research that supports the existence of a specific form of puerperal psychosis does not find an association with menstrual psychosis [2]. This leads to the conclusion that menstrual psychosis is probably related to bipolar spectrum syndromes, and that shares with "classic" puerperal psychosis the symptoms we have described as nonspecific.

In both classic texts and contemporary studies, it has also been described post-abortion or after hydatidiform mole psychosis [27].

21.4 Epidemiology

Postpartum psychosis is not highly prevalent. The incidence is approximately 1–2 cases per 1,000 births [19]. The period after childbirth is the phase of a woman's life in which there is the greatest probability of psychosis. During the postpartum period, there is a risk of psychosis onset 22 times higher than in the 2 years prior to delivery. It should be noted that we refer to many different forms of psychosis and from all spectra (schizophrenic psychosis, bipolar mania, cycloid psychosis, etc.). Therefore, there must be numerous precipitating (and numerous forms of illness) to explain this dramatic increase in the number of cases.

Psychosis is a serious condition that can compromise the safety of the mother and baby, and seriously affect the subsequent mother–child relationship. It must be considered of great importance to know and properly treat severe postpartum psychiatric disorders. In a study conducted in the UK, suicide was the leading cause of maternal death. Suicide accounted for 28 % of maternal deaths, over any other medical cause [28]. Over 50 % of women with puerperal psychosis have delusions that their baby is being harmed or killed, and approximately 4 % commit infanticide [29]. Although infanticide is rare, it is a serious consequence (that often results in the mother's suicide [30]) to be prevented by close monitoring. In addition, obstetric and perinatal complications are more common in children of mothers suffering from psychosis, probably because of poorer self-care by these patients. There is a significant tendency to stigmatize women diagnosed with psychosis, and a tendency to consider that they are not able to conduct proper care of the baby. However, a recent study suggests that, in children of mothers with psychosis, physical health indicators are not different from matched baby controls [31]. The risk factors most closely associated with puerperal psychosis are the presence of obstetric complications and primiparity [5, 32].

Concerning the legal status of puerperal psychosis, there are countries like Canada, Great Britain, Australia, and Italy that recognize postpartum mental illness as a mitigating factor in cases of infanticide. In the United States, it is not accepted as a mitigating criminal cause. Britain has had the Infanticide Act since 1922, which considers that, if a mother commits infanticide in the first months after birth, the crime is considered less serious than homicide.

The risk of recurrence of puerperal psychosis is around 20 %, and up to 50 % if the depressive episodes are included [33]. Moreover, it is also important to note the importance of both maternal and paternal mental health before birth because, in many cases, childbirth unleashes a psychosis that is the crystallization of a pre-existing mental illness, or a new episode of disease. Some studies indicate that the degree of parental well-being before birth affects more than the post-natal health the adequate care of the neonate [34]. With a correct treatment, the episodes usually cease within a few weeks. Mild to moderate cases can be treated without hospitalization and continuous monitoring of the patient.

21.5 Etiology and Pathogenesis

The postpartum period is a time when there is an exceptionally high risk of recurrence of mental imbalance. There is a high frequency of anxiety disorders, depression, mania, and other psychoses, especially in women with bipolar disorder [35].

Two complementary hypotheses about the etiology of postpartum psychosis are considered. On the one hand, an abrupt life change occurs, and, on the new mother many requirements and environmental stressors converge. On the other hand, many physical changes that affect brain function happen, causing increased vulnerability to the development of mental illness.

The time period surrounding the birth, probably involves major changes in the life of a woman. The new mother faces many stressors [36]. In a short time, she must manage the physical effects of childbirth (anemia, fatigue, and pain), sleep deprivation, bodily changes, the care of the newborn and other children, loss of libido and possible couple problems, economic and labor conditions, isolation at home, and breastfeeding [37]. In addition to the summation of these factors, motherhood itself is a social requirement and a moral imperative, the great sign of feminine identity [38] and a challenge in which she cannot fail. However, the various psychosocial stressors associated with childbirth seem to have more influence on the occurrence of postpartum depression than in psychosis. In classical medicine, the health of women was considered by their reproductive activity. It is noteworthy that puerperal psychosis is more common after the first birth. Since hormonal changes should be similar in all births, and life changes are most pronounced after the first, they make conceivably a significant contribution to psychogenic etiology.

There are a variety of biological alterations after childbirth. Many of these changes have been associated with the occurrence of psychotic symptoms both postpartum and at other life stages.

Some studies show evidence indicating a genetic component. A family association of puerperal psychosis has been described in bipolar women [39]. Molecular studies provide evidence of alterations in chromosome 16 [40].

Regarding biological hypotheses contemplating puerperal psychosis, the most commonly known and accepted refers to the role of regulation of sex hormones. The sharp decrease in the concentrations of sex steroids after delivery is undoubtedly one of the most unique and relevant biological factors in the postpartum, and one of its distinctive features. A widely accepted explanation is that the sudden drop in estrogen levels alters dopaminergic function, and this alteration facilitates the emergence of psychotic (and affective) symptoms that occur postpartum [41, 42]. Treatments with estrogen supplements have been tried, with varying results, but generally favorable [14, 43].

In recent decades, other biological changes related to the onset of psychosis have been described. Among them all, we will list the following.

1. Women with **postpartum** psychosis are at a higher risk not only of autoimmune thyroid dysfunction but also of clinical thyroid failure. Some authors consider thyroid dysfunction to be a potentially strong etiological factor [44].
2. Changes in immune response, manifested as a lack of T cell activation and overactivation of the monocyte/macrophage arm of the immune system [45]. During pregnancy, the immunity is modified in order to avoid an immune response against the fetus, and to transmit the immunoglobulins to the neonate. These changes could lead to autoimmune responses against hormone or neurotransmitter receptors (e.g., NMDA [46]), and favor the development of psychosis.
3. Decrease in brain activity in prefrontal areas and changes in the cingulated cortex [47].

4. Alteration of other hormonal axes. Increases in the levels of cortisol were observed [48], and parathyroid hormone has been related to psychoses (with improvement correcting calcium levels) [49].
5. Psychosis as a symptom of paraneoplastic encephalitis [50].
6. Decreased levels of indolamines.
7. Sleep disturbance [51].

The confluence of these biological and psychosocial factors determines the onset of a wide range of disorders of varying severity [52, 53] whose incidence increases after delivery [52]. There have been cases of puerperal psychosis in men, but they are rare and have unspecific characteristics. These male psychoses probably respond to stressors, as there is no evidence of hormonal change in men after the birth of a child [54]. Overall, unlike other postpartum disorders, puerperal psychosis seems to be more influenced by biological than by psychosocial factors. This may be because most cases respond to bipolar disorder and schizophrenia, whereas other forms of psychosis ("classic" and others), with greater psychological component, are much less frequent.

21.6 Treatment and Prognosis

Prognostic and therapeutic elements help to define the essential aspects of a disease. If puerperal psychosis were a single-cause disease, it would be expected a high recurrence rate after subsequent pregnancies and a low incidence of episodes of nonpuerperal mental illness. That is not the case. Patients with puerperal psychosis have a high rate of previous psychiatric illness (25 %) and of disease in relatives [55, 56]. Also, a close association seems to exist between the presence of a first contact with psychiatry in postpartum and the subsequent diagnosis of bipolar disorder [57]. In the study of Klompenhouwer, where he conducted extensive monitoring of patients with associated symptoms of classical puerperal psychosis, up to 40 % required subsequent hospitalization, and half of them because of mood disorders. The total numbers of patients requiring treatment for any reason rose to 57 %, and 60 % of them were treated for an affective disorder. Therefore, there is a close association between classical puerperal psychosis and affective disorders. This association can be interpreted within the context of a life-time vulnerability to affective disorders, with childbirth as the precipitating factor. No prognostic differences between classical puerperal psychosis group and the group that includes other forms of psychosis were found.

Studies agree that the mainstay of treatment of postpartum psychosis is drug therapy [58, 59]. They recommend the use of atypical antipsychotics as treatment and prophylaxis with mood stabilizers (lithium) in high-risk cases.

The joint hospitalization of the mother and the baby seems to be the best therapeutic option. There are day hospitals for the mother and newborn. The joint admission allows, first, to evaluate the interaction between mother and child, and second to avoid the presence of feelings of guilt or detachment in the mother.

21.7 Discussion

In the nineteenth century, many classic authors described the existence of a form of postpartum psychosis. From then until now, two schools of thought survive: one that states that it is a specific pathology, and another that considers that it is symptomatic variation framed in other form of psychosis. The "classic" puerperal psychosis seems to exist, at least, as a syndrome or as a group of symptoms. This is a much less common clinical picture than other forms of psychosis, which also experience a dramatic increase in incidence after childbirth. Although it shows a relatively definite group of symptoms, it often overlaps with other diagnoses. As in many other psychiatric syndromes, an spiral of silence effect occurs, which, not having been recognized in the consensus taxonomies, is avoided by most of the research and statistical studies.

However, in recent decades the debate about postpartum psychosis has resurfaced. From the studies reviewed in this paper, it can be concluded that this is a stable clinical condition, which predicts future episodes of psychosis (with the same or different characteristics) or the development of an affective illness.

Postpartum psychosis, whether understood in either direction, is a serious disease that affects women in a period of life in which a large number of biological and psychosocial stressors are added. Such is the multiplicity of etiological factors and different forms of puerperal psychosis that it could be argued that if science managed to understand it, it would have attained complete knowledge about psychosis (nowadays, a too distant aspiration).

Regarding psychosocial factors, movements in defense of the rights of women have traditionally asked to what extent are cultural and social constructions. Social roles of women have been built and cultivated around motherhood, and the fact of motherhood, in turn, is strongly influenced by the historical and cultural tradition. Since Simone de Beauvoir [60] said that motherhood was the basis of gender inequality, it has been theorized broadly and deeply about this. Apart from other considerations, which are not the subject of this chapter, it is evident that many of the stressors that are considered causative agents of puerperal psychosis affect, for customary reasons only, women.

A widely held explanation for this asymmetry is what might be called the hormonal hypothesis, which serves as the basis of the explanation of all puerperal psychiatric disorders. Owing to the rise of biological paradigms, there is a marked tendency to attribute most of female pathologies to hormonal changes. This hormonal hypothesis, just as other reductionist assumptions (such as the aminergic theory of depression), explains part of the problem while denying another.

First, because the hormonal changes could be due to environmental stress. Second, because, assuming a fundamentally biological cause, a biological solution arises (that is centered on drug treatment), even though studies show that social support is the most important prognostic factor of puerperal psychosis.

Postpartum psychosis is an epiphenomenon that arises from the interaction of many underlying factors, and should be interpreted as a complex phenomenon. Hopefully, in the coming years, advances in biological knowledge and the improvement of living conditions of women may mitigate the dramatic effect of this serious disease.

The occurrence of postpartum psychosis in a male patient after the birth of his first child is described in some case reports. An association with the phenomenon of the Couvade syndrome that is observed in all cultures has been made in other case reports [61]. The stressful life event of pregnancy in a partner related to the onset and development of a first psychotic episode is reported. The term Couvade syndrome is used in psychiatry to describe psychic manifestations in men during their partner's pregnancy or during the postpartum period. Not many studies make reference to this syndrome, but it has described a wide range in its prevalence (13–97 %). Therefore, it may be more useful to think that almost all parents manifest any of the symptoms, but not the syndrome *per se,* which would imply that we are facing a dimensional phenomenon [62]. Although no one knows for sure what its causes are, different theories have been proposed. In any case, this phenomenology is interesting because the need to understand these events leads us beyond the purely biological aspects that have been used to justify the psychopathological disturbances of women. We should consider the stressful and emotional connotations and sociocultural aspects of what it means to be a mother and father in society [2]. A psychotic episode represents the extreme end of that spectrum and suggestions are made for early identification and treatment in both male and female patients.

Couvade is a well-documented phenomenon in which the man, at the time of the birth of his child, retires to his bed and goes through the motions of labor and receives attention appropriate to someone in labor. Couvade was known in ancient Greece and was observed by Marco Polo in Chinese Turkistan [63]. It has been found in China, India, Vietnam, Borneo, Thailand, Africa, and the Americas. Among the Mohave Indians, the transvestite men mimic pregnancy and childbirth and go aside from the camp to be ceremonially delivered of stones [64].

References

1. Hamilton JA. Postpartum psychiatric problems. St. Louis: Mosby; 1962.
2. Klompenhouwer JL. Puerperal psychosis. PhD thesis. University of Rotterdam; 1992.
3. Klompenhouwer J, van Hulst A, Tulen J, Jacobs M, Jacobs B, Segers F. The clinical features of postpartum psychoses. Eur Psychiatry. 1995;10:355–67.
4. Katona CLE. Puerperal mental illness: comparisons with non-puerperal controls. Br J Psychiatry. 1982;141:447–52.
5. Brockington IF, Cernik KF, Schofield EM, et al. Puerperal psychosis: phenomena and diagnosis. Arch Gen Psychiatry. 1981;38:829–33.
6. Dean C, Williams RJ, Brockington IF. Is puerperal psychosis the same as bipolar manic-depressive disorder? A family study. Psychol Med. 1989;19(3):637–47.
7. Berrios GE. The history of mental symptoms. Descriptive psychopathology since the nineteenth century. Cambridge: Cambridge University Press; 1996. p. 238–9.
8. Laín Entralgo P. Historia de la Medicina. Barcelona: Elsevier, Masson; (1978, reimpresión 2006).

9. Esquirol J. Des maladies mentales considerées sous le rapport medical hygienique et medico-legal, Paris; 1838.
10. Henry Ey, Bernard P, Brisset Ch. Tratado de psiquiatría. Barcelona: Masson; 1965. p. 708–16.
11. Bonhoeffer K. Die exogenen Reactionstypen. Archiv. f. Psychiatrie und Nervenkrankheiten; 1917.
12. Dean C, Kendell RE. The symptomatology of puerperal illnesses. Br J Psychiatry. 1981;139:128–33.
13. Kohl C. Postpartum psychoses: closer to schizophrenia or the affective spectrum? Curr Opin Psychiatry. 2004;17:87–90.
14. Kumar C, McIvor RJ, Davies T, et al. Estrogen administration does not reduce the rate of recurrence of affective psychosis alter childbirth. J Clin Psychiatry. 2003;64:112–8.
15. American Psychiatric Association. Diagnostic and statistical manual of mental disorders. 3rd ed., revised. Washington, DC: APA; 1987.
16. The ICD-10 Classification of Mental and Behavioral Disorders: clinical descriptions and diagnostic guidelines. Geneva: World Health Organization; 1992.
17. McGorry P, Connell S. The nosology and prognosis of puerperal psychosis: a review. Compr Psychiatry. 1990;31(6):519–34.
18. Klompenhouwer JL, van Hulst AM. Classification of postpartum psychosis: a study of 250 mother and baby admissions in the Netherlands. Acta Psychiatr Scand. 1991;84:255–61.
19. Kendell RE, Chalmers JC, Platz C. Epidemiology of puerperal psychoses. Br J Psychiatry. 1987;150:662–73.
20. Alberto Monchablon Espinoza, María Inés Peralta. Psicosis puerperales. Alcmeon, Revista Argentina de Clínica Neuropsiquiátrica. Núm 15.
21. Hays P, Douglas A. A comparison of the puerperal psychosis and the schizophreniform variant of manic depression. Acta Psychiatr Scand. 1984;69(3):177–81.
22. Muñoz RA. Postpartum psychosis as a discrete entity. J Clin Psychiatry. 1985;46:5.
23. Amard T. Traité analytique de la folie et des moyens de la guérir. Lyon: Imp. de Ballanche; 1807.
24. Krafft-Ebing R. Psychosis Menstrualis. Eine klinisch-forensische Studie. Stuttgart: Enke; 1902 (Ger).
25. Brockington I. Menstrual psychosis. World Psychiatry. 2005;4:9–17.
26. Jolly P. Menstruation und Psychosen. Arch Psychiatrie Nervenkr. 1914;55:637–86 (Ger).
27. Hopker SW, Brockington IF. Psychosis following hydatidiform mole in a patient with recurrent puerperal psychosis. Br J Psychiatry. 1991;158:122–3.
28. Oates M. Perinatal psychiatric disorders: a leading cause of maternal morbidity and mortality. Br Med Bull. 2003;67:219–29.
29. Doucet S, Jones I, Letourneau N, Dennis CL, Blackmore ER. Interventions for the prevention and treatment of postpartum psychosis: a systematic review. Arch Womens Ment Health. 2011;14(2):89–98.
30. Brockington IF. Infanticide. Motherhood and mental health. Oxford: Oxford University Press; 1996.
31. Howard LM, Goss C, Leese M, Thornicroft G. Medical outcome of pregnancy in women with psychotic disorders and their infants in the first year after Barth. Br J Psychiatry. 2003;182:63–7.
32. Blackmore ER, Jones I, Doshi M, Haque S, Holder R, Brockington I, Craddock N. Obstetric variables associated with bipolar affective puerperal psychosis. Br J Psychiatry. 2006;138:32–6.
33. Robertson E. Risk of puerperal and non-puerperal recurrence of illness following bipolar affective puerperal (post-partum) psychosis. Br J Psychiatry. 2005;186(3):258.
34. Parfitt Y, Pike A, Ayers S. The impact of parents' mental health on parent-baby interaction: a prospective study. Infant Behav Dev. 2013;36(4):599–608.
35. Chaudron LH, Jefferson JW. Mood stabilizers during breastfeeding: a review. J Clin Psychiatry. 2000;61:79–90.

36. Gelder MG, López-Ibor JJ, Andreasen N. Tratado de Psiquiatría. Barcelona: Ars Medica; 2003. p. 1434–5.
37. Marks M, Lovestone S. The role of the father in parental postnatal mental health. Br J Med Psychol. 1995;68(Pt 2):157–63.
38. Mead M. Sexo y Temperamento. Paidós: México; 1990.
39. Jones I, Craddock N. Familiality of the puerperal trigger in bipolar disorder: results of a family study. Am J Psychiatry. 2001;158(6):913–7.
40. Jones I, Hamshere M, Nangle JM, Bennett P, Green E, Heron J, Segurado R, Lambert D, Holmans P, Corvin A, Owen M, Jones L, Gill M, Craddock N. Bipolar affective puerperal psychosis: genome-wide significant evidence for linkage to chromosome 16. Am J Psychiatry. 2007;164(7):1099–104.
41. Rapkin AJ, Mikacich JA, Moatkef-Imani B, Rasgon N. The clinical nature and formal diagnosis of premenstrual, postpartum, and perimenopausal affective disorders. Curr Psychiatry Rep. 2002;4:419–28.
42. Glover V. Do biochemical factors play a part in postnatal depression? Prog Neuropsychopharmacol Biol Psychiatry. 1992;16(5):605–15.
43. Ahokas A, Aito M. Role of estradiol in puerperal psychosis. Psychopharmacology (Berl). 1999;147:108–10.
44. Bergink V, Kushner SA, Pop V, Kuijpens H, Lambregtse-van den Berg MP, Drexhage RC, Wiersinga W, Nolen WA, Drexhage HA. Prevalence of autoimmune thyroid dysfunction in postpartum psychosis. Br J Psychiatry. 2011;198(4):264–8.
45. Bergink V, Burgerhout KM, Weigelt K, Pop VJ, de Wit H, Drexhage RC, Kushner SA, Drexhage HA. Immune system dysregulation in first-onset postpartum psychosis. Biol Psychiatry. 2013;73(10):1000–7.
46. Shaaban HS, Choo HF, Sensakovic JW. Anti-NMDA-receptor encephalitis presenting as postpartum psychosis in a young woman, treated with rituximab. Ann Saudi Med. 2012;32 (4):421–3.
47. Salmaso N, Nadeau J, Woodside B. Steroid hormones and maternal experience interact to induce glial plasticity in the cingulate cortex. Eur J Neurosci. 2009;29(4):786–94.
48. Magiakou MA, Mastorakos G, Rabin D, Dubbert B, Gold PW, Chrousos GP. Hypothalamic corticotropin-releasing hormone suppression during the postpartum period: implications for the increase in psychiatric manifestations at this time. J Clin Endocrinol Metab. 1996;81 (5):1912–7.
49. Patil NJ, Yadav SS, Gokhale YA, Padwa N. Primary hypoparathyroidism: psychosis in postpartum period. J Assoc Physicians India. 2010;58:506–8.
50. Yu AY, Moore FG. Paraneoplastic encephalitis presenting as postpartum psychosis. Psychosomatics. 2011;52(6):568–70.
51. Sharma V. Role of sleep loss in the causation of puerperal psychosis. Med Hypotheses. 2003;61(4):477–81.
52. Terp IM, Mortensen PB. Post-partum psychoses. Clinical diagnoses and relative risk of admission after parturition. Br J Psychiatry. 1998;172:521.
53. Brockington I. Postpartum psychiatric disorders. Lancet. 2004;363:303.
54. Shahani L. A father with postpartum psychosis. BMJ Case Rep. 2012; 2012. pii: bcr1120115176. doi:10.1136/bcr.11.2011.5176.
55. Latz C, Kendell RE. A matched-control follow-up and family study of "puerperal psychoses". Br J Psychiatry. 1988;153:90–4.
56. Davidson J, Robertson E. A follow-up study of postpartum illness, 1946-1978. Acta Psychiatr Scand. 1985;71:451–7.
57. Munk-Olsen T, Laursen TM, Meltzer-Brody S, Mortensen PB, Jones I. Psychiatric disorders with postpartum onset: possible early manifestations of bipolar affective disorders. Arch Gen Psychiatry. 2012;69(4):428–34.

58. Bergink V, Bouvy PF, Vervoort JSP, Koorengevel KM, Steegers EAP, Kushner SA. Prevention of postpartum psychosis and mania in women at high risk. Am J Psychiatry. 2012;169:609–15.
59. Yonkers KA, Wisner KL, Stowe Z, Leibenluft E, Cohen L, Miller L, Manber R, Viguera A, Suppes T, Altshuler L. Management of bipolar disorder during pregnancy and the postpartum period. Am J Psychiatry. 2004;161:608–62.
60. Beauvoir, Simone de. El Segundo Sexo. Trad. Juan María Puente. Buenos Aires: Sudamericana; 1999.
61. Shapiro S, Nass J. Postpartum psychosis in the male. Psychopathology. 1986;19:138–42.
62. Maldonado-Durán M, Lecanne EF. El padre en la etapa perinatal. Perinatol Reprod Hum. 2008;22:145–54.
63. Couvade. Encyclopaedia Britannica. Chicago: University of Chicago Press; 1958. p 690.
64. Devereux G. Institutionalized homosexuality of the Mohave Indians. Hum Biol. 1937;9:498–527.

Psychopathological Symptoms and Treatment of Menopause

22

Sonia Ruiz de Azua and Sara Barbeito

Abstract

Menopause is a period in which women stop menstruating and experience changes in their body that mark the end of their reproductive period. We noted that symptoms are not the same in all women. There are some biological and socioeconomic factors that affect the form and appearance of symptoms, such as anxiety, depression, hot flashes, sleep disorder, incontinence, and sexual difficulties. We must state that these symptoms do not affect all women, and they do not affect them to the same degree. We explained variables that have been related to a greater risk and greater protection; for example, it has been found that attitude or belief about the menopause is an important factor related to this experience. Nowadays, this cycle in the lives of women is an issue of concern for those who suffer from it and for the scientific community. The principal treatments for these symptoms are reviewed in this chapter to explain the principal findings found in the literature. In conclusion, there are some types of treatments that have been proven effective and should be included, such as coadjuvant treatment to improve the quality of life of women with these problems. Hence, multidisciplinary and preventive treatment could be the key.

S. Ruiz de Azua (✉)
Department of Psychiatry, Alava University Hospital, Vitoria, Spain

University of the Basque Country UPV/EHU, Leioa, Spain

CIBERSAM, Madrid, Spain
e-mail: SARA.BARBEITORESA@osakidetza.net

S. Barbeito
Department of Psychiatry, Alava University Hospital, Vitoria, Spain

CIBERSAM, Madrid, Spain
e-mail: SONIA.RUIZDEAZUAGARCIA@osakidetza.net

M. Sáenz-Herrero (ed.), *Psychopathology in Women*,
DOI 10.1007/978-3-319-05870-2_22

22.1 Introduction

Menopause is a period in which women stop menstruating and experience changes in their body that mark the end of their reproductive period. Menopause usually appears between 45 and 54 years of age, with a mean age at onset of around 51 years [1].

Biologically, all women are born with a finite number of eggs, which are stored in the ovaries. The ovaries regulate ovulation and menstruation using hormones such as estrogen, progesterone, and monotropic follicle-stimulating hormone. Menopause begins with some variations in the menstrual cycle (shorter duration, irregular periods), hot flashes, and mood changes.

The process of menopause is not sudden; it happens gradually in approximately three stages:

- Perimenopause: this stage can range from 2 to 10 years before the start of menopause. The ovaries gradually produce less estrogen; however, at this stage the ovaries are still releasing eggs and menopause symptoms start.
- Menopause: the period with absence of menstruation for 12 months.
- Postmenopause: the 3 years after menopause. At this stage, the symptoms of menopause decrease.

22.2 Causes

All women suffer menopause at around 50 years old, but the symptoms of menopause are different. Menopause is a natural process in the life of all women. When a girl is born, she has around one to three million eggs. Throughout her life, the eggs are gradually lost through ovulation and through atresia. Menopause occurs when the ovaries produce less estrogen and progesterone and the follicle-stimulating hormone stops egg production.

Therefore, changes in the balance of sex hormones cause menopause. Usually, these changes are natural and progressive, although sometimes the menopausal process is not natural and is caused by medical treatments that produce a lowering of estrogen.

22.3 Symptoms

There are individual and cultural differences in the symptoms of menopause [2]. Some biological and socioeconomic factors affect the form and appearance of symptoms [3, 4].

It is therefore considered appropriate to create special programs to manage the symptoms associated with menopause that take into account ethnic differences in the treatment of menopausal symptoms [5].

Some of the most common symptoms of the menopause are the following:

- Vasomotor symptoms. Hot flashes, cold sweats, bouts of pounding, or irregular heartbeat (75 % of women suffer from them, some authors even put this figure at 85 %) [6, 7]. The irregular heartbeat scares women because for them it is very difficult to remain calm. There are other causes of this symptom such as stress, anxiety, and caffeine and nicotine consumption, and it is very important to discriminate from several other pathologies.
- Sleep disorders. Insomnia, waking many times during the night and turning are the most frequent disturbances; almost 40 % of women suffer from them [8, 9]. Usually, the sleep is less restful and it is very difficult for the women to get to sleep.
- Vaginal dryness. When estrogen levels drop, the vaginal tissue becomes drier, thinner, and less elastic. The reduction in lubrication leads to uncomfortable intercourse and decreased sexual interest (over 55 % of women) [10]. These symptoms can affect women emotionally and it is very important to treat them if they affect quality of life.
- Incontinence. There are three types of incontinence. Stress incontinence happens because the internal muscles fail when the woman laughs, coughs or sneezes. Urge incontinence is when the bladder contracts and empties at any time, despite efforts to resist. Overflow incontinence is when the individual does not realize that the bladder is full (76 % of women suffer from incontinence) [11]. There is a relationship between the number of pregnancies and the prevalence of incontinence [12].
- Mood lability. The most common changes in the mood are irritability, depression, and anxiety [13], which are caused by the sudden drop in levels of estrogen affecting the neurotransmitters that regulate the mood in the brain, such as serotonin and dopamine. Sometimes, if the problems are not treated well panic attacks can occur.
- Cognitive difficulties. It is very usual for women in the menopause to have trouble remembering things or to suffer mental blocks. The estrogen deficiency and the age and sleep disorders can increase the concentration difficulties. Memory problems can affect the functioning of the women, such as forgetting important meetings [14].
- Headaches. This symptom could be related to the hormonal imbalance in the menopause. When the body begins slowing down its production of estrogen the women suffer more frequent and worse headaches.
- Hair loss or thinning and brittle nails. The estrogen deficiency weakens the hair follicles and is very usual on the head and other parts of the body. The appearance of nails could indicate nutritional deficiency or hormonal imbalance. In the menopause the nails are softer and crack, split or break more frequently, and called brittle nails.
- Weight gain. Some authors have said that weight gain is not related to menopause; however, fewer estrogen hormones can retain more fat cells and lower testosterone levels, leading to a decreased metabolic rate; thus, women need fewer calories daily and changes in diet and exercise are necessary.

All these symptoms clearly affect the quality of life of women. It has been found that women who suffer from vasomotor symptoms during menopause experience a decreased perception of their health; thus, it is very important to find the correct hormone treatment to try to reduce the symptoms [15].

Symptoms may last several years, with a mean duration between 5 and 10 years [16]. We should note that psychological factors (anxiety, self-esteem, negative beliefs and thoughts) will influence the testing of hot flashes [17].

22.4 Changes After Menopause

After menopause, several changes can happen more frequently, such as osteoporosis [18], an increased risk of chronic cardiovascular disease [19], and the risk of metabolic syndrome increases by 60 % [20]. Data have even been found that associate this period with a greater vulnerability to a cognitive decrease and to depressive symptoms and disorders [14]. Nevertheless, these results cannot necessarily be generalized beyond the studies included in this review.

22.5 Early Menopause

Premature ovarian failure is when the menopause appears before 40 years of age. The prevalence of this disorder is uncommon but not rare, between 1 and 3 % [21]. In most women there are no signs that precede the cessation of periods; they have a normal menstrual history, menarche, and fertility prior to the onset of premature ovarian failure [22].

The diagnosis of early menopause is difficult; however, most clinicians make it when women have had amenorrhea for 3–6 months, the FSG concentrations are above 40 mIU/ml, and estrogen levels are low [22].

There are some variables that can predict the age at menopause: higher educational level, prior oral contraceptive use, and higher weight at baseline, as well as being employed, not smoking, consuming alcohol, having less physical activity, and having better self-rated health over the follow-up, were all significantly associated with later age at the final menstrual period [23]. Other studies have shown that socioeconomic status is not menopause-related and that women smokers with lower body mass index reached their menopause earlier [24].

The main problems of women who suffer early menopause were worries about fertility, bones, and emotional well-being; 49 % of women requested psychological support because they felt a negative impact on their self-esteem [21].

The early menopause accelerates physical aging [25], and is related to the onset of diabetes [26] and to a higher risk of venous thromboembolism [27].

22.6 Emotional Symptoms

22.6.1 Beliefs About Symptoms

The beliefs that women have regarding menopause influence the way in which they make this transition to menopause [28]. Some psychological factors influence the perception and cognition of the hot flashes and the night sweats [29]. Hunter and Rendall [17] note that there are two different points of view with regard to menopause. First, there are women with a positive view of menopause, who think that menopause is a cessation of menstruation and pregnancy risk, and second, there are others who associate the menopause with aging and a negative image.

Women who have negative attitudes toward menopause are more likely to suffer severe menopausal symptoms during the transition [30, 31]. However, the belief of the women is not only important for the symptomatology, the severity of menopausal complaints may also be related to the attitudes of their husbands toward menopause [31].

22.6.2 Anxiety and Depression

The transition to menopause is often accompanied by negative physical and emotional changes that can significantly affect the quality of life of women. Menopausal women are four times more likely to experience a major depressive episode [32]. Women with low anxiety before menopause, early or late perimenopause, or postmenopause were more likely to report high-anxiety symptoms, independent of life events, financial strain, and perceived health problems including vasomotor symptoms [33].

Several studies have found an association among menopause, anxiety, and depression, suggesting that depressive mood is related to the severity of menopausal symptoms [34].

The intensity of depression depended on the type of menopause; women with natural menopause developed moderate and severe depression and those who had undergone ovariectomy had mild symptoms of depression. The women with essential hypertension and without nocturnal variations in blood pressure had the highest level of depression [35].

The factors that have been found to be associated with depression in menopause were personal history of psychological problems [36], the socio-educational status [28], life events [37], prior poor health [38], body mass index, smoking [24, 39], and attitude toward menopause [17].

However, other studies found that there is no clear evidence that only the transition to menopause increases the risk of emotional disorders, and only women who have psychosocial stress, severe vasomotor symptoms, and a history of mood disorders experience anxiety and depression [40]. Therefore, depressive mood should not automatically be attributed to the transition to menopause [17].

22.7 Treatments

There are some pharmacological treatments that reduce the physical symptoms of menopause. However, the psychological symptoms can influence the severity of these symptoms. Thus, there are no other pharmacological treatments that may be of benefit to women to improve the experience of menopause, to treat the associated symptoms, and to improve function and quality of life [41, 42].

22.7.1 Yoga

Evidence of yoga as a therapy in women with menopause is not clear. There were five randomized controlled clinical trials using yoga in menopausal women. In one, there was moderate evidence for the short-term effects on psychological symptoms (depression, anxiety, sleep disorders). No evidence was found for total menopausal symptoms, somatic symptoms, vasomotor symptoms or urogenital symptoms [43]. Conversely, a recent study concluded that 3 months of yoga is effective in reducing total menopausal symptoms, psychological symptoms, somatic symptoms, and urogenital symptoms [44]. However, other studies did not find enough evidence to suggest that yoga might be an effective therapy for reducing the symptomatology of menopause [45–47]. Yoga was not associated with adverse events; thus, this therapy can be used as an adjuvant treatment.

22.7.2 Physical Exercise

Some clinical trials on the effectiveness of physical exercise programs in postmenopausal women did not find evidence reducing vasomotor symptoms [48, 49]; nevertheless, other studies found that 6 months' aerobic exercise training improves sleep quality and reduces hot flashes [50]. There is evidence that the exercise improves bone density [49] and skeletal muscle mass index [51] being useful to prevent osteoporosis. Pelvic floor training is useful to improve urinary stress incontinence and thus the quality of life in postmenopausal women [52].

22.7.3 Diet

Whiteman [53] conducted an observational study with 1,087 women, 56 % of them refer to hot flashes, but women who smoke and who have a high body mass index (BMI) had a greater probability of experiencing hot flashes and these were more intense and more frequent.

A clinical trial about exercise and/or diet with 118 postmenopausal women found that the combination between diet and exercise is more effective than either one of them alone at improving quality of life, psychological symptoms, and general health [54]. Other authors note the importance of combining diet at this stage of life with isoflavones, calcium, and vitamin D [55].

22.7.4 Psychological Treatments

There are few studies of psychological interventions in the climacteric, the period between before and after menopause [56, 57].

22.7.4.1 Cognitive Behavioral Therapy

Keefer, in 2005, performed a pilot study with 19 women and found that in 48 % of women who enrolled in cognitive behavioral therapy (CBT) vasomotor symptoms reduced significantly; however, the findings should be treated with caution because the sample was very small [58].

Cognitive behavioral therapy has been found to be effective at reducing menopausal symptoms such as hot flashes, night sweats, sleep problems, sexual difficulties, muscle aches, anxiety, depression, and at improving quality of life [17, 55–57, 59–61]. Also, favorable results have been found for CBT and physical exercise in women with breast cancer treatment-induced menopause with regard to endocrine symptoms, sexuality, and physical function [62].

Among the cognitive behavioral techniques that have proven effective in women who suffer mild symptoms are relaxation techniques, psychoeducation, nutrition, fitness exercises, Kegel exercises, and problem-solving techniques [17, 56, 57, 59–63].

One of the key points in improving the general health of menopausal women is to work with the knowledge of the physical and psychological changes of the menopausal period, with destigmatization, improved social interaction, and support, and to teach to women to cope with this stage [60].

However, we must take into account the importance of the perception of women who have symptoms [17] and therefore this factor works to improve the quality of life of these women.

22.7.4.2 Mindfulness

The aim of mindfulness therapy is to help patients to recognize and differentiate thoughts, sensations, and feelings as events in the mind without over-identifying with them [64].

In a study with 110 late perimenopausal and early postmenopausal women experiencing severe hot flashes and night sweats a clinically significant reduction in the degree of bother and distress was found in women who participate in mindfulness-based stress reduction therapy [65]. Mindfulness is related to sleep disorders in postmenopausal women; women who suffer from insomnia are less mindful than those without insomnia and these interventions may be beneficial [66].

22.7.4.3 Psychoeducation

Education, in general, is beneficial and contributes to improvement of symptoms and adherence to other treatments, especially in menopause [67]. Psychoeducation improves attitudes toward menopause, reduces the severity of symptoms [58], changes the perception of women, and improves quality of life and autonomic nervous system activity [68]. Tremblay [69] carried out a systematic review about the effectiveness of psychoeducation in postmenopausal women and breast cancer survivors and found that psychoeducational interventions alleviate hot flashes and vasomotor symptoms in general; however, there are not enough studies and more research is necessary.

The lifestyle and perception of women with regard to the menopause affect the severity and frequency of symptoms; however, these factors can be modified with educational sessions that may help to prevent symptoms changing these variables.

22.7.4.4 Holistic Approach

Menopause has a significant impact in several areas of life of women, affecting them physically, psychologically, and socially. Some authors [55] emphasized that the best care in menopause is to treat all the factors together that could affect a women's life. This approach includes several clinical specialists who are involved in the treatment: gynecologists, endocrinologists, mental health, physical activity, etc.; collaboration with the woman's family is also necessary. Overall, there is an association between hormonal changes and climacteric symptomatology, and the association is modulated by cultural factors. There is a considerable variation in the prevalence and pattern of symptoms in different countries, a variation probably due to diversity in cultural norms and traditions as well as in diet and other lifestyle factors.

There are important social implications of becoming menopausal that vary from one society to another [70]. The definition of menopause for any culture is derived from the meaning and consequences of menopause and from the way in which women's roles are defined in that society. Women are aware of these stereotypes and interpret their bodily changes in accordance with what they have learned. The experience of menopause is associated with a woman's health history as well as with a wide range of variables, such as genetic factors, diet, education, marital status, number of pregnancies, the kind of work she has carried out, social support, and access to health care [71].

On the other hand, medicalization of the menopause in cultures in which the menopause is not perceived as a problem is an important issue that should be debated. Some critics have questioned the role of the pharmaceutical industry in influencing health care through product promotion [72].

Conclusions

The aim of this chapter is to learn more about the symptomatology of menopause and the best method to treat it correctly. We need to realize that menopause is a normal process for all women. Menopause should be "demedicalized" and treated as a normal phase of women's lives instead of as a disease in the general population.

On the other hand, it is necessary to focus more attention on the symptoms and on the real problems of these women, who form a significant proportion of the population. To date, insufficient attention has been paid to them and treatment is inadequate.

In the menopause many biological changes occur; however, they are not the most important changes. There is some evidence that other treatments (psychotherapy, diet, and physical activity) can help women to improve their symptoms and their quality of life.

As noted, the attitude of women to this transition, this new stage, experiencing varying symptoms, therefore affects their quality of life to a smaller or larger extent. Major risk factors are associated with greater emotional and physical symptoms; thus, early detection in this population could bring earlier treatment to even prevent risk factors and enhance protection such as information and support. Therefore, a multidisciplinary and preventive treatment perspective could be the key to reducing both dysfunctional beliefs about menopause and reducing stress and negative coping strategies as well as obtaining and reducing many of the symptoms associated with this period of transition in the lives of women.

Cross-cultural comparisons fuel the debate by showing that the relation between hormones and symptoms is, indeed, complex. There are significant differences in the patterns and prevalence of symptoms between countries and, interestingly, in the types of symptom reported in different ethnic groups within countries. It is difficult, however, to draw firm conclusions from available cultural and ethnographic comparison studies because of a number of limitations. Among these are differences among cultures in the language used to describe symptoms and in women's inclination to report symptoms; use of different methodologies in study design and instruments used to measure symptoms; and differences in diet and other lifestyle factors that make it difficult to establish cultural versus biological reasons for symptom expression.

The reality is that women need education and balanced information to make personal decisions regarding their health.

References

1. World Health Organisation. Research on menopause. Report of a WHO scientific group. WHO technical report N670. WHO Geneva; 1981.
2. Jones EK, Jurgenson JR, Katzenellenbogen JM, Thompson SC. Menopause and the influence of culture: another gap for Indigenous Australian women? BMC Womens Health. 2012;12:431.
3. Winterich JA, Umberson D. How women experience menopause: the importance of social context. J Women Aging. 1999;11(4):57–73.
4. Melby MK, Lock M, Kaufert P. Culture and symptom reporting at menopause. Hum Reprod Update. 2005;11:495–512.

5. Im EO, Ko Y, Hwang H, Chee W. Symptom-specific or holistic menopausal symptom management. Health Care Women Int. 2012;33(6):575–92.
6. Avis NE, Crawford SL, McKinlay SM. Psychological behavioural, and health factors related to menopause symptomatology. Womens Health. 1997;3:103–20.
7. Kadakia KC, Loprinzi CL, Barton DL. Hot flashes: the ongoing search for effective interventions. Menopause. 2012;19(7):719–21.
8. Dennerstein L, Dudley EC, Hopper JL, Guthrie JR, Burger HG. A prospective population-based study of menopausal symptoms. Obstet Gynecol. 2000;96:351–8.
9. Ameratunga D, Goldin J, Hickey M. Sleep disturbance in menopause. Intern Med J. 2012;42 (7):742–7.
10. van Geelen JM, van de Weijer PH, Arnolds HT. Urogenital symptoms and resulting discomfort in non-institutionalized Dutch women aged 50 to 75 years. Ned Tijdschr Genesk. 1996;140:713–6.
11. Trutnovsky G, Rojas RG, Mann KP, Dietz HP. Urinary incontinence: the role of menopause. Menopause. 2013;21(4):399–402.
12. Findik RB, Unluer AN, Sahin E, Bzkurt OF, Karakaya J, Unsal A. Urinary incontinence in women and its relation with pregnancy, mode of delivery, connective tissue disease and other factors. Adv Clin Exp Med. 2012;21(2):207–13.
13. Cohen LS, Soares CN, Vitonis AF, Otto MW, Harlow BL. Risk for new onset of depression during the menopausal transition: the Harvard study of moods and cycles. Arch Gen Psychiatry. 2006;63:385–90.
14. Weber MT, Maki PM, McDermott MP. Cognition and mood in perimenopause: a systematic review and meta-analysis. J Steroid Biochem Mol Biol. 2014 Jul;142:90–8.
15. Dibonaventura MD, Chandran A, Hsu MA, Bushmakin A. Burden of vasomotor symptoms in France, Germany, Italy, Spain, and the United Kingdom. Int J Womens Health. 2013;5:261–9.
16. Woods NF, Mitchell ES. Symptoms during the perimenopause: prevalence, severity, trajectory, and significance in women's lives. Am J Med. 2005;118(Suppl 12B):14–24.
17. Hunter M, Rendall M. Bio-psycho-socio-cultural perspectives on menopause. Best Pract Res Clin Obstet Gynaecol. 2007;21(2):261–74.
18. Riggs BL, Khosla S, Melton III J. Sex steroids and the construction and conservation of the adult skeleton. Endocr Rev. 2002;23(3):279–302.
19. Ramezani Tehrani F, Behboudi-Gandevani S, Ghanbarian A, Azizi F. Effect of menopause on cardiovascular disease and its risk factors: a 9-year follow-up, population-based, cohort study. Climacteric. 2014;17(2):164–72.
20. Eshtiaghi R, Esteghamati A, Nakhjavani M. Menopause is an independent predictor of metabolic syndrome in Iranian women. Maturitas. 2010;65(3):262–6.
21. Singer D, Mann E, Hunter MS, Pitkin J, Panay N. The silent grief: psychosocial aspects of premature ovarian failure. Climacteric. 2011;14(4):428–37.
22. Woad KJ, Watkins WJ, Prendergast D, Shelling AN. The genetic basis of premature ovarian failure. Aust N Z J Obstet Gynaecol. 2006;46(3):242–4.
23. Gold EB, Crawford SL, Avis NE, Crandall CJ, Matthews KA, Waetjen LE, Lee JS, Thurston R, Vuga M, Harlow SD. Factors related to age at natural menopause: longitudinal analyses from SWAN. Am J Epidemiol. 2013;178(1):70–83.
24. Hardy R, Kuh D, Wadsworth M. Smoking, body mass index, socio-economic status and the menopausal transition in a British national cohort. Int J Epidemiol. 2000;29:845–51.
25. Li S, Rosenberg L, Wise LA, Boggs DA, Lavalley M, Palmer JR. Age at natural menopause in relation to all-cause and cause-specific mortality in a follow-up study of US black women. Maturitas. 2013;75(3):246–52.
26. Monterrosa-Castro A, Blümel JE, Portela-Buelvas K, Mezones-Holguín E, Barón G, Bencosme A, Benítez Z, Bravo LM, Calle A, Chedraui P, Flores D, Espinoza MT, Gómez G, Hernández-Bueno JA, Laribezcoa F, Lima S, Martino M, Mostajo D, Ojeda E, Onatra W, Sánchez H, Navarro D, Tserotas K, Vallejo MS, Witis S, Zuñiga MC; for the

Collaborative Group for Research of the Climacteric in Latin America (REDLINC). Type II diabetes mellitus and menopause: a multinational study. Climacteric. 2013;16(6):663-72.
27. Canonico M, Plu-Bureau G, O'Sullivan MJ, Stefanick ML, Cochrane B, Scarabin PY, Manson JE. Age at menopause, reproductive history, and venous thromboembolism risk among postmenopausal women: the Women's Health Initiative hormone therapy clinical trials. Menopause. 2013;21(3):214–20.
28. Hunter MS. Editorial: depression and the menopause. BMJ. 1996;313:1217–8.
29. Hunter MS, Chilcot J. Testing a cognitive model of menopausal hot flushes and night sweats. J Psychosom Res. 2013;74(4):307–12.
30. Ayers B, Forshaw M, Hunter MS. The impact of attitudes towards the menopause on women's symptom experience: a systematic review. Maturitas. 2010;65(1):28–36.
31. Aksu H, Sevinçok L, Kücük M, Sezer SD, Oğurlu N. The attitudes of menopausal women and their spouses towards menopause. Clin Exp Obstet Gynecol. 2011;38(3):251–5.
32. Bromberger JT, Kravitz HM, Chang Y, Cyranowski JM, Brown C, Matthews KA. Major depression during and after the menopausal transition: Study of Women's Health Across the Nation (SWAN). Psychol Med. 2011;41:1879–88.
33. Bromberger JT, Kravitz HM, Chang Y, Randolph Jr JF, Avis NE, Gold EB, Matthews KA. Does risk for anxiety increase during the menopausal transition? Study of women's health across the nation. Menopause. 2013;20(5):488–95.
34. Pérez-López FR, Pérez-Roncero G, Fernández-Iñarrea J, Fernández-Alonso AM, Chedraui P, Llaneza P; for The MARIA (MenopAuse Risk Assessment) Research Group. Resilience, depressed mood, and menopausal symptoms in postmenopausal women. Menopause. 2013;21(2):159-64.
35. Larëva NV, Govorin AV. Psychosomatic relationships in postmenopausal women. Ter Arkh. 2013;85(3):86–9.
36. Hunter MS. Psychological and somatic experience of the menopause: a prospective study. Psychosom Med. 1990;52:357–67.
37. Cooke DJ, Greene JG. Types of life events in relation to symptoms at the climacterium. J Psychosom Res. 1981;25:5–11.
38. Hunter M, Liao K. Evaluation of a four-session cognitive-behavioural intervention for menopausal hot flushes. Br J Health Psychol. 1996;1:113–25.
39. Dennerstein L, Lehert P, Burger H, et al. Mood and the menopause transition. J Nerv Ment Dis. 1999;187:685–91.
40. Hickey M, Bryant C, Judd F. Evaluation and management of depressive and anxiety symptoms in midlife. Climacteric. 2012;15(1):3–9.
41. Tom SE, Cooper R, Patel KV, Guralnik JM. Menopausal characteristics and physical functioning in older adulthood in the National Health and Nutrition Examination Survey III. Menopause. 2012;19(3):283–9.
42. Mann E, Singer D, Pitkin J, Panay N, Hunter MS. Psychosocial adjustment in women with premature menopause: a cross-sectional survey. Climacteric. 2012;15(5):481–9.
43. Cramer H, Lauche R, Langhorst J, Dobos G. Effectiveness of yoga for menopausal symptoms: a systematic review and meta-analysis of randomized controlled trials. Evid Based Complement Alternat Med. 2012;2012:863905.
44. Joshi S, Khandwe R, Bapat D, Deshmukh U. Effect of yoga on menopausal symptoms. Menopause Int. 2011;17(3):78–81.
45. Lee MS, Kim JI, Ha JY, Boddy K, Ernst E. Yoga for menopausal symptoms: a systematic review. Menopause. 2009;16(3):602–8.
46. Elavsky S, McAuley E. Exercise and self-esteem in menopausal women: a randomized controlled trial involving walking and yoga. Am J Health Promot. 2007;22(2):83–92.
47. Chattha R, Nagarathna R, Padmalatha V, Nagendra HR. Effect of yoga on cognitive functions in climacteric syndrome: a randomised control study. BJOG. 2008;115(8):991–1000.
48. Daley A, Stokes-Lampard H, Macarthur C. Exercise for vasomotor menopausal symptoms. Cochrane Database Syst Rev. 2011;11(5), CD006108.

49. Babatunde OO, Forsyth JJ, Gidlow CJ. A meta-analysis of brief high-impact exercises for enhancing bone health in premenopausal women. Osteoporos Int. 2012;23(1):109–19.
50. Mansikkamäki K, Raitanen J, Nygård CH, Heinonen R, Mikkola T, EijaTomás LR. Sleep quality and aerobic training among menopausal women–a randomized controlled trial. Maturitas. 2012;72(4):339–45.
51. Aragão FR, Abrantes CG, Gabriel RE, Sousa MF, Castelo-Branco C, Moreira MH. Effects of a 12-month multi-component exercise program on the body composition of postmenopausal women. Climacteric. 2014;17(2):155–63.
52. Pereira VS, de Melo MV, Correia GN, Driusso P. Vaginal cone for postmenopausal women with stress urinary incontinence: randomized, controlled trial. Climacteric. 2012;15(1):45–51.
53. Whiteman MK, Staropoli CA, Lengenberg PW, McCarter RJ, Kjerulff KH, Flaws JH. Smoking, body mass, and hot flashes in midlife women. Obstet Gynecol. 2003;101:264–72.
54. Imayama I, Alfano CM, Kong A, Foster-Schubert KE, Bain CE, Xiao L, Duggan C, Wang CY, Campbell KL, Blackburn GL, McTiernan A. Dietary weight loss and exercise interventions effects on quality of life in overweight/obese postmenopausal women: a randomized controlled trial. Int J Behav Nutr Phys Act. 2011;8:118.
55. Kalra B, Agarwal S, Magon S. Holistic care of menopause: understanding the framework. J Midlife Health. 2012;3(2):66–9.
56. Alder J, Eymann Besken K, Armbruster U, Decio R, Gairing A, Kang A, Bitzer J. Cognitive-behavioural group intervention for climacteric syndrome. Psychother Psychosom. 2006;75 (5):298–303.
57. Larroy García C, Gómez-Calcerrada SG. Cognitive-behavioral intervention among women with slight menopausal symptoms: a pilot study. Span J Psychol. 2011;14(1):344–55.
58. Keefer L, Blanchard EB. A behavioral group treatment program for menopausal hot flashes: results of a pilot study. Appl Psychophysiol Biofeedback. 2005;30(1):21–30.
59. Ayers B, Smith M, Hellier J, Mann E, Hunter MS. Effectiveness of group and self-help cognitive behavior therapy in reducing problematic menopausal hot flushes and night sweats (MENOS 2): a randomized controlled trial. Menopause. 2012;19(7):749–59.
60. Balabanovic J, Ayers B, Hunter MS. Cognitive behaviour therapy for menopausal hot flushes and night sweats: a qualitative analysis of women's experiences of group and self-help CBT. Behav Cogn Psychother. 2013;41(4):441–57.
61. Green SM, Haber E, McCabe RE, Soares CN. Cognitive-behavioral group treatment for menopausal symptoms: a pilot study. Arch Womens Ment Health. 2013;16(4):325–32.
62. Duijts SF, van Beurden M, Oldenburg HS, Hunter MS, Kieffer JM, Stuiver MM, Gerritsma MA, Menke-Pluymers MB, Plaisier PW, Rijna H, Lopes Cardozo AM, Timmers G, van der Meij S, van der Veen H, Bijker N, de Widt-Levert LM, Geenen MM, Heuff G, van Dulken EJ, Boven E, Aaronson NK. Efficacy of cognitive behavioral therapy and physical exercise in alleviating treatment-induced menopausal symptoms in patients with breast cancer: results of a randomized, controlled, multicenter trial. J Clin Oncol. 2012;30(33):4124–33.
63. Larroy García C, Gutiérrez G-CS. Cognitive-behavioral intervention in menopausal symptomatology: short-term effects. Psicothema. 2009;21(2):255–61.
64. Carmody J. Evolving conceptions of mindfulness in clinical settings. J Cogn Psychother. 2009;23(3):270–80.
65. Carmody JF, Crawford S, Salmoirago-Blotcher E, Leung K, Churchill L, Olendzki N. Mindfulness training for coping with hot flashes: results of a randomized trial. Menopause. 2011;18(6):611–20.
66. Garcia MC, Pompéia S, Hachul H, Kozasa EH, de Souza AA, Tufik S, Mello LE. Is mindfulness associated with insomnia after menopause? Menopause. 2014;21(3):301–5.
67. Catalbiano ML, Holzheimer M. Dispositional factors, coping and adaptation during menopause. Climacteric. 1999;2:21–8.
68. Senba N, Matsuo H. Effect of a health education program on climacteric women. Climacteric. 2010;13(6):561–9.

69. Tremblay A, Sheeran L, Aranda SK. Psychoeducational interventions to alleviate hot flashes: a systematic review. Menopause. 2008;15(1):193–202.
70. Kaufert PA. Myth and the menopause. Sociol Health Illn. 1982;4:141–66.
71. Kaufert PA. The social and cultural context of menopause (review). Maturitas. 1996;23 (2):169–80.
72. Coney S, Seaman B. The menopause industry: how the medical establishment exploits women. Alameda, CA: Hunter House; 1994.

Part IV

Gender in Psychiatric Disorders

Affective Disorders

23

Patricia Pérez and Jon Gaviña

Abstract

Women are typically 2–3 times more likely to develop depressive disorders than men. Although depression is a multifactorial disorder, its etiology cannot be dissociated from the socioeconomic and cultural environment. The current construct of role has a great importance in the etiology of depression. Despite the fact that genetic vulnerability and sex hormones have been considered the main causal factors of this difference, nowadays some other factors are taken into account, such as emotion regulation strategies (women are more likely to ruminate, whereas men tend to suppress or avoid their emotions) and changes in the classical personality features attributed to men and women ("depressive temperament") and in the sex role (chronic stresses associated with traditional female roles lead to a higher prevalence of depression). Attending to the way of presentation, depressed women are more likely to exhibit "atypical" symptoms and more anxiety and somatization.

There is a huge controversy regarding pharmacological treatment according to different sexes, but not psychotherapy; cognitive behavioral theory has been the most empirically demonstrated to be effective on both sexes.

23.1 Introduction

Affective disorders have plagued womankind since the earliest documentation of human experience. In this chapter, depressive disorders, the group of clinical conditions included in the recent *Diagnostic and Statistical Manual of Mental Disorders, Fifth Edition* [1], are described: disruptive mood dysregulation disorder;

P. Pérez (✉) • J. Gaviña
Alava University Hospital, Vitoria, Spain
e-mail: PATRICIA.PEREZMARTINEZDEARRIETA@osakidetza.net; JON.GAVINAARENAZA@osakidetza.net

M. Sáenz-Herrero (ed.), *Psychopathology in Women*,
DOI 10.1007/978-3-319-05870-2_23

major depressive disorder, single and recurrent episodes; persistent depressive disorder (dysthymia); premenstrual disorder; substance/medication-induced depressive disorder; depressive disorder due to another medical condition; other specified depressive disorder; unspecified depressive disorder.

The depressive disorders are characterized by lifelong vulnerability to episodes of disease involving depressed mood or loss of interest and pleasure in activities, experienced as a feeling of sadness, irritability, dejection, despair, with neurovegetative or biological signs such impairment in sleep, appetite, energy level, libido, and psychomotor activity, and marked impairment in concentration with increased distractibility, and the presence of guilty preoccupation. All these symptoms result in a change from the person's previous functioning [2].

Depression affects the person's environment, time spent in leisure activities, economy, and social relationships, and it has been reported that major unipolar depression is the main source of disease-related disability for women all over the world [3, 4].

Although depression is a multifactorial disorder, its etiology cannot be dissociated from the social contexts that frame our lives. The last three decades have been characterized by a redefinition of identities and gender relations in many societies, but although it has different nuances and particular manifestations, the gender gap has not been eliminated.

Depression has become a modern and globalized disease, largely because of unfavorable living conditions in the contemporary world. Job insecurity, professional competence, poverty, and migration are problems that affect women more than men, and they are part of the phenomenon of globalization, which has an impact not only on the economy and social development but also on the cultural sphere and on the definition and redefinition of identities and gender roles.

We live in a world of social changes and in a historical transition period marked by advances in education and technology, accompanied by the massive incorporation of women into the labor market and economic changes and periods of crisis that promote instability and job insecurity. These elements affect other complex phenomena such as gender relations and promote new cultural constructions about what it means to be male or female in contemporary societies. The gender perspective is a useful analytical tool for explaining sex-differentiated distribution of psychopathology, with a special interest in depression.

The concept of gender role in the health sciences did not appear until 1955, proposed by Money [5] to refer to social behavior attributed to men and women. Thus, gender identity is defined as the private experience of gender role, and gender role as the public expression of gender identity. Gender identity is not a completed sociocultural construction; it is built dynamically over time and according to the type of relationships that people establish with themselves, with others, and with culture.

The concept of femininity is defined in terms that go far beyond biology and anatomy, taking into account the diversity of environmental and psychological factors that influence the development of the person.

Gender is a social construct that refers to cultural characteristics assigned to each sex. It is the system of beliefs, attitudes, values, personality characteristics and cognitions that are culturally determined about men and women [6]. These are the values that are considered more desirable for one sex than another within a given culture and that are assimilated into a socialization process by individuals belonging to this cultural context.

Throughout this chapter we discuss in detail the differential issues regarding both the epidemiology of depression, the risk factors that can produce it, the clinical characteristics and comorbidity, and, of course, the commonly used therapeutic approaches. We also analyze in depth these differences to shed some light on the reasons behind them. To do this, we rely on the point of view of gender—not only the biological but also the socio-cultural construct—and its implications for affective disorders.

23.2 Epidemiology

Each year 6 % of adults will experience an episode of depression, and over the course of a person's lifetime more than 15 % of the population will have an episode. Depression is the leading cause of suicide and currently the fourth highest disease burden on society in terms of its treatment costs, its effect on families and careers, and its impact on productivity in the workplace. Depression can be disabling and distressing and, for many people, it can become a chronic disorder, especially if it is inadequately treated [4].

Women are typically twice to three times more likely to develop depressive disorders than men, although this ratio has been reported to vary across different types of depressive disorders. There has been a roughly five-fold increase in the lifetime prevalence of depression in the USA over the four decades between the early 1950s and early 1990s, according to research [7,8]. This fact could be related to sex role theories, which will be extensively developed later in this chapter.

There is an enormous variation in the prevalence of major depression, with lifetime prevalence estimated between 6 and 25 % for women and 5 and 12 % for men, with the prevalence of major depression disorder (MDD) for adults in community samples ranging from 5 to 9 % for women and from 2 to 3 % for men [7–10].

A substantial number of epidemiological studies have also examined gender differences in chronic minor depression or dysthymia. These studies have consistently found female:male prevalence ratios of around 2:1. Lifetime prevalence estimates of dysthymia are typically in the range of 6–8 % when diagnostic hierarchy rules are not made and 2–3 % when they are [8, 9, 11].

Epidemiological surveys suggest that the prevalence of major depression has increased dramatically over the past few decades among both women and men; neither the population distribution of sex hormones nor the gene pool changes this quickly, which means that the influence of changing environmental conditions must account for these dramatic increases.

The explanation for this higher prevalence of depression in women has been the subject of intense theoretical speculation that has led to very different hypotheses.

Gender differences in the estimated prevalence of depression might be due, to *self-report bias* because women may be more willing than men to admit their depression to an interviewer [8, 9, 12].

However, the available evidence is inconsistent with this hypothesis because a higher prevalence of current depression among women than men is found in studies that rely on self-report, but also in those that use informant reports. In addition, a number of methodological studies using standard psychometric methods to assess potential biasing factors such as social desirability, expressivity, lying, and dichotomic questions (yes/no) have found no evidence that the gender difference in self-reported psychological distress is due to these biasing factors [13]. On the other hand, symptom-level assessments are inconsistent with the response–bias argument. Specifically, response bias should make women more likely than men to admit ever having a period of being sad, blue, or depressed lasting 2 weeks or longer, but should not affect reports of the less stigmatizing symptoms associated with depressed mood, such as sleep disturbance, eating disturbance, and lack of energy. It is also possible that recall bias existed, that is to say, the man tended to minimize the impact of the depressive episode and the presented symptoms during it. Thereby, it was found in some studies that men tended to communicate their past depressive episodes in an incomplete way, while women tended to exaggerate them. However, this fact could only justify the differences found in studies conducted retrospectively [14]. In conclusion, in the light of these studies, we found that gender differences regarding the prevalence of depression are not an artifact of epidemiological studies. Thus, if we assume these differences, we should hypothesize about possible explanations, which will be developed in the etiology section.

23.2.1 Depression in Young People

The presence of depressive disorders has progressively increased in recent decades, perhaps because adolescence begins earlier nowadays, or because young people are currently facing even earlier a greater number of stressful situations. Among children of pre-school age major depression is rare, around 0.3 % in the general population, and 0.9 % among children in psychiatric consultation. At school age, the rate increases to 2 %. In prepubertal individuals, gender differences in the prevalence of depression have not been described, or, if any, depression is more prominent in men, but since puberty the frequency of depressive disorders is much higher in women, a difference that is maintained in adulthood.

It is believed that this difference emerges between 15 and 18 years of age [15], but the highest prevalence in women seems to be related to the time of puberty rather than age itself. The pubertal status seems to predict the expected sex ratio better than the age; only after the transition to mid-puberty (Tanner stage II and above), adolescent girls are at a greater risk for depression than adolescent boys because before Tanner stage III, it was adolescent boys who are the ones who have a higher rate of depression [16]. The hypothesis that the increased risk of depression in adolescent girls might be linked to factors such as changes in body morphology, which would adversely affect the self-image and social interaction has not been validated in studies linking alterations at hormones and risk of depression [17].

Puberty not only involves various hormonal changes, but also implies important changes in terms of cognition and stressful experiences that significantly influence the onset of depression. Various studies show prevalence rates of depression in adolescents ranging from less than 1 to 6 % [18] nearer to 1 % in the case of diagnosis of major depression. Including all types of depressive disorders, the prevalence increases to 10 %. As we mentioned before, the rate of depression in adolescent girls increases markedly; it even it doubles the rate in boys.

In the case of dysthymia, considered a risk factor for the development of a major depressive episode, it is more common than major depression in children, with rates of around 2.5 %, and less common than major depression in adolescents, 3.3 %, also being more prevalent among women and girls [19].

23.2.2 Depression in the Elderly

In women, menopause is associated with an evolution of estrogen deficiency, and this postmenopausal estrogen depletion has been associated with vasomotor symptoms, urogenital changes, atrophy, decreased cognition, and greater vulnerability to major depressive disorder (MDD), as well as dysthymia and even dysphoria in the setting of physical illness and other stressful life events. The examination of depression in the elderly shows similar hypothalamic–pituitary–adrenal axis abnormalities as seen in younger adults with serious depressive disorders and significantly different from nondepressed elderly controls [20].

Recent studies have suggested that older women manifest lower rates of MDD in comparison to younger women [21], and that the greater prevalence of MDD in women relative to men diminishes somewhat with increasing age [22]. It is considered that rates of depression in men could remain stable or increases during the life span whereas women could have decreasing rates of depression thereby explaining the similar rates of depression in older adult men and women [23].

23.3 Etiology and Pathophysiology

Greater understanding of the underlying etiology and pathophysiology of MDD is the focus of genetic, neurobiological, and psychosocial investigation. We will not develop the pathogenesis of depressive disorder in this chapter, but we will try to highlight the most notable differences that exist with regard to gender.

Surveys of depression among children and adolescents show that the gender differences first emerge in the age range 11–14. This raises obvious questions about the role of sex hormones in the high prevalence of depression among women, especially as many women report changes in depressed mood associated with other experiences that cause changes in levels of sex hormones, such as menopause, use of oral contraceptives and use of hormone replacement therapy; however, systematic reviews consistently fail to find that rates of major depression are associated with any of these experiences. Furthermore, the emergence of the gender difference in depression is not constant across all race–ethnic groups in the US samples, further suggesting another etiopathogenic factor different from the hormonal effects. The only other case where rates of major depression related to hormones increasing substantially is during the postpartum period.

23.3.1 Environmental Effect (Risk Factors of Depression)

A number of consistently significant risk factors have been found, including family history, childhood adversity, various aspects of personality, social isolation, and exposure to stressful life experiences [9]. It is important to note that the family history results have generally shown little specificity; that is, family histories of anxiety or alcoholism or other psychiatric disorders have often been just as important as a family history of mood disorders in predicting depression.

In comparison, some specificity has been found in the effects of stressful life experiences. Stressors involving loss are strongly related to risk of depression, stressors involving danger are related to risk of anxiety, and stressors involving a combination of danger and loss are related to risk of mixed anxiety–depression [24,25]. There are some differential effects of stress on episode onset of major depression among women and men, which we will develop later.

Some studies have concluded that individuals with low socio-economic status demonstrate higher risk for depression than individuals who are financially well-off.

Studies on the effect of work on mental illness do not give conclusive results [26]. In women, the fact of being married, having three or more young children at home, being unemployed, being of a low social class, and the loss of her mother in childhood are risk factors for developing depression. In a reverse way, in rural areas, a lack of employment outside home and the caring of young children represent a protective factor [27, 28]. In men, unemployment is a clear risk factor for depression [29].

Regarding the educational level it is described from the 1970s that women with less cultural training have a lower risk of mental illness [30], although among students, the psychiatric morbidity between men and women was similar in another study [31]. Therefore, the findings in terms of educational level are not very clear with regard to depression, other social factors being most notable in its pathogenesis.

In terms of marital status, some authors consider that marriage has a protective effect against depression in men, whereas in women it is a significant source of stress [32–34]. In addition, lower morbidity was found among unmarried than among married, divorced, and separated men and women [35, 36] Among the elderly population, men who live alone or outlive their spouses are particularly vulnerable to depression, in contrast to women, who may be more resilient, if they are widowed or live alone [29].

23.3.2 Sexual Hormones and Maturation

Sex hormones appear to play a key role in both aspects of cognitive functioning, as in behavior and mood. Thus, the appearance of a mood disorder would be related to their decrease, as in pre-menstrual dysphoric disorder and postpartum depression. Consequently, they could not explain the increase in mood disorders at the beginning of the childbearing age of women, when the hormonal explosion occurs [17].

For this reason, the emergence of the gender difference in depression during puberty, following cohorts of prepubescent boys and girls through puberty using direct measures of sex hormones from blood samples. These studies found that the increase in depression among girls relative to boys occurs sharply at mid-puberty and that change in body morphology is more important than increase in age in predicting the gender difference in depression. A subsequent report showed that statistical control for changes in sex hormones eliminated the effects of body morphology. This led to the argument that the effect is due to biology rather than to societal reactions to physical maturation, but this conclusion may be premature. It was also related that girls who matured physically early experience more psychological distress than their counterparts who matured on time or late. This elevated distress is exacerbated by having mixed-sex friends rather than same-sex friends [37] and these results suggest that environmental stresses related to sex roles might potentiate the effects of sex hormones. Several investigations have been conducted about why adolescent girls are more prone to depression than men, finding risk factors, in addition to hormonal differences, such as personality traits in pre-adolescence (excessive emotionality, trend toward self-incrimination), which may favor the development of depression in response to typical biological and social experiences in adolescence [38].

Sex hormones may also play an indirect role through the modulation of neurotransmitters. Estrogens reduce the activity of monoamine oxidase (MAO), an effect that is associated with a decrease in depressive symptoms [39]. They also produce changes in the serotonergic and noradrenergic system by increasing their availability in synapses, as well as increasing the number of 5-HT$_2$ receptors [40]. In contrast, progesterone appears to increase the activity of MAO and catechol-O-methyltransferase (COMT) [41]. Estrogen and progesterone also seem to have a direct effect on serotonergic function: estrogen increases serotonin reuptake and influences the circadian variation [42], while progesterone causes an increase in its metabolism [43].

According to psychoanalytical theory and recent trauma theories [44] the distinction between global self-esteem and an experience of the self, which has been altered by past traumatic experiences, must be emphasized. This duality of the self may persist into later years in women, making them vulnerable to depression when exposed to loss. Because of this, it has been suggested that patterns of socialization and upbringing of girls contribute to strengthening women's emotional dependence and fear of being alone, low self-esteem, and a subordinate position.

The concept of gender in psychoanalysis [45] proposes that guilt is the feeling that underlies much of the female universe. This is manifested by the continuous self-reproach and self-referential disqualification resulting from the attributed social devaluation of women's emotionality, which is associated with weakness, lack of control, and dependency. This author also points to the mothering relationships as the dominant motivation in women, and the need for attachment, establishing care links.

Disruption of these mechanisms may be the result of the onset of disease, in this case, depressive illness and therefore the target for psychotherapeutic approaches [29].

Emotion regulation strategies are a range of activities that allow an individual to monitor, evaluate, and modify the nature and course of an emotional response, in order to pursue his or her goals and appropriately respond to environmental demands. The inability to use these strategies to downregulate negative emotions makes them more uncontrollable, severe and chronic, and can lead to depression [46–49]. The gender differences in emotion regulation strategies may contribute to the gender differences in psychopathology [50–52]. Rumination of negative thoughts, suppression of emotional expression and of unwanted thoughts, and avoidance of emotions are three processes that predict the diagnosis of major depression [53–55].

Rumination theory suggests that women are more likely than men to dwell on problems and, because of this, to let transient symptoms of dysphoria grow into clinically significant episodes of depression. That is to say that more rumination in women compared with men accounts for greater depression [56,57]. In the other hand, men are more likely to suppress or avoid their emotions. It is also important at this point to note that in the case of women, their greater tendency to engage in reappraisal, problem-solving, acceptance or seeking social support, compared with men, may mitigate the gender differences in depression.

Men are more likely to engage in automatic and unconscious emotion regulation, like automatic reappraisal, for example, comparing themselves with others to reduce reactivity to negative stimuli [58]. Men also seek support from male friends through shared activities, which protects them from depression. Men appear to engage in angry rumination more than women and this is associated with an increase in angry feelings and thoughts and more aggressive behavior.

In the case of women, seeking social support is one of their most important protective factors from depression, but co-rumination is a potential risk: discussing the same problem repeatedly, mutual encouragement of discussing problems, speculating about problems and focusing on negative feelings [59]. This is the reason why social support in women is not strongly related to improvements in mood in women.

The cognitive styles of autonomy and sociotropy predispose individuals to developing depression. As a result of socialization, women are more likely to develop sociotropic structures, while men are more likely to develop autonomous structures. Apart from this, women usually are presented with higher scores for harm avoidance than men.

A number of personality features have been proposed as vulnerability factors for the development and maintenance of depression. These include neuroticism, introversion, interpersonal dependency, self-criticism, and perfectionism. Clinically depressed women are significantly more likely to have a "depressive temperament," which includes features of self-criticism and preoccupation with inadequacy and failure. They also report higher levels of conscientiousness and of sociotropy. Thus, men and women have a similar frequency of brief episodes of sadness, but women, because of their tendency toward rumination, internalization of feelings, and amplification of this mood, allow these episodes to frequently crystallize in a major depressive episode, that is to say, the female sex, by their personality features, would be more likely to suffer depression after a stressful life event [60]. In housewives the probability of depression increases as the children grow up and leave the house, which can cause depression, fear of loneliness, and loss of sense of life. The so-called empty nest syndrome is a good example of this situation [61, 62] and empirical studies link low self-esteem and dependency traits of women with depression [63, 64].

One of the most controversial sociological explanations for the higher prevalence of depression in women is based on the social position of women as a risk factor for depression. Sex-role theories suggest that the chronic stresses associated with traditional female roles lead to a higher prevalence of depression among women than men [65].

The family as a social institution has undergone enormous changes throughout history; women have been traditionally dedicated to housework (private sphere, expressive–reproductive role), while men have been developed in the world of paid work (public sphere, instrumental–productive role) [43].

For several decades a dramatic and rapid social change has been taking place that has implicated the renovation and restructuring of these roles, having a particular impact on women, but not less on the male role. The influence of different aspects of the traditional female role in the psychic development of women should be analyzed, such as housewife occupation, femininity, and traditionalism in beliefs about the role of women. While it is clear that in recent decades there has been a trend toward flexibility in gender roles and toward equal opportunities for people regardless of their sex, it is also clear that men and women still socialize with different rules and expectations regarding the expression of feelings, the pressure of success in studies or work, participation in domestic tasks, commitment to the care and concern for relationships, and caring for others [66], which has meaningful psychological consequences. The traditional female role is primarily characterized by being focused in the private circle and the interest and care of intimate relationships. Femininity as a personality characteristic includes not only aspects such as kindness, loyalty, sensitivity to the needs of others, the ability of understanding, tenderness, but also dependency, impressionability, lack of assertiveness, tendency toward emotional expression, etc. Socially, the female role has been constrained to the private sphere, particularly in the care of family members and the care of the housework.

It has been known for over two decades that women report higher levels of depressed mood than men in community surveys and that this gender difference is stronger for married people than for the unmarried. According to the sex role explanation, women are more depressed than men because of the higher levels of stress and lower levels of fulfillment in female versus male sex roles. The specification by marital status, according to this account, is because married women are more strongly exposed to traditional sex-role experiences than single women. This could be because of both the presence of a greater number of stressors (family demands, overload of both domestic and nondomestic work, negative marital experiences, etc.). A non-equitable distribution of social and family responsibilities between men and women contributes to creating additional sources of stress for women who are already subject to the performance of multiple roles [62]. Recent studies show that job stress accompanied by an overload of activities in the home increases the rates of depression among women [67].

However, return to work has been a major achievement for a large number of women in terms of their personal and professional fulfillment and financial independence. The literature has reported that breaking social isolation and creating new relationships improves the physical and emotional wellbeing of women working outside the home compared with those who are housewives [68, 69]. Both paid work and having sufficient financial resources are associated with better physical and mental health in both sexes.

Studies comparing mental health of married women who work and those who are housewives, show contradictory results. Some authors [70] found that women who even after having children continue working away from home have less depression than housewives. It is believed that employment encourages self-esteem as it helps them feel useful and provides stimuli to overcome challenges and the opportunity to be accompanied by other adults. Only when these working mothers do not have help in caring for their children, if they suffer from a deficiency, or when their children are at preschool age, are they more prone to suffering stress than housewives [71].

However, other authors believe that while housewives demand more treatment and subjective index of disease is higher than those of working mothers, the differences do not become significant; thus, it is concluded that there is little evidence of more psychiatric disorders among housewives [72].

Regarding femininity and masculinity, there is considerable evidence that in both men and women, masculinity tends to be associated with an index of personal adjustment, including higher self-esteem and a tendency toward having lower levels of depression [65,73–75].

On the other hand, femininity relates to certain aspects of personal and social adjustment such as the perception of self-efficacy, satisfaction in personal relationships and self-esteem components that relate to social relationships [76, 77]. Other works [78] find lower self-esteem, lower life satisfaction, and higher anxiety in more traditional women compared with those who manifest more progressive attitudes to their role as women, taking into account that this role has been characterized by their limitations and inferiority to men. Thus, certain traits that describe femininity (sensitivity, complacency, passivity, obedience, the need for emotional contact, lack of aggression and competence) appear to hinder the psychological well-being of women because they easily result in situations of passivity, dependency, lack of assertiveness and low self-esteem, which often lead to presentation of depressive symptoms [79].

Although all these assumptions may be valid to explain more recurrences or chronicity of depression, it cannot explain the increased risk in women of presenting a first depressive episode and that, if true, epidemiological studies should begin to detect differences from men in adulthood and not in puberty, as previously described [80].

23.3.3 The Conflict of Role: Repercussions on Women and Men

Recent changes in women's roles have redefined male roles, creating new tensions and ambiguities, but also opening up new opportunities for self-realization (greater cooperativeness in the parenting and domestic work, greater expressiveness, greater support for women's work activities, and greater appreciation of women's contribution in the family) [81, 82].

Several hypotheses have been developed and described the phenomenon of conflict that can be generated by performing the male role, defining the gender role conflict as a psychological state in which socialized gender roles have negative consequences for the health of the person or those who interact with it; conflict appears when the roles are played in a sexist, rigid or restricted way that determines the restriction, devaluation and the violation of themselves or others.

The men educated into the framework of these societies express an obsessive preoccupation with power, success and competition, with a restrictive emotionality that makes it difficult to express, understand, and manage emotions, generating homophobia and fear of the feminine and conflicts between the work role and the family role or other areas of life.

Conflicts with gender role appear mainly when masculinity is questioned by others (friends, parents, and teachers). Men can be mistreated or be violent with others when they are unable to satisfy the expectations of the stereotypes of gender role or their own expectations. Consequently, men who experience a fear of failing as a man are vulnerable to developing depression, anxiety, abuse of medication, drugs, and alcohol and can suffer from disorders involving overeating or practicing compulsive exercise [83].

23.3.4 Relationship and Depression

The partner relationship is a privileged context to study whether depressive symptoms in women are associated with a lack of intimacy or emotional connection and social inequalities, reflected in the differences in the power sharing between spouses [84–89].

There are several theoretical models and plentiful empirical evidence that explains and evaluates the impact of the lack of emotional support in the family on women [85, 90–93].

With regard to inequalities of power, analyzing the relationship from a gender perspective, they connect the welfare of the female partner with the distribution of resources, burdens and privileges between spouses. From this perspective it is argued that there is a parallel, which is especially significant for women with children and more traditional roles, between the level of power of the woman in the relationship and the depressive symptomatology [85,94,95].

From a systemic point of view, hypotheses that interpret clinical depression of one spouse as a reflection of imbalances or power struggles are formulated. Depression is considered to be an expression of helplessness or weakness and simultaneously, a protest or rebellion, that is to say, an indirect way of questioning this asymmetry and gaining power over the spouse. Women are at a higher risk of being depressed because they are socially determined to carry the weakened role in the relationship, must sacrifice "me" in terms of "us" [96]. If a woman is not able to question her position in the relationship, she could attribute her discomfort to the couple, and it would be difficult for her to challenge the balance of the relationship, which she herself also helps to maintain [88, 97].

23.3.5 Gender Violence

In recent years, the attention to domestic violence has been a primary focus of attention, concerning not only the justice, but also the political world and the mental health services because of the psychological consequences that this implies. Patriarchy has been considered as generating structure of inequality and inequity, based on a supposed father–male power legitimized as an actor that does violence to the other dependent members; there are also significant primary socialization patterns that involve children in the reproduction of gender inequalities and the internalization of violent actions as a form of conflict resolution [98]. It seems that the main factors that predispose men to violence against women are: the socialization in the gender role, distorted patterns, conflicts with gender roles and mechanisms of defense, and strategies for self-protective defense.

If we focus on the acute psychological injuries of domestic abuse, we can find a first reaction of self-protection and self-survival instinct, with frequent occurrence of reactions of shock, denial, confusion, sadness, dizziness, and fear. In response to this potential danger, some battered women may develop intense anxiety and even a post-traumatic stress disorder. Other associated disorders include dissociative disorders, eating disorders, substance abuse, and persistent personality alterations. With regard to the topic at hand, depression is another prevalent diagnosis among populations of battered women [99, 100]. The depression can remain a long time after leaving the relationship, even with a higher prevalence [101,

102]. Furthermore, there is a subgroup with a higher incidence of depression after the abandonment of the violent relationship in which women tend to blame themselves for the abuse they experience [29, 103].

23.4 Course of Illness

23.4.1 Onset

One of the most consistent findings across studies is the female preponderance of major depressive disorder (MDD) and its emergence in adolescence. Studies of adolescents have reported gender differences consistent with adult populations, about twice as many girls as boys meet the criteria for MDD at some time in their lives [104,105]. The change in the sex ratio usually emerges around puberty [106–108], with the greatest increase in gender difference occurring between ages 15 and 18 [15].

Mechanisms underlying this shift in prevalence are still unclear; however, it may reflect the interplay of gender socialization, gonadal hormonal mechanisms [109], stressful events associated with adolescence [110] such as higher rates of physical and sexual abuse [111] or childhood adversity, the experience of more interpersonal stressors [112], and the greater tendency to ruminate [113].

Studies among adults [80, 114] and adolescents [115] have also reported a greater number of first onsets of depression in women than in men.

In concordance with these studies, recently the ABC model has been proposed to explain the emergence of gender difference in depression in adolescence. According to this model, affective (emotional reactivity), biological (genetic vulnerability, pubertal hormones, and pubertal timing and development), and cognitive (cognitive style, objectified body consciousness, rumination) factors confer vulnerability to depression. These factors interact with negative life events or stress, leading to significantly more girls than boys having depression in adolescence. Why men and women differ in most of these factors, which in turn have contributed to gender differences in depression, is still unclear and should be the main objective of study for future research [43, 50].

23.4.2 Chronicity and Recurrence

Considering the number of episodes presented, women are two times more likely to develop a single episode unipolar depression and they are even four times more likely to develop recurrent unipolar depression in community samples. However, according to research, results on gender differences in the duration or recurrence of depression are somewhat inconsistent. Some evidence exists that women have a more chronic course of depression than men. However, methodological studies show fairly convincingly that this is due to a differential recall bias, for instance. The environmental experiences that are associated with chronicity and recurrence are different for women and men; for example, financial pressures are more depressogenic for men than women while family problems are more depressogenic for women than men.

According to many studies, in women compared with men with a history of depression subsequent depressive episodes are more likely to be developed [116–118], not only in childhood or adolescence but also in adulthood [106].

However, some other studies failed to find gender differences in the recurrence of depression among adolescents [115] or adults [114]. However, because the participants in studies among adolescents are still young, it is possible that greater female recurrence may emerge at a later age. Similarly, in another study, that gender difference in recurrence in major depression in adults was interpreted as a greater number of first onsets of depression in women compared with men, but without gender differences in the duration or recurrence of depression [80].

In both genders, an earlier onset of depression was significantly correlated with a higher number of depressive episodes. Interestingly, lower age at onset predicts a worse course of depression in women, but not in men. The finding that an earlier age of onset increased the chances of experiencing depressive episodes can be interpreted as supporting previous findings that an early onset MDD is more severe than those with a later onset [119]. The finding that an earlier onset is associated with a worse course in women only could have important theoretical implications. It seemed to suggest that depressive episodes tend to leave "scars" or residual effects [120], on an individual, which may serve to increase the likelihood of future depressive episodes. This effect is more likely to be experienced by women because of their greater tendency to ruminate in response to their depressed moods [121], which activate and strengthen the associative networks of negative cognitions [122], the greater genetic effects on MDD in women [123,124], and their interpersonal orientation that overvalues relationships as sources of self-worth [125].

Another line of argument may be biologically oriented. Depression may increase biological reactivity to stress by sensitizing the neurotransmitter and neuroendocrine systems linked to depression [126]. This in turn lowers the threshold for new depressive episodes, such that even mild stressors can trigger a new episode. It could be further argued that women are more reactive to stress than men. Support of this hypothesis comes from a recent study [112] that showed that adolescent girls compared with boys were also more reactive to both total and interpersonal stress and consequently, were more likely to become depressed [43].

23.4.3 Duration of Episodes

The duration of the depressive episodes showed a trend toward being lengthier in women [106,127].

Apart from this fact, it is important to highlight that the presence of a comorbid disorder prolongs the duration of MDD episodes in men predominantly. The exact reason for this gender difference is unclear; however, it could be the case that among men, major depression is secondary to other conditions such as substance use disorders, which men are more prone to having [128–130]. Studies have also indicated that protracted substance abuse was associated with more severe depression and health problems in men than in women [131].

23.5 Symptomatology

If human brain is developed in a different way in men and women and if it is influenced by the action of sex hormones, it is logical that differences will arise in the presentation of psychopathology. But although it is widely held that there are no significant differences between men and women in terms of the symptoms that they experience during depressive episodes, the simple observation of our patients suggests that there might be different characteristics in the clinical manifestations of this condition in women. which underlies biological and cultural differences rather than the classic male–female sexual dimorphism. Recent research suggests that subtle differences in symptom profile may exist and may point to fundamental gender differences in the pathophysiology of depressive states.

A number of studies have found that depressed women tend to exhibit more "atypical" depressive symptoms, with a frequency more than twice as high as men (excessive fatigue, overeating, and oversleeping) and more anxiety and somatization symptoms compared with men [132–136]. Besides those mentioned above, we have found anger and psychomotor retardation [43].

Higher levels of atypical symptoms in women could reflect a pathophysiological difference between male and female depression. For example, it has been suggested that this atypical depression is associated with under-activity of the hypothalamic–pituitary–adrenal (HPA) axis [137]. Given that female gonadal steroids are known to modulate factors such as corticotrophin-releasing hormone (CRH) secretion, serotonergic activity [138], and gamma-aminobutyric acid (GABA) transmission [139], it is possible that the clinical syndrome of atypical depressive symptoms is at least in part a consequence of the action of female hormones on the HPA axis [140]. A finding like this may have important implications for the treatment of depression, as we will mention later.

Women with clinical depression may tend to experience a greater severity of depressive symptoms, and their depression is often associated with a greater functional impairment [141, 142]. Women with sub-threshold depression have also been reported to endorse a greater overall number of depressive symptoms in comparison to men. Gender differences are especially prominent in the self-reported severity of depressive symptoms compared with interview-based measures of depression severity, which implies that women express their psychic distress.

23.6 Comorbidity

Women are shown to have higher rates of both threshold and sub-threshold co-morbid *anxiety*. As mentioned before, it is proposed that the gender difference in depression might be partly due to a difference in prior anxiety [43,143,144]; this claim has been supported by showing that the odds ratio (OR) of gender predicting major depression substantially attenuates when controls are introduced for the prior existence of anxiety. That is to say, in studies in adolescents, this temporal sequence of anxiety and depression in women would occur not because of an increased vulnerability for depression after an anxiety disorder, which is observed similarly in both sexes, but because of the higher prevalence of these anxiety disorders in relation to men.

It has to be outstanding that this finding is limited in that it focuses on a predictor that is characteristic of women while ignoring other comparable predictors that are more characteristic of men (e.g., alcohol or drug abuse, antisocial personality disorder, and conduct disorder). Thus, it has been demonstrated [145] that the gender differences in OR increased when another model was estimated that controlled for prior substance use disorders and conduct disorder (more often found among men than women) rather than for prior anxiety disorders; when the design of the model controlled simultaneously prior anxiety disorders, substance use disorders, and conduct disorder, the observed difference in OR was found to be exactly the same as the model that had no controls.

These results clearly show that history of prior psychiatric disorders does not play an important part in explaining the observed gender difference in the onset risk of major depression.

As mention before, the presence of a comorbid disorder prolongs the duration of MDD episodes in men predominantly. The exact reason for this gender difference is unclear; however, it could be that among men, major depression is secondary to other conditions such as substance use disorders, which men are more prone to have [129, 130]. This condition in men is also associated with more severe depression and health problems in men than in women [131].

23.7 Heritability

Depression is also an illness that aggregates in families. Family studies have observed an increase in the risk of developing major depressive disorder in the relatives of individuals with major depressive disorder, although the magnitude of risk differed between reports [146, 147]. On the other hand, twin studies have consistently supported genetic effects in the development of depression [148,149]. Studies of twins recruited from psychiatric treatment centers demonstrated strong genetic influences on the development of depression (with heritability between 60 and 70 %).

The influence of genetic factors, however, may not be equal for men and women. As part of the National Institute of Mental Health Collaborative Program on the

Psychobiology of Depression, subjects with depression and their first-degree relatives were studied and the "transmissibility" of depression, which encompasses both environmental and genetic factors that are passed from parents to offspring, was examined. Women were found to have significantly greater transmissibility of depression than men. However, twin studies [150, 151] did not find any sex differences in the magnitude of genetic and environmental contributions to depression. In conclusion, the results document that in women genetic factors play a substantial, but not overwhelming, role in depression; the tendency for depression to aggregate in families results largely from shared genetic and environmental factors [152].

Genetic factors, however, do not seem to contribute to the increased risk to women by a direct mechanism. Instead, genetic factors may indirectly increase vulnerability to depression in women through other mechanisms, such as how the different sexes handle stress. In fact, higher depression rates have been reported in adolescent girls, suggesting that the genetic predisposition to depression and to stressful events might be turned on at puberty in women [153,154].

Some studies have set out to answer why stressful experiences lead to depression in some people but not in others. They reported that a functional polymorphism in the promoter region of the serotonin transporter gene was found to moderate the influence of stressful life events on depression. This important epidemiological study provides evidence of a gene-by-environment interaction, in which an individual's response to environmental stress is moderated by his or her genetic make-up [155–157].

23.8 Pharmacological Treatment

All epidemiological data indicate that depression is more prevalent in women than in men. However, until recently, research has paid little attention to gender differences in antidepressant treatment. In this regard, studies show that there are gender differences in the enzymatic metabolism of some antidepressants and currently various studies are being carried out to see how these differences would reflect on clinical efficacy [158].

Gender differences in the pharmacokinetics and pharmacodynamics of antidepressants suggest that men and women might differ in their response to treatment. These effects may be particularly marked in women of childbearing age given the influence of estrogen, but there is a huge controversy about the differences in response to antidepressants according to gender [159–161].

It is known that sex differences in the presentation of depression, lie in atypical symptoms that may have important implications for treatment because patients with atypical depression are more likely to respond to monoamine oxidase inhibitors (MAOIs) than tricyclic antidepressants (TCAs) [162, 163].

According to studies, MAOIs are superior in effectiveness in men, compared with SSRIs, which are better in women and TCAs are less effective than SSRIs [164].

Nowadays, MAOIs are not very extensively used and this is the reason why other types of new antidepressants have been studied in terms of effectiveness. SSRIs have been demonstrated to be equally as effective as MAOIs in the treatment of atypical depression [165] and TCAs would be less effective than SSRIs; thus, women should respond well to either an SSRI or MAOI, but poorly to TCAs [157].

Moreover, further analyses of treatment trials of MAOIs in atypical depression suggest that a good response to this drug might not be the result of atypical features *per se*, but rather the early age of onset and chronicity often associated with atypical depression [166].

There is some evidence that women respond more poorly than men to tricyclic antidepressants (TCAs), with imipramine studied the most. In contrast, we found other studies indicating that both men and women are equally likely to respond to TCAs.

In the case of chronic depression, recent studies have found that men respond more favorably to imipramine than women, while the latter show a more favorable response to sertraline and fluoxetine than men [161].

Other reports have suggested that anxious depression is associated with poorer response to all antidepressants [167, 168] or treatment resistance. The largest of these, based on the STAR*D sample, suggested that those with anxious depression might be less likely to respond to citalopram and more likely to report adverse events (STAR*D) [169]. It has been suggested that MAOIs may be more effective than TCAs in these patients and more recently that SNRIs are more effective than TCAs. A recent report suggested that the SSRI escitalopram might be more efficacious than the TCA nortriptyline in relieving the anxious symptoms of depression. In another study it was observed that in patients with melancholic depression treated with clomipramine, citalopram, paroxetine or moclobemide, men and women respond equally well to treatment. However, a number of large meta-analyses have failed to identify such differences. If, as these epidemiological studies suggest, women are more likely to report co-morbid anxiety, it is possible that women also respond overall more poorly to antidepressants than men. Although this hypothesis is in line with a number of findings, it remains to be rigorously tested.

A more recent study combining data from 15 randomized trials of six antidepressants suggested that women responded better to SSRIs than SNRIs such as venlafaxine [170].

It has been reported that in postmenopausal women not undergoing HRT, high levels of LH were associated with a poor response to antidepressants and they also showed that HRT, which decreased LH and FSH and increased estradiol, improved response to antidepressants in postmenopausal women [171]. A similar study suggested that both postmenopausal status and high levels of FSH might be associated with a poorer response to SSRIs [172]. These results are in line with other studies reporting an antidepressant effect of estrogen in peri- and postmenopausal women [173]. They are also consistent with studies that show increased efficacy of SSRIs in peri- and postmenopausal women when combined with HRT or estrogen replacement therapy (ERT) [174, 175].

With regard to plasma concentrations there appears to be some agreement that tricyclics are higher in women than in men. However, not all studies support this hypothesis.

Women generally have a lower body weight and organ size and a higher percentage of fat, all of which are known to affect both the absorption and distribution of drugs, and it is known that lighter patients respond preferentially to the SSRI fluoxetine [176, 177].

According to many studies, differential responses in different sexes may be the result of differential percentage of body fat and body fat distribution between men and women because obese men respond more poorly than thinner men in comparison to overweight women [178].

P-glycoprotein (P-gp) is a drug transporter, which plays a critical role in the absorption and distribution of antidepressants. It has been reported that a gender difference exists in the expression of P-gp such that women express only one-third to one-half of protein compared with men [179], which implies an increase in the concentration of drugs and therefore a higher toxicity in women. With regard to plasma concentrations there appears to be some agreement that in tricyclics they are higher in women than in men. However, not all studies support this hypothesis. It is very important to pay attention to the dosage of antidepressants in women to prevent adverse effects. Women need lower doses owing to their physiological characteristics as they reach higher plasma concentrations.

The most important CYPs in antidepressant metabolism are CYP2D6, CYP2C, CYP3A, and CYP1A [180]. Animal studies suggest that there is a differential expression of CYPs in men and women [181]. CYP3A4 activity is higher in women. CYP1A2 activity appears to be higher in men than women and this may be the result of its inhibition of CYPA2 by estrogens in women [182–185]; indeed, the contraceptive pill has been shown to inhibit the enzyme [186]. Similarly, CYP2C19 activity has also been shown to be reduced in women and it has also been suggested that this may be a direct result of inhibition by estrogen [183] and oral contraceptives [185–187]. In CYP2D6 activity, some studies report slightly higher activity in women [185] and others no difference [188].

Consistent with lower P-gp activity at absorption and lower activity of CYP1A2 and CYP2C19, plasma levels of imipramine, of TCA nortriptyline, and of desipramine are reportedly higher in women than men [189–191].

The effects of gender on plasma levels of SSRIs are, however, less clear. Plasma levels of sertraline have been shown to be higher in older women [192], which is consistent with the inhibitory effects of estrogen on both CYP1A2 and CYP2C19 activity. Similarly, plasma levels of the SSRIs citalopram and paroxetine may also be higher in women than men [193, 194], although inconsistent findings have been reported.

In terms of differences in adverse effects, the existing literature is very limited. Findings that suggest that women are more likely to experience adverse events to TCAs are in line with evidence from pharmacokinetic studies, which suggest that women have higher plasma levels of these drugs than men. With respect to the sexual side effects, patients are not generally informed about them. This undesirable effect has been specially focused on men, but it can affect women negatively. Even though there are specific drugs to treat erectile dysfunction in men, their effectiveness is questionable in the case of women. More research should be carried out in relation to this topic in order to analyze significant differences between men and women.

Suicidal ideation is considered not only a symptom of depression, but also a common side effect in antidepressant treatment as a result of an exacerbation of the irritable symptoms, which are observed more often in men with depression. It has long been recognized that gender differences exist in suicidal behavior [195], and it has also been shown that suicidal ideation was both drug- and gender-dependent; specifically, men treated with nortriptyline were more likely to suffer an increase in suicidal ideation during treatment [196], suggesting that this the gender-specific effects of nortriptyline on suicidal ideation might be the result of the worsening of the irritable symptoms.

Genetic variation also affects both the pharmacokinetics and pharmacodynamics of antidepressants [197] and a number of recent studies suggest that the effects of genetic polymorphisms may differ in men and women. A well studied pharmacogenetic candidate, which affects the pharmacodynamics of SSRIs, is the gene encoding the serotonin transporter (SLC6A4); three polymorphisms in this gene have been associated with response to antidepressants. Concretely, the short variant of the 5-HTTLPR has been associated with poor response and nonremission to antidepressants [198] and these findings were subsequently replicated in STAR*D, after considering the ethnicity of the study population [199]. Given the interaction between estrogen and the serotonin transporter, it has been suggested that the effects of genetic variation in the gene encoding the transporter may be moderated by gender. Consistent with this hypothesis in the GENDEP study the "S" allele of the 5-HTTLPR was associated with poorer response to escitalopram in men but not women [200].

23.9 Psychotherapy in Depression According to Gender

Women use psychotherapy to resolve their psychological conflicts rather more often than men. In addition, they ask for help and are committed to treatment with far less difficulty than men.

Psychotherapy and the idea of femininity have been historically linked. Thus, Freud described the psychology of women in terms of the observed shortcomings by comparing it with male psychology, which was taken as a model, referring to the narcissistic inferiority or "penis envy" [201]. Soon, however, new concepts were promoted because these ideas did not reflect the experiences of women, shifting the focus to the interpersonal and maternal determinants of mental development [5]. As early as the 1980s the debate about gender identity that associates psychoanalytical teaching to biology and sociology had begun.

Chodorow describes how the basic feminine sense of self is seen to be connected to the world, whereas the basic sense of self in man is conceived as apart from the world. These different relationship skills and the type of identification is what prepares women to assume the role of adult.

Bleichmar explains the presence of guilt as a characteristic element of the female psyche, which regulates the relationship of women herself and her environment. She also proposes the hypothesis that fear of loss of love is the most dangerous situation that promotes anxiety in women, the reassurance of emotional ties being the main organizer of femininity.

Psychotherapy cannot have a position free from values of the therapist and the psychotherapeutic model used. Therefore, it seems essential to be aware of our ideology and gender bias when performing psychotherapy. Failure to observe these biases can cause variations in the perception of the problem, in the diagnosis, in the objectives to be treated and in the etiological explanations of symptoms, according to the sex of the patient.

With regard to gender, it is crucial for the development of psychotherapy to take into account certain aspects and to promote an egalitarian relationship between therapist and patient. The main objective would be to help the patient, male or female, to become aware of gender inequalities, analyzing the processes of socialization and considering the sources of internal and external issues when addressing them. We should encourage the person to develop by themselves a process of questioning the assessments generally associated with the man or woman. And as mentioned above, it is imperative to note that individual female development is guided through a relational experience.

For all these reasons, it is essential to take into account all these different characteristics of female gender identity in order to structure the most appropriate therapy for each patient, following the lines of evidence-based recommendations for the treatment of major depression [29].

Specific depression-based psychological treatment for MDD is available [44] and this supportive psychotherapeutic management of depression facilitates the pharmacological response.

These treatments have included: cognitive behavioral therapy, interpersonal psychotherapy, brief dynamic psychotherapy, and marital and family therapy.

Cognitive behavioral theory [202] is the most empirically examined psychosocial theory in relation to the management and treatment of the depressed patient, and emphasizes a number of dysfunctional attitudes, cognitions, and images associated with depressive symptomatology; Beck posited that cognitive distortions (negative self-schemas) cause depression and are associated with maintenance of the disorder; the cognitive perspective is elaborated further by learned helplessness models, and hopelessness theory [203, 204]. In cognitive behavioral therapy [205], education, behavioral assignments, and cognitive retraining form the active components of psychotherapy [206]. This cognitive therapy has been demonstrated to be an effective short-term psychotherapy for depression [207].

Interpersonal psychotherapy of depression (IPT), which is demonstrated to be effective in acute treatment trials [16], addresses interpersonal difficulties such as interpersonal loss or grieving, role transitions, interpersonal disputes, and social deficits. The depressed female older adult, who could be struggling with the loss of a spouse or a change in marital status, or transition from workplace to retirement, or from having raised a family to an empty home, benefits from IPT.

Brief dynamic psychotherapy, which was not specifically designed for treatment of MDD, addresses current conflicts as manifestations of difficulty in early attachment.

From a psychoanalytical perspective, the pathology is due to the lack of integration of the feminine and masculine and therefore, its goal is the aggregation of both poles, while recognizing the vulnerability of female patients.

Similarly, research is needed to determine the efficacy of marital and family therapy in individuals with MDD. However, marital distress is a major event associated with the development of a depressive episode, marital discord will often persist after the remission of depression, and subsequent relapses are frequently associated with disruptions of marital relationships.

Conclusion

Affective disorders are multifactorial diseases well delimited from the scientific and medical point of view, but the current process of globalization and the socio-economic and cultural environment begin to have great importance and influence on them, especially the current gender construct.

In the past three decades we have experienced great changes related to the redefinition of gender identity (basically related to female gender identity), with major changes in social, cultural, and economic levels, but not from a medical and psychopathological point of view, where gender identity is kept subordinated to the historical and traditional "masculinity" of the symptomatology described from the past.

Depression has also been affected by these changes, becoming a global disease with the peculiarities of the socio-cultural context where it appears, being influenced differently by the current gender perspective (incorporation of women into work, changes in the classic roles of identity, periods of crisis, and financial problems).

Nowadays, women must respond to classic and current roles: housewives, taking care of the family, caregiver role, the double workday (at the office, at home) often without any support from their partners and without social appreciation of themselves as autonomous agents. This stressful environment can result in a disease, especially depression. Because of this process of transformation around gender identity, a new perspective of psychopathology must be made.

Currently, the need to reconcile family and working life is emphasized, but this is only possible with an equitable distribution of social and family responsibilities between men and women; otherwise, they will continue to contribute to creating additional sources of stress for women who are already subjected to performing multiple roles. Recent studies show that job stress accompanied by an overload of activities at home increases the rates of depression among women.

At the same time, we must emphasize the role of caregiver usually assigned to the woman, which leads to overload and increases the likelihood of developing depression, because the psychological burden that affects caregivers, usually women, which makes them develop feelings of fear, helplessness, responsibility, insecurity, and anxiety.

From a purely epidemiological point of view we know that women are typically 2–3 times more likely to develop depressive disorders than men; some authors claim that "depression is more unacceptable for men because it disagrees with the male stereotype," because it is difficult for men to recognize it, and even harder to show it openly because it does not correspond with the masculine ideals of success in our society; thus, men often deny having depressive symptoms and the collected data in research about prevalence do not agree with the clinical reality. The male stereotype is characterized by competence, strength, and avoidance of anything that denotes femininity, while depression would be a manifestation of little value, weakness, vulnerability, emotional expressiveness, and crying, aspects traditionally associated with women.

The etiology and pathophysiology of depression should be considered as a construct that includes genetic, neurobiological, and psychosocial aspects.

The value of hormonal function in the different developmental stages of women and the particular environmental factors that result in a psychopathological process (traumatic childhood experiences, low socio-economic status, social isolation, family dynamics, particular aspects of personality) is well known, but we must take greater account of the traditional role of women established since ancient times and its current definition as a source of pathology.

The prevalent symptomatology in depressive women differs substantially from that which prevails in men, guiding us to underlying biological and cultural issues; it is shown that depressed women tend to have greater number of atypical symptoms than men (excessive fatigue, hypersomnia and hyperorexia, more frequent anxiety symptoms, and somatic symptoms). The prevalence of atypical depression is twice as high in women as in men, with the consequent higher clinical severity and higher comorbidity that influences the onset of the disorder at an earlier age, the higher frequency of recurrent episodes, and longer duration of symptoms. All these specific events in women and the subjective opinion of excessive severity of symptoms, could reflect a depressogenic cognitive style associated with the female identity.

Regarding the pharmacological treatment, there are significant differences between women and men in the enzymatic metabolism of some of the antidepressants used (mainly related to the lower expression of P-gp in women), with the consequent differences in the clinical response to treatment; we also know that the response to antidepressants in depression with high anxiety comorbidity is lower; thus, it seems that antidepressant use in women is generally less effective.

If we focus on psychotherapy, it is crucial to take into account an egalitarian relationship between therapist and patient and to become aware of gender inequalities, analyzing the processes of socialization and questioning the assessments generally associated with men or with women, cognitive behavioral therapy having been the most empirically tested.

References

1. American Psychiatric Association. Diagnostic and statistical manual of mental disorders. 5th ed. American Psychiatric Association; Arlington, VA: Masson; 2013.
2. Sadock BJ, Kaplan HI, Sadock VA. Kaplan & Sadock Synopsis of Psychiatry. s.l.: Wolters Kluwer España; 2009.
3. Murray CJL, Lopez AD. The Global Burden of Disease: a comprehensive assessment of mortality and disability from diseases, injuries and risk factors in 1990 and projected to 2020. Cambridge: Harvard University Press; 1996. p. 325–95.
4. Kessler RC. Epidemiology of women and depression. J Affect Disord. 2003;74(1):5–13.
5. Barbieri NB. Psychoanalytic contributions to the study of gender issues. Can J Psychiatry. 1999;44(1):72–6.
6. Rodríguez Vega B. Proceso terapéutico y género. In: II Symposium Nacional. Tratamiento de adicción en la mujer, Oviedo; 2002.
7. Weissman MM, Bland R, Joyce PR, Newman S, Wells JE, Wittchen HU. Sex differences in rates of depression: cross-national perspectives. J Affect Disord. 1993;29(2–3):77–84.
8. Kessler RC, McGonagle KA, Nelson CB, Hughes M, Swartz M, Blazer DG. Sex and depression in the National Comorbidity Survey. II: Cohort effects. J Affect Disord. 1994;30(1):15–26.
9. Kessler RC, Zhao S, Blazer DG, Swartz M. Prevalence, correlates, and course of minor depression and major depression in the National Comorbidity Survey. J Affect Disord. 1997;45(1–2):19–30.
10. Ezcurra J, González Pinto A, Gutiérrez-Fraile. Psiquiatría y mujer. s.l.: Aula médica; 2006.
11. Angst J, Merikangas K. The depressive spectrum: diagnostic classification and course. J Affect Disord. 1997;45(1–2):31–9.
12. Young MA, Fogg LF, Scheftner WA, Keller MB, Fawcett JA. Sex differences in the lifetime prevalence of depression: does varying the diagnostic criteria reduce the female/male ratio? J Affect Disord. 1990;18(3):187–92.
13. Gove WR, Geerken MR. Response bias in surveys of mental health: an empirical investigation. AJS. 1977;82(6):1289–317.
14. Wilhelm K, Parker G. Sex differences in lifetime depression rates: fact or artefact? Psychol Med. 1994;24(1):97–111.
15. Hankin BL, Abramson LY, Moffitt TE, Silva PA, McGee R, Angell KE. Development of depression from preadolescence to young adulthood: emerging gender differences in a 10-year longitudinal study. J Abnorm Psychol. 1998;107(1):128–40.
16. Angold A, Costello EJ, Worthman CM. Puberty and depression: the roles of age, pubertal status and pubertal timing. Psychol Med. 1998;28(1):51–61.
17. Angold A, Costello EJ, Erkanli A, Worthman CM. Pubertal changes in hormone levels and depression in girls. Psychol Med. 1999;29(5):1043–53.
18. Fleming JE, Offord DR, Boyle MH. Prevalence of childhood and adolescent depression in the community. Ontario Child Health Study. Br J Psychiatry. 1989;155:647–54.
19. Garrison CZ, Waller JL, Cuffe SP, McKeown RE, Addy CL, Jackson KL. Incidence of major depressive disorder and dysthymia in young adolescents. J Am Acad Child Adolesc Psychiatry. 1997;36(4):458–65.
20. Seidman SN. The neuroendocrine system in late life. In: Roose SP, Sackeim HA, editors. Late-life depression. New York: Oxford University Press; 2004. p. 167–81.

21. Jeste DV, Alexopoulos GS, Bartels SJ, Cummings JL, Gallo JJ, Gottlieb GL, Halpain MC, Palmer BW, Patterson TL, Reynolds III CF, Lebowitz BD. Consensus statement on the upcoming crisis in geriatric mental health: research agenda for the next 2 decades. Arch Gen Psychiatry. 1999;56(9):848–53.
22. Barefoot JC, Mortensen EL, Helms MJ, Avlund K, Schroll M. A longitudinal study of gender differences in depressive symptoms from age 50 to 80. Psychol Aging. 2001;16(2):342–5.
23. Rokke PD, Klenow DJ. Prevalence of depressive symptoms among rural elderly: examining the need for mental health services. Psychotherapy. 1998;35(4):545–58.
24. Brown GW. Genetics of depression: a social science perspective. Int Rev Psychiatry. 1996;8(4):387–401.
25. Nazroo JY, Edwards AC, Brown GW. Gender differences in the onset of depression following a shared life event: a study of couples. Psychol Med. 1997;27(1):9–19.
26. Brown G, Harris T. Social origins of depression: a study of psychiatric disorder in women. London: Tavistock; 1978.
27. Vázquez-Barquero JL, Díez-Manrique JF, Peña C, Aldama J, Samaniego Rodríguez C, Menéndez Arango J, et al. A community mental health survey in Cantabria: a general description of morbidity. Psychol Med. 1987;17:227–41.
28. De Santiago A, Vázquez JL, Díez JF. [Article in Spanish] [The feminine role as a determinant of mental health among the women of the general population of Cantabria]. Actas Luso Esp Neurol Psiquiatr Cienc Afines. 1993;21(5):168–80.
29. Ferrando Bundío L. Salud Mental y Género en la práctica clínica. Ars Médica s.l.; 2007.
30. Mas Hesse J, Tesoro Amate A. Women and mental health, myths and realities. Madrid: s.n.; 1993, Spanish Association of Neuropsychiatry.
31. Holmström R, Koivisto RL, Niemi P. Differences in adjustment among university-educated men and women. Acta Psychiatr Scand Suppl. 1988;343:1–109.
32. Gove WR. The Relationship between sex roles, marital status, and mental illness. Soc Forces. 1972;51(1):34–44.
33. Ballinger CB, Smith AH, Hobbs PR. Factors associated with psychiatric morbidity in women: a general practice survey. Acta Psychiatr Scand. 1985;71:272–80.
34. Surtees PG, Dean C, Ingham JG, Kreitman NB, Miller P, Sashidharan SP. Psychiatric disorder in women from an Edinburgh community: association with demographic factors. Br J Psychiatry. 1983;142:238–46.
35. Finlay-Jones RA, Burvill PW. Contrasting demographic patterns of minor psychiatric morbidity in general practice and the community. Psychol Med. 1984;8:455–66.
36. Pinilla B, Salcedo M. Sintomatología psíquica en pacientes de medicina general: avance de hipótesis. Actas Luso Espa Neurol Psiquiatr. 1987;15:320–6.
37. Ge X, Lorenz FO, Conger RD, Elder GH, Simons RL. Trajectories of stressful life events and depressive symptoms during adolescence. Dev Psychol. 1994;30(4):467–83.
38. Nolen-Hoeksema S, Girgus JS. The emergence of gender differences in depression during adolescence. Psychol Bull. 1994;115(3):424–43.
39. Klaiber EL, Broverman DM, Vogel W, Kobayashi Y. Estrogen therapy for severe persistent depressions in women. Arch Gen Psychiatry. 1979;36(5):550–4.
40. Biegon A, McEwen BS. Modulation by estradiol of serotonin receptors in brain. J Neurosci. 1982;2(2):199–205.
41. Pajer K. New strategies in the treatment of depression in women. J Clin Psychiatry. 1995;56 Suppl 2:30–7.
42. Cohen IR, Wise PM. Effects of estradiol on the diurnal rhythm of serotonin activity in microdissected brain areas of ovariectomized rats. Endocrinology. 1988;122(6):2619–25.
43. Piccinelli M, Wilkinson G. Gender differences in depression. Critical review. Br J Psychiatry. 2000;177:486–92.
44. Gruenberg AM, Goldstein RD. Mood disorders: depression. In: Rasman A, Kay J, Lieberman JA, editors. Psychiatry, vol. 2. 2nd ed. Chichester: Wiley; 2003. p. 1207–36.
45. Levinton NE. superyó femenino. La moral en las mujeres. Madrid: Biblioteca Nueva; 2000.

46. Susan Nolen-Hoeksema S, Wisco BE, Lyubomirsky S. Rethinking rumination. Perspect Psychol Sci. 2008;3(5):400–24.
47. Mennin DS, Holaway RM, Fresco DM, Moore MT, Heimberg RG. Delineating components of emotion and its dysregulation in anxiety and mood psychopathology. Behav Ther. 2007;38 (3):284–302.
48. Nolen-Hoeksema S. Emotion regulation and psychopathology: the role of gender. Annu Rev Clin Psychol. 2012;8:161–87.
49. Campbell-Sills L, Barlow DH. Incorporating emotion regulation into conceptualizations and treatments of anxiety and mood disorders. In: Gross JJ, editor. Handbook of emotion regulation. New York: Guilford; 2007. p. 542–60.
50. Hyde JS, Mezulis AH, Abramson LY. The ABCs of depression: integrating affective, biological, and cognitive models to explain the emergence of the gender difference in depression. Psychol Rev. 2008;115(2):291–313.
51. Zahn-Waxler C, Shirtcliff EA, Marceau K. Disorders of childhood and adolescence: gender and psychopathology. Annu Rev Clin Psychol. 2008;4:275–303.
52. Zahn-Waxler C, Crick NR, Shirtcliff EA, Woods KE. The origins and development of psychopathology in females and males. In: Cohen D, Cicchetti D, editors. Handbook of developmental psychopathology. Hoboken, NJ: Wiley; 2006. p. 76–139.
53. Aldao A, Nolen-Hoeksema S, Schweizer S. Emotion-regulation strategies across psychopathology: a meta-analytic review. Clin Psychol Rev. 2010;30(2):217–37.
54. Gross JJ. The emerging field of emotion regulation: an integrative review. Rev Gen Psychol. 1998;2(3):271–99.
55. Wenzlaff RM, Wegner DM. Thought suppression. Annu Rev Psychol. 2000;51:59–91.
56. Barrett LF, Bliss-Moreau E. She's emotional. He's having a bad day: attributional explanations for emotion stereotypes. Emotion. 2009;9(5):649–58.
57. Barret LF, Lane RD, Sechrest L, Schwartz GE. Sex differences in emotional awareness. Personal Soc Psychol Bull. 2000;26:3–29.
58. Williams LE, Bargh JA, Nocera CC, Gray JR. The Unconscious regulation of emotion: nonconscious reappraisal goals modulate emotional reactivity. Emotion. 2009;9(6):847–54.
59. Rose AJ, Carlson W, Waller EM. Prospective associations of co-rumination with friendship and emotional adjustment: considering the socioemotional trade-offs of co-rumination. Dev Psychol. 2007;43(4):1019–31.
60. Nolen-Hoeksema S. Sex differences in unipolar depression: evidence and theory. Psychol Bull. 1987;101(2):259–82.
61. Lazarevich I, Mora-Carrasco F. Depresión y género: factores psicosociales de riesgo. Salud Problema, segunda época. 2008;1(4):9–18.
62. Barberá E, Martínez-Benlloch I. Psicología y género. Madrid: Pearson Prentice Hall; 2004.
63. Díaz-Loving R, Rocha Sánchez TE, Rivera AS. La instrumentalidad y la expresividad desde una perspectiva psico-socio-cultural. México: Porrúa y Facultad de Psicología; 2007.
64. Lara-Cantú MA. Inventario de Masculinidad y Femineidad. IMAFE. México: Manual Moderno; 1993.
65. Pérez Blasco J, Serra DE. Influencia del rol tradicional femenino en la sintomatología ansiosa en una muestra de mujeres adultas. Anales de Psicología. 1997;13(2):155–61.
66. Poal MG. Entrar, quedarse, avanzar: aspectos psicosociales de la relación mujer-mundo laboral. Madrid, España: Siglo XXI; 1993.
67. Medina-Mora ME, Borges G, Lara C, Benjet C, Blanco J, et al. Prevalencia de trastornos mentales y uso de servicios: Resultados de la Encuesta Nacional de Epidemiología Psiquiátrica en México. Salud Mental. 2003;26:1–16.
68. Lara M, Acevedo M. Incorporación de la mujer al trabajo remunerado: repercusiones para su salud reproductiva. In: Langer A, Tolbert K, editors. Mujer: sexualidad y salud reproductiva en México. México, DF: EDAMEX; 1996. p. 119–51.

69. Walters V, McDonough P, Strohschein L. The influence of work, household structure, and social, personal and material resources on gender differences in health: an analysis of the 1994 Canadian National Population Health Survey. Soc Sci Med. 2002;54(5):677–92.
70. Hoffman LW. Effects of maternal employment in the two-parent family. Am Psychol. 1989;44(2):283–92.
71. Hoffman LW, Youngblade LM. Mothers at work: effects on children's well-being. New York: Cambridge University Press; 1999.
72. Rodríguez Vega B, Bayón C, Franco B, Cañas F, Graell M, Salvador M. Parental rearing and intimate relations in women's depression. Acta Psychiatr Scand. 1993;88(3):193–7.
73. Adams CH, Sherer M. Sex-role orientation and psychological adjustment: comparison of MMPI profiles among college women and housewives. J Pers Assess. 1982;46(6):607–13.
74. Bassoff ES, Glass GV. The relationship between sex roles and mental health: a meta-analysis of twenty-six studies. Couns Psychol. 1982;10:105–12.
75. Taylor MC, Hall JA. Psychological androgyny: theories, methods, and conclusions. Psychol Bull. 1982;92(2):347–66.
76. O'Heron CA, Orlofsky JL. Stereotypic and nonstereotypic sex role trait and behavior orientations, gender identity, and psychological adjustment. J Pers Soc Psychol. 1990;58 (1):134–43.
77. Flaherty JF, Dusek JB. An investigation of the relationship between psychological androgyny and components of self-concept. J Pers Soc Psychol. 1980;38:984–92.
78. Kleimplatz P, McCarrey M, Kateb C. The impact of gender-role identity on women's self-esteem, lifestyle satisfaction and conflict. Can J Behav Sci. 1992;24(3):333–47.
79. Dio Bleichmar E. La Depresión en la Mujer. Madrid: Ediciones Temas de Hoy; 1991.
80. Kessler RC, McGonagle KA, Swartz M, Blazer DG, Nelson CB. Sex and depression in the National Comorbidity Survey. I: Lifetime prevalence, chronicity and recurrence. J Affect Disord. 1993;29(2–3):85–96.
81. Gómez OV. Relaciones de conflicto con el rol de género masculino y la actitud sexista con la violencia familiar, la ansiedad, la depresión y la calidad de vida de una muestra bogotana de hombres. Suma Psicológica. 2003;10(1):1–24.
82. Bird GW, Melville K. Families and intimate relationships. New York: McGraw-Hill; 1994.
83. O'Neil JM, Nadeau RA. Men's gender-role conflict, defense mechanism, and self protective defensive strategies: explaining men's violence against women from a gender role socialization perspective. In: O'Neil JM, Harway M, editors. What causes men's violence against women? Thousand Oaks, CA: Sage; 1999. p. 89–116.
84. Goldner V. Generation and gender: normative and covert hierarchies. In: Anderson C, Walsh F, McGoldrick M, editors. Women in families. New York: Norton; 1989.
85. Moreno Fernández A, Rodríguez Vega B, Carrasco Galán MJ, Sánchez Hernández JJ. Relación de pareja y sintomatología depresiva de la mujer: implicaciones clínicas desde una perspectiva de género. Apuntes de Psicología. 2009;27:489–506.
86. Carter NM, Williams M, Reynolds PD. Discontinuance among new firms in retail: the influence of initial resources, strategy, and gender. J Bus Ventur. 1997;12:125–45.
87. Knudson-Martin C. The politics of gender in family therapy. J Marital Fam Ther. 1997;23 (4):421–37.
88. Byrne M, Carr A. Depression and power in marriage. J Fam Ther. 2000;22:408–27.
89. Steil JM. Contemporary marriage: still an unequal partnership. In: Hendrick SS, Hendrick C, editors. Close relationships: a sourcebook. Thousand Oaks, CA: Sage; 2000. p. 125–52.
90. Coyne JC, Thompson R, Palmer SC. Marital quality, coping with conflict, marital complaints, and affection in couples with a depressed wife. J Fam Psychol. 2002;16(1):26–37.
91. Heene E, Buysse A, Van Oost P. An interpersonal perspective on depression: the role of marital adjustment, conflict communication, attributions, and attachment within a clinical sample. Fam Process. 2007;46(4):499–514.

92. Hollist CS, Miller RB, Falceto OG, Fernandes CL. Marital satisfaction and depression: a replication of the Marital Discord Model in a Latino sample. Fam Process. 2007;46(4):485–98.
93. Whiffen VE, Foot ML, Thompson JM. Self-silencing mediates the link between marital conflict and depression. J Soc Pers Relat. 2007;24(6):993–1006.
94. Halloran EC. The role of marital power in depression and marital distress. Am J Fam Ther. 1998;26(1):3–15.
95. Byrne M, Carr A, Clark M. Power in relationships of women with depression. J Fam Ther. 2004;26(4):407–29.
96. Simonds SL. Depression and women: an integrative treatment approach. New York, NY: Springer; 2001.
97. Jones E, Asen E. Systemic couple therapy and depression. London: Karnac Books; 2002.
98. Viveros M, Bernal M, Gómez F, Serna G. Masculinidades y violencia intrafamiliar en Colombia. Texto final de la consultoría presentada a la Consejería para la Política Social-Política de Construcción de Paz y Conciencia Familiar. Santafé de Bogotá: s.n.; 2000.
99. Campbell JC. A test of two explanatory models of women's responses to battering. Nurs Res. 1989;38(1):18–24.
100. Echeburúa E, de Corral P, Amor PJ, Sarasua B, Zubizarreta I. Repercusiones psicopatológicas de la violencia doméstica en la mujer: un estudio descriptivo. Revista de Psicopatología y Psicología Clínica. 1997;2(1):7–19.
101. Andrews B, Brown GW. Marital violence in the community. A biographical approach. Br J Psychiatry. 1988;153:305–12.
102. Walker LEA. The battered woman syndrome. New York: Springer; 1984/2000.
103. Andrews B, Brewin CR. Attributions of blame for marital violence. A study of antecedents and consequences. J Fam Marriage. 1990;52:757–67.
104. Lewinsohn PM, Hops H, Roberts RE, Seeley JR, Andrews JA. Adolescent psychopathology: I. Prevalence and incidence of depression and other DSM-III-R disorders in high school students. J Abnorm Psychol. 1993;102(1):133–44.
105. Galambos NL, Leadbeater BJ, Barker ET. Gender differences in and risk factors for depression in adolescence: a 4-year longitudinal study. Int J Behav Dev. 2004;28:16–25.
106. Essau CA, Lewinsohn PM, Seeley JR, Sasagawa S. Gender differences in the developmental course of depression. J Affect Disord. 2010;127(1–3):185–90.
107. Essau CA, Conradt J, Petermann F. Frequency, comorbidity, and psychosocial impairment of depressive disorders in adolescents. J Adolesc Res. 2000;15:470–81.
108. Cohen P, Cohen J, Kasen S, Velez CN, Hartmark C, Johnson J, Rojas M, Brook J, Streuning EL. An epidemiological study of disorders in late childhood and adolescence–I. Age and gender-specific prevalence. J Child Psychol Psychiatr. 1993;34(6):851–67.
109. De Rose LM, Wright AJ, Brooks-Gunn J. Does puberty account for the gender differential in depression? In: Keyes CLM, Goodman SH, editors. Women and depression: a handbook for the social, behavioral, and biomedical sciences. Cambridge, NY: Cambridge University Press; 2006. p. 89–128.
110. Cyranowski JM, Frank E, Young E, Shear MK. Adolescent onset of the gender difference in lifetime rates of major depression: a theoretical model. Arch Gen Psychiatry. 2000;57(1):21–7.
111. Weiss EL, Longhurst JG, Mazure CM. Childhood sexual abuse as a risk factor for depression in women: psychosocial and neurobiological correlates. Am J Psychiatry. 1999;156(6):816–28.
112. Shih JH, Eberhart NK, Hammen CL, Brennan PA. Differential exposure and reactivity to interpersonal stress predict sex differences in adolescent depression. J Clin Child Adolesc Psychol. 2006;35(1):103–15.
113. Nolen-Hoeksema S. Gender differences in depression. Curr Dir Psychol Sci. 2001;10:173–6.
114. Eaton WW, Anthony JC, Gallo J, Cai G, Tien A, Romanoski A, Lyketsos C, Chen LS. Natural history of Diagnostic Interview Schedule/DSM-IV major depression. The Baltimore Epidemiologic Catchment Area follow-up. Arch Gen Psychiatry. 1997;54 (11):993–9.

115. Kovacs M. Gender and the course of major depressive disorder through adolescence in clinically referred youngsters. J Am Acad Child Adolesc Psychiatry. 2001;40(9):1079–85.
116. Amenson CS, Lewinsohn PM. An investigation into the observed sex difference in prevalence of unipolar depression. J Abnorm Psychol. 1981;90(1):1–13.
117. Lewinsohn PM, Zeiss AM, Duncan EM. Probability of relapse after recovery from an episode of depression. J Abnorm Psychol. 1989;98(2):107–16.
118. Lewinsohn PM, Pettit JW, Joiner Jr TE, Seeley JR. The symptomatic expression of major depressive disorder in adolescents and young adults. J Abnorm Psychol. 2003;112(2):244–52.
119. Barnett RC, Brennan RT, Marshall NL. Gender and the relationship between parent role quality and psychological distress: a study of men and women in dual-earner couples. J Fam Issues. 1995;15:229–52.
120. Rohde P, Lewinsohn PM, Seeley JR. Are adolescents changed by an episode of major depression? J Am Acad Child Adolesc Psychiatry. 1994;33(9):1289–98.
121. Nolen-Hoeksema S. The role of rumination in depressive disorders and mixed anxiety/depressive symptoms. J Abnorm Psychol. 2000;109(3):504–11.
122. Teasdale JD. Cognitive vulnerability to persistent depression. Cogn Emot. 1988;2:247–74.
123. Jansson M, Gatz M, Berg S, Johansson B, Malmberg B, McClearn GE, Schalling M, Pedersen NL. Gender differences in heritability of depressive symptoms in the elderly. Psychol Med. 2004;34(3):471–9.
124. Kendler KS, Gatz M, Gardner CO, Pedersen NL. A Swedish national twin study of lifetime major depression. Am J Psychiatry. 2006;163(1):109–14.
125. Joiner T, Coyne JC, editors. The interactional nature of depression: advances in interpersonal approaches. Washington, DC: American Psychological Association; 1999.
126. Post RM, Weiss SRB. Neurobiology of treatment-resistant mood disorders. In: Bloom FE, Kupfer DJ, editors. Psychopharmacology. The fourth generation of progress. New York: Raven; 1994. p. 1155–70.
127. Birmaher B, Williamson DE, Dahl DE, Axelson DA, Kaufman J, Dorn LD, Ryan NR. Clinical presentation and course of depression in youth: does onset in childhood differ from onset in adolescence? J Am Acad Child Adolesc Psychiatry. 2004;43:63–70.
128. Merikangas KR, Cs G. Comorbidity for alcoholism and depression. Psychiatr Clin North Am. 1990;13(4):613–32.
129. Perkonigg A, Lieb R, Wittchen HU. Dependence of illicit drugs among adolescents and young adults in a community sample. Eur Addict Res. 1998;4:58–66.
130. Swendsen JD, Merikangas KR. The comorbidity of depression and substance use disorders. Clin Psychol Rev. 2000;20:173–89.
131. Kinnier RT, Metha AT, Okey JL, Keim L. Adolescent substance abuse and psychological health. J Alcohol Drug Educ. 1994;40:51–5.
132. Agosti V. QFSJMP. Somatization as a predictor of medication discontinuation due to adverse events. Int Clin Psychopharmacol. 2002;17:311–24.
133. Bennett DS, Ambrosini PJ, Kudes D, Metz C, Rabinovich H. Gender differences in adolescent depression: do symptoms differ for boys and girls? J Affect Disord. 2005;89(1–3):35–44.
134. Silverstein B. Gender differences in the prevalence of somatic versus pure depression: a replication. Am J Psychiatry. 2002;159:1051–2.
135. Moskvina V, Farmer A, Swainson V, O'Leary J, Gunasinghe C, Owen M. Interrelationship of childhood trauma, neuroticism, and depressive phenotype. Depress Anxiety. 2007;24(3):163–8.
136. Moskvina V, et al. Sex differences in symptom patterns of recurrent major depression in siblings. Depress Anxiety. 2008;25(6):527–34.
137. Gold PW, Chrousos GP. Organization of the stress system and its dysregulation in melancholic and atypical depression: high vs low CRH/NE states. Mol Psychiatry. 2002;7:254–75.
138. Klink R, Robichaud M, Debonnel G. Gender and gonadal status modulation of dorsal raphe nucleus serotonergic neurons. Part I: effects of gender and pregnancy. Neuropharmacology. 2002;43:1119–28.

139. Herbison AE. Estrogen regulation of GABA transmission in rat preoptic area. Brain Res Bull. 1997;44:321–6.
140. Antonijevic IA. Depressive disorders-is it time to endorse different pathophysiologies? Psychoneuroendocrinology. 2006;31(1):1–15.
141. Angst J, Dobler-Mikola A. The Zurich Study: a prospective epidemiological study of depressive, neurotic and psychosomatic syndromes. IV. Recurrent and nonrecurrent brief depression. Eur Arch Psychiatry Neurol Sci. 1985;234(6):408–16.
142. Benazzi F. Prevalence and clinical features of atypical depression in depressed outpatients: a 467-case study. Psychiatry Res. 1999;86:259–65.
143. Breslau N. SLPE. Sex differences in depression: a role for preexisting anxiety. Psychiatry Res. 1995;58:1–12.
144. Wilhelm K, Parker G, Hadzi-Pavlovic D. Fifteen years on: evolving ideas in researching sex differences in depression. Psychol Med. 1997;27(4):875–83.
145. Kessler RC. Gender differences in major depression: epidemiological findings. In: Frank E, editor. Gender and its effects on Psychopathology. Washington, DC: American Psychiatric Press; 2000. p. 61–84.
146. Weissman MM, Kidd KK, Prusoff BA. Variability in rates of affective disorders in relatives of depressed and normal probands. Arch Gen Psychiatry. 1982;39(12):1397–403.
147. Bierut LJ, Heath AC, Bucholz KK, Dinwiddie SH, Madden PA, Statham DJ, Dunne MP, Martin NG. Major depressive disorder in a community-based twin sample: are there different genetic and environmental contributions for men and women? Arch Gen Psychiatry. 1999;56(6):557–63.
148. Lyons MJ, Eisen SA, Goldberg J, True W, Lin N, Meyer JM, Toomey R, Faraone SV, Merla-Ramos M, Tsuang MT. A registry-based twin study of depression in men. Arch Gen Psychiatry. 1998;55(5):468–72.
149. Kendler KS, Prescott CA. A population-based twin study of lifetime major depression in men and women. Arch Gen Psychiatry. 1999;56(1):39–44.
150. Kendler KS, Neale MC, Kessler RC, Heath AC, Eaves LJ. A population-based twin study of major depression in women. The impact of varying definitions of illness. Arch Gen Psychiatry. 1992;49(4):257–66.
151. Kendler KS, Neale MC, Kessler RC, Heath AC, Eaves LJ. A longitudinal twin study of 1-year prevalence of major depression in women. Arch Gen Psychiatry. 1993;50(11):843–52.
152. Silberg J, Pickles A, Rutter M, Hewitt J, Simonoff E, Maes H, Carbonneau R, Murrelle L, Foley D, Eaves L. The influence of genetic factors and life stress on depression among adolescent girls. Arch Gen Psychiatry. 1999;56(3):225–32.
153. Accortt EE, Freeman MP, Allen JJ. Women and major depressive disorder: clinical perspectives on causal pathways. J Womens Health (Larchmt). 2008;17(10):1583–90.
154. Caspi A, Sugden K, Moffitt TE, Taylor A, Craig IW, Harrington H, McClay J, Mill J, Martin J, Braithwaite A, Poulton R. Influence of life stress on depression: moderation by a polymorphism in the 5-HTT gene. Science. 2003;301(5631):386–9.
155. Eley TC, Sugden K, Corsico A, Gregory AM, Sham P, McGuffin P, Plomin R, Craig IW. Gene-environment interaction analysis of serotonin system markers with adolescent depression. Mol Psychiatry. 2004;9(10):908–15.
156. Bundío BL, Rahola GJ. Trastornos depresivos en la mujer. In: Leal C, editor. Tratamiento de los trastornos afectivos en la mujer. Barcelona: Masson; 1999. p. 189–234.
157. Kornstein SG, Sloan DM, Thase ME. Gender-specific differences in depression and treatment response. Psychopharmacol Bull. 2002;36(4 Suppl 3):99–112.
158. Quitkin FM, Stewart JW, McGrath PJ, Taylor BP, Tisminetzky MS, Petkova E, Chen Y, Ma G, Klein DF. Are there differences between women's and men's antidepressant responses? Am J Psychiatry. 2002;159(11):1848–54.
159. Hildebrandt MG, Steyerberg EW, Stage KB, Passchier J, Kragh-Soerensen P. Danish University Antidepressant Group. Are gender differences important for the clinical effects of antidepressants? Am J Psychiatry. 2003;160(9):1643–50.
160. Keers R, Aitchison KJ. Gender differences in antidepressant drug response. Int Rev Psychiatry. 2010;22(5):485–500.

161. Davidson J, Pelton S. Forms of atypical depression and their response to antidepressant drugs Psychiatry Res. 1986;17(2):87–95.
162. Kornstein SG, Schatzberg AF, Thase ME, Yonkers KA, McCullough JP, Keitner GI, Gelenberg AJ, Davis SM, Harrison WM, Keller MB. Gender differences in treatment response to sertraline versus imipramine in chronic depression. Am J Psychiatry. 2000;157 (9):1445–52.
163. Henkel V, Mergl R, Allgaier AK, Kohnen R, Möller HJ, Hegerl U. Treatment of depression with atypical features: a meta-analytic approach. Psychiatry Res. 2006;141(1):89–101.
164. Joyce PR, Mulder RT, Luty SE, Sullivan PF, McKenzie JM, Abbott RM, Stevens IF. Patterns and predictors of remission, response and recovery in major depression treated with fluoxetine or nortriptyline. Aust N Z J Psychiatry. 2002;36(3):384–91.
165. Stewart JW, McGrath PJ, Quitkin FM. Do age of onset and course of illness predict different treatment outcome among DSM IV depressive disorders with atypical features? Neuropsychopharmacology. 2002;26(2):237–45.
166. Fava M, Rush AJ, Alpert JE, Balasubramani GK, Wisniewski SR, Carmin CN, et al. Difference in treatment outcome in outpatients with anxious versus nonanxious depression: a STAR*D report. Am J Psychiatry. 2008;165(3):342–51.
167. Olgiati P, Bajo E, Bigelli M, Montgomery S, Serretti A. C.E.A.P group. Challenging sequential approach to treatment resistant depression: cost-utility analysis based on the Sequenced Treatment Alternatives to Relieve Depression (STAR D) trial. Eur Neuropsychopharmacol. 2013;23(12):1739–46.
168. Khan A, Brodhead AE, Schwartz KA, Kolts RL, Brown WA. Sex differences in antidepressant response in recent antidepressant clinical trials. J Clin Psychopharmacol. 2005;25 (4):318–24.
169. Zanardi R, Rossini D, Magri L, Malaguti A, Colombo C, Smeraldi E. Response to SSRIs and role of the hormonal therapy in post-menopausal depression. Eur Neuropsychopharmacol. 2007;17(6–7):400–5.
170. Pae CU, Mandelli L, Kim TS, Han C, Masand PS, Marks DM, Patkar AA, Steffens DC, De Ronchi D, Serretti A. Effectiveness of antidepressant treatments in pre-menopausal versus post-menopausal women: a pilot study on differential effects of sex hormones on antidepressant effects. Biomed Pharmacother. 2009;63(3):228–35.
171. Schmidt PJ, Murphy JH, Haq N, Danaceau MA, St CL. Basal plasma hormone levels in depressed perimenopausal women. Psychoneuroendocrinology. 2002;27(8):907–20.
172. Morgan ML, Cook IA, Rapkin AJ, Leuchter AF. Estrogen augmentation of antidepressants in perimenopausal depression: a pilot study. Clin Psychiatry. 2005;66(6):774–80.
173. Nagata H, Nozaki M, Nakano H. Short-term combinational therapy of low-dose estrogen with selective serotonin re-uptake inhibitor (fluvoxamine) for oophorectomized women with hot flashes and depressive tendencies. J Obstet Gynaecol Res. 2005;31(2):107–14.
174. Papakostas GI, Thaseb ME, Favaa CM, Nelsond JC, Sheltone RC. Are antidepressant drugs that combine serotonergic and noradrenergic mechanisms of action more effective than the selective serotonin reuptake inhibitors in treating major depressive disorder? A meta-analysis of studies of newer agents. Biol Psychiatry. 2007;11(62):1217–27.
175. Papakostas GI, McGrath P, Stewart J, Charles D, Chen Y, Mischoulon D, Dording C, Fava M. Psychic and somatic anxiety symptoms as predictors of response to fluoxetine in major depressive disorder. Psychiatry Res. 2008;161(1):116–20.
176. Khan A, Schwartz KA, Kolts RL, Brown WA. BMI, sex, and antidepressant response. J Affect Disord. 2007;99(1–3):101–6.
177. Schuetz EG, Furuya KN, Schuetz JD. Interindividual variation in expression of P-glycoprotein in normal human liver and secondary hepatic neoplasms. J Pharmacol Exp Ther. 1995;275(2):1011–8.
178. Niznik HB, Tyndale RF, Sallee FR, Gonzalez FJ, Hardwick JP, Inaba T, Kalow W. The dopamine transporter and cytochrome P45OIID1 (debrisoquine 4-hydroxylase) in brain: resolution and identification of two distinct [3H] GBR-12935 binding proteins. Arch Biochem Biophys. 1990;276(2):424–32.

179. Cheung C, Yu AM, Ward JM, Krausz KW, Akiyama TE, Feigenbaum L, Gonzalez FJ. The cyp2e1-humanized transgenic mouse: role of cyp2e1 in acetaminophen hepatotoxicity. Drug Metab Dispos. 2005;33(3):449–57.
180. Relling MV, Lin JS, Ayers GD, Evans WE. Racial and gender differences in N-acetyltransferase, xanthine oxidase, and CYP1A2 activities. Clin Pharmacol Ther. 1992;52(6):643–58.
181. Tantcheva-Poór I, Zaigler M, Rietbrock S, Fuhr U. Estimation of cytochrome P-450 CYP1A2 activity in 863 healthy Caucasians using a saliva-based caffeine test. Pharmacogenetics. 1999;9(2):131–44.
182. Han XM, Ouyang DS, Chen XP, Shu Y, Jiang CH, Tan ZR, Zhou HH. Inducibility of CYP1A2 by omeprazole in vivo related to the genetic polymorphism of CYP1A2. Br J Clin Pharmacol. 2002;54(5):540–3.
183. Jin Y, Pollock BG, Frank E, Cassano GB, Rucci P, Müller DJ, et al. Effect of age, weight, and CYP2C19 genotype on escitalopram exposure. J Clin Pharmacol. 2010;50(1):62–72.
184. Granfors MT, Backman JT, Laitila J, Neuvonen PJ. Oral contraceptives containing ethinyl estradiol and gestodene markedly increase plasma concentrations and effects of tizanidine by inhibiting cytochrome P450 1A2. Clin Pharmacol Ther. 2005;78(4):400–11.
185. Hägg S, Spigset O, Dahlqvist R. Influence of gender and oral contraceptives on CYP2D6 and CYP2C19 activity in healthy volunteers. Br J Clin Pharmacol. 2001;51(2):169–73.
186. Laine K, Tybring G, Bertilsson L. No sex-related differences but significant inhibition by oral contraceptives of CYP2C19 activity as measured by the probe drugs mephenytoin and omeprazole in healthy Swedish white subjects. Clin Pharmacol Ther. 2000;68(2):151–9.
187. Tamminga WJ, Wemer J, Oosterhuis B, Wieling J, Wilffert B, de Leij LFMH, de Zeeuw RA, Jonkman JHG. CYP2D6 and CYP2C19 activity in a large population of Dutch healthy volunteers: indications for oral contraceptive-related gender differences. Eur J Clin Pharmacol. 1999;55:177–84.
188. Funck-Brentano C, Boëlle PY, Verstuyft C, Bornert C, Becquemont L, Poirier JM. Measurement of CYP2D6 and CYP3A4 activity in vivo with dextromethorphan: sources of variability and predictors of adverse effects in 419 healthy subjects. Eur J Clin Pharmacol. 2005;61(11):821–9.
189. Preskorn SH, Dorey RC, Jerkovich GS. Therapeutic drug monitoring of tricyclic antidepressants. Clin Chem. 1988;34(5):822–8.
190. Dahl ML, Bertilsson L, Nordin C. Steady-state plasma levels of nortriptyline and its 10-hydroxy metabolite: relationship to the CYP2D6 genotype. Psychopharmacology. 1996;123(4):315–9.
191. Abernethy DR, Greenblatt DJ, Shader RI. Imipramine and desipramine disposition in the elderly. J Pharmacol Exp Ther. 1985;232(1):183–8.
192. Hiemke C, Härtter S. Pharmacokinetics of selective serotonin reuptake inhibitors. Pharmacol Ther. 2000;85:11–28.
193. Gex-Fabry M, Eap CB, Oneda B, et al. CYP2D6 and ABCB1 genetic variability: influence on paroxetine plasma level and therapeutic response. Ther Drug Monit. 2008;30:474–82.
194. Reis M, Lundmark J, Bengtsson F. Therapeutic drug monitoring of racemic citalopram: a 5-year experience in Sweden, 1992-1997. Ther Drug Monit. 2003;25:183–91.
195. Perroud N, Aitchison KJ, Uher R, Smith R, Huezo-Diaz P, Marusic A, et al. Genetic predictors of increase in suicidal ideation during antidepressant treatment in the GENDEP project. Neuropsychopharmacology. 2009;34:2517–28.
196. Perroud N, Uher R, Marusic A, Rietschel M, Mors O, Henigsberg N, et al. Suicidality during treatment of depression with escitalopram and nortriptyline in GENDEP: a clinical trial. BMC Med. 2009;7:60.
197. Gupta B, Keers R, Uher R, McGuffin P, Aitchison KJ. Pharmacogenetics of antidepressant response. In: Pariante C, Nesse RM, Nutt D, Wolpert L, editors. Understanding depression: a translational approach. New York: Oxford University; 2009.
198. Serretti A, Kato M, De Ronchi D, Kinoshita T. Meta-analysis of serotonin transporter gene promoter polymorphism (5-HTTLPR) association with selective serotonin reuptake inhibitor efficacy in depressed patients. Mol Psychiatry. 2007;12:247–57.

199. Mrazek DA, Rush AJ, Biernacka JM, et al. SLC6A4 variation and citalopram response. Am J Med Genet B Neuropsychiatr Genet. 2008;150:341–51.
200. Huezo-Diaz P, Uher R, Smith R, Rietschel M, Henigsberg N, Marus A, et al. Moderation of antidepressant response by the serotonin transporter gene in the GENDEP study. Br J Psychiatry. 2009;195:30–8.
201. Phyllis T. A developmental line of gender identity role and choice of love of subject. J Am Psychoanal Assoc. 1986;30:61–86.
202. Beck AT. Cognitive therapy and the emotional disorders. New York, NY: Meridian; 1976.
203. Abramson LY, Metalsky GI, Alloy LB. Hopelessness depression: a theory-based subtype of depression. Psychol Rev. 1989;96:358–72.
204. Seligman MEP. Helplessness: on depression, development, and death. San Francisco: W.H. Freeman; 1975.
205. DeRubeis RJ, Evans MD, Hollon SD, Garvey MJ, Grove WM. y Tuason VB. How does cognitive therapy work? Cognitive change and symptom change in cognitive therapy and pharmacotherapy for depression. J Consult Clin Psychol. 1990;58:862–9.
206. Agency for Health Care Policy and Research Depression Guideline Panel. Depression in primary care: Vol. 2. Treatment of major depression (Clinical Practice Guideline No. 5; ACHPR Publication No. 93"0551). Rockville, MD: U.S. Department of Health and Human Services, Public Health Service; 1993.
207. Elkin I, Shea MT, Watkins JT, Imber SD, Sotsky SM, Collins JF, Glass DR, Pilkonis PA, Leber WR, Docherty JP, et al. National Institute of Mental Health Treatment of Depression Collaborative Research Program. General effectiveness of treatments. Arch Gen Psychiatry. 1989;46(11):971–82.

Anxiety Disorders

24

Ane Eizaguirre, Karim Haidar, and Margarita Sáenz-Herrero

Abstract

Anxiety disorders are more prevalent among women than men. A higher prevalence of anxiety in women compared with men has been repeatedly reported in the literature. The disorders include agoraphobia, post-traumatic stress disorder (PTSD), and generalized anxiety disorder (GAD). Similar data between the two sexes have been obtained for social phobia and obsessive compulsive disorder (OCD). This suggests that biological, psychosocial, and cultural factors are related. The aim of this review is to incorporate sex and gender considerations into anxiety disorders, including current psychological theories and treatment of anxiety disorders.

Lower levels of assertiveness and self-support in women compared with men and men's lower levels of inclination toward dependency and helplessness contribute to the higher prevalence of reported anxiety in women. Gendered aspects of daily life can play a role as well. The relationship between psychopathology and femininity is itself a matter of discussion because it is assumed that masculine behavior is taken as the standard for mental health. From our point of view and because the methodological problems in research did not

A. Eizaguirre
Department of Psychiatry, Alava University Hospital, Vitoria, Spain
e-mail: ANE.EIZAGUIRREGARCIA@osakidetza.net

K. Haidar
Department of Psychiatry, Alava University Hospital, Vitoria, Spain
e-mail: MAHMOUD.KARIMHAIDAR@osakidetza.net

M. Sáenz-Herrero (✉)
Department of Psychiatry, Alava University Hospital, Vitoria, Spain

University of the Basque Country UPV/EHU, Vitoria, Spain
e-mail: margarita.saenzherrero@osakidetza.net

M. Sáenz-Herrero (ed.), *Psychopathology in Women*,
DOI 10.1007/978-3-319-05870-2_24

permit an objective review of this kind of complex causation, this could only result in speculation with regard to the available data. To explore the role of culture and ethnicity, future research is needed. The World Health Organization has identified gender as a critical determinant of mental Health and mental illness and suggested that integrating gender considerations in health research contributes to better science and consequently to more effective and efficient mental health programs.

24.1 Introduction

It is increasingly defended that being a man or woman influences not only the prevalence of mental disorders but also the manifestation and expression of symptoms, the willingness to request medical and psychological assistance, the course of the disease, and even the response to treatment [1, 2]. The WHO considers that not enough attention was being paid to the specific determinants of each sex in the mechanisms that promote and protect mental health and boost resistance to stress and adversity [3]. Whereas widespread attention has been paid to sex differences in the prevalence of anxiety disorders and their possible origins, limited research has been carried out on the gender perspective of these differences, which could influence treatment provided to these patients.

We define sex as the biological features distinguishing male and female animals and human beings, whereas gender consists of the socio-cultural aspects of defining people's identity in relation to sex.

It is interesting to dedicate a separate section to the subject of gender and its relationship with anxiety. Understanding the construct of gender from a wide point of view, which we do not delve into here, but distinguishing it from differences between the sexes from anatomical and purely biological perspectives, we can reach numerous conclusions, which are named specifically in subsequent sections with regard to anxiety, which is the subject at hand.

Therefore, from the gender point of view, certain attributes have historically been given to women and men; these inexorably represent the roles of each, circumscribed on the basis of these attributes. While male sex is related to public space, the abstract, the word, the active, female sex is related to the private, passive, to submission. In this way the social, economic, political roles, among others, to which each gender is assigned are different and lie below a dichotomy construct between opposites [4].

From an anthropological perspective Marilyn Strathern and Carol Cormack [5, 6] have stated a discourse about nature and culture that usually portrays nature as feminine; it must be subordinated to a culture that is constantly presented as active and abstract. Mind and reason are related to masculinity, whereas the body and nature are associated with femininity, awaiting significance provided by an opposing subject.

Thus, so-called symbolic domination is produced, which often adopts the form of bodily emotions—shame, humiliation, shyness, anxiety, and guilt—or passions and feelings—love, admiration, respect—and sometimes more painful emotions when they become more visible manifestations such as flushing, verbal confusion, clumsiness, shaking, anger, or impotent rage, all of which are ways of being subjected, although it may be despite oneself, to the subterranean complicity of the guidelines of the conscience and willpower, which maintain social structures with inherent censure.

Although a specific section is devoted to each anxiety entity, the influence of gender, and its role in the distinct psychopathological expression between men and women, we can advance or propose their possible influence. For example, on the genesis of phobia and the rate of prevalence, where the woman, by being subjugated to the private space, fundamental to the household, could have greater difficulty, from this perspective, to be exposed to the public, both in presence and in manifestations (posture, language, etc.).

The different roles could influence the psychopathological expression of different mental diseases to such an extent that our own social dynamic is influenced by them. This can be observed thanks to transgenerational changes that represent changes in the expression of the different roles and changes in representations, perceptions, appreciations, and opinions of society in general and the individual in particular. To this fact we should add the transcultural differences observable in gender roles, with significant ethnographic differences. Global analysis of these and other variables could bring us closer to understanding the influence of gender on different psychopathological expressions as a whole and, consequently, attempt to understand what these differences are caused by, explain the different prevalences of the various pathologies and their symptomatology, and therapeutic alternatives based on this analysis.

24.2 Epidemiological Data

In several research studies of anxiety disorders of different population and cultural samples, women present prevalence figures that are substantially higher than those observed among men [7, 8]. It has been detected that women usually present a subjective perception of lower psychological welfare, worse quality of life, and worse state of health than men [9, 10]. The existence of anxiety disorders complicates or increases the risk of significant disability in the population that suffers from it, a disability similarly serious to that observed in other chronic diseases [11]. In general terms there are predisposing factors (genetics, somatic diseases, psychological traumas during development, absence of coping mechanisms, thought, beliefs, and distorted cognitive processing) and other precipitating factors (somatic or toxic problems, external and intense long-lasting stress, stress that affects vulnerability, and other factors [12, 13].

Other factors that suggest differences between sexes with regard to anxiety disorders in general are previous comorbidity, genetic predisposition, personality traits, sexual hormones, endocrine reactivity to stress, the systems of neurotransmission, and neuropsychological determinants [14, 15].

Despite the lack of studies, there is more and more solid evidence that differences exist between the two sexes with regard to cerebral anatomy, neurochemistry, and activation and response patterns to environmental stimuli, as well as differences in the physiology and physiopathology of other body systems, differences that might influence the etiology and course of psychiatric disorders [16].

Over the menopausal period, different conditions have been proposed that could contribute to the genesis of anxiety symptomatology such as children leaving home ("empty nest"), the termination of work activity, changes in roles within the family, the appearance of diseases, loss of interpersonal relationships, and changes in physical appearance [17].

Anxiety disorders are more prevalent among women than among men according to a literature review. Most data on the prevalence of anxiety disorders are based on self-reports and various authors have hypothesized that observed sex differences are due, at least partly, to less willingness in men to report symptoms of anxiety [18, 19].

Traditional masculine sex-role stereotypes may make it difficult for men to openly display weakness in general (crying) One may argue that the data regarding social phobia 1:1 do not support this assumption. Again the possibility that the true proportion of men with social phobia is higher than that of women cannot be ruled out because of the role that shame may play in men.

From a methodological point of view, prevalence differences may be an artifact associated with men's inhibition with regard to reporting symptoms, again ensuing from masculinity standards. The type of self-report measure used may influence the degree to which sex differences emerge. Furthermore, the relationship between psychopathology and femininity is itself a matter of discussion, because one may assume that masculine behavior is often, but erroneously, taken as the standard for mental health [20].

24.3 Psychological Models of Anxiety Disorders

Bekker and Van Mens-Verhulst [20] explain the psychological theories of anxiety disorders. They begin with the learning perspective, which is the theory that is most extensively studied in the field of anxiety disorders, then sex-role theories, and finally attachment and schema theory.

24.3.1 Learning Perspective

From this perspective one could question why more women than men develop phobic fear responses and/or phobic avoidance behavior. Using the terms conditioning or learning and gender or sex differences provides few clues. Authority works on anxiety disorders do not offer gender-specific viewpoints on the etiology of learned behavior, even if they consider the prevalence and possible background of sex differences.

It has been hypothesized that women are more vulnerable to being conditioned to fear responses. There is evidence supporting an exposure hypothesis (women compared with men are more frequently exposed to anxiety-evoking traumas and a vulnerability to anxiety disorders). Women's more frequent exposure to sexual violence has repeatedly been mentioned, as well as domestic violence against women, and poverty, all of which support the exposure hypothesis.

In addition to women being exposed to the trauma of sexual violence more often than men, other aversive stimuli occur more frequently in women's lives and/or may provoke more fear in them (lack of affirmation of one's personal identity, going out "unprepared" not in line with existing norms, not having acquired the skills needed in public, anonymous situations. Future research could focus on the gender-specific meanings of the situations being feared and avoided and relate these to their significance for specific demographic and individual differences and also for various subgroups of women [20].

24.3.2 Sex/Gender Role Perspective

From the sex-role perspective, phobic avoidance behavior is an inevitable product of Western culture. The traditional feminine sex role discourages assertiveness and self-supportive behavior in women and prescribes them to react to stress with dependence and helplessness [21–26].

This sex-role perspective on anxiety disorders has been studied since the 1970s, mainly in relation to agoraphobia. Agoraphobia in women was expected to decrease in frequency as Western culture placed more demands on women to be employed outside the home and to be self-reliant and assertive. From this perspective the sex role not only comprises the gender role, but also the socioeconomic positions society expects women and men to take. Two epidemiological studies supplied evidence for the hypothesis that the frequency of phobia among women might decrease as their employment increased. However, to our knowledge this relationship has not been investigated during the past decade.

Another approach within the sex-role perspective is to focus on a culture's masculinity and femininity. Based on the aforementioned assumption that sex roles and phobia within Western culture are frequently related, the degree of masculinity/femininity in 11 countries was compared (in countries with high masculinity, social gender roles are clearly distinct; in those with low masculinity/high femininity, gender differentiation is weak) High masculinity predicted higher national levels of agoraphobia and several specific fears, but not cross-national differences in social fears.

Another individual-level, gender-role approach to anxiety and other disorders focuses on gender role stress (GRS). This approach places more emphasis on the stressful side of the gender role than does the sex role model, which uses more neutral feminine and masculine characteristics. The original authors defined GRS as stress resulting from a rigid commitment to gender roles, together with inherently dysfunctional coping. Masculine GRS components are (fear of) physical inadequacy, emotional expressiveness, subordination to women's intellectual inferiority, and performance failure. However, this study lacked both a measure of feminine GRS and a stress measure that may be more neutral. Therefore, it remains unknown whether the association would have been found for stress regardless of gender-bound nature, or whether it is specifically for masculine GRS.

24.3.3 Attachment and Schema Theory: Gender Neutral and Gender Specific

Schemata are the inner working models to others that children develop in relation to their primary caregivers. If children experience their primary caregivers as insufficiently available or responsive to their needs, they develop a condition of insecure attachment. In the case of anxiety disorder, the insecure attachment may predominantly involve a fearful or avoidant attachment style. Most studies on attachment and anxiety disorders failed to report sex differences in the patterns of insecure attachment styles. This may have occurred because the original theory on attachment (as well as the schema theory) is gender neutral. With feminist neopsychoanalytical theory, a gender-specific version of the attachment theory has become available [27]. Authors consider the fact that the primary attachment person in children's lives is usually a woman—their mother—which provides a source of sex differences in autonomy development [28–30].

Considered from this perspective, the early same-sex mother–daughter relationship would imply that the symbiotic phase with the mother is longer, more enduring, and more intense for girls than it is for boys. As a result, girls would meet more problems with individuation and separation, boys with commitment and displaying their dependency needs.

The fact that insecure attachment may be expressed in sex-specific insecure attachment styles and patterns of autonomy connectedness may contribute to the unequal prevalence of many mental disorders, including anxiety disorders between the sexes.

24.3.4 Clarification Remarks and Proposals

One explanation refers to the lower levels of assertiveness and self-support in women compared with men, and men's lower levels of inclination toward dependency and helplessness, all factors that contribute to anxiety complaints. Also, alcohol abuse appeared to be a masculine (thus gendered) masking strategy. On the other hand, using anxiolytics and engaging in binging can be assumed to be feminine masking strategies. Gendered aspects of daily life can play a role as well. However, neither the role of feminine gender role stress nor the interaction with gender-neutral stress has been studied in relation to these factors.

Sexual and physical assaults must be acknowledged as etiological factors with the unchallenged fact that the percentage of female survivors surpasses that of men by almost tenfold.

There are those who defend the theory that despite sociocultural determinants influencing the psychopathological differences in anxiety between the two sexes, they do not explain the differences in the prevalence of anxiety disorders. Nor do the processes of socialization and sexual roles determine those differences [31, 32].

It is plausible that other psychological and biological factors are also important, such as a more feminine pattern of reacting to bodily sensations in interaction with specific attachment styles. More research remains to be done in these areas.

The relationship between psychopathology and femininity is in itself a matter of discussion, because one may assume that masculine behavior is often, but erroneously, taken as the standard for mental health.

There are deficiencies in sex-specific information on the prevalence of the common Diagnostic and Statistical Manual of Mental Disorders (DSM) anxiety disorders in specific ethnic groups, as well as prevalence in non-Western anxiety disorders in and outside of Western countries, including their gender distribution. To explore the role of culture and ethnicity, future research should determine whether and to what extent changes are occurring in the distribution of specific subtypes of anxiety disorders.

From our point of view gender roles should be given more attention in therapy research. More data should be collected on the gender characteristics of patients, therapists, and therapeutic relationships, instead of sex characteristics only.

24.4 Biological Factors

A common genetic vulnerability exists for panic disorder, generalized anxiety, agoraphobia, and affective disorders [33]. This vulnerability consists of a neurobiological response of hyperactivity to stress, with a chronic increase in the function of the neurochemical systems (corticotropin- and adrenaline-releasing factor) that mediate in the response to stress, and that act on determined cerebral regions (hippocampus and medial prefrontal, temporal, parietal, and cingulate cortex) [34].

When the activity of the amygdala, which is crucial for subjects in remembering the emotional events after viewing slides of disturbing images, was assessed, men who showed an intense emotional response exhibited greater activity in the right amygdala, while women exhibited greater activity in the left amygdala [35, 36]. Whereas anxiety due to separation from the mother increased the concentration of serotonin receptors in the amygdala of boys, the same situation decreased the concentration of these receptors in girls. If we add to this theory that the production of serotonin is 52 % higher in the male subject than in the female [37, 38], it turns out to be a very interesting and promising line of research to be able to understand the predisposition of women to developing anxiety and mood disorders.

24.4.1 Sexual Hormones

For many years, the differences between the sexes and the role that the gonadal hormones played in these differences were studied by focusing exclusively on sexual conduct. Currently, apart from controversies, it is accepted that sexual differentiation implies diverse structural, chemical, and functional variants between the brain of the male and that of the female, that affect all the areas of the subject [37, 38]. With regard to differences in response to stress that are seen in both sexes, the possible influence of sexual hormones has been described [39]. It has been reported that estrogens could influence the response to stress mediated by noradrenalin. These are important facilitators of the serotonergic response in humans [40].

Women of reproductive age are more vulnerable to developing anxiety disorders than men, between 2 to 3 times more. In fact, 17.5 % of women compared with 9.5 % of men suffered some kind of anxiety disorder during their lifetime, while 8.7 % of women compared with 3.8 % of men had suffered an anxiety disorder over the last year [41, 42].

If we also take into account that the changes introduced by reproductive hormones during the intrauterine phase and puberty, the menstrual cycle, pregnancy, and the menopause, clearly modify the cerebral structure and function, all of which suggest that sexual hormones play a deciding role in etiology and in the clinical manifestations of these pathological conditions [16, 43]. It has been speculated that a primary post-puberty effect of the gonadal hormones on the stimulation of the limbic system might predispose women to higher rates of anxiety and affective disorders [32].

To be precise, anxiety diminishes during pregnancy [44] and the luteal phase of the woman's menstrual cycle. A deterioration of the symptoms of many anxiety disorders following birth is observed and seems to indicate that progesterone may play an important role in the differences between sexes with regard to anxiety disorders. Sutter-Dallay [45] observed that a quarter of women with an anxiety disorder suffered a probability of depression during the postpartum period three times greater than the general population [45]. Similarly, it is noticeable that information existing about anxiety disorders in the menopause is scarce and a high level of prescription and self-medication of anxiolytics is observed at this stage of life [17].

Hormonal changes that occur during the menstrual cycle could also influence the anxiety symptomatology present in the context of a premenstrual dysphoric disorder, which is usually pronounced [46, 47], as well as in the context of anxiety disorders. It is known that anxiety disorders tend to deteriorate over the premenstrual period [48], when ovarian hormones are at their lowest level in the cycle.

Hsiao et al. [49] observed that a significant percentage of women with generalized anxiety disorder (GAD) and panic disorder (PD) together with the premenstrual disorder syndrome also suffered exacerbation of their symptomatology in the premenstrual phase, which we consider to be the possible influence of the hormonal cycle of a woman with anxiety symptoms. The exacerbation of the symptomatology in the premenstrual and follicular phase that women with GAD and associated premenstrual tension syndrome mention does not appear in the phase that only presents GAD [48].

The syndrome of premenstrual tension has been associated with anxiety disorders, especially with GAD and PD, with which on occasions a differential diagnosis is proposed [50]. But a separate chapter in the same book is dedicated to the dysphoric premenstrual syndrome; therefore, we do not analyze the possible analogies and common influences of the two disorders here. We tackle changes related to the gonadal influence in each subtype of anxiety disorder in subsequent epilogues that will deal with the differential characteristics between the two sexes in each corresponding entity

24.5 Subtypes of Anxiety Disorders

The diagnostic categorical criteria usually used are subject to continual modifications in the different versions of international classifications such as the DSM. The DSM-5 [51] comprises disorders that share features of excessive fear and anxiety and related behavioral disturbances. Fear is the emotional response to real or perceived imminent threat, whereas anxiety is anticipation of future threat.

Anxiety disorders in DSM-5 are arranged developmentally, with disorders sequenced according to the typical age at onset. DSM-5 contains specific phobia, social anxiety disorder (social phobia), panic disorder, agoraphobia without a history of panic disorder, generalized anxiety disorder, anxiety disorder due to a medical disease, anxiety disorder induced by substances, and unspecified anxiety disorder [51]. This edition also includes separation anxiety disorder and selective mutism. Obsessive compulsive disorder (OCD) and related disorders are in another section of DSM-5 classification.

We try hereby to explain the different subtypes, emphasizing the anxiety disorders that from a gender perspective deserve particular attention.

24.5.1 Separation Anxiety Disorder

The individual with separation anxiety disorder is fearful or anxious about separation from attachment figures to a degree that is developmentally inappropriate. There is persistent fear or anxiety about harm coming to attachment figures and events that could lead to loss of separation from attachment figures, and reluctance to be parted from attachment figures, as well as nightmares and physical symptoms of distress. Although the symptoms often develop in childhood, they can be expressed throughout adulthood as well [51].

24.5.2 Selective Mutism

Selective mutism is characterized by a consistent failure to speak in social situations in which there is an expectation to speak (e.g., school) even though the individual speaks in other situations. The failure to speak has significant consequences for achievement in academic or occupational settings or otherwise interferes with normal social communication [51].

24.5.3 Phobia

The word phobia derives from the Greek term "*phobos*," which means fear, panic or terror. The term social phobia was introduced by Janet in 1903 and acquired its own identity with the classification of Marks in 1969 [20]. Anxiety acquired a core importance as the pathogenic origin of the phobic disorder, whose presence contributes to its self-perpetuation. According to Lepine and Chignon [52] the diagnosis of this entity requires the presence of the feared object and situation, anxious manifestations, which, as we say, are of special relevance, an anti-phobic reaction and difficulties in functioning well for the sufferer.

Although there is a predominance of phobic disorders in the female, there appear to be differences according to the type of phobia. These differences are explained by the diverse mechanisms that could have an influence such as ideological factors, the social facilitation of aggressive behavior and courage in the male, and the greater tendency in men to not admit fear, because it damages self esteem and social consideration. The DSM-5 [51] distinguishes social phobia, specific phobia, and agoraphobia as the main entities that make up phobic disorders in general.

24.5.4 Social Anxiety Disorder (Social Phobia)

We can briefly sum up social phobia as an acute and persistent fear of one or more social situations or events in public in which the subject feels exposed to persons that do not belong to the family environment or to possible assessment by others [13].

We distinguish between social phobia, generalized (referring to most social situations) and nongeneralized social phobia, where the phobia is particularly about speaking in public; the DSM-5 specifies performance only: if the fear is restricted to speaking or performing in public. Although this classification may seem not to be definitive. There are those who defend the idea that it is a continuum of gravity that deals with different aspects of a same spectrum of social anxiety [53]. According to other authors the distinction between social phobia and personality disorder by avoidance is not even conclusive, postulating the fact that they form part of the same psychopathological context [54–56].

According to DSM-5 [51], hypersensitivity to criticism of the assessment of others, the difficulty in self-affirmation, low self-esteem, and feelings of inferiority are some of the characteristics of this type of phobia.

Over recent years, numerous publications on this subject have given an idea of the growing attention that this entity receives [57, 58], partly because of great comorbidity, 70–80 % with other psychiatric disorders, above all from the anxiety series, depression, substance abuse, panic disorders, and personality disorders [59]. Yonkers et al. [60] observed a greater tendency toward substance abuse in men; women, on the other hand, tended to present agoraphobia [60]. In the same study they described how women, who had backgrounds of attempted suicide and a worse premorbid adjustment, had a worse prognosis.

It has been observed that diagnosed women usually present deterioration in symptoms in the premenstrual phase of the cycle, the same as pregnant women, who exhibit an increase in social anxiety levels during the first 3 months of pregnancy [61].

It appears that several authors agree that both environmental and genetic factors influence social phobia [13, 62, 63]. Psychosocially, childhood environmental factors have been reported (imitation of parental phobia conduct, overprotection, anxious parents, etc.); conflicts during adulthood are also identified as contributing to their appearance (fundamentally traumatic situations) [13, 64]. Personality in general shows characteristics of introversion (shyness and dependence), which some authors defend, and is linked equally to the evasive personality disorder [13, 54]. Other environmental factors that we could mention are the lack of social support, low educational level, and single status [13, 65].

24.5.5 Specific Phobia

These are acute and persistently irrational, excessive, out of control fears and occur in the presence or anticipation of specific objects or situations that the subject tries to avoid [13].

Specific phobias are considered to constitute the third most frequent psychiatric disorder, with a prevalence throughout a lifetime of 12.5 %. Women have a greater tendency to present social phobia [13, 66]. The age at appearance is very early; it is considered one of the most precocious psychiatric pathological conditions, with an average onset around the age of 7, according to studies [67]. Women have a greater frequency of a phobia of animals and men of heights (acrophobia) [68].

Comorbidity in social phobia is relatively frequent; the most accredited disorders are social phobia, substance abuse, and depression [69]. Among women, comorbidity has been reported in 28.3 % of anxiety disorders, 13.7 % of affective disorders, 3.2 % of somatoform disorders, 2.2 % of substance-related disorders, and 4 % of food disorders [68].

With regard to etiopathogenesis, it seems that the genetic load could have a greater influence in men; among women societal family factors have had greater relevance [70]. Genetic polymorphism of catechol-O-methyltransferase (COMT) has been linked to specific phobia [71].

24.5.6 Panic Disorder

Panic (*angustia* in Spanish, *angst* in English (borrowed from the German), and the verb *ängstigen* in German) is defined by an affliction, distress or oppressive fear without a precise cause. Etymologically, it shares the same Greek root as the verb *anjo*, which actively means to press, asphyxiate, while in its passive sense it means to drown, with other terms such as *anjoné*, *agón*, *agoniates*, *angere*, *angustus* [72].

Panic disorder appears in sudden episodes, during the daytime or at night, characterized by a neurovegetative discharge, intense moral panic, frequent feeling of impending death, anxiety, and eventual psychomotor unrest, with a duration of approximately 15–30 min [13].

It is not our aim to carry out a nosographic revision of the term, although it is interesting to mention that several of the symptoms previously mentioned were described in the twentieth century BC, in the Kahun papyrus, attributing it to the uterus. In addition, Hippocrates named these anxious manifestations, presented in paroxysmal form, under the term "hysteria," explaining them with mechanistic reasoning, where the uterus is displaced by the body pressing on the chest and the throat, a fact that was linked to unsatisfactory sexual relations [72].

Life prevalence is estimated to be 4.7 %; epidemiological studies speak of an incidence that is twice as high among women as among men [41, 66, 73, 74]. Marked differences have been described in the age at presentation of the panic disorder; it is estimated that in women it appears between the ages of 25 and 34, and in men the onset is described as being later at around 35–44 [75].

With regard to the clinical aspects, women speak of more psychological symptoms of the panic disorder with greater frequency [76]. Among women anticipatory anxiety is more frequent [75], whereas men exhibit greater worries at the somatic clinic [77]. Somatic manifestations also show differences: in women the presence of respiratory symptoms and dizziness is more frequent [78], whereas among men the most frequent are gastrointestinal symptoms [79].

Comorbidity of panic disorder with other psychiatric pathological conditions of the anxiety spectrum (OCD, GAD, social phobia), mood disorders (depression and dysthymia), impulse control, and substance abuse exists [80, 81]. The course of the disease is chronic, with periods of variable remission [82, 83]; women have a worse evolution of the disease, a factor of bad prognosis being identified for women [84]. Among women higher rates of relapse are observed [85, 86], and it is a more disabling pathological condition [73, 81]. High rates of cardiovascular mortality and suicide have been detected among individuals with panic disorder [87]; suicide has been related to depression, substance abuse, and personality disorders [88]. In women suicide rates are three times higher than those of men [89]. In women with panic disorder a higher rate of smoking has been observed at the start and during the disease than for men [90].

With regard to etiology, panic disorder has been related to a background of trauma during infancy; this relation, which is also present in other anxiety disorders, is more intense in panic disorder [91].

A greater predisposition of women to traumatic events that evoke anxiety disorders has been mentioned, such as sexual abuse, domestic violence, and poverty [20].

The debate on genetic influence in panic disorder is still open [92]. Genetic polymorphism of the COMT has been linked (Val 158met), with panic disorder among women. Recently, this polymorphism has been related to a greater activation of the amygdala and prefrontal cortex in panic disorder [93, 94].

Other neuroimaging studies identify that men show a higher reduction in the right amygdala and in the bilateral insular cortex, whereas women showed a more marked decrease in the right temporal lobe, in the dorsolateral prefrontal and ventrolateral cortex, in the parietal cortex, and in the thalamus [95].

It is known that the progesterone metabolites may have anxiolytic effects owing to their agonist action on γ-aminobutyric acid/benzodiazepine (GABA/BZD) receptors [96], by which a possible alteration in this complex receptor could explain the factors that link panic responses, reproductive female cycle, and premenstrual tension (PMT) [79]. In particular, women with panic disorder presented a reduction in receptor sensibility that was not observed among men [97]. It has been observed that women with PMT tend to have panic following exposure to different panicogenic agents such as lactate, CO_2, or the antagonists of cholecystokinin [98].

24.5.7 Agoraphobia

The DSM-IV subordinates this entity to panic disorder, although it contemplates agoraphobia without a panic crisis. Agoraphobia is diagnosed in DSM-5 irrespective of the presence of panic disorder. If an individual's presentation meets criteria for panic disorder and agoraphobia, both diagnoses should be assigned [51].

Agoraphobia is defined as "irrational fear of places or public places," although this extends to the fear of not being able to escape inmediately from a place in which it is difficult to ask for help. Both entities, panic disorder with or without agoraphobia according to NCS-R 2007, are more frequent among women [66].

Expulsion from public places condemns women to separate spaces, this provokes that their approach to a masculine place, through a socially imposed agoraphobia, leads women to voluntary and exclude themselves from the *agora* [4].

The division of social and socioeconomic roles between the sexes may lead to women not being employed, having greater representation in the private sphere, and carrying out the main tasks within the home [20].

Bekker et al. [7, 20, 35], refers to the enumeration of several characteristics that predispose to an significant fear of agoraphobic situations in women such as the lack of affirmation of their own identity, not having acquired the necessary abilities for anonymous public situations, a poor adjustment to existing norms, etc.

Latas et al. [99] reported a greater subjective perception in women of agoraphobic avoidance; men on the other hand, were more liable to anticipate the physical consequences of panic attacks. It has been observed that the lower rate of recovery between panic crises increases the severity of the disorder and facilitates the appearance of agoraphobia [100].

According to various studies a 3–4 % prevalence among men has been observed compared with 7–9 % among women; at the same time, a greater severity of the condition for women has been observed, as well as a worse quality of life [101, 102].

Comorbidity between panic disorder and agoraphobia moves within the range 22.5–58.2 % [73]. In both entities there is comorbidity with disorders such as depression, dysthymia, generalized anxiety, social phobia, and OCD [81]. In panic disorder with agoraphobia a greater degree of association has been identified with the following entities, bipolar disorder I, specific phobia, generalized anxiety, personality disorders, and substance dependence [103]. Alcohol abuse is more frequent in men, and in women there is a greater tendency toward depression [81, 102, 104]. Alcohol abuse seems to be a male disguising strategy. By analogy, the use of tranquilizers represents a female disguising strategy [20].

24.5.8 Generalized Anxiety Disorder

The DSM-IV and DSM-5 define the generalized anxiety disorder as excessive anxiety and worry about different events or activities during most days, over a period of at least 6 months. The worry is difficult to control and is associated with somatic symptoms such as muscular tension, irritability, and sleep and worry disorders. It excludes the presence of Axis I disorder and is neither caused by consumption of substances nor by organic disease and implies a great deterioration in the life of the individual [105].

The nosological situation of this disorder is subject to criticism, as well as its neurobiological and therapeutic bases [13, 106]. Initially, the DSM-III-R included the demand that the anxiety symptomatology must be of at least 1 month's duration as a diagnostic element, a prerequisite that was modified in the DSM-IV, after which it was proposed that the symptomatology should be present continuously over 6 months. Therefore, when generalized anxiety disorder prevalence figures are examined, they show great variability, which makes it necessary to consider the time criteria employed to characterize the disease. Now it seems that the DSM-V is also going to propose changes with regard to time, where the symptomatology is reduced to period of 3 months.

A different focus for persons with a different degree of affectation of the anxiety disorder does not sustain the idea that they all should be encompassed under the same diagnostic category. In fact, the patient who does not have very intense clinical symptoms could benefit from a "step by step" diagnosis [107].

A reduction in the symptomatology duration of GAD, may contribute to a greater difficulty between the distinction of the latter from other situations such as maladaptive and nonpathological anxiety disorders. Thus, it loses its category as a chronic disease [108].

A lifetime prevalence of 5.7 % of GAD is estimated, which is twice as frequent in women, appearing at around the start of the second decade of life [66, 109]. Although this diagnosis is not very frequent in clinical practice, the discrepancy is attributed to the lack of attention given to this diagnosis, secondary to scarce recognition shown by practitioners [110, 111]. Some authors doubt the diagnosis of this clinical condition, as many times GAD coexists with other conditions as in Axis I [112]. Generalized anxiety disorder has been labeled a "comorbid" disease [113].

Some authors defend that excessive worry (pathological) is a vague term, and more clarity and rigor is required to define it. What does it really mean? Most women have excessive worry related to social aspects: social inequality, glass ceiling, domestic violence, lower salaries in the same jobs within the labor market, etc.

The amount of time dedicated to domestic work is the most evident element of gender inequality in the use of daily time. The increasing participation of women in paid work has modified the gender division of domestic tasks; nonetheless, women still carry the heaviest load in terms of working hours spent on care work. Women have less free time because they spend more time in domestic and child care. This brings psychological distress and it can explain per se the "excessive worry" they are involved in from our point of view in some way. What is normal or healthy is very close to what is unhealthy or abnormal. In some way the disease does not exist until we have accorded its existence, when we name it, we perceive it, and we act on it, from our viewpoint.

To describe excessive worry as nervous expectation is not sufficient to distinguish it from normal worry. Intolerance of uncertainty is not specific for pathological worry in GAD, as it has also been associated with the symptoms of obsessive compulsive disorder and depression [114, 115].

The lifetime prevalence rate is 4 % in men, compared with 7 % in women [66, 101, 102]. This divergence between the sexes begins at an early age and continues into adolescence and adulthood [116].

The clinical course of GAD is usually the same in men as in women, as is the risk of remission and relapses [117]; women present greater associated comorbidity [118].

The prevalence of personality disorders from clusters B and C, poor interpersonal relationships, and comorbidity with another psychiatric pathology are factors that are related to a limited remission of the symptomatology [119].

Very frequently, the comorbidity of depression is accompanied by anxiety disorders, especially with GAD, which could us lead to question the primacy of depression or anxiety in women [32].

A dimensional relationship between depression and GAD has been proposed; those who support this idea based their belief on multiple suggestions that speak in favor of both entities presenting with a greater frequency based on personality in which "neuroticism" predominates [120].

Women may experience and/or report more psychological perturbation and alteration of behavior following panic attacks and other acute aversive events than men. This may be explained by Nolen-Hoeksema and Jackson [34, 121] and Bekker et al. [18, 20, 27] who report that owing to higher levels of rumination in women than in men and following the proposal that women respond to body sensations with the cognitive response more than men, this implies a lack of control over their bodies.

24.5.9 Substance/Medication-Induced Anxiety Disorder and Anxiety Due to Another Medical Condition

Substance/medication-induced anxiety disorder involves anxiety due to substance intoxication or withdrawal or to a medication treatment. In anxiety disorder due to another medical condition, anxiety symptoms are the physiological consequences of the other medical condition [51].

24.5.10 Other Specified Anxiety Disorder

This category applies in DSM-5 to presentations in which symptoms characteristic of an anxiety cause significant distress. Examples of presentations that can be included are: limited-symptom attacks; generalized anxiety occurring more days than not; *khyâi cap* (wind attacks); and *ataque de nervios* (attack of nerves) [51].

24.5.11 Obsessive Compulsive Disorder

In DSM-IV-TR, OCD was encompassed in the spectrum of panic disorders; a reclassification of this diagnosis entity into a new dimension has been included in the recent DSM-5. However, we will try to describe the differential aspects between the two genders, regardless of whether or not their future conceptualization should remain outside the field of anxiety disorders. The main objective is gender differences in OCD.

In DSM-5 OCD and related disorders that are included are body dysmorphic disorder, hoarding disorder, trichotillomania (hair pulling disorder), excoriation (skin-picking) disorder, substance/medication-induced obsessive compulsive and related disorder, and unspecified obsessive compulsive and related disorder (e.g., body-focused repetitive behavior disorder, obsessional jealousy) [51].

According to Lochner et al. [122] some studies do not show differences with regard to sex in the prevalence rates of OCD whereas others, such as those carried out by the CSN-R 2007, report rates of prevalence of 2.3 % with a probability twice as high for women as for men; nevertheless, numerous studies have reported differences in age at the appearance of symptoms, where the early onset of symptoms is more frequent among men, a high percentage of whom started before the age of 25; while among women the age at onset is before the age of 20, and the acute onset and episodic course of the disease are frequent [123]. Between 13 and 36 % of women with obsessive disease refer to the onset during the pregnancy or postpartum period; 30 % suffered deterioration of the disease during the postpartum period [11].

Differences have also been described in the course of the disease and response to treatment [124]. However, more similarities than differences have been described in the clinical condition of the disorder [125]. With regard to symptoms, women show more harmful compulsions regarding cleanliness and checking things, while men present more nervous tics, a greater severity of the symptoms in general, and a worse prognosis [122].

Sexual repression in female subjectivity history can be avoided in the construction of this disorder. Most religions have focused on the repression of female sexuality and polarization.

In OCD over half the women reported symptoms relating to the baby during the perinatal period, with obsessive thoughts of harming their child, these feelings becoming more intense following birth [126]; in fact, it was concluded that in 20–30 % of cases the deterioration occurs in the postpartum period [40], and it has also been observed that this fact would increase the risk of postpartum depression among women [127].

In a not insignificant number of women with OCD, their condition was abruptly initiated in the immediate postpartum period, which was attributed to serotonergic dysfunction, causing a manifest drop in ovaric hormones over this period [128].

The age at onset of the earliest symptoms is associated with nervous tics, anxiety, food, somatoform, and impulse control disorders; a prolonged duration of the disease is associated with a lower number of nervous tics with depressive comorbid disorder [129, 130].

Women with OCD show a greater tendency to be married and have children and there is also a greater tendency to have a background of food disorders and depression, while men present anxious personality characteristics [123, 131]. Women are more prone to presenting anxiety and food and impulse control disorders [130].

Some women reported stressful symptoms with more intensity and the course of the disease for them is more difficult and has a worse result than for men [122, 123]. In addition, there is a greater frequency of sexual abuse during childhood [122].

With regard to the associated comorbidity of the disorder, among women the appearance of food behavior disorders, depression or panic crises is more frequent [40], while among men phobias and nervous tics are more frequent [123].

The course of the disease tends toward chronicity [132]. Individuals who present OCD show a deterioration in their quality of life and the severity of the clinical condition is fundamentally related to the intensity of obsessive symptoms [133].

Concrete changes have been observed in the symptoms of women with OCD, both in the premenstrual/menstrual phase and following pregnancy and menopause; the interrelation between cyclical menstrual/reproductive changes and relapses and fluctuations in the symptoms of this disorder is confirmed [122]. Women with OCD refer to a deterioration in symptomatology during the menopause and premenstrual phase [126, 127, 134]. A greater prevalence of OCD in women was reported in the prenatal and postpartum period than in the population in general [135].

24.6 Treatment

Women tend to present higher concentrations of psychotropic drugs [136]; this makes it interesting to carry out a general vision of the differential characteristics of pharmacological treatment, where the joint use of benzodiazepines and antidepressants for all anxiety disorders is widespread. In this section we will try to explain the distinctive characteristics with regard to metabolization and differential response to treatment or factors that influence it; subsequently, in each space reserved to analyze each anxiety disorder, reference will be made, when considered suitable, to the particular differences described for each disorder in question.

Women have rates of anxiolytic prescription that are twice as high as men, despite not being diagnosed with an anxiety disorder; in fact the diagnosis probably passes unnoticed for a long period of time during which the symptoms are patent [137, 138].

Studies suggest a lower hepatic metabolization of benzodiazepines, which are thinned by combining with lorazepam and oxacepam; these differences have not been reported for oxidative metabolization of benzodiazepines such as diazepam. It has been reported how women who suspended contraceptive treatment and who consumed these drugs in combination with benzodiazepines underwent deterioration in their cognitive performance and slowing down of the psychomotor processes. Thus, oral contraceptives could produce a reduction in the hepatic metabolism of benzodiazepines [139].

Some antidepressants may present oscillations in plasma levels through the menstrual cycle of the woman; in the luteal phase a reduction in plasma values of desipramine and trazodone has been described [140]. Various studies have reported higher plasma levels for imipramine among women than men; a lower rate of hepatic thinning for clomipramine has also been determined, as well as amitryptiline, nortriptyline, and desipramine. These drugs, which belong to the tricyclics group and whose efficiency with anxiety disorders is proven, effect an increase in plasma levels among women; this is seen following the combined use of oral contraceptives [141].

With regard to ISRS, higher concentrations have been observed among women for fluvoxamine and sertraline, which could explain the higher incidence of diarrhea with the use of the latter among women. Differences have been seen in the metabolism of trazodone, where, in a sample that compares women and men of an advanced age, hepatic thinning among women is lower.

The overall assessment that both pharmacological therapy and cognitive behavioral therapy (CBT) contribute to improvement of anxiety disorders seems to be effective for women and men. However, there is a remarkable lack of information regarding the sex-specific effects, not to mention the gender-specific effects, of treatments.

Regrettably, the available sex-specific studies of psychosocial treatment are lacking in at least two respects. From a gender point of view, they lack a thorough reflection on possible gender bias in sampling procedures, measurement, and analysis, and they disregard the gender-specific context. From a treatment research point of view, they do not meet one of the criteria for inclusion in a meta-analysis: that of being a randomized controlled trial. Moreover, most of the available meta-analyses appear to fail to systematically consider the sex distribution of the studies included, much less the calculation of possible sex differences in effect sizes [20].

Butler et al. [142] highlighted this deficiency in their review of meta-analyses. Butler also mentioned inattention to possible moderator variables (gender differences) as a frequent limitation of the meta-analysis procedure.

Conclusions

Gender and social, cultural, and economic factors affect health. Women have a substantially higher risk of developing lifetime anxiety disorders compared with men. In addition, research evidence has generally observed an increased symptom severity, chronic course, and functional impairment in women with anxiety disorders in comparison to men. However, the reasons for the increased risk in developing an anxiety disorder in women are still unknown and have yet to be adequately investigated including a gender perspective. Not only genetic factors and female reproductive hormones may play important roles in the expression of these gender differences but . sex and gender affect who we are, what we do, and how we are treated. Evidence of gender differences in treatment response to different anxiety disorders are varying and remain largely inconclusive. Future research in gender perspective is needed to do good science.

References

1. Phillips KA, First MB. Introduction. In: Narrow WE, First MB, Sirovatka PJ, Regier DA, editors. Diary research for DSM-V. Considerations on the age and gender in psychiatric diagnosis. Barcelona: Elsevier Masson; 2009. p. 3–6.
2. Wisner KL, Dolan-Sewell R. Why is gender important? In: Regier DA, editor. Considerations on the age and gender in psychiatric diagnosis. Diary research for DSM-V. Barcelona: Elsevier Masson; 2009. p. 7–17.
3. WHO. Women's mental health: an evidence based review. Report on the world health. 2000.
4. Bourdieu P. Masculine domination. Barcelona: Anagrama; 2000.
5. MacCormack C, Strathern M. Nature, culture and gender. New York: Routledge; 1990.
6. Marylin Strathern M. An anthropological perspective. In: Harris O, Young K, editors. Feminist anthropology. Barcelona: Anagrama; 1979.
7. Wasserman GA, McReynolds LS, Ko SJ, Laura M. Gender differences in psychiatric disorders at juvenile probation intake. Am J Public Health. 2005;95:131–7.
8. Robins LN, Helzer JE, Weissman NM, Orvaschel H, et al. Lifetime prevalence of specific disorders in three sites. Arch Gen Psychiatry. 1984;41:949–58.

9. Linzer M, Spitzer R, Kroenke K, et al. Gender, quality of life, and mental disorders in primary care: results from the PRIME-MD 1000 study. Am J Med. 1996;101:526–33.
10. Gamma A, Angst J. Concurrent psychiatric comorbidity and multimorbidity in a community study: gender differences and quality of life. Eur Arch Psychiatry Clin Neurosci. 2001; 251 Suppl 2:S1143–1146.
11. Cloitre M, Yonkers KA, Pealstein T, Aletmus M, Davidson KW, Pigott A. Women and anxiety disorders: implications for diagnosis and treatment. CNS Spectr. 2004;9 Suppl 8: S1–16.
12. Stein MB, et al. Childhood physical and sexual abuse in patients with anxiety disorders and in a community sample. Am J Psychiatry. 2004;153:275–7.
13. Ballús-Creus C, Bernardo M, Bioque Alcazar M, et al. Introduction to psychopathology and psychiatry. 7th ed. Vallejo Ruiloba J, editor. Spain: Elsevier Masson; 2011.
14. Grant BF, Weissman MM. Gender and prevalence of psychiatric disorders. In: Narrow WE, First MB, Sirovatka PJ, Regier DA, editors. A research agenda for DSM5. Arlington, VA: American Psychiatric Publishing; 2007. p. 31–45.
15. Eaton W, Kessler RC, Wittchen HV. Panic and panic disorder in the United States. Am J Psychiatry. 1994;151:413–20.
16. Altemus M. Neurobiology, sex and gender. In: Narrow WE, First MB, Sirovatka PJ, Regier DA, editors. Considerations on the age and gender in psychiatric diagnosis. Barcelona: Elsevier Masson. Diary research for DSM-V 2009. p. 47–62.
17. Forero J. Anxiety disorders. In: Gaviria S, Luna I, Corra E, editors. Climacteric. An integrative vision. Medellín: CES; 2003.
18. Bekker MH. Agoraphobia and gender: a review. Clin Psychol Rev. 1996;16:129–46.
19. MacKinaw-Koons B, Vasey MW. Considering sex differences in anxiety and its disorders across life span: a construct-validation approach. Appl Prev Psychol. 2000;9:191–209.
20. Bekker M, van Mens-Verhulst J. Anxiety disorders: sex differences in prevalence, degree, and background, but gender-neutral treatment. Gend Med. 2007;4(Suppl B):S178–93.
21. Al-Ilssa I. The psychopathology of women. Englewood Cliffs, NJ: Prentice-Hall; 1980.
22. Chambless DL, Goldstein AJ, editors. Agoraphobia. Multiple perspectives on theory and treatment. New York: Wiley; 1982.
23. Fodor IG. The phobic syndrome in women. In: Franks V, Burtle V, editors. Women in therapy. New York: Brunner/Mazel; 1974.
24. Gelfond M. Reconceptualizing agoraphobia: a case study of epidemiological bias in clinical research. Fem Psychol. 1991;1:247–62.
25. Symonds A. Phobias after marriage. Women's declaration of dependence. Am J Psychoanal. 1971;31:14–152.
26. Wolfe BE. Gender ideology and phobias in women. In: Spatz Widom C, editor. Sex roles and psychopathology. New York, NY: Plenum; 1984. p. 51–72.
27. Bekker MH. The development of an autonomy scale based on recent insights into gender identity. Eur J Pers. 1993;7:177–94.
28. Chodorw NJ. The reproduction of mothering: psychoanalysis and the sociology of gender. Berkeley: University of California Press; 1978.
29. Chodorw NJ. Feminism and psychoanalytic theory. Cambridge, MA: Pility Press; 1989.
30. Jordan JV, Kaplan AG, Miller JB, et al. Women's growth in connection: writings from the stone center. New York: Guildford; 1991.
31. Klose M, Jacobi F. Can gender differences in the prevalence of mental disorders be explained by sociodemographic factors? Arch Womens Ment Health. 2004;7:133–48.
32. Nolen Hoek-sema S. Emotion regulation and psychopathology: the role of gender. Annu Rev Clin Psychol. 2012;8:161–87.
33. Hettema JM, Prescott CA, Myers JM, Neale MC, Kendler KS. The structure of genetic and environmental risk factors for anxiety disorders in men and women. Arch Gen Psychiatry. 2005;62:182–9.

34. Barlow DH. Behavioral and cognitive models of post-traumatic stress disorder. Sante Ment Que. 1996;21(1):129–44 [Review] [57 refs] [French].
35. Cahill L, Haier RJ, White NS, Fallon J, Kilpatrick L, et al. Sex-related difference in amygdale activity during emotionally influenced memory storage. Neurobiol Learn Mem. 2001;75:1–9.
36. Cahill L. Sex-and hemisphere-related influences on the neurobiology of emotionally influenced memory. Prog Neuropsychopharmacol Biol Psychiatry. 2003;27:1235–41.
37. Cahill L. Why sex matter for neuroscience. Nat Rev Neurosci. 2006;7:477–84.
38. Cahill L. Brain sexual dimorphism. Sexual instinct. Tems 56: Sexual instinct. Sexual instinct. Res Sci. 2009;56:62–70.
39. Mitev YA, Darwish M, Wolf SS, Holsboer F, Almeida OF, Patchev VK. Gender differences in the regulation of 3 alpha-hydroxysteroid dehydrogenase in rat brain and sensitivity to neurosteroid-mediated stress protection. Neuroscience. 2003;20:541–9.
40. Piggot TA. Gender differences in the epidemiology and treatment of anxiety disorders. J Clin Psychiatry. 1999;60 Suppl 18:S4–15.
41. Alonso J, Angermeyer MC, Bernert S, Bruffaerts R, Brugha TS, Bryson H, et al. Prevalence of mental disorders in Europe: results from the European Study of the Epidemiology of Mental Disorders (ESEMED) project. Acta Psychiatr Scand Suppl. 2004;109(420):S21–27.
42. Carrasco-Galán I, Espinar-Fellmann I. Anxiety disorders and gender. Mind Brain. 2008;31: 12–21.
43. Horst GJ, Wichmann R, Gerrits M, Westenbroek C, Lin Y. Sex differences in stress responses: focus on ovarian hormones. Physiol Behav. 2009;97:239–49.
44. Heron J, et al. The course of anxiety and depression through pregnancy and the postpartum in a community sample. J Affect Disord. 2004;80:65–73.
45. Sutter-Dallay AL, et al. Women with anxiety disorders during pregnancy are at increased risk of intense postnatal depressive symptoms: a prospective survey of the MATQUID cohort. Eur Psychiatry. 2004;19:459–63.
46. Johnson SR. The epidemiology and social impact of premenstrual symptoms. Clin Obstet Gynecol. 1987;30:369–84.
47. Woods NF, Most A, Dery GK. Prevalence of perimenstrual symptoms. Am J Public Health. 1982;72:1257–64.
48. McLeod D, Hoehn-Saric R, Foster G, Hipsley P. The influence of premenstrual syndrome on rating of anxiety in woman with generalized anxiety disorder. Acta Psychiatr Scand. 1993;88: 248–51.
49. Hsiao MC, et al. Premenstrual symptoms and premenstrual exacerbation in patients with psychiatric disorders. Psychiatry Clin Neurosci. 2004;58:186–90.
50. Freeman EW. Premenstrual syndrome and premenstrual dysphoric disorder: definitions and diagnosis. Psychoneuroendocrinology. 2003;28 Suppl 3:S25–37.
51. Diagnostic and statistical manual of mental disorders. 5th ed. Arlington, VA: American Psychiatric Association; 2013.
52. Sanchez PMG, Eguiluz UI. Thought content. In: Eguiluz UI, Segarra RE, editors. Introduction of the psychopathology, a integrative view. 3rd ed. Madrid: Panamericana; 201[illegible]. p. 98.
53. Marteinsdottir I, Furmark T, Tillfors M, et al. Personality traits in the social phobia. Eur Psychiatry. 2001;8:283–90.
54. Reich J. The relationship of social phobia to avoidant personality disorder: a proposal to reclassify avoidant personality disorder based on clinical empirical findings. Eur Psychiatry. 2000;15:151–9.
55. Chambless D, Fydrich T, Rodebaugh T. Generalized social phobia and avoidant personality disorder: meaning the distinction or useless duplications? Depress Anxiety. 2006;0:1–12.
56. Hummelen B, Wilberg T, Pedersen G, Karterud S. The relationship between avoidant personality disorder and social phobia. Compr Psychiatry. 2007;48:348–56.
57. Cervera S, Roca M, Bobes J. Social phobia. Barcelona: Masson; 1998.
58. Heimberg R, Liebowitz M, Hope D, Scheneider F. Social phobia: diagnosis, prognosis and treatment. Barcelona: Martinez Roca; 2000.

59. Liebowitz M. Easing the burden of social anxiety disorder. J Clin Psychiatry. 2008;69(9): 1485–96.
60. Yonkers KA, et al. An eight-year longitudinal comparison of clinical course and characteristics of social phobia among men and women. Psychiatr Serv. 2001;52:637–43.
61. Peer M, Soares C, Steiner M. The complex interrelationships of menstrual cyclicity and anxiety disorders. Psychiatr Times. 2008;25:1–14.
62. Chavina D, Stein M. Phenomenology of social phobia. In: Estein A, Hollander E, editors. Anxiety disorders treaty. Barcelona: Ars Medica; 2004.
63. Marcin M, Nemeroff C. The neurobiology of social anxiety disorder: the relevance of fear and anxiety. Acta Psychiatr Scand Suppl. 2003;108(417):S51–64.
64. Ballenger JC, Davidson JR, Lecrubier Y, Nutt DJ, Baldwin DS, Kasper S, et al. Consensus statement on panic disorder from the International Consensus Group on Depression and Anxiety. J Clin Psychiatry. 1998;59 Suppl 8:S47–54.
65. Furmark T. Social phobia: overview of community surveys. Acta Psychiatr Scand. 2000;105: 84–93.
66. NCS-R. Lifetime prevalence of GSM-IV/WMH-CIDI disorders by de sex and cohort. NCS-Update. Jun 17 2007.
67. Kessler RC, et al. Prevalence, severity, and comorbidity of 12-month DSM-IV disorder in the National Comorbidity Survey Replication. Arch Gen Psychiatry. 2005;62:617–27.
68. Becker ES, et al. Epidemiology of specific phobia subtypes: findings from the Dresden Mental Health Study. Eur Psychiatry. 2007;22:69–74.
69. Wythilingun B, Stein D. Specific phobia. In: Stein D, editor. Clinical manual of anxiety disorders. Washington: American Psychiatric Public; 2004.
70. Turk CL, et al. An investigation of gender differences in social phobia. J Anxiety Disord. 1998;12:209–23.
71. Hajudk A. A search for psychobiological determinants of anxiety disorders. Ann Acad Med Stetin. 2004;50:65–75.
72. Burcazo JA, Caballero R, Cabranes JA, Montero I, Ruiz, I. Gender and mental health. In: López-Ibor JJ, Leal C, Carbonell C, editors. Images of Spanish psychiatry, Chap 34. 1st ed. Barcelona: Glosa; 2004, p. 423–433.
73. Weissman M, Bland R, Canino G, Faravelli C, et al. The cross-national epidemiology of panic disorder. Arch Gen Psychiatry. 1997;54(4):305–9.
74. Eaton W, Kramer M, Anthony JC. The incidence of specific DIS/DSM-III mental disorders: data from the NIMH Epidemiologic Catchment Area Program. Acta Psychiatr Scand. 1989; 79(2):163–78.
75. Scheibe G, Albus M. Age at onset, precipitating events, sex distribution, and co-occurrence of anxiety disorders. Psychopathology. 1992;25:11–8.
76. Sheikh JI, et al. Gender differences in panic disorder: findings from the National Comorbidity Survey. Am J Psychiatry. 2002;159:55–8.
77. Turgeon L, Marchand A, Dupuis G. Clinical features in panic disorder with agoraphobia: a comparison of men and women. J Anxiety Disord. 1998;12(6):539–42.
78. Dick CL, et al. Epidemiology of psychiatric disorders in Edmonton. Panic disorder. Hum Mol Genet. 2004;8:621–4.
79. Leskin GA, Sheikh JI. Gender differences in panic disorder. Psychiatr Times. 2004;21:1–6.
80. Kressler RC, et al. The epidemiology of panic attacks, panic disorder and agoraphobia in the National Comorbidity Survey Replication. Arch Gen Psychiatry. 2006;62:415–24.
81. Starcevic V, Djordjevic A, Latas M, Bogojevic G. Characteristics of agoraphobia in woman and men with panic disorder with agoraphobia. Depress Anxiety. 1998;8:8–13.
82. Keller M, Hanks D. Course and outcome in panic disorder. Prog Neuropsychopharmacol Biol Psychiatry. 1993;17(4):551–70.
83. Keller M, Yonkers K, Warshaw M, Pratt LA, et al. Remission and relapse in subjects with panic disorder and panic with agoraphobia: a prospective short-interval naturalistic follow-up. J Nerv Ment Dis. 1994;182(5):290–96.

84. Kendler K, Walters E, Neale M, Kessler R, et al. The structure of genetic and environmental risk factors for six major psychiatric disorders in women. Phobia, generalized anxiety disorder, panic disorder, bulimia, major depression, and alcoholism. Arch Gen Psychiatry. 1995;52(5):374–83.
85. Yonkers KA, et al. Chronicity, relapse, and illness-course of panic disorder, social phobia, and generalized anxiety disorder: findings in men and women from 8 years of follow-up. Depress Anxiety. 2003;17:173–9.
86. Yonkers KA, Zlotnick C, Allsworth J, et al. Is the course of panic disorder the same in men and women? Am J Psychiatry. 1998;155:596–602.
87. Hagood J, De Leo D. Anxiety disorders and suicidal behavior: an update. Curr Opin Psychiatry. 2008;21:51–64.
88. Diaconu G, Turecki G. Panic disorder and suicidality: is comorbidity with depression the key? J Affect Disord. 2007;104(1–3):203–9.
89. Weissman M, Klerman G, Markowitz J, Quellette R. Suicidal ideation and suicide attempts in panic disorder and attacks. N Engl J Med. 1989;321:1209–14.
90. Pohl R, Yeragani VK, Balon R, Lycaki H, et al. Smoking in patients with panic disorder. Psychiatry Res. 1992;43(3):253–62.
91. Zlotnik C, et al. Childhood trauma, trauma in adulthood, and psychiatric diagnoses: results from a community sample. Compr Psychiatry. 2008;49:16316–9.
92. Kendler KS, et al. Panic syndromes in a population-based sample of male and female twins. Psychol Med. 2001;31:989–1000.
93. Domschke K, et al. Meta-analysis of COMT vall158met in panic disorder: ethnic heterogeneity and gender specificity. Am J Med Genet B Neuropsychiatr Genet. 2007;144B:567–3.
94. Domschke K, et al. Influence of the catechol-O-methyltransferase val158met genotype on amygdala and prefrontal cortex emotional processing in panic disorder. Psychiatry Res. 2008; 163:13–20.
95. Asami T, Yamasue H, Hayano F, Nakamura M, Uehara K, Otsuka T, et al. Sexually dimorphic gray matter volume reduction in patients with panic disorder. Psychiatry Res. 2009;173: 128–34.
96. Seeman MV. Psychopathology in women and men: focus on female hormones. Am J Psychiatry. 1997;154:1641–7.
97. Kim IR, Min SK, Yu BE. Differences in beta-adrenergic receptor sensibility between women and men with panic disorder. Eur Neuropsychopharmacol. 2004;14:515–20.
98. Le Melledo JM, Van Driel M, Coupland NJ, Lott P, Jhangri GS. Response to flumazenil in women with premenstrual dysphoric disorder. Am J Psychiatry. 2000;157:821–3.
99. Latas M, et al. Gender differences in psychopathologic features of agoraphobia with panic disorder. Vojnosanit Pregl. 2006;63:569–74.
100. Francis JL, et al. Characteristics and course of panic disorder and panic disorder with agoraphobia in primary care patients. Prim Care Companion J Clin Psychiatry. 2007;9: 173–9.
101. Altemus M, Epstein L. Sex differences in anxiety disorders. In: Becker JB, Berkley KJ, Geary N, Hampson E, Herman JP, Young EA, editors. Sex differences in the brain. New York: Oxford University Press; 2008. p. 397–404.
102. Kessler RC, McGonagle KA, Zhao S, et al. Lifetime and 12 month prevalence of DSM-III-R psychiatric disorders in the United States: results from the national comorbidity survey. Arch Gen Psychiatry. 1994;51(1):8–19.
103. Grant BF, et al. The epidemiology of DSM-IV panic disorder and agoraphobia in the United States: results from the National Epidemiologic Survey on Alcohol and Related Conditions. J Clin Psychiatry. 2006;67:363–74.
104. Cox BJ, Swinson RP, Shulman ID, et al. Gender effects and alcohol use in panic disorder with agoraphobia. Behav Res Ther. 1993;31(4):413–16.
105. Sadock BJ, Sadock VA. Kaplan and Sadock's synopsis of psychiatry. 10th ed. New York, NY: Wolters Kluwer; 2012.

106. Davidson J. Pharmacotherapy social anxiety disorder. J Clin Psychiatry. 1998;59 Suppl 17: S47–51.
107. Batstra L, Frances A. Holding the line against diagnostic inflation in psychiatry. Psychother Psychosom. 2012;81:5–10.
108. Van der Heiden C, Methortrst G, Muris P, van der Molen HT. Generalized anxiety disorder: clinical presentation, diagnostic features, and guidelines for clinical practice. J Clin Psychol. 2011;67:58–73.
109. Kessler RC, et al. The epidemiology of generalized anxiety disorder. Psychiatr Clin North Am. 2001;24:19–39.
110. Somers JM, Goldner EM, Waraich P, Hsu L. Prevalence and incidence studies of anxiety disorders: a systematic review of the literature. Can J Psychiatry. 2006;51:100–13.
111. Beesdo-Braun K, Winkel S, Pine KS, Hoyer J, Höfler M, Lieb R, Wittchen HU. The diagnostic threshold of generalized anxiety disorder in the community: a develop perspective. J Psychiatr Res. 2011;45:962–72.
112. Yonkers KA, Warshaw MG, Massion AO, Keller MB. Phenomenology and course of generalized anxiety disorder. Br Psychiatry. 1996;168(3):308–13.
113. Nutt D, Argyropoulos S, Hood S, Potokar J. Generalized anxiety disorder: a comorbid disease. Eur Neuropsychopharmacol. 2006;16:109–18.
114. Gentes EL, Ruscio AM. A meta-analysis of the relation of intolerance of uncertainty to symptoms of generalized anxiety disorder, major depressive disorder, and obsessive-compulsive disorder. Clin Psychol Rev. 2011;31:923–33.
115. Kertz SJ, Bigda-Peyton JS, Rosmarin DH, Björgvinsson T. The importance of worry across diagnostic presentations: prevalence, severity and associated symptoms in a partial hospital setting. J Anxiety Disord. 2012;26:126–33.
116. McLean CP, Anderson ER. Brave men and timid women? A review of the gender differences in fear and anxiety. Clin Psychol Rev. 2009;29:496–505.
117. Yonkers KA, Kidner CL. Sex differences in anxiety disorders. In: Lewis-Hall F, Williams TS, Panetta JA, Herrera JM, editors. Psychiatric illness in women. Washington: American Psychiatric Publishing; 2002. p. 5–30.
118. Howell HB, Brawman-Mintzer O, Monnier J, Yonkers KA. Generalized anxiety disorder in women. Psychiatr Clin North Am. 2001;24:165–78.
119. Yonkers KA, Dyck I, Warshaw M, et al. Factors predicting the clinical course of generalized anxiety disorder. Br J Psychiatry. 2000;176:544–50.
120. Kendler KS, et al. The sources of co-morbidity between mayor depression and generalized anxiety disorder in a Swedish national twin sample. Psychol Med. 2007;37:453–62.
121. Hoek-sema Susan N. Emotion regulation and psycopathology: the role of gender. Annu Rev Clin Psychol. 2012;8:161–87.
122. Lochner C, Hemmings SM, Kinnear CJ, Moolman-Smook JC, Corfield VA, Knowles JA, et al. Gender in obsessive-compulsive disorder: clinical and genetic findings. Eur Neuropsychopharmacol. 2004;14:105–13.
123. Bogetto F, Venturello S, Albert U, Maina G, Gand L, Ravizza A. Gender-related clinical differences in obsessive-compulsive disorder. Eur Psychiatry. 1999;14:434–41.
124. Torresan RC, Ramos-Cerqueira AT, De Mathis MA, Diniz J-B, Ferrão YA, Miguel EC, Torres AR. Sex differences in the phenotypic expression of obsessive-compulsive disorder: an exploratory study from Brazil. Compr Psychiatry. 2009;50:63–9.
125. Tukel R, Polat A, Genc A, Bozkurt O, Atli H. Gender-related differences among Turkish patients with obsessive-compulsive disorder. Compr Psychiatry. 2004;45:362–6.
126. Labad J, et al. Female reproductive cycle and obsessive-compulsive disorder. J Clin Psychiatry. 2005;66:428–35.
127. Williams KE, Koran LM. Obsessive-compulsive disorder in pregnancy, the puerperium, and the premenstruum. J Clin Psychiatry. 1997;58:330–4.
128. Sichel DA, Cohen LS, Rosenbaum JF, Driscoll J. Postpartum onset of obsessive-compulsive disorder. Psychosomatics. 1993;34:277–9.

129. Diniz JB, et al. Impact of age at onset and duration of illness on the expression of comorbidities in obsessive. Compulsive disorder. J Clin Psychiatry. 2004;65:22–7.
130. De Mathis MA, et al. Obsessive-compulsive disorder: influence of age at onset comorbidity patterns. Eur Psychiatry. 2008;23:187–94.
131. Castle DJ, et al. Gender differences in obsessive compulsive disorder. Aust N Z J Psychiatry. 1995;29:114–17.
132. Alonso P, et al. Long-term follow up and predictors of clinical outcome in obsessive-compulsive patients treated with serotonin reuptake inhibitors and behavioral therapy. J Clin Psychiatry. 2001;62:535–40.
133. Eisen JL, et al. Impact of obsessive-compulsive disorder on quality of life. Compr Psychiatry. 2006;47:270–5.
134. Vulink NC, et al. Female hormones affect symptom severity in obsessive-compulsive disorder. Int Clin Psychopharmacol. 2006;21:171–5.
135. Ross LE, Mclean LM. Anxiety disorders during pregnancy and the postpartum period: a systematic review. J Clin Psychiatry. 2006;67:1285–98.
136. Hamilton J, Yonkers K. Sex differences in pharmacokinetics of psychotropic medications. In: Jensvold M, Halbreich U, Hamilton J, editors. Psychopharmacology and woman. Washington, DC: American Psychiatric Press; 1996.
137. Van der Waals FW, et al. Sex differences among recipients of benzodiazepines in Dutch general practice. Br Med J. 1993;307:363–6.
138. Wang PS, et al. Failure and delay in initial treatment contact after first onset of mental disorders in the National Comorbidity Survey Replication. Arch Gen Psychiatry. 2005;62: 603–13.
139. Ellinwood EH, Easler ME, Linnoila M. Effects of oral contraceptives on diazepam induced psychomotor impairment. Clin Pharmacol Ther. 1994;35:360–6.
140. Kimmel S, Gonsalves L. Fluctuating level of antidepressants premenstrually. J Psychosom Obstet Gynaecol. 1992;13:277–80.
141. Abernethy DR, Greenblatt DJ, Shader RI. Imipramine and desipramine disposition in the elderly. J Pharmacol Exp Ther. 1985;232:183–8.
142. Butler AC, Chapman JE, Forman EM, Beck AT. The empirical status of cognitive-behavioral therapy: a review of meta-analyses. Clin Psychol Rev. 2006;26:17–31.

Gender Differences in Post-traumatic Stress Disorder

25

Ana Villamor and Estibaliz Sáez de Adana

Abstract

Post-traumatic stress disorder (PTSD) was first described in situations of war in ancient Greece. For this reason the female gender was practically excluded for decades from this diagnosis because of a gender issue. Epidemiological differences point to the predominance of PTSD in women over men; even with the highest prevalence of trauma in men, women are more likely to develop this condition. It is possible that these figures belie an oversimplification of epidemiological studies that do not consider certain traumas or certain predispositions determined by the female gender role. In this chapter we review the psychopathological differences that can be found in this syndrome by gender, based on the few studies that address the issue, because we have found a scientific vacuum that is yet to be explored.

Gender violence is a major source of trauma, whether acute or chronic, occurring much more frequently in women than in men and that has been silenced for many years; for this reason it has not been recorded or studied by experts as a focus of PTSD.

The way in which men and women channel and manage emotions is different, and these strategies that we use as men or women can determine the presence or absence of PTSD. The question is whether this is due to biological differences or to assimilating how to behave, adjusting to the expectations that society has invested in us according to our male or female gender.

A. Villamor (✉) • E. Sáez de Adana
Alava University Hospital, Vitoria, Spain
e-mail: ANARESURRECCION.VILLAMORGARCIA@osakidetza.net

M. Sáenz-Herrero (ed.), *Psychopathology in Women*,
DOI 10.1007/978-3-319-05870-2_25

25.1 History

The first mention of post-traumatic stress disorder (PTSD) can be traced back to 400 years BC and was made by Herodotus in describing the battle of Marathon. About 40 centuries ago the Egyptian papyrus Kunyus observed the reaction of many people to severe flooding caused by the overflowing of the Nile River delta [1]. Classical Greek authors such as Hippocrates and Herodotus referred to stories of nightmares and other PTSD symptoms in surviving soldiers who conducted battle. Also found in the Old Testament, allusion was made to soldiers being withdrawn from battle for emotional breakdowns, and it also described that their reactions could be contagious [2].

Historically, trauma has been associated with war situations, which is why it has been linked mainly with physical trauma and with the male condition. It must be remembered that the term *trauma* is of Greek origin and refers to a wound. Trauma is remembered later when the psyche becomes relevant.

In one review it is tracked accurately from classical antiquity and mentions all those people with serious mental disorders as a result of participating in fighting, as well as descriptions of individuals who, in situations that today would be called psychically traumatic, react with symptoms of anxiety, and chronic disorganization of behavior may persist [3].

Pinel [4] describes what we would now call PTSD in people affected by military actions that took place around the French Revolution, describing for the first time a post-traumatic picture in a person affected by an accident (the philosopher Pascal, after a carriage accident). Psychopathology was considered by authors like Charcot, Janet, and Freud centuries later.

After Pinel, Erichsen in 1866 and Page in 1885 described some cases of traumatic consequences of railway accidents. In the early twentieth century there was an increasing interest in trying to define and describe this condition.

Oppenheim in 1884 first used the term *traumatic neurosis* in his comments on railway accidents and labor; in 1907, Honigman coined the term *shell shock* from case studies in the Russo-Japanese War, and emphasized the similarities of the observations to the cases studied by Oppenheim. In 1915, during World War I, British authorities opened a unit specializing in the treatment of what was beginning to be called shell shock. This term was first used by Myers [5] for patients who experienced dropping bombs near them. In 1917 Salmon [6] was a military doctor who formulated the five key principles for the care of these patients. The Vietnam War was a decisive turning point in the consideration of these disorders.

Throughout the history of psychiatry, women have been involved in a significant part of mental health problems. They were ignored in the concept of PTSD because the concept only included war victims (mostly men), and physical situations such as rape, sexual abuse, were ignored for many years. This could have changed the way that psychic symptomatology was differently expressed as a function of gender.

Culture as a benchmark for understanding PTSD is inexcusable, in that it represents a set of unique patterns of adaptation to a specific context, involving the response to threats that may arise. Clearly, there are certain universal threats that are perceived as such in all groups, but the average modulation capability and very important cultural values introduce variations in the way the individual processes a specific threat and presents her concrete trauma. Culture includes gender, ethnicity, and social and economical status too.

Although it is clear that in recent decades there has been a trend toward flexibility in gender roles and toward equal opportunities for people regardless of gender, it is also clear that men and women are still socialized with different rules and expectations regarding the expression of feelings, the pressure to succeed in academic tasks or work, participation in domestic work, commitment to the care and concern for relationships and caring for others, etc., and this leads to significant psychological consequences. For many authors, the gender socialization gives rise ultimately to different trends in men and women with regard to their mental health [7].

There is considerable evidence that the incidence of various forms of psychopathology, as well as the demand for psychotherapeutic care services, differs between men and women. The most notable differences were observed in rates of depression, neurosis, somatic disorders and anorexia nervosa, with a clear female predominance, and, depending on various drugs, sociopaths and paranoia, which were more frequent among men [8].

As for anxiety disorders, which are the most prevalent psychological disorders in both the general population and in psychiatric settings, although the difference in rates between genders is less well established, in general, we can say that women are, on the whole, at a much greater risk of suffering than men. The question is: why is that happening?

Another important aspect linked to the traditional role of women is femininity. Numerous studies have investigated the relationship among masculinity, femininity, and androgyny on the one hand and the various indices of mental health on the other. There is considerable evidence that in both men and women, masculinity tends to be associated more than femininity with personal adjustment indices, including increased self-esteem and a tendency to have lower levels of anxiety and depression [9–11].

Other studies have found a relationship, in people of both sexes, between femininity and such aspects of personal and social adjustment as the perception of self-efficacy, satisfaction in personal relationships, and self-esteem components that relate to communal aspects [12, 13].

Studies that analyze the relationship among masculinity, femininity, and androgyny anxiety indicate that in addition to higher levels of anxiety existing in women than in men, individuals with a female typing also exhibit a greater tendency toward anxiety than men or androgynous individuals [14–17]. The question is, if the sociocultural aspects are essential in the presentation of symptoms in the general population, why does it have an important influence on the presentation of clinical symptoms in women?

25.2 Neuroendocrine Stress Response

Stress is the specific and stereotyped body's response to any stressor, it can result in various symptoms and clinical or may favor an adaptive response to the situation. The stressor may be objective or subjective, single or repeated, and trigger an acute or chronic response. Psychological stress in the cognitive and emotional component of the response will be different, depending on the overall assessment made by the subject of the threatening situation.

In the acute response of the amygdala stress is one of the structures that plays a very important role. The activation of the hypothalamic–pituitary–adrenal (HPA) from the release of adrenocorticotropic hormone (ACTH), and catecholamine and immune systems, among others, forms the biological response of stress; gonadal hormones participate as modulating factors.

In this way one can understand the role of estrogen in the differential response between the sexes coping with stress. Estrogens determine a specific organization of neural circuits that regulate gonadotropin release and sexual behavior, and also participate in the regulation of the HPA axis.

However, women have greater neuroendocrine response activation than men in a stressful situation, which has been expressed in higher levels of ACTH and prolactin. The action of estrogen can partially explain PTSD in women but also the abuse exploitation, psychical and sexual abuse, denial of rights, etc. We cannot forget that until the early twentieth century women had no rights, they could not vote, they could not have an equal education; the only way was to marry and have children. They were much more frequently abused inside the family and this was socially accepted. This must lead to chronic stress in the brain [18].

Early estrogen facilitates the stress response with increased cortisol, but then decreased estrogen produces a state equivalent to the follicular phase of the menstrual cycle, which favors a PTSD-type response.

Sex steroids are not only involved in development of the brain architecture but also affect brain function through interaction with different neurobiological systems, influencing the expression and development of sexual behavior and modulating effects through the levels, metabolism, and receptors of 5-HT (serotonin).

Estrogens promote the response of 5-HT 1A receptors in the hippocampus and progesterone modulates responses sensitivity in 5-HT 1A receptors. Progesterone can act as a glucocorticoid antagonist, thereby regulating stress resistance.

Under stress cortisol is released, glucocorticoid directly inhibits the function of 5-HT 1A receptors, progesterone sensitivity modulates responses in the 5-HT 1A, altering its effects. Women presented higher levels of 5-HT and its metabolite 5-HIAA (5-hydroxyindoleacetic acid) and greater imipramine binding in the right orbital cortex. The difference in sensitivity to the stimulation of 5-HT, due to the different modulation by sex steroid receptors, may constitute the basis of differences in the behavior, aggression, impulsivity, and mood regulation of some mental disorders.

25.2.1 Neurotransmitters and PTSD

A threatening situation is detected by the subject through the sense organs, which in turn generates a memory register for both the actual facts and the emotional component. Hormonal response to stress begins with the release of the hypothalamic peptides corticotropin-releasing hormone (CRH) and arginine vasopressin, which leads to an increase in the release of ACTH and cortisol.

Post-traumatic stress disorder is characterized by peripheral system hyporesponsiveness of the hypothalamic hypophyseal adrenal axis (HHA; hypocortisolemia) with high concentrations of CRH in the cerebrospinal fluid and more negative feedback inhibition of cortisol [19, 20]. There is therefore a hypersensitive HPA that translates ACTH response to decreased CRH (which may be the result of hyper-responsiveness of the pituitary to feedback of cortisol and increased glucocorticoid receptors in the pituitary) [21]. Through the dexamethasone suppression test, which is a requirement for the HPA, it has been found that PTSD causes greater suppression in ACTH and cortisol release. The HPA axis has a number of effects on the female hormonal cycle and, in turn, changes in estrogen and progesterone can influence changes in PTSD symptoms.

The relative hypercortisolemia in the third trimester of pregnancy may facilitate transient adrenal suppression in the postpartum period, which could affect PTSD symptoms in late pregnancy or postpartum in women with this diagnosis.

The role of context is important, i.e., how hormones are involved in a person susceptible to a particular psychiatric disorder, and also as context-dependent hormones. The context for hormone action includes current physiological conditions, the external environment, previous experiences, and history of exposure to specific stimuli and genetics. Of course, the sociocultural context also plays a major role in the development of PTSD, so that lives at risk (poverty, low education, etc.) can be a defining factor for the presence of this disease. Ultimately it is the set of biological and sociocultural factors that determines the development of PTSD [22].

In PTSD associated with a history of child abuse accompanied by alterations in brain development, sex differences in brain maturation were found; in men there was a smaller brain volume and corpus callosum and a greater increase in the volume of the lateral ventricles in women [23].

The structure and function of the hippocampus were compared in women with a history of sexual abuse with and without PTSD, using MRI and CT. The results showed a failure of the hippocampus to activate and a lower volume of this component in women with PTSD, also presenting decreased activity of the prefrontal cortex (the medial and anterior cingulate areas), as well as visual and parietal cortices [24].

Shin and colleagues have shown by PET and provocation of symptoms that women with a history of sexual abuse and PTSD have an increased blood flow concentrated in the orbitofrontal cortex and anterior temporal pole.

Post-traumatic stress disorder has a profile in which the value of corticotropin-releasing factor is high, whereas cortisol levels are reduced. Hyper-responsiveness to the dexamethasone suppression test (PTSD patients are hypersuppressors), increased the concentration and sensitivity of glucocorticoid receptors in lymphocytes and increased response to adrenocorticotropic hormone (ACTH) stimulation before metyrapone [25].

There seems to be a difference in response to traumatic situations in both genders. Women report fewer traumatic experiences throughout life, but they are more vulnerable to them, so that these experiences will generate more serious psychiatric morbidity [26]. The difference between the sexes in the neurobiological response to stress is considered the mediating action of sex hormones [27].

25.3 Epidemiology

Recent reviews finding that the range of lifetime prevalence in the general population is between 1.0 and 12.3 % state that the overall risk of developing PTSD in people who have suffered some type of trauma must be estimated to be about 9.2 % (Table 25.1) [28]. PTSD figures reached 23.6 % of those who suffered some kind of trauma, and within these, sex appears as a determinant: 30.7 % of the exposed women develop PTSD compared with only 14 % of the exposed group of people as a whole [29]. In other studies such as by Stein [30, 31] figures for the general population vary: 6.0 % in women and 1.4 % in men.

There are distinguishing aspects that remain, however, throughout cultures, and persist despite their development, for example, the higher frequency of emotional problems in women from adolescence. As in gender violence and sexual assaults on children, and in sexual abuse, being a woman or a girl is one of the circumstances that has traditionally been regarded as a high risk factor for victimization. In fact, different studies agree that the highest incidence of sexual abuse is in girls (2–3 girls per child). Sexual abuse is committed in all walks of life, against all cultural backgrounds or and to all races.

Sexual assault is a traumatic event, as in the case of other negative events, and can produce negative psychological effects. Consider the consequences of sexual abuse as a form of PTSD. About 15 % of the female population suffer from a sexual assault at some point in their lifetime [32].

Table 25.1 Lifetime prevalence of post-traumatic stress disorder (PTSD; %) in the general population

Year	Author	Women	Men
1987	Helzer	1.3	0.5
1991	Davidson	1.7	0.9
1991	Breslau	11.3	6.0
1992	Norris	8.5	6.1
1994	Rioseco	5.1	2.7
1995	Kessler	10.4	5.0
1998	Breslau	18.3	10.8
2002	Perkonning	2.2	1.0
2002	Vicente	6.2	2.5

It is remarkable that the most common diseases in women correspond to the realm of the spirits. The two main risk factors for PTSD are sex and a history of previous trauma (especially violence in childhood).

Among the demographic factors in the prevalence of PTSD it was found that the age of women was not a factor, that race did not influence the risk of PTSD; however, the educational and economic levels have an inverse association with the prevalence of PTSD.

Women's risk of developing PTSD in most of the literature is twice that of men and one study even reported a risk three times higher [33]. The risk of developing PTSD is different depending on the trauma. In women the traumas more associated with the risk of PTSD are rape and child abuse. The frequency of PTSD in women after an episode of rape varies according to authors between 35 and 65 %. Other situations of violence, such as assaults, are accompanied by an increased risk of PTSD in women compared with men (54.1 % vs 15.4 %).

Pulcino et al. [34] proposed that in women biographical and behavioral factors are specifically responsible for the increased likelihood of PTSD after a disaster. Women traffic accident victims with peritraumatic dissociation at the time of the accident are at an increased risk of acute PTSD compared with men [35]. In women who have been victims of rape in childhood it has been observed that the failure to disclose what happened within a month reduces the rate of PTSD [36].

Pregnancy can be a condition facilitating the emergence of PTSD, even at the stage close to parturition [37]. Also, spontaneous abortion may be associated with PTSD in 25 % of patients at a month and 7 % at 4 months [38]. A woman facing the probable diagnosis of breast cancer may experience traumatic reactions with symptoms of PTSD in 4–7 % of cases [39].

Female victims of domestic assault are at a higher risk of PTSD, which would not be associated directly with the severity of aggression or with physical injuries, but rather with the intensity of the perceived threat [40].

25.4 Trauma

In DSM-IV trauma is defined as "an event that poses a threat to the physical integrity of the self or others". This definition supports a clear subjectivity (often a disparity between the perceived threat and the real threat), including traumatic events of variable gravity.

The types of trauma can be classified as natural disasters (floods, earthquakes), accidents (fires, traffic accidents or occupational), and trauma caused deliberately by man (physical abuse and/or sexual abuse and neglect, gender violence, assault, rape, terrorism, war, captivity, torture). The traumatic event can be unique (traffic accident) or repeated (child abuse, war experience) and produce an emotional impact that lasts from minutes to days, months or years. The trauma acquires a meaning for each person, and this meaning determines the type of response, which involves the type and intensity of the traumatic event, personality, and biography of the subject, and the biological and the social context [41].

The risk of a person being exposed throughout their lives to a traumatic situation can reach about 70 %. These figures seem to be on the rise in accordance with the conditions of modern city life, in which both gender violence in the community increases, and accidents (especially traffic) in some countries, causing an alarming increase in fatalities and a large number of people with physical and psychological scars. Resnick et al. [42, 43] found that from 4,008 women 36 % had been victim of a criminal situation, 33 % had suffered criminal trauma, 27 % sexual assault or rape, and 10 % had been assaulted.

In the US population, the most frequent precipitating situations for men were participating in combat and witnessing death or serious injury, and especially women reported assaults or physical or sexual threats and witnessed a life-threatening event [44].

A clear example of how studies conducted in environments have a section on female statistics is a recent documentary that shows that 15 % of recruits entering the army have committed or have attempted to commit a violation (usually to a partner in his company), which is double the percentage of the civilian population. In addition, these crimes committed in military settings allow the perpetrator to get away with it because in 33 % of cases the person who must report the incident is a friend of the rapist and in 25 % of cases is the same rapist. Therefore, after a war PTSD is not a disorder of a single cause, and the poor performance may be determined by social factors linked to a particular gender role [45].

Although women have a slightly lower average lifetime exposure to trauma, developing PTSD may depend on the type of trauma and its meaning. Rape and sexual abuse occur more commonly in women. Women have higher PTSD rates after childhood trauma than men, which suggests that trauma exposure in women at a young age might be a risk factor.

Women are also at a greater risk of developing PTSD later on in life as a result of a minor traumatic event if they have experienced a prior violent assault (Table 25.2). The effect of previous trauma suggests a kindling effect, with initial insults causing damage at the early developmental stages and influencing the perception of later trauma, thus increasing the likelihood of PTSD [46, 47].

A breakdown of the results of studies of lifetime prevalence of mental disorders in the USA, conducted by Kessler et al. [48] in the National Comorbidity Survey (NCS; Table 25.3), women have significant gender differences regarding the number of traumas experienced. Three traumas occur in 9.5 % of men and 5.0 % of women, and four or more traumas in 10.2 % of men and 6.4 % of women. Included in the type of traumatic event in men are frequently the atrocities of war, violent crime, and kidnapping and captivity, whereas in women the highest frequencies correspond to physical abuse and rape. Men have more accidents in childhood or serious physical injury than women (28 % vs 11 %) [48, 49].

Another study reported that the rates of PTSD are similar among men and women after events such as accidents (6.3 vs 8.8 %), natural disasters (3.7 vs 5.4 %), or the sudden death of a loved one (12.6 vs 16.2 %). Although women are more than 10 times more likely than men to be raped, the incidence of PTSD after rape is higher in men (65 vs 46 %). The rate of PTSD is lower in men than in

Table 25.2 Exposure to traumatic events by sex

Author	Men (%)	Women (%)
Kessler et al. (1995)[a]	60.7	51.2
Breslau et al. (1991)[b]	43.0	36.7
Kessler et al. (1995)[c]	35.6	14.5
Kessler et al. (1995)[d]	10.0	6.0
Breslau et al. (1998)[e]	5.3	4.3

[a, b]Lifetime prevalence of at least one traumatic event
[c]Witness to a death
[d]Exposure to four traumas
[e]Average traumatic events throughout urban life

Table 25.3 Significant sex differences for different traumatic events experienced by the general US population (Kessler et al. 1995)

Traumatic event type	Women (%)	Men (%)
Natural disaster	15.2	18.9
Life-threatening accident	13.8	25.0
Sexual abuse	12.3	2.8
Violation	9.2	0.7
Physical attack	6.9	11.1
Threatened with a weapon	6.8	19.0
Combat	0.0	6.4

women after events such as molestation (12.2 vs 26.5 %) and physical assault (1.8 vs 21.3 %) [50].

Whereas most traumatic events involving personal violence against men result from urban violence, women are more frequently victimized by domestic and sexual violence. For both men and women, the most frequent cause of PTSD is the sudden, unexpected death of a loved one, accounting for 34 % of all PTSD cases, followed by being mugged or threatened with a weapon among women (13.3 %), and being beaten up as a child by a caregiver among men (10 %). The exposure to rape and sexual assault constitutes the highest conditional risk for PTSD, both for men (20.1 %) and women (40 %) [51]. The risk of a woman developing PTSD after traumatic exposure is twice that of men, and some studies point to a risk of PTSD up to four times higher [47, 52].

The highest rates of PTSD in women have been attributed to higher rates of exposure to sexual trauma in women [53], but this seems to offer only a partial explanation of the differences between men and women. These differences found may also be due in part to the preexistence of anxiety disorders and major depression because they are more prevalent in women.

A study found that even among people who have not been exposed to sexual trauma, PTSD rates following exposure to other serious forms of trauma (i.e., aggressive violence) are several times higher in women than in men. The reasons for this differential susceptibility remain unknown, and may involve biological–genetic factors or sociocultural factors, or a combination [34].

25.5 Risk Factors for Trauma

In the female population the risk factors for developing this disorder include: suffering the trauma at an age below 15 years, more severe trauma, a history of behavioral or psychological problems, a family history of psychiatric disorder, parental poverty, child abuse, and separation or divorce of parents before the age of 5. In any case, these risk factors may not be specific only to women, as they are part of the wide range of vulnerability factors for psychiatric disorders in general.

In turn, victims of traumatic events are at an increased risk of separation or divorce, unemployment, and poverty, thus creating a vicious circle. Urban life increases the risk of adolescents experiencing more traumatic events (both community violence and gender violence) compared with the general population: between 8 and 55 situations for urban living vs 28 for the general population [54]. In a general population sample of 2,863 women found by a prospective study of 3 years, poverty status, single status or recently separated or divorced, and a lower educational level than their mothers or caregivers predisposed them to violence [55].

25.6 Gender Violence

One study found that PTSD was present in half of the subjects abused, which is a similar percentage to that in sexual assault. The forms of gender violence, psychological or physical, did not lead to changes in the prevalence of PTSD. In fact, among the victims of abuse and sexual assault there are also differences in other psychopathological variables (anxiety and depression), except for global maladjustment to everyday life, which is more pronounced in battered women. In any case, anxiety tends to appear more frequently in sexual assault victims; the depression, in the abuse, perhaps results from the feeling of helplessness with regard to a chronic aversive situation. Otherwise, a higher risk of experiencing adult lifetime partner violence among women with depressive disorders, anxiety disorders, and PTSD was found compared with women without mental disorders [56, 57].

A study of 1,952 women attending primary care found that 1 in 20 women had suffered gender violence in the last year, either as a child or as an adult, and an increased risk factors for violence (such as single or separate living, substance abuse, physical symptoms, and psychopathology) was found. It is estimated that more than 50 % of the women in Latin America and the Caribbean suffer some type of family violence [58, 59]. We also found that 21–34 % of women were victims of sexual abuse by their male partners over their lifetime [60, 61] and Polusny et al. [62], when they studied the general population, found that 15–33 % of women and 13–16 % of the men had been victims of childhood sexual abuse.

Gender violence, assessed in 422 households in Temuco (an urban community of southern Chile) determined that 49 % of women suffered psychological aggression, 13 % physical violence, and 5.5 % sexual abuse at the hands of her husband or partner and 8.5 % experienced physical violence during pregnancy. As factors associated with gender violence, anxiety and depressive symptoms were found.

There were also significant records of victims witnessing violence between parents, having a low level of education, having no gainful employment, abusing alcohol, and lacking a support network of neighbors. Violent men were characterized as being victims of violence in childhood, having a low level of education, having only occasional work, and drinking heavily [63].

In abused women during pregnancy, because of domestic violence, the risk of spontaneous abortion, pregnancy hypertension, intrahepatic cholestasis, and intrauterine growth retardation increased [64].

Moreover, women can also be the aggressor, but it is men who accumulate the highest figures relating to aggression. Child sexual abuse is committed in 96 % of cases by men (who usually have some kinship with the victims) and 4 % by women (who usually are the mothers of the victims) [65]. One percent of US violations are committed by a woman, according to Justice Department data [66].

In relation to the specific psychopathological profile of PTSD in different types are subjects, re-experiencing is very high in the victims of sexual assault, terrorism, and abuse; avoidance is very strong in almost all categories of patients and affects hyperactivation in all victims, except for people diagnosed with a serious illness. In the latter case symptoms of hopelessness are predominantly present [33, 61].

25.7 Clinic

The good assimilation and adaptation to psychological trauma is called resilience, the ability of the subject to respond adequately to a traumatic event. The concept of resilience is the opposite of vulnerability. A traumatic event can cause many different reactions from a few isolated emotional symptoms to the complete picture of PTSD, including even psychotic reactions, which are sometimes difficult to manage. Along with the psychological consequences, trauma can also be expressed in medical conditions such as smoking, cancer, ischemic heart disease, sexually transmitted disease or stroke [67].

25.8 Emotional Expression and Regulation

Expressing emotions is more common in the female gender. Several studies suggest greater verbal and written expression of emotions, whether positive or negative, in women, as they more frequently show a positive correlation between verbal and nonverbal expression than men. For some authors, men are used to avoiding criticism and conflict and stonewalling; this involves inhibition and minimizing facial expression and eye contact [68].

The trend in women is to externalize emotions. In fact, when PTSD symptoms have been present in the past 12 months, women are more willing to seek help than men, according to results of the NCS [69]. For all emotions except anger, women are superior at recognizing and decoding emotional facial, nonverbal, and vocal expressions.

Male anger is expressed through vocal modalities, facial and behavioral; however, women express anger of greater intensity and longer duration than men [70]. Women scored higher than men on variables of empathy and sympathy [71]; positive emotions collected included more intense or more frequent joy, affection, love, warmth, and good feelings [72]. The more dominant emotions that men tend to express are loneliness, contempt, arrogance, confidence, and guilt, scoring higher on the scales of irritability and anger.

A possible reflection of this is that this greater vocal and emotional recognition of women would make them more vulnerable to anxiety and affective disorders. Another thought is that women, being more prone to rumination as an emotional regulation strategy, experience greater depression and anxiety compared with men [32, 73].

The term "emotional regulation" has been used to refer to the variety of activities that allow individuals to monitor, evaluate, and modify the nature and course of emotional response, to pursue their goals, and respond appropriately to environmental demands.

There seem to be some gender differences in the relationships between emotional regulation strategies and psychopathology. Some theories suggest that gender differences in emotional regulation might contribute to gender differences in certain types of psychopathology [74–76].

Following this line, several theories suggest that psychopathology might result from the inability to downregulate negative emotions through strategies such as reappraisal, acceptance, troubleshooting or attentional redeployment. The reassessment is to find powers or negative and positive interpretations of an event to prevent or reduce negative mood about the event. Acceptance involves recognizing emotions without judging them. Problem solving includes active attempts to overcome or prevent a problem [77]. Finally, redistribution involves diverting attention from one of the positive or benign stimuli to change the mood (for example, avoiding watching a frightening scene) [78–81].

Some people not only fail to downregulate negative emotions, but also develop processes that exacerbate and prolong these emotions. Rumination, defined as perseverance, a proactive approach to negative emotions and the causes and consequences thereof, without participating in the resolution of problems, prospectively predicts the symptoms and diagnosis of major depression and anxiety [82–92]. Among the specific anxiety disorders, rumination is associated with an increased risk for social phobia [93], PTSD [94, 95], and generalized anxiety [77, 96, 97].

Psychopathology may also result from excessive attempts to downregulate negative emotions through strategies such as removal or avoidance [84, 98]. The various forms of repression and avoidance have been implicated in psychopathology, including suppression of emotional expression and unwanted thoughts [99].

The stereotypical view that the female sex is more emotional tends to be dominant in most cultures. In the majority of studies women have more emotional intensity than men and are more expressive. In one study carried out [100] only 3 of the 37 countries analyzed did not predominantly attribute the more emotional profile to women.

Women are widely viewed as the "more emotional sex" with a greater tendency to express and experience their emotions [101–106]. Men, on the other hand, are seen to have been designed to eliminate or avoid both experiencing and expressing emotions.

According to these views, some theories about gender roles suggest that women might use more introspection-focused responses, passive responses to their emotions, such as rumination, whereas men are more likely to use suppression or avoidance. Because the male gender role is to be more active, women are more likely to use strategies concerning emotional regulation like problem-solving, acceptance, distraction, seeking social support (or religion) and reassessment to try to control or change the situations that are directing their emotions [107].

Much of the emotional regulation in men can be automatic and unconscious. Also, the way men use social support to regulate their emotions may be different from that in women. Among women coping or emotional regulation through seeking social support predominates. Men often seek support from male relatives through shared activities and also have this predisposition to ruminate when they are angry, contributing to their higher rates of aggressive or antisocial activity.

This type of automatic, nonconscious engagement in emotional regulation may be more efficient and effective at reducing emotion arousal than conscious emotional regulation [108]. Thus, to the extent that men are especially likely to engage in nonconscious emotional regulation compared with women, they may be benefiting from strategies such as reappraisal even more than women. These gender differences in nonconscious emotional regulation and rumination may explain men's lower rates of disorders such as depression and PTSD compared with women.

Men may engage in more automatic, nonconscious emotional regulation, and the types of social support that men provide to one another may be different from those that women provide. In addition, men may engage in more anger rumination than women [79].

A study of women who had experienced civilian war-related trauma and women who had not suffered found that positive coping strategies related to civil war may be related to overcoming traumatic stress symptoms. Avoidance coping strategy is an important factor in maintaining PTSD symptoms that are consistent with the disorder itself [109].

25.8.1 Diagnostic Criteria

The DSM-IV-R classified PTSD into the group of anxiety disorders, but now the new classification, published in May 2013 (DSM-5), places it in a separate category called trauma and stressor-related disorders. All conditions included in this classification require exposure to a stressful or traumatic event as diagnostic criteria. The rationale for the creation of this new class is based on the clinical recognition of variable expressions of distress as a result of the traumatic experience. Trauma and stressor-related disorders include reactive attachment disorder, disinhibited social engagement disorder, PTSD, acute stress disorder, and adjustment disorders.

The necessary exposure criteria unify the tables included in this class: homogeneous expression of anxiety- or fear-based symptoms, anhedonia and dysphoric symptoms, aggressive symptoms, the dissociative, or some combination of those diagnoses listed differentiate this category.

The PTSD is defined by three symptom clusters in DSM-5: intrusive reexperiencing of the event, persistent avoidance of stimuli associated with the traumatic event, and the state of hyperarousal. These symptoms must last more than a month for the diagnosis of PTSD to be considered. The criteria apply for adults, adolescents, and children older than 6 years. Symptoms must cause clinically significant distress or impairment in social, occupational, or other important areas of functioning.

Intrusive phenomena include recurrent and intrusive recollections of the event, nightmares and feelings about them, behaviors or feelings, and sudden reliving of the traumatic event. Such situations, events, objects, and memories are correlated with abnormal or exaggerated physiological reactivity (sweating, tachycardia, tachypnea, tremor, piloerection, etc.). In many cases a stimulus, which can be an image, a tone of voice, a smell, a color or a word, can trigger the onset of these intrusive phenomena, which act as "triggers" or precipitants of the clinical symptoms.

Sometimes the syndrome presents with partial or complete amnesia episodes; thus, in the absence of a head injury the focus is on dissociative amnesia. We can also encounter other dissociative symptoms such as depersonalization, derealization, perceptual disturbances, and dissociative leakage, but these dissociative symptoms represent poor prognostic factors. The DSM-5 includes a clinical subtype "dissociative symptoms," which is applicable to individuals who meet the criteria for PTSD with the additional experience of depersonalization and derealization.

The second group of symptoms is related to the persistent avoidance of stimuli associated with the trauma; thus, the patient is able to minimize or prevent the onset of symptoms and autonomic invaders, which may involve avoidance of places, people, commemorative dates, conversations, etc.

The DSM-IV included here another group of symptoms: blunted affect. This consists of a reduction of the individual's ability to express emotions, which may give a wrong depressive aspect. The DSM-5 considers emotional numbing to be a specific group of symptoms.

Finally, the third group of symptoms is exaggerated startle response, hypervigilance, and concentration problems. There is an increased activation of a general state of hyperarousal. This group also includes insomnia and irritability.

The three groups of symptoms of the DSM-IV are divided into four groups in the DSM-5: intrusion, avoidance, negative alterations in cognition and mood, and changes in arousal and reactivity. It has broken up criterion C of the DSM-IV, avoidance and numbing, into two criteria: criterion C (avoidance) and criterion D (negative alterations in cognition and mood).

There are two forms of presentation of this entity. The acute form in where the remission of symptoms occurs in the first 3 months. If the clinical symptoms persist beyond 6 months we have a chronic presentation of the disorder. When the clinical picture does not emerge immediately after the traumatic event but appears after 6 months it is called delayed onset PTSD.

25.9 Clinical Features in Women

Women are about five times more likely to report symptoms of avoidance and four times more likely to have a state of hyper-alertness, loss of interest in significant activities, and sleep, concentration, and startle response problems [110]. Often the disease is complicated by depressive disorders, suicidal behavior and attempts, and alcohol abuse in women. Men more often have behavioral disorders. Women are more likely to become chronic [111].

Post-traumatic stress disorder is more common in women than in men. Sex role orientation will influence the way in which, from childhood, fear reactions are perceived in both sexes, so that children who see themselves as more masculine report fewer intensity fears associated with failure and criticism, less fear of the unknown and medical problems. However, there has been a positive relationship between femininity and fears. It is thought that these differences in children of either sex with regard to the reaction to stress may influence the spectrum of anxiety pathology at later ages. In the same vein, men express less anxiety than women, and they also seem to perceive their relationships and those of others in a less reliable manner than women, compared with an outside observer [112–114].

25.10 Comorbidity

Post-traumatic stress order is often associated with other mental pathological conditions such as major depression, anxiety disorders, substance use disorders, somatoform disorders, dissociative disorders, eating disorders, and borderline personality disorders [49, 115].

The extensive research of Kessler et al. [48] identified that 17 % of women had a diagnosis associated with PTSD compared with 12 % of men, but when three or more diagnoses were included men outnumbered women (59 % vs 44 %). These data suggest a possible induction of an underlying neurobiological diathesis given in youth adverse environments, and an effect on the development, causing increased susceptibility to the deleterious effects of future trauma.

Alternative explanations have been proposed for the association between PTSD and these disorders. First, preexisting psychiatric disorders may increase the likelihood of PTSD by increasing the risk for the exposure to traumatic events of the type that lead to PTSD or increase victims' susceptibility to the PTSD-inducing effects of trauma. Second, PTSD may be a causal risk factor for other psychiatric disorders. Use of alcohol or drugs to relieve the distressing symptoms of PTSD may increase the likelihood of dependence; major depression may develop as a complication of PTSD and its associated impairment. Third, the associations may be noncausal, reflecting shared genetic or environmental factors [48, 116].

To assess the comorbidity of PTSD it should be considered whether the variety is acute (up to 3 months' duration) or chronic PTSD. In chronic PTSD comorbidity has been described that can reach 80 % [117]. In contrast, in acute PTSD Carvajal et al. [118] found comorbidity of 38 % and it was the most frequent diagnosis of personality disorder.

Post-traumatic stress disorder also increases the risk in women of presenting a first depressive episode, dysthymia, mania, other anxiety disorders, and of developing substance abuse and dependence between three and four times that of people without PTSD. Conversely, in women who abuse substances, the frequency of PTSD is between 43 and 59 % [119, 120].

Both men and women with PTSD are more than twice as likely to have an associated medical pathological condition compared with subjects without PTSD. Depression and low income were risk factors for the medical comorbidity of PTSD in women, but not in men, according to data from the NCS [121].

A group of women who had been raped or had experienced an assault were evacuated within 2 weeks of the traumatic event and 3 months later, PTSD was diagnosed in 76 % and 49 % respectively. Also, comorbid depression was found in 29 % and 13 % [122]. The association between a history of sexual abuse and somatic symptoms in women attending primary care were studied and it was found that of 219 women, 43.9 % reported one or more traumatic events. More somatic symptoms and a history of abuse were a good predictor of more days of rest and further consultation in the 6 months prior to the study [123].

The PTSD diagnosis was proportionally more frequent among men than among women veterans; however, the risk of PTSD after combat exposure would be similar in both sexes. The problem is that there is probably a misdiagnosis of PTSD among women, as they have more medical problems and there would be a continuing relationship between hyperarousal symptoms and physical discomfort [124].

Dobie et al. [125] studied 1,259 veterans and found 21.0 % with PTSD. Patients with PTSD also had higher scores for psychiatric problems, substance abuse, and exposure to domestic violence. They also had a higher risk of physical problems (obesity, smoking, irritable bowel syndrome, fibromyalgia, chronic pelvic pain, polycystic ovary syndrome, asthma, cervical cancer, and stroke).

Personality disorder comorbid with PTSD in women with a history of sexual or nonsexual abuse in adulthood or childhood sexual abuse was not a factor that determines a higher percentage of PTSD at the end of treatment; however, women with disorder personality still had more symptoms at the end of therapy compared with those who only had PTSD. Hembree et al. [126] attributed this finding to the fact that patients with personality disorder treatment initiated were more symptomatic than the control group.

In the Canadian general population it was found that a history of childhood physical abuse was accompanied by an increased risk of developing a comorbid form of alcohol abuse and dependence with PTSD. Physical abuse reached a frequency of 51.4 % in PTSD vs 31.4 % in those without PTSD [72, 127].

One study examined the lifetime prevalence of trauma exposure and PTSD in patients with a first psychiatric admission for psychosis. The prevalence of trauma exposure was 68.5 %. Female gender and substance abuse were risk factors for trauma exposure. The prevalence of PTSD was 14.3 % in the full sample and 26.5 % in those with trauma exposure. Other significant risk factors were younger age and trauma exposure that was repeated and ongoing or that involved childhood victimization [128].

25.11 Discussion

Post-traumatic stress disorder is a relatively recent diagnosis. What really forced American psychiatry to consider this new diagnosis was the frequency and severity of cases observed in soldiers repatriated from the Vietnam War. For many years it has been a diagnosis exclusive to the battlefield, a field in which women were under-represented, so that indirectly they were excluded from the diagnosis. There are few studies that include women in the context of war; therefore, at least in this aspect, it is difficult to make an analysis of gender differences. Also, in most of the literature reviewed the concept of biological sex equates to that of gender.

Psychopathological differences that we found between the men and women differ in different studies, but primarily there has been a predominance of hyper-arousal and avoidance symptoms in women. It is possible that these differences, as well as the increased susceptibility of women to developing PTSD, may be based on the different strategies used by men and women when it comes to regulating their emotions.

Women are more prone to rumination, while men often employ strategies unaware that they decrease the risk of developing PTSD. These findings may be closely related to the gender role that is socially assimilated by a person who is either male (less expression of emotions, less likely to empathize, etc.) or female (increased expression of emotions, greater ability to talk and think about how she feels, etc.), which is not given by a biological fact but is associated with a way of being or being in the world that is largely determined by gender.

Despite the many studies reviewed, the reality is that these gender differences are determined by an unexplored world, a variable that today is not included in epidemiological studies and is therefore an important bias in determining the prevalence and the mode that presents the clinical expression of PTSD.

References

1. Alarcón R. Posttraumatic stress disorder. Studies in American veterans and their relevance for Latin America. Rev Chil Neuro-Psiquiat. 2002;40 Suppl 2:35–47.
2. Deuteronomy 20:1–9. The Holly Bible
3. Crocq MA, Crocq L. From shell shock and war neurosis to posttraumatic stress disorder: a history of psychotraumatology. Dialogues Clin Neurosci. 2001;2:47–55.
4. Pinel Ph. Nosographie Philosóphique. Paris: Bailliére; 1978.
5. Merskey H. Posttraumatic stress disorder and shell shock. In: Berrios GE, Porter R, editors. A history of clinical psychiatry. London: Athlone Press; 1995.
6. Salmon TW. Care and treatment of mental diseases and war neuroses (shell shock) in the British army. Ment Hyg. 1917;1:509–54.
7. Poal G. Enter, stay, move. Psychosocial aspects of the relationship between women and employment. Madrid: Siglo XXI; 1993.
8. Buenaventura Saez C. Gender socialization and psychopathology: a hypothesis for reflection. In: Gonzalez de Chavez MA (ed) Body and female subjectivity. Health and gender. Madrid: Siglo XXI; 1993.
9. Adams CH, Sherer M. Sex-role orientation and psychological adjustment: comparison of MMPI profiles among college women and housewives. J Pers Assess. 1982;46:607–13.
10. Bassoff ES, Glass GV. The relationship between sex roles and mental health: a meta-analysis of twenty-six studies. Couns Psychol. 1982;10:105–12.
11. Taylor MC, Hall JA. Psychological androgyny: theories, methods, and conclusions. Psychol Bull. 1982;92:347–66.
12. Orlofsky JL, O'Heron CA. Stereotypic and nonstereotypic sex role trait and behavior orientations: implications for personal adjustment. J Pers Soc Psychol. 1987;52(5):1034–42.
13. Flaherty JF, Duse JB. An investigation of the relationship between psychological androgyny and components of self-concept. J Pers Soc Psychol. 1980;38:984–92.
14. Gallacher F, Kieger DM. Sex role orientation and fear. J Psychol. 1995;129(1):41–9.
15. Thoronton B, Leo R. Gender typing, importance of multiple roles, and mental health consequences for women. Sex Roles. 1992;27(5–6):307–17.
16. Ward LC, Dillon EA. Psychiatric symptom correlates of the Minnesota multiphasic personality inventory masculinity-femininity scale. Psychol Assess. 1990;2(3):286–8.
17. Pérez Blasco J, Serra Desfilis E. Influence of traditional female role in anxiety symptoms in a sample of adult women. J Psychol. 1997;13(2):155–61.
18. Jezova D, Jurankova E, Mosnarova A, Kriska M, et al. Neuroendocrine response during stress with relation to gender differences. Acta Neurobiol Exp. 1996;56:779–85.
19. Yehuda R, Southwich SM, Nussbaum G, Wahby V, et al. Low urinary cortisol excretion in patients with posttraumatic stress disorder. J Nerv Ment Dis. 1990;178:366–9.
20. Bremner J, Licinio J, Darness A, Krystal JM, et al. Elevated CSF corticotropin-releasing factor concentrations in post-traumatic stress disorder. Am J Psychiatry. 1997;154:624–9.
21. Carvajal C. Neurobiological bases and pharmacotherapy of posttraumatic stress disorder. Rev Chil Neuropsiquiatr. 2002;40 Suppl 2:48–68.
22. Rubinow DR, Schmidt PJ. Gonadal steroids, brain and behavior: role of context. Dialogues Clin Neurosci. 2002;4:123–37.
23. De Bellis MD, Keshavan MS. Sex differences in brain maturation in maltreatment-related pediatric posttraumatic stress disorder. Neurosci Biobehav Rev. 2003;27:103–17.
24. Bremner JD, Vythiliogam M, Vermetten E, Southwick SM, et al. MRI and PET study of deficits in hippocampal structure and function in women with childhood sexual abuse and posttraumatic stress disorder. Am J Psychiatry. 2003;160:924–32.
25. Ferrando Bundío L, Álvarez Segura M. Salud mental y género en la práctica clínica. Ars Medica Psiquiatría. 2007;21:19–23.

26. Punamaki RL, Komproe IH. The role of peritraumatic dissociation and gender in the association between trauma and mental health in a Palestinian community simple. Am J Psychiatry. 2005;162:545–51.
27. Mitev YA, Dawish M, Wolf SS, Holsboer F, Almeida OF, Patchev VK. Gender differences in the regulation of 3 alpha-hydroxysteroid dehydrogenase in rat brain and sensitivity to neurosteroid-mediated stress protection. Neuroscience. 2003;20:541–9.
28. Fairbank J. Posttraumatic stress disorder. London: M. Dunitz; 2000.
29. Breslau N, Davis GC, Andreski P, Peterson EL, Schultz LR. Sex differences in posttraumatic stress disorder. Arch Gen Psychiatry. 1997;54(11):1044–8.
30. Stein MB, Walker JR. Findings from a community survey. Am J Psychiatry 1997.
31. Ezkurra J, Glez Pinto A, Gutierrez M. Psychiatry and women. Madrid: Grupo Aula Médica, SL; 2006.
32. Wolfe VV, Gentile C, Wolfe DA. The impact of sexual abuse on children: a PTSD formulation. Behavior Therapy. 1989;20(2):215–28.
33. Stein MB, Walker JR, Forde DR. Gender differences in susceptibility to posttraumatic stress disorder. Behav Res Ther. 2000;38:619–28.
34. Pulcino T, Galea S, Ahern J, Resnick H, et al. Posttraumatic stress in women after the September 11 terrorist attacks in New York City. J Womens Health. 2003;12:809–20.
35. Fullerton C, Ursano R, Epstein R, Crowley B, et al. Gender differences in posttraumatic stress disorder after motor vehicle accidents. Am J Psychiatry. 2001;158:1486–91.
36. Ruggiero KJ, Smith DW, Hanson RF, Resnick HS, et al. Is disclosure of childhood rape associated with mental health outcome? Results from the National Women's Study. Child Maltreat. 2004;9:62–77.
37. Soderquist J, Wijma K, Wijma B. Traumatic stress in late pregnancy. J Anxiety Disord. 2004;18:127–42.
38. Engelhard IM, van der Hount MA, Arntz A. Posttraumatic stress disorder after pregnancy loss. Gen Hosp Psychiatry. 2001;23:62–6.
39. Lindberg NM, Wellisch DK. Identification of traumatic stress reactions in women at increased risk of breast cancer. Psychosomatics. 2004;45:7–16.
40. Sutherland C, Bybee D, Sullivan C. The long-term effects of battering on women's health. J Womens Health. 1998;4:41–70.
41. Ursano RJ, Kao T, Fullerton CS. PTSD and meaning: human structuring chaos. J Nerv Mental Dis. 1992;180:756–9.
42. Resnick HS, Kilpatrick DG, Dansky BS, Saunders BE, et al. Prevalence of civilian trauma and posttraumatic stress disorder in a representative national sample of women. J Consult Clin Psychol. 1993;61:984–91.
43. Davidson JR. Trauma: the impact of posttraumatic stress disorder. J Psychopharmacol. 2000;14(2 Suppl):S5–12.
44. Rock Bennasar M. Neurotic disorders. Barcelona, Spain: Spanish Society of Psychiatry and Spanish Society of Biological Psychiatry. Editors Psychiatry S. L. 2002.
45. Dick K. "The Invisible War" United States; 2012.
46. Breslau N, Davis GC, Peterson EL, Schultz L. Psychiatric sequelae of posttraumatic stress disorder in women. Arch Gen Psychiatry. 1997;54:81–7.
47. Kohen D. Women and mental health. New York: Oxford University Press; 2010.
48. Kessler RC, Sonnega A, Bromet E, Hughes ME, et al. Posttraumatic stress disorder in the national comorbidity survey. Arch Gen Psychiatry. 1995;52:1048–60.
49. Breslau N, Davis GC, Peterson EL, Schultz L. Trauma and posttraumatic stress disorder in the community: the 1996 Detroit area survey of trauma. Arch Gen Psychiatry. 1996;1998 (55):626–32.
50. Cienachanowski P, Katon W. Last updated 30 Nov 2012. Posttraumatic stress disorder. Uptodate.com. Available at http://www.uptodate.com/contents/posttraumatic-stress-disorder
51. Viana MC, de Souza Dantas H, Farid Gattaz W, Andrade LH. Gender differences in exposure to traumatic events and post-traumatic stress disorder in the São Paulo megacity mental

health survey, Brazil: prevalence, distribution and conditional risk. In: 5th World Congress on women's mental health. 2013.
52. Vieweg WV, Julius DA, Fernandez A, Beatty-Brooks M, Hettema JM, Pandurangi AK. Posttraumatic stress disorder: clinical features, pathophysiology, and treatment. Am J Med. 2006;119(5):383.
53. Macmillan HL, Fleming JE, Trocme N, Boyle MJ, Wong M, Racine UA, Beardslee WR, Offord DR. Prevalence of child physical and sexual abuse in the community: results from the Ontario Health Supplement. Am J Med. 1997;278:131–5.
54. Horowitz K, Weine S, Jekel J. PTSD symptoms in urban adolescent girls: compounded community trauma. J Acad Child Adolesc Psychiatry. 1995;34:1353–61.
55. Byrne CA, Resnick HS, Kulpatrick DG, Best CL, et al. The socioeconomic impact of interpersonal violence on women. J Consult Clin Psychol. 1999;67:362–6.
56. Howard LM. Domestic violence and mental health. In: 5th World Congress on women's mental health. 2013.
57. Echeburúa E, de Corral P, Amor PJ. Differential profiles of PTSD in different types of victims. Analysis and behavior modification, vol 24, no. 96; 1998.
58. Silvia Gaviria. Violence against women in South America. In: 5th World Congress on women's mental health. 2013.
59. McCauley J, Kern DE, Kolodner K, Hill L, et al. The battering syndrome: prevalence and clinical characteristics of domestic violence in primary care internal medicine practices. Ann Intern Med. 1995;123:737–46.
60. Browne A. Violence against women by male partners: prevalence, outcomes, and policy implications. Am Psychol. 1993;48:1077–87.
61. Sassetti MR. Domestic violence. Prim Care. 1993;20:289–305.
62. Polusny MA, Follette VM. Long-term correlates of child sexual abuse: theory and review of the empirical literature. Appl Prev Psychol. 1995;4:143–66.
63. Vizcarra MB, Cortes J, Bustos L, Alarcon M, et al. Violencia married in the city of Temuco: a study of prevalence and associated factors. Chile Rev Med. 2001;129:1405–12.
64. Arcos E, Uarac M, Molina I, Repossi A, et al. Impact of domestic violence on reproductive and neonatal health. Rev Med Chile. 2003;131:1454–62.
65. Russell DE. The incidence and prevalence of intrafamilial and extrafamilial sexual abuse of female children. Child Abuse Negl. 1982;7:133–46.
66. Greenfeld LA. Sex offenses and offenders: an analysis on data on rape and sexual assault. Washington, DC: U.S. Department of Justice; 1997: Publication # NCH 163 392.
67. Felliti VJ, Anda RF, Nordenberg D, Williamson DF, et al. Relationship of childhood abuse and household dysfunction to many of the leading causes of death in adults: the adverse childhood experiences (ACE) study. Am J Prev Med. 1998;14:145–58.
68. Levenson R, Carstensen L, Gottman J. The influence of age and gender on affect, physiology, and their interrelations: a study of long-term marriages. J Pers Soc Psychol. 1994;67:56–68.
69. Kessler RC. Posttraumatic stress disorder: the burden to the individual and to society. J Clin Psychiatry. 2000;61 Suppl 5:4–12.
70. Brody LR. On understanding gender differences in the expression on emotion: gender roles, socialization an language. In: Ablon S, Brown D, Khantzian E, Mack J, editors. Human feelings: exploration in affect development and meaning. Hillsdale, NJ: Analytic Press; 1993. p. 89–121.
71. Gross JJ. The emerging field of emotion regulation: an integrative review. Rev Gen Psychol. 1998;2:271–99.
72. Lennon R, Eisenberg N. Gender and age differences in empathy and sympathy. In: Eisenberg N, Strayer J, editors. Empathy and its development. Cambridge: Cambridge University Press; 1987. p. 195–217.
73. Nolen-Hoeksema S. Emotion regulation and psychopathology: the role of gender. Annu Rev Clin Psychol. 2012;8:161–87.

74. Hyde JS, Mezulis AH, Abramson LY. The ABCs of depression: integrating affective, biological, and cognitive models to explain the emergence of the gender difference in depression. Psychol Rev. 2008;115:291–313.
75. Nolen-Hoeksema S. Responses to depression and their effects on the duration of depressive episodes. J Abnorm Psychol 1991;100:569–82.
76. Zahn-Waxler C, Shirtcliff EA, Marceau K. Disorders of childhood and adolescence: gender and psychopathology. Annu Rev Clin Psychol. 2008;4:275–303.
77. Hayes SC, Wilson KG, Gifford EV, Follette VM, Strosahl KD. Experiential avoidance and behavioral disorders: a functional dimensional approach to diagnosis and treatment. J Consult Clin Psychol. 1996;64:1152–68.
78. Billings AG, Moos RH. The role of coping responses and social resources in attenuating the stress of life events. J Behav Med. 1981;4(2):139–57.
79. Eisenberg N, Hofer C, Vaughan J. Effortful control and its socioemotional consequences. *Handbook of emotion regulation*: 2007:287–306
80. Kochanska G, Murray KT, Harlan ET. Effortful control in early childhood: continuity and change, antecedents, and implications for social development. Dev Psychol. 2000;36:220–32.
81. Rothbart MK, Bates JE. Temperament. In: Damon W, Eisenberg N, editors. Handbook of child psychology: vol 3. Social, emotional and personality development. New York: Wiley; 2006. p. 105–76.
82. Aldana A, Nolen-Hoeksema S, Schweizer S. Emotion regulation strategies across psychopathology: a meta-analytic review. Clin Psychol Rev. 2010;30:217–37.
83. Mor N, Winquist J. Self-focused attention and negative affect: a meta-analysis. Psychol Bull. 2002;128:638–62.
84. Rood L, Roelofs J, Bogels SM, Nolen-Hoeksema S, Schouten E. The influence of emotion-focused rumination and distraction on depressive symptoms in non-clinical youth: a meta-analytic review. Clin Psychol Rev. 2009;29:607–16.
85. Watkins ER. Constructive and unconstructive repetitive thought. Psychol Bull. 2008;134:163–206.
86. Clohessy S, Ehlers A. PTSD symptoms, response to intrusive memories and coping in ambulance service workers. Br J Clin Psychol. 1999;38:251–65.
87. Fresco DM, Frankel AN, Mennin DS, Turk CL, Heimberg RG. Distinct and overlapping features of rumination and worry: the relationship of cognitive production to negative affective states. Cogn Ther Res. 2002;26:179–88.
88. Harrington JA, Blankenship V. Ruminative thoughts and their relation to depression and anxiety. J Appl Soc Psychol. 2002;32:465–85.
89. Mayou RA, Ehlers A, Bryant B. Posttraumatic stress disorder after motor vehicle accidents: 3-year follow-up of a prospective longitudinal study. Behav Res Ther. 2002;40:665–75.
90. Nolen-Hoeksema S. The role of rumination in depressive disorders and mixed anxiety/depressive symptoms. J Abnorm Psychol. 2000;109:504–11.
91. Schwartz JAJ, Koenig LJ. Response styles and negative affect among adolescents. Cogn Ther Res. 1996;20:13–36.
92. Segerstrom SC, Tsao JCI, Alden LE, Craske MG. Worry and rumination: repetitive thought as a concomitant and predictor of negative mood. Cogn Ther Res. 2000;24:671–88.
93. Mellings TMB, Alden LE. Cognitive processes in social anxiety: the effects of self-focus, rumination, and anticipatory processing. Behav Res Ther. 2000;38:243–57.
94. Ehlers A, Mayou RA, Bryant B. Psychological predictors of chronic posttraumatic stress disorder after motor vehicle accidents. J Abnorm Psychol. 1998;107:508–19.
95. Murray J, Ehlers A, Mayou RA. Dissociation and post-traumatic stress disorder: two prospective studies of road traffic accident survivors. Br J Psychiatry. 2002;180:363–8.
96. McLaughlin KA, Nolen-Hoeksema S. Rumination as a transdiagnostic factor in depression and anxiety. Behav Res Ther. 2011;49:186–93.
97. Watkins ER. Depressive rumination and co-morbidity: evidence for brooding as to transdiagnostic process. J Ration Emot Cogn Behav Ther. 2009;27:160–75.

98. Wenzlaff RM, Wegner DM. Thought suppression. Annu Rev Psychol. 2000;51:59–91.
99. Fischer AH, Rodriguez Mosquera AM, van Vianen AE, Manstead AS. Gender and culture differences in emotion. Emotion. 2004;1:87–94.
100. Barrett L, Bliss-Moreau E. She's emotional. He's having a bad day: attributional explanations for emotion stereotypes. Emotion. 2009;9:648–58.
101. Brody LR, Hall JA. Gender and emotion in context. In: Lewis M, Haviland JM, Barrett LF, editors. Handbook of emotions. New York: Guilford; 1993. p. 89–121.
102. Deaux K, Major B. Putting gender into context: an interactive model of gender-related behavior. Psychol Rev. 1987;94:369–89.
103. Fabes RA, Martin CL. Gender and age stereotypes of emotionality. Staff Soc Psychol Bull. 1991;17:532–40.
104. Fischer AH, Manstead ASR. The relation between gender and emotions in different cultures. In: Fischer AH, editor. Gender and emotion: social psychological perspectives. New York: Cambridge University Press; 2000. p. 71–94.
105. LaFrance M, Banaji M. Toward a reconsideration of the gender-emotion relationship. In: Clark MS, editor. Emotion and social behavior. Newbury Park, CA: Sage; 1992. p. 178–201.
106. Shields SA. Women, men, and the dilemma of emotion. In: Shaver P, Hendrick C, editors. Sex and gender: review of personality and social psychology. Thousand Oaks, CA: Sage; 1987. p. 229–50.
107. Tamres LK, Janicki D, Helgeson VS. Sex differences in coping behavior: a meta-analytic review and an examination of relative coping. Staff Soc Psychol Rev. 2002;6:2–30.
108. Mauss IB, Evers C, Wilhelm FH, Gross JJ. How to bite your tongue without blowing your top: implicit evaluation of emotion regulation predicts affective responding to anger provocation. Personal Soc Psychol Bull. 2006;32:589–602.
109. Franciskovic T, Stevanovic A, Colic M. Coping strategies and PTSD among female civilian victims of war. In: 5th World Congress on women's mental health. 2013.
110. Howell HB, Brawman-Mintzer O, Monnier J, Yonkers KA. Generalized anxiety disorder in women. Psychiatr Clin North AM. 2001;24:165–78.
111. Breslau N, Davis G. Posttraumatic stress disorder in an urban population of young adults: risk factors for chronicity. Am J Psychiatry. 1992;149:671–5.
112. Ginsburg GS, Silverman WK. Gender role orientation and fearfulness in children with anxiety disorders. J Anxiety Disord. 2000;14:57–67.
113. Roy K, Brownhill S. Gender differences in depression risk and coping factors in a clinical sample. Acta Psychiatr Scand. 2002;106:45–53.
114. Laura Ferrando Bundio. Mental health and gender in clinical practice, 1st ed. Group Communication Ars XXI, SL; 2007.
115. Brady KT, et al. Comorbidity of psychiatric disorders and posttraumatic stress disorder. J Clin Psychiatry. 2000;61:22–32.
116. Breslau N. Epidemiologic studies of trauma, Posttraumatic stress disorder and other psychiatric disorders. Can J Psychiatry. 2002;47:923–9.
117. Brady KT. Posttraumatic stress disorders and comorbidity: recognizing the many faces of PTSD. J Clin Psychiatry. 1997;58 suppl 9:12–5.
118. Carvajal C, González M, Carbonell CG, Trucco M. PTSD in work accidents. Rev Chil Neuropsiquiatr. 1997;35:161–5.
119. Brown PJ, Recupero PR, Stout R. PTSD substance abuse comorbidity and treatment utilization. Addict Behav. 1995;20:251–4.
120. Danky BS, Roitsch JC, Brady KT, Saladin ME. Posttraumatic stress disorder. Posttraumatic stress disorder and substance abuse. Use of research in a clinical setting. J Trauma Stress. 1997;10:141–8.
121. Kimerling R. An investigation of sex differences in non psychiatric morbidity associated with posttraumatic stress disorder. J Am Med Womens Assoc. 2004;59:42–7.
122. Resnick P. An exploration of PTSD and MDD comorbidity. In: Presented at the 150th annual meeting. New York: American Psychiatric Association; 2004.

123. Stein MB, Lang AJ, Lafaye C, Satz L, et al. Relationship of sexual assault history to somatic symptoms and health anxiety in women. Gen Hosp Psychiatry. 2004;26(3):178–83.
124. Kimerlin R, Clum G, Wolfe J. Relationships among trauma exposure, chronic posttraumatic stress disorders symptoms and self reported health in women: replication and extension. J Trauma Stress. 2000;13:115–28.
125. Dobbie DJ, Kivlahan DR, Maynard C, Bush K, et al. Posttraumatic stress disorder in female veterans: association with self-reported health problems and functional impairment Arch Intern Med. 2004;164:394–400.
126. Hembree EA, Cachil SP, Foa EB. Impact of personality disorder on treatment outcome form female assault survivors with chronic posttraumatic stress disorder. J Personal Disord. 2004;18:117–27.
127. Van Ameringen MA, Mancini CL, Pipe B, Oakman D, et al. Child abuse and the development of PTSD in a Canadian epidemiological sample. Presented at the 157th annual meeting. New York: American Psychiatry Association; 2004.
128. Neria Y, Bromet EJ, Sievers S, Lavelle J, Fochtmann LJ. Trauma exposure and post-traumatic stress disorder in psychosis: findings from a first admission cohort. J Consult Clin Psychol. 2002;70:246–51.

Gender and First Psychotic Episodes in Adolescence

26

Beatriz Payá-González, Jose López-Gil, Emma Noval-Aldaco, and María Ruiz-Torres

Abstract

Gender-related differences in epidemiological and clinical variables of psychosis have long been recognized; however, data in first episodes of psychosis (FEPs) in subjects younger than 18 years old are scarce. Before the onset of psychosis, women are more likely to have a history of suicide attempts and depression, and they are more likely to have depressive symptoms. In samples of FEPs, a female preponderance for specific traumatic events such as sexual abuse and bullying is found.

Men have a longer duration of untreated illness and poorer premorbid adjustment than women. Men also have substance use problems that were evident before admission and have a poorer response to antipsychotic medications and a poorer outcome than women.

Overall findings suggest different pathways to the development of psychosis between adolescent men and women and point to the influence of gender over some of the predisposing factors in this age range. In addition to biological differences, gender seems to have an effect on the impact of individual risk factors or on the possibility of exposure to specific life events. Men seem to have more susceptibility to neurodevelopmental abnormalities as well as a predisposition to substance abuse. However, traumatic experiences as a risk factor for psychosis may carry greater weight in the female gender. For this reason, we should consider a female predominance in psychotic disorders associated with trauma.

B. Payá-González (✉) • J. López-Gil
Valdecilla University Hospital, Santander, Spain
e-mail: bpaya@humv.es

E. Noval-Aldaco • M. Ruiz-Torres
Department of Psychiatry, Valdecilla University Hospital, Santander, Spain

M. Sáenz-Herrero (ed.), *Psychopathology in Women*,
DOI 10.1007/978-3-319-05870-2_26

26.1 Introduction

Gender-related differences in prevalence, clinical expression, and outcome of psychosis have long been recognized. However, epidemiological data in first episodes of psychosis (FEPs) are scarce, and even more so for FEPs in subjects younger than 18 years old.

Some studies of FEPs in young adult subjects [1] replicate the male preponderance found in adult samples. Generally, women are older than men and have a shorter duration of untreated psychosis (DUP).

In samples of patients with FEPs [2] it was observed that before the onset of psychosis, women were more likely to have a history of suicide attempts and depression and they are more likely to have depressive symptoms. Conversely, men had a longer DUP and marked substance use problems that were evident before admission and persisted throughout treatment. In addition or moreover, follow-up studies of FEPs in people younger than 25 years [3] reveal that female sex, an older age at the onset of psychosis, and shorter DUP predicted symptomatic remission at the end of follow-up. These findings reveal the existence of differences between men and women in the clinical characteristics and outcome of the FEP that point to the role of gender as a relevant variable to take into account in the study of FEPs and that may help to better understand some of the etiopathogenic mechanisms of the illness.

Throughout this chapter we review and discuss current findings regarding this topic in adolescents with FEPs of adolescent onset.

26.2 Gender Differences in the Early Phases of the Psychotic Illness: Premorbid Adjustment and DUP

A large body of research has focused interest on the period that precedes the onset of the psychosis because it could help us to understand the underlying mechanisms that predispose to the illness [4–7]. Some of these studies, focusing on the level of functioning before the onset of the illness, find gender differences in premorbid adjustment [8]. Men exhibit more severe premorbid impairment with a faster deterioration than women. The impairment of premorbid adjustment has been associated with poorer outcome in samples of FEPs in both adults [9] and at early onset [10].

Overall, a pattern of poor and deteriorated premorbid adjustment indicates that a process of asymptomatic deficit precedes the onset of the psychosis by some period. Based on this, some authors propose that the existence of premorbid deficits supports a neurodevelopmental model in the genesis of the psychosis. The neurodevelopmental model has long been dominant for childhood-onset neuropsychiatric disorders and posits that the illness is the end state of an abnormal neurodevelopmental process that started years before the illness onset.

According to the findings of better premorbid adjustment in women, some authors suggest that estrogens, with effects on both neurodevelopment and neurotransmission, might play a neuroprotective role in women [11, 12].

Studies with rodents also find specific differences by sex in genetic expression [13] and neurochemical response of brain following brain injury (hypoxia–ischemia) in the neonatal period [14]; these findings also support the female gender possibly having better mechanisms for cerebral neuroprotection compared with the male.

In general samples of FEPs, another variable linked to the early phases of the illness is the DUP; this variable was also found to be longer in men than in women [15]. Recent studies of DUP in adolescent-onset psychosis, found that DUP is approximately twice the length of DUP amongst adults. In adolescent samples, the longer DUP was associated with younger age at onset of the psychosis and with greater life-time cannabis use [16].

Interestingly, different studies [17, 18] have reported that substance abuse is more prevalent in adolescent men than in women before the onset of the psychosis. In adolescent FEP samples, there are no comparisons in DUP by gender; however, the higher prevalence of substance abuse between adolescent men may predispose to a longer duration of untreated psychosis between men compared with women as happens in adult samples.

26.3 The Role of Gender in Risk Factors of Psychosis

26.3.1 Substance Abuse

Different drugs, such as alcohol, cannabis, amphetamines, cocaine, and psychedelics have been linked to psychosis in adolescents [19, 20]. However, the relationship between cannabis and psychosis is the most extensively studied in the literature. Cannabis use has been associated with different mental disorders, particularly psychotic disorders. Cannabis intoxication can produce acute and transient psychotic symptoms and exacerbation of pre-existing psychotic symptoms [21].

Different meta-analyses have consistently found an association between cannabis use and psychosis [22, 23]; however, the mechanism by which cannabis predisposes to psychotic disorders is yet to be clarified. Findings of follow-up studies suggest that continued use of cannabis might increase the risk of developing a psychotic disorder through the persistence of symptoms [24]. Cannabis is the most commonly used drug worldwide, especially in the adolescence and it is also the most frequently used illicit substance in FEP patients. In this population, a greater proportion of men than women have a current illicit substance use disorder (SUD) at the onset of the illness [18].

Some research [23] supports the notion that the risk of experiencing psychotic symptoms with cannabis is higher in younger ages (less than 14 years); thus, its relevance as a predisposing factor for psychosis must be considered in this age population, especially in male subjects.

26.3.2 Traumatic Life Events

Exposure to childhood adverse experiences is strongly associated with an increased risk of psychosis [25]. Several large population-based studies have found associations between various types of early trauma (such as sexual, physical, emotional abuse, and neglect) and psychotic symptoms in adolescence as well as full-blown psychotic disorders in adulthood [26–28].

Some studies have also explored this issue in FEP [29]. In the studies mentioned a high percentage of patients with FEP had been exposed to stressful events before psychosis onset and a considerable percentage of them had been exposed to sexual and physical abuse (SPA).

The group of patients exposed to SPA was more likely to have presented other psychiatric disorders before psychosis onset. Three specific diagnoses that include post-traumatic stress disorder, substance abuse, and suicide attempts were significantly more prevalent in the past history of abused compared with non-abused patients. Another type of childhood trauma, that of being a victim of bullying, has also been associated with a wide range of mental health problems in adolescence [30], as well as subclinical psychotic symptoms [31–34]. Some authors have also shown an interest in studying gender differences in the rates of childhood trauma [29] in samples of FEPs, finding a female preponderance for sexual but not for physical abuse.

In samples of FEP, gender differences were additionally found for bullying; compared with men, a larger proportion of women had been bullied.

A first explanation for the female preponderance observed in sexual abuse and bullying may be sociocultural values that predispose adolescent girls to exposure to higher stress levels than men and to specific life events such as sexual abuse. In fact, several studies have shown that women experience more depressogenic and a greater number of negative life events than men, such as violence and sexual abuse [35]. A stronger effect or a deeper impact of bullying than other forms of early victimization in women [36] with regard to men could be another explanation for the phenomena observed.

Accordingly, it has been postulated that there is a female cognitive predisposition to higher levels of negative affect upon the occurrence of negative life events. Different studies have also confirmed a greater female tendency toward rumination in both adolescents [37–39] and adults [40–43]. A ruminative response style, defined by Nolen-Hoeksema [44] as a response to negative life events characterized by excessive focus on negative emotions, increased the likelihood of developing psychopathological disorders.

It is known that girls are more prone to develop internalizing difficulties, whereas boys tend to respond by exhibiting externalizing behavior or substance abuse [36, 45]. Furthermore, internalizing problems have been found to mediate the association between bullying exposure and psychotic symptoms [46], which may therefore put girls at greater risk of developing psychosis in specific stress situations.

26.4 Risk Factors, Gender, and Subtypes of Psychotic Disorders

In the etiology of psychosis, monocausal models have been replaced by multidisciplinary perspectives that integrate psychosocial interactions as well as neurobiological predispositions. In this way, biological vulnerabilities could make some individuals more susceptible to specific environmental factors and potentially lead to the development of the psychotic illness. Shah et al. [47] also highlight the influence of the social factors on an ecological level in the way that they can change the risk of a population basis or change environmental risk in a multifaceted and complex interplay between individual and ecological dimensions. In this sense, and in addition to differences in biological variables, gender, understood to be the cultural construct on which society elaborates on anatomical sex, could also modulate in an ecological dimension, at least to some extent, the predisposition to the psychotic illness, either by decreasing the impact of individual risk factors or by reducing the possibility of exposure to individual social risks.

As mentioned above, regarding environmental risk factors, increasing evidence supports the role of cannabis and other drugs and childhood trauma in the etiology of psychosis, but underlying mechanisms as well as their implication in the different types of psychotic disorders are poorly understood.

Substance use disorders (SUD), postulated as one of the predisposing factors for psychosis, constitute a more frequent clinical condition among men than among women at the onset of the FEP. Studies show that patients with SUD at the debut of the illness are more likely to be men with a lower age at onset than those patients without SUD [17, 18].

Naninck et al. [48] propose that there is a greater tendency of men to cope with sadness or stress in different ways than women, having a greater tendency to increase toxic consumption in stressful situations. Based on this thinking it is reasonable to believe that the younger the subject, the fewer psychological strategies to manage stress they have; therefore, the use of drugs of abuse as a mechanism to manage emotional distress may be a more common coping mechanism in this age range.

Follow-up studies show that cannabis-induced psychotic disorders turn into other types of psychotic disorders in the follow-up, schizophrenia spectrum disorders constituting a significant percentage [49]. Available data [17] also suggest that substance use disorders, especially cannabis use disorders, are common in FEP patients and appear to be linked to a longer duration of untreated psychosis, a poor response to antipsychotic medications, and a poor outcome; thus, the existence of cannabis use disorder seems to have a negative effect on the level of severity and outcome of the psychosis. Interestingly, some of these clinical and outcome variables are more usually linked to men than women in clinical studies of FEPs.

In summary, these findings point to the existence of an interrelation between male gender and substance abuse. In addition, this particular gender–environmental interaction seems to predispose to a specific clinical profile with a worse outcome of the FEP in men.

Although exposure to childhood adverse experiences is strongly associated with an increased risk of psychosis [25], more questions arise about the role of trauma at the different psychotic disorders (the role or the weight that trauma have in the genesis of each of the different psychotic disorders). A review by Bendall and colleagues [50] pointed out the lack of evidence for a stronger effect of childhood trauma on schizophrenic psychosis than on affective psychosis. According to this review, preliminary studies on small adolescent samples did not support any specific association with either schizophrenia or bipolar disorders, but reported a higher prevalence of early adversities in subjects with atypical psychosis. In this type of psychosis, dissociative symptoms and context-specific hallucinations and delusions are usual clinical symptoms.

The association between trauma and atypical clinical presentation of psychotic episodes has also been supported by other authors [51] , who report dissociative symptoms in psychotic patients with early maltreatment. These authors find a positive association between severity of childhood trauma and dissociative symptoms. Emotional abuse showed the strongest associations with dissociation in both chronic patients and FEP patients. Higher levels of depression, anxiety, and a poorer sense of self [52] have also been reported in those subjects who had experienced past trauma and bullying.

Testing theories of the relationship between childhood traumatic experiences and atypical clinical presentation in FEP, Bendall et al. [53] found that those subjects with FEP and childhood sexual abuse (CSA) had more severe hallucinations and delusions than those with FEP and without CSA. The results are consistent with the post-traumatic intrusions account of hallucinations and delusions in those with CSA and psychosis.

Studies in early onset psychotic disorders also find differences in premorbid antecedents between groups of psychotic disorders. Meanwhile, social withdrawal and peer problems are specific to youths with schizophrenia; the psychotic disorder not otherwise specified (PsyNOS) has higher rates of abuse histories and post-traumatic stress disorder. The PsyNOS is a diagnostic entity that involves the presence of at least one positive psychotic symptom that does not fulfill the criteria for schizophrenia or schizoaffective disorder, a psychotic mood disorder, delusional disorder, acute psychotic disorder, schizophreniform disorder, or a psychotic disorder secondary to a medical disorder or substance use [54]. In clinical practice, the diagnosis of PsyNOS is often used in atypical psychotic presentations. The abuse antecedents in the psychosis NOS group may explain the atypical nature of their reported psychotic symptoms, which in many cases likely represent a post-traumatic phenomenon.

Conclusions

The findings presented throughout this chapter reveal gender differences in adolescent onset FEPs that may suggest different pathways to the development of psychosis. Data also point to the influence of gender over some predisposing factors for psychosis in adolescents. In this sense, and in addition to differences in biological variables, gender seems to modulate the predisposition to the psychotic illness either by its effect on the impact of individual risk factors or in the possibility of exposure to individual social risks.

Biological differences between men and women interacting with the predisposing factors that may in turn be influenced by social and cultural factors may explain differences in the etiopathogenesis and clinical expression of psychosis between men and women.

First, most of the studies support the notion that women exhibit better premorbid adjustment than men, less deterioration in premorbid functioning from childhood to late adolescence than men, and shorter DUP. On the other hand, male gender tends to be linked to variables of worse outcome.

The impairment and the deterioration of premorbid functioning have been proposed as neurodevelopmental markers in schizophrenia [6, 7, 55–57]. The poorer and more deteriorated premorbid adjustment among men supports a male vulnerability to suffer psychosis with a neurodevelopmental origin. In fact, a higher frequency of neurodevelopmental disorders such as dyslexia or autism is more commonly diagnosed in boys than in girls.

This hypothesis is also supported by animal studies that reveal gender differences in the expression of genes as well as in neurochemical mechanisms involved in neurodevelopment. These studies also find a different brain response in male and female subjects after perinatal insults.

In addition to a hypothetical, gender-specific, biological vulnerability to certain types of psychosis, another highlight is how gender itself may have an influence on the predisposing factors for psychosis.

Whereas women may translate the traumatic experiences first into anxiety, depression, and nonclinical psychotic symptoms, and then contribute to the development of an at-risk state for psychosis, men may be more likely to manage traumatic life events through substance abuse.

The etiology of psychosis is complex and requires explanatory models that include gene by environment interactions. In this sense the male gender could lead to increased susceptibility to neurodevelopmental abnormalities as well as to a predisposition to substance abuse. The interaction of the two factors could confer to the male gender greater vulnerability to suffering more severe psychosis of neurodevelopmental origin, such as schizophrenia spectrum disorders, and with a worse prognosis.

On the other hand, the stress and traumatic experiences as a risk factor for psychosis may carry greater weight in the female gender in two ways. First, because the fact of being a woman increases the probability of being exposed to certain traumatic experiences such as sexual abuse, and partly because there seems to be evidence supporting the interaction of sociocultural pressure with biological factors, which may determine that one traumatic experience can have a greater impact on women than men.

Therefore, we should consider the possible predominance of the female gender in psychotic disorders associated with trauma, such as the brief psychotic disorder or psychosis with atypical clinical expressions and dissociative symptoms.

The prevalence of this type of psychosis in women may explain, together with increased resistance to possible perinatal brain insults, the better outcome found in FEPs in women. However, more studies are needed to clarify all these questions that may have n significant implication for implementing specific prevention strategies and individualized treatments based on the gender of the adolescent.

References

1. Cocchi A, Lora A, Meneghelli A, La Greca E, Pisano A, Cascio MT, Preti A. Sex differences in first-episode psychosis and in people at ultra-high risk. Psychiatry Res. 2014;215(2):314–22.
2. Cotton SM, Lambert M, Schimmelmann BG, Foley DL, Morley KI, McGorry PD, Conus P. Gender differences in premorbid, entry, treatment, and outcome characteristics in a treated epidemiological sample of 661 patients with first episode psychosis. Schizophr Res. 2009;114 (1–3):17–24.
3. Chang WC, Tang JY, Hui CL, Lam MM, Chan SK, Wong GH, Chiu CP, Chen EY. Prediction of remission and recovery in young people presenting with first-episode psychosis in Hong Kong: a 3-year follow-up study. Aust N Z J Psychiatry. 2012;46(2):100–8.
4. Addington J, Addington DA. Patterns of premorbid functioning in first episode psychosis: relationship to 2-year outcome. Acta Psychiatr Scand. 2005;112(1):40–6.
5. McClellan J, Breiger D, McCurry C, Hlastala SA. Premorbid functioning in early-onset psychotic disorders. J Am Acad Child Adolesc Psychiatry. 2003;42(6):666–72.
6. Monte RC, Goulding SM, Compton MT. Premorbid functioning of patients with first-episode nonaffective psychosis: a comparison of deterioration in academic and social performance, and clinical correlates of premorbid adjustment scale scores. Schizophr Res. 2008;104(1–3): 206–13.
7. Payá B, Rodríguez-Sánchez JM, Otero S, Muñoz P, Castro-Fornieles J, Parellada M, Gonzalez-Pinto A, Soutullo C, Baeza I, Rapado-Castro M, Sáenz-Herrero M, Moreno D, Arango C. Premorbid impairments in early-onset psychosis: differences between patients with schizophrenia and bipolar disorder. Schizophr Res. 2013;146(1–3):103–10.
8. Larsen TK, McGlashan TH, Johannessen JO, Vibe-Hansen L. First-episode schizophrenia: II. Premorbid patterns by gender. Schizophr Bull. 1996;22(2):257–69.
9. Chang WC, Tang JY, Hui CL, Wong GH, Chan SK, Lee EH, Chen EY. The relationship of early premorbid adjustment with negative symptoms and cognitive functions in first-episode schizophrenia: a prospective three-year follow-up study. Psychiatry Res. 2013;209(3):353–60.
10. Hassan GA, Taha GR. Long term functioning in early onset psychosis: two years prospective follow-up study. Behav Brain Funct. 2011;7:28.
11. Pregelj P. Neurobiological aspects of psychosis and gender. Psychiatr Danub. 2009;1:128–31.
12. Kulkarni J, Gavrilidis E, Worsley R, Van Rheenen T, Hayes E. The role of estrogen in the treatment of men with schizophrenia. Int J Endocrinol Metab. 2013;11(3):129–36.
13. Ziats MN, Rennert OM. Identification of differentially expressed microRNAs across the developing human brain. Mol Psychiatry. 2014;19(7):848–52.
14. Weis SN, Toniazzo AP, Ander BP, Zhanm X, Careagam M, Ashwood P, Wyse AT, Netto CA, Sharp FR. Autophagy in the brain of neonates following hypoxia-ischemia shows sex- and region-specific effects. Neuroscience. 2014;256:201–9.
15. Chang WC, Tang JY, Hui CL, Lam MM, Wong GH, Chan SK, Chiu CP, Chung DW, Law CW, Tso S, Chan K, Hung SF, Chen EY. Duration of untreated psychosis: relationship with baseline characteristics and three-year outcome in first-episode psychosis. Psychiatry Res. 2012;198 (3):360–5.
16. Dominguez MD, Fisher HL, Major B, Chisholm B, Rahaman N, Joyce J, Woolley J, Lawrence J, Hinton M, Marlowe K, Aitchison K, Johnson S, Hodes M. Duration of untreated

psychosis in adolescents: ethnic differences and clinical profiles. Schizophr Res. 2013;150 (2–3):526–32.
17. Green AI, Tohen MF, Hamer RM, Strakowski SM, Lieberman JA, Glick I, Clark WS, HGDH Research Group. First episode schizophrenia-related psychosis and substance use disorders: acute response to olanzapine and haloperidol. Schizophr Res. 2004;66(2–3):125–35.
18. Lange EH, Nesvåg R, Ringen PA, Hartberg CB, Haukvik UK, Andreassen OA, Melle I, Agartz I. One year follow-up of alcohol and illicit substance use in first-episode psychosis: does gender matter? Compr Psychiatry. 2014;55(2):274–82.
19. McClellan J, Stock S. Practice parameter for the assessment and treatment of children and adolescents with schizophrenia. J Am Acad Child Adolesc Psychiatry. 2013;52(9):976–90.
20. Kuzenko N, Sareen J, Beesdo-Baum K, Perkonigg A, Höfler M, Simm J, Lieb R, Wittchen HU. Associations between use of cocaine, amphetamines, or psychedelics and psychotic symptoms in a community sample. Acta Psychiatr Scand. 2011;123(6):466–74.
21. Minozzi S, Davoli M, Bargagli AM, Amato L, Vecchi S, Perucci CA. An overview of systematic reviews on cannabis and psychosis: discussing apparently conflicting results. Drug Alcohol Rev. 2010;29(3):304–17.
22. Moore TH, Zammit S, Lingford-Hughes A, Bames TR, Jones PB, Burke M, et al. Cannabis use and risk of psychotic or affective mental health outcomes: a systematic review. Lancet. 2007;370:319–28.
23. Stefanis NC, Delespaul P, Henquet C, Bakoula C, Stefanis CN, Van Os J. Early adolescent cannabis exposure and positive and negative dimensions of psychosis. Addiction. 2004;99:1333–41.
24. Kuepper R, van Os J, Lieb R, Wittchen HU, Höfler M, Henquet C. Continued cannabis use and risk of incidence and persistence of psychotic symptoms: 10 year follow-up cohort study. BMJ. 2011;342:d738.
25. Varese F, Smeets F, Drukker M, Lieverse R, Lataster T, Viechtbauer W, Read J, van Os J, Bentall RP. Childhood adversities increase the risk of psychosis: a meta-analysis of patient-control, prospective- and cross-sectional cohort studies. Schizophr Bull. 2012;38(4):661–71.
26. Morgan C, Fisher H. Environment and schizophrenia: environmental factors in schizophrenia: childhood trauma–a critical review. Schizophr Bull. 2007;33(1):3–10.
27. Read J, van Os J, Morrison AP, Ross CA. Childhood trauma, psychosis and schizophrenia: a literature review with theoretical and clinical implications. Acta Psychiatr Scand. 2005;112 (5):330–50.
28. Schäfer I, Fisher HL. Childhood trauma and psychosis—what is the evidence? Dialogues Clin Neurosci. 2011;13(3):360–5.
29. Conus P, Cotton S, Schimmelmann BG, McGorry PD, Lambertm M. Pretreatment and outcome correlates of sexual and physical trauma in an epidemiological cohort of first-episode psychosis patients. Schizophr Bull. 2010;36(6):1105–14.
30. Arseneault L, Bowes L, Shakoor S. Bullying victimization in youths and mental health problems: 'much ado about nothing'? Psychol Med. 2010;40(5):717–29.
31. Arseneault L, Cannon M, Fisher HL, Polanczyk G, Moffitt TE, Caspi A. Childhood trauma and children's emerging psychotic symptoms: a genetically sensitive longitudinal cohort study. Am J Psychiatry. 2011;168(1) 65–72.
32. Campbell ML, Morrison AP. The relationship between bullying, psychotic-like experiences and appraisals in 14-16-year olds. Behav Res Ther. 2007;45(7):1579–91.
33. Kelleher I, Keeleym H, Corcoran P, Ramsay H, Wasserman C, Carli V, Sarchiapone M, Hoven C, Wasserman D, Cannon M. Childhood trauma and psychosis in a prospective cohort study: cause, effect, and directionality. Am J Psychiatry. 2013;170(7):734–41.
34. Mackie CJ, O'Leary-Barrett M, Al-Khudhairy N, Castellanos-Ryan N, Struve M, Topper L, Conrod P. Adolescent bullying, cannabis use and emerging psychotic experiences: a longitudinal general population study. Psychol Med. 2013;43(5):1033–44.
35. Kendler KS, Gardner CO, Prescott CA. Clinical characteristics of mayor depression that predict risk of depression in relatives. Arch Gen Psychiatry. 1999;56:322–7.

36. Fisher H, Morgan C, Dazzan P, Craig TK, Morgan K, Hutchinson G, Jones PB, Doody GA, Pariante C, McGuffin P, Murray RM, Leff J, Fearon P. Gender differences in the association between childhood abuse and psychosis. Br J Psychiatry. 2009;194(4):319–25.
37. Nolen-Hoeksema S. Responses to depression and their effects on the duration of depressive episodes. J Abnorm Psychol. 1991;100:569–82.
38. Broderick PC. Early adolescent gender differences in the use of ruminative and distracting coping strategies. J Early Adolesc. 1998;18:173–91.
39. Hart IB, Thompson JM. Gender role characteristics and depressive symptomatology among adolescents. J Early Adolesc. 1996;16:407–26.
40. Schwartz JAJ, Koenig LJ. Response styles and negative affect among adolescents. Cognit Ther Res. 1996;20:13–36.
41. Butler LD, Nolen-Hoeksema S. Gender differences in responses to depressed mood in a college sample. Sex Roles. 1994;30:331–46.
42. Nolen-Hoeksema S, Morrow J. Effects of rumination and distraction on naturally-occurring depressed mood. Cognit Emot. 1993;7:561–70.
43. Nolen-Hoeksema S, Larson J, Grayson C. Explaining the gender differences in depressive symptoms. J Pers Soc Psychol. 1999;77:1061–72.
44. Nolen-Hoeksema S. Sex differences in depression and explanatory style in children. J Youth Adolesc. 1991;20:233–45.
45. McFadyen-Ketchum SA, Bates JE, Dodge KA, Pettit GS. Patterns of change in early childhood aggressive-disruptive behavior: gender differences in predictions from early coercive and affectionate mother-child interactions. Child Dev. 1996;67(5):2417–33.
46. Fisher HL, Schreier A, Zammit S, Maughan B, Munafò MR, Lewis G, Wolke D. Pathways between childhood victimization and psychosis-like symptoms in the ALSPAC birth cohort. Schizophr Bull. 2013;39(5):1045–55.
47. Shah J, Mizrahi R, McKenzie K. The four dimensions: a model for the social aetiology of psychosis. Br J Psychiatry. 2011;199(1):11–4.
48. Naninck EFG, Lucassen PJ, Bakker J. Sex differences in adolescent depression: do sex hormones determine vulnerability? J Neuroendocrinol. 2011;23:383–92.
49. Schwartz JE, Fennig S, Tanenberg-Karant M, Carlson G, Craig T, Galambos N, Lavelle J, Bromet EJ. Congruence of diagnoses 2 years after a first-admission diagnosis of psychosis. Arch Gen Psychiatry. 2000;57:593–600.
50. Bendall S, Jackson HJ, Hulbert CA, McGorry PD. Childhood trauma and psychotic disorders: a systematic, critical review of the evidence. Schizophr Bull. 2008;34(3):568–79.
51. Braehler C, Valiquette L, Holowka D, Malla AK, Joober R, Ciampi A, Pawliuk N, King S. Childhood trauma and dissociation in first-episode psychosis, chronic schizophrenia and community controls. Psychiatry Res. 2013;210(1):36–42.
52. Addington J, Stowkowy J, Cadenhead KS, Cornblatt BA, McGlashan TH, Perkins DO, Seidman LJ, Tsuang MT, Walker EF, Woods SW, Cannon TD. Early traumatic experiences in those at clinical high risk for psychosis. Early Interv Psychiatry. 2013;7(3):300–5.
53. Bendall S, Hulbert CA, Alvarez-Jimenez M, Allott K, McGorry PD, Jackson HJ. Testing a model of the relationship between childhood sexual abuse and psychosis in a first-episode psychosis group: the role of hallucinations and delusions, posttraumatic intrusions, and selective attention. J Nerv Ment Dis. 2013;201(11):941–7.
54. American Psychiatric Association. Diagnostic and statistical manual of mental disorders. 4th ed. Washington, DC: American Psychiatric Association; 1994.
55. Allen DN, Frantom LV, Strauss GP, van Kammen DP. Differential patterns of premorbid academic and social deterioration in patients with schizophrenia. Schizophr Res. 2005;75 (2–3):389–97.
56. Fuller R, Nopoulos P, Arndt S, O'Leary D, Ho BC, Andreasen NC. Longitudinal assessment of premorbid cognitive functioning in patients with schizophrenia through examination of standardized scholastic test performance. Am J Psychiatry. 2002;159(7):1183–9.
57. Gunnell D, Harrison G, Rasmussen F, Fouskakis D, Tynelius P. Associations between premorbid intellectual performance, early-life exposures and early-onset schizophrenia. Cohort study. Br J Psychiatry. 2002;181:298–305.

Schizophrenia and Gender

27

Iñaki Zorrilla, Saioa López-Zurbano, Ana Isabel Cano,
and Ana González-Pinto

Abstract

The existence of significant differences in schizophrenia is an issue that has been discussed extensively. There are differences in the prognosis, marked by the age at onset, treatment adherence, or drug use. Another aspect is the clinical pattern (particularly cognitive symptoms), the response to treatment, and side effects. These differences can be explained on the basis of biological and psychosocial hypotheses. Schizophrenia is a very heterogeneous disorder if we consider its basic clinical characteristics. That heterogeneity is shown by the vast variability in the onset and clinical presentation, the course of the illness, and response to both pharmacological and psychosocial treatment. That heterogeneity may be due to gender-related features, or at least gender variables may help to understand those differences. For this reason, gender differences in schizophrenia have been widely studied in past few decades. Unfortunately, research for many of those differences has not been conclusive.

I. Zorrilla (✉)
Alava University Hospital, Vitoria, Spain
e-mail: INAKI.ZORRILLAMARTINEZ@osakidetza.net

S. López-Zurbano • A.I. Cano
Department of Psychiatry, Alava University Hospital, Vitoria, Spain

A. González-Pinto
Department of Psychiatry, Alava University Hospital, Vitoria, Spain

University of the Basque Country UPV/EHU, Guipúzcoa, Spain
e-mail: anamaria.gonzalezpintoarrillaga@osakidetza.net

M. Sáenz-Herrero (ed.), *Psychopathology in Women*,
DOI 10.1007/978-3-319-05870-2_27

27.1 Introduction

The existence of gender differences in the incidence of schizophrenia has been a controversial issue. Traditionally, it has been thought that the incidence and prevalence of the disorder is the same for both men and women. More recently, however, studies have shown that, when using more restrictive criteria for diagnosis, fewer women fulfill them. For example, if using the Feighner restrictive criteria the female-to-male ratio is 0.41:1, and if using International Classification of Diseases criteria, it is 0.92:1 [1]. A current meta-analysis studying an incidence population found a higher incidence in men (ratio, 1.42) [2]. However, prevalence studies of the general population do not find gender differences. Maybe this is because men have lower adherence to pharmacological treatment and a higher suicide rate. Another explanation may be the study designs, which are focused on epidemiological information for prevalence or on clinical data for studying incidence [1].

One of the most relevant pieces of data in the research into gender differences in schizophrenia refers to the age at onset. It is higher in women, regardless of culture, onset criteria defining diagnosis, or sex correlation in the population. It is also noteworthy that women have better premorbid adjustment with a higher educational level and social functioning, with fewer behavioral disorders, less aggression, and fewer neurocognitive deficits. These gender differences are not seen in first-episode patients, but they are obvious in chronic patients [3], which leads to a hypothesis that there is a different course of the illness in men and women.

The clinical features of the disease are also different in women, who have a greater affective component and more positive psychotic symptoms. This explains why the most common schizophrenia subtype in women is the paranoid subtype [3]. They also experience more schizoaffective disorders and brief psychoses.

The prognosis of the disorder seems to be better for women, who have fewer readmissions, less drug abuse, and greater functionality in several areas such as work, social, and occupational status [1–3]. Thus, we can conclude that women have a better quality of life.

Because there is gender bias in clinical trials, with a disproportion of men in the samples, the response to treatment is still a poorly studied area. However, women have greater adherence to treatment and better response to psychosocial treatment. Based on the results of the CATIE study, women are at a higher risk of metabolic syndrome, cardiac events, diabetes, and obesity in the context of use of antipsychotics [4].

Another differential pattern is the cognitive deficits observed with disease progression. Women tend to have better results in attention, immediate memory, and delayed memory. On the other hand, men have more cognitive impairment but better results in visuospatial function [3]. According to the results of some authors [5], there are no differences in executive functioning.

Trying to explain these differences and the protective role attributed to gender, various biological and psychosocial theories have been proposed. We summarize most of the biological theories [6], especially those on the protective role of estrogen in the dopaminergic system. Psychosocial theories are still pending generalization and replication because these factors may be subjected to contextual changes (increased demand and expectations in adolescents vs adults). Other hypotheses to be confirmed and replicated are those involving specific neural circuits.

27.2 Clinical Differences

27.2.1 Age of Onset

Several studies indicate that men tend to develop the disorder at the age of 14–24, an average of 3 years before women, whose mean age at onset is 25–35. However, women appear to have two peaks in the age of the illness onset: the first is after menarche, and the second is between 45 and 54, the menopause-related years [7].

Nevertheless, the first group (after menarche) seems to be similarly distributed between the genders [1].

27.2.2 Obstetric History

Traditionally, perinatal complications have been associated with an earlier onset and with a worse course of the disease. The data obtained in the study of gender differences for obstetric history complications in schizophrenia is inconclusive [1]; some research reports an obstetric complication history to be more common among men [8], others in women [9], and others do not find gender differences [10]. We find the same circumstance when analyzing influenza virus exposure in the second trimester of pregnancy: the data are not conclusive [11].

27.2.3 Family Risk

One of the first analyzed gender differences in schizophrenia was the family risk [12], showing a higher familial risk for schizophrenia, schizophreniform disorder, and schizoaffective disorder in women's relatives than in relatives of men. These differences were attenuated when the spectrum of psychosis was widened. Pulver's group found that relatives of men with the disease who have an age at onset under 17 are at a significantly higher risk of schizophrenia. On the other hand, they also found an association between age at onset and familial risk in women [13].

Other research groups have not found an association among gender, familial risk, and age at onset [14].

27.2.4 Substance Use

The prevalence of substance abuse is higher in people with schizophrenia and first-episode psychosis than in the general population. Overall, men have higher rates of substance abuse, both in the general population and in the population suffering from mental illness.

Another factor related to gender differences is cannabis abuse. The use of cannabis is related both to male sex and to earlier age at onset. Thus, it has been proposed that some of the differences between men and women with regard to age at onset are mediated by cannabis use [15].

In a schizophrenic population, rates indicated that men consume more cannabis than women [16–18]. Moreover, Rodríguez-Jiménez et al. [18] found that men have a higher comorbidity of cocaine, hallucinogenics, and cannabis use than women. In the case of alcohol abuse, the data showed that men presented higher levels of consumption than women [19].

In addition, Arendt et al. [20] demonstrate that the risk of developing psychosis is higher in men who consume cannabis than in women under the same circumstances. The study assessed a total of 535 people with a cannabis-induced psychosis over 3 years, and the rates for developing schizophrenia were 47.6 % in men vs 29.8 % in women.

Men presented higher prevalence of a second diagnosis of substance abuse [21] and higher levels of comorbidity than women. Moreover, it seems that substance abuse could be a greater risk factor for developing psychosis in men than in women [20].

Women also have more difficulties in quitting tobacco use than men, when they use tobacco and cannabis together [22].

27.2.5 Premorbid Functioning

The premorbid functioning is associated with the prognosis of the schizophrenic illness; thus, finding gender differences in this particular area can make a big difference to the evolution of the illness. Most studies that have analyzed the role of the gender variable in premorbid adjustment found less severe deficits in women than in men [23, 24].

Women have a better global outcome than men [25] because they are better educated, have held jobs more often, and their functionality is better than in men [3, 26, 27]. It seems that, with a later onset of the disease, women are more often married than men, with a better social adjustment and support at baseline and in their lifetime [1, 3]. Furthermore, men tend to have more negative symptoms, with poorer cognitive and social functioning [21].

27.2.6 Cognitive Functioning

Cognitive deficits in schizophrenia are considered by many psychiatrists to be a prominent symptom that requires attention, adequate treatment, and rehabilitation. There are various factors that could affect neuropsychological functioning of schizophrenic patients, within which were included medication, toxic abuse, and gender.

This is also a controversial domain in gender differences in schizophrenia. Most of the studies agree that men have worse cognitive functioning than women. However, there is some controversy about what neuropsychological areas are more affected in men [28].

It seems that women perform cognitively better for attention, immediate and delayed memory, verbal abilities, and executive function [1, 3]. On the other hand, men have better visuospatial functioning, as it happens with healthy controls [29]. These differences are more significant in chronic schizophrenia than in first episodes of psychosis [3].

A recent study by Abu-akel et al. [30] showed that women are better mentalizers than men, these differences being regardless of intelligence level or clinical or demographical variables. Their finding was that, apart from their better cognitive functioning, schizophrenic women also have a better social cognition. They can employ both cognitive and affective mentalizing, particularly to identify emotions of other people. That means that women can appreciate other people's mental state better than male patients.

As the illness develops, men present more and more severe negative symptoms than women [1, 3, 21, 31], the incidence of negative schizophrenia in premenopausal women being lower than in men at the same age.

An inverse relationship has been established between energy and 17B estradiol levels [32] that reinforces the minor presence of negative symptoms in premenopausal women or in treatment with hormone replacement therapy [33, 34]. This links the hormonal condition with the absence of neuronal atrophy and neuronal loss frequent in negative symptoms [35].

Furthermore, women with schizophrenia have lower serum estradiol 17B than controls, which means that serum 17B estradiol levels correlate with the severity of symptoms [32].

Regarding cognitive symptoms, recent research has also indicated that estrogen plays an essential role in enhancing executive functions in action at the prefrontal cortex level [36].

In a more recent review, conducted by Krysta et al. [37], and based on analysis of several studies, it is shown that cognitive differences found between tests applied to men and women with schizophrenia, postulated poorer performance on neuropsychological tests in male patients. Like others who had similar findings, in the latter study, the male schizophrenic patients showed more deficits in cognitive functioning compared with female patients in domains such as attention, verbal memory, and executive functions. Moreover, this review also found no sex-specific differences in the cognitive functioning of schizophrenic patients or that such differences are not clinically significant. Hence, the need arises for more research on the issue of gender differences in cognitive functioning in patients with schizophrenia [28].

27.2.7 Social Functioning

Studies found that women perform better in social functioning; they are better adapted and have fewer disabilities than men. These differences are found both during the prodromal phase and in the psychotic phase of schizophrenia [3]. Women have higher scores on a GAF functioning scale during a 5-year follow-up [21].

One of the most robust indicators of social functioning is marital status. The percentage of single or never married and childless schizophrenic men is much greater than the percentage of women [1, 3, 21]. However, there is no significant difference in marriage and having children in first-episode patients. This means that as the disease goes on, more women get married and become parents than men [21].

Furthermore, men seem to be more vulnerable than women to develop psychotic features when stressful life events take place [38]. Thus, it is likely that women show a higher resilience than men in managing stress [1].

About schizophrenic patient's social needs, Ochoa et al. found that men presented more basic (food, daily activities) and functional needs (education, money, personal care), whereas women had more service needs (information about illness, benefits, transport, etc.) [39].

27.3 Course of Illness

The course of schizophrenia shows different patterns in men and women. We have already explained how the onset of the illness is earlier in men, and this is linked to a worse cognitive prognosis [40].

Early in the 1990s, in an 8-year follow-up [41], it was revealed that women had a better course of hospital treatment, with a shorter hospital stay, and survived for longer in the community after their first hospital admission.

Later, these results have been confirmed. Being men predicts a higher risk of institutionalization [3, 42], and men have higher relapse rates and took longer to recover [22].

Men have a worse prognosis as their clinical parameters deteriorate; while at the beginning of the illness women have multiple and worse symptoms, as it develops this changes to just the opposite. Therefore, men do not just have more positive symptoms as the disorder progresses, but also more negative symptoms and more comorbid substance abuse. It is not only the clinical features, but their social network is also weaker; they tend to live alone, have less education and less access to work, and they also have problems asking for help. All this is linked to the fact that more schizophrenic men than women die, with a suicide rate seven times higher in men [22].

Most studies conclude that gender influences both clinical variables (number of episodes, length of stay, relapse, symptoms during follow-up) and social variables (global adaptation, occupational status); women present better results than men.

However, other studies of long-term monitoring (over 10 years) found no significant differences [43, 44].

We have widely described how men have more and worse negative symptoms, especially as the disease develops.

With regard to psychotic symptoms, women score higher results on positive [21] and general psychopathology scales [3]. Thus, if women experience more hallucinations, delusions [3], illogical thinking, inappropriate affect and bizarre behavior [1] it is understandable why they are more often diagnosed with the paranoid subtype of schizophrenia. Women also tend to experience more affective symptoms [3].

Men, on the other hand, experience more negative symptoms, such as, asociality, anhedonia or affective flattening; therefore, they are more frequently diagnosed with the residual subtype [1, 3].

27.3.1 Neuroimaging

Studies conducted to determine gender differences have structural and functional variables and are controversial.

Several NMR studies suggest that ventricular enlargement found in patients with schizophrenia is more prevalent in men [45, 46], although other, less abundant results have been published that demonstrate that the increase occurs in female patients compared with control women, and that there are no significant differences in men with schizophrenia compared with controls [47].

Another common finding is the presence of a greater number of structural abnormalities in male patients [46–48], focusing on the region of the corpus callosum [49].

Researchers have also tried to analyze the differences in the temporal lobe disorders, but the results have been mixed.

Although there is a relative abundance of evidence of brain abnormalities in schizophrenia, it remains unclear to what extent these changes, such as brain volume, present before antipsychotic treatment, an important consideration in the current debate about what structural effects antipsychotics can cause in the brain of schizophrenic patients.

In some meta-analyses that have combined principles of CT and MRI [50] intracranial volume is an important variable, since it has been suggested that a reduction in the volume is one of the root causes of brain abnormalities in schizophrenia.

In a meta-analysis by Haijima et al. [51], where data on brain volume are collected from 317 MRI studies in schizophrenia from 1 September 1998 until

1 January 2012, data are collected from 18,000 patients and controls. In this meta-analysis 33 studies were included with 771 patients treated with antipsychotics and 939 controls, and changes in brain volume present before antipsychotic treatment is initiated can be assessed. Besides the use or not of antipsychotics, it was addressed to what extent the volumes were affected by the disease duration and sex, among other factors. In this study, we believe that loss of brain volume in schizophrenia is related to a combination of decreased intracranial volume reflecting early neurodevelopmental processes, together with the effect of the progression of the disease. As for the authors' conclusions regarding sex and intracranial volume reduction, associated reductions were found in men.

In a pair of studies in which pituitary volume was assessed, one in a first episode of schizophrenia [52], which identified a significant effect of sex on pituitary volume at both the initial time point and at later tracking. A higher volume was found in women, with data being consistent with the findings of previous studies. Although the functional significance of the increased pituitary volume in women is still unknown, it is believed to have connotations for sex differences in psychiatric disorders implicated in hypothalamic–pituitary–adrenal (HPA) axis dysregulation. The other study [53] in which pituitary volume in schizophrenia spectrum disorders is equally valued on the basis that there is growing evidence suggesting that the hyperactivity of the HPA axis is present in schizophrenia spectrum disorders, as well as the ability to respond to stress, both closely related to schizophrenia. All study participants met the criteria for age (18–55 years), IQ over 75 and normal brain MRI assessed by a clinical neuroradiologist, with no history of seizures, head trauma with loss of consciousness, neurological disorder, and any antecedent or addiction. The results showed a main effect of gender ($p = 0.001$), indicating an increased pituitary volume in women compared with men, independent of the group analyzed.

The regional neuropathology and association with specific symptoms of schizophrenia appear to be dependent on gender. Thus, Cowell et al. [54] found that in women greater frontal volume was associated with more severe disorganization and suspicion, while in men there was a lower volume, which was associated with disorganization (but no correlation with suspicion). Malla et al. [55] published a study that found that diffuse cerebral atrophy was associated with positive psychotic symptoms in women, but not in men.

27.4 Different Response to Treatment

Given the differences observed and reported in the literature regarding treatment response mediated by gender, different protocols should be carried out.

Young women on maintenance treatment (20–39 years) require lower doses of antipsychotics than men [56, 57], which is reversed after the age of 40 years.

Other studies suggest that better treatment response rates can be obtained in a phase cycle in which estrogen levels are higher [58].

There are many factors responsible for these differences. First, we must consider the pharmacokinetic differences [59] such as slower gastric emptying in women (greater absorption of antipsychotics in women as results suggest [60] and a more efficient cerebral blood flow in women [61].

Also, we cannot forget the greater proportion of adipose tissue in women, a factor in the distribution of antipsychotics (lipophilic) with a slower release in the case of women, who could protect them in times of noncompliance with treatment [62].

There have been few studies examining gender differences in response to psychosocial treatments. Haas et al. [63] and Davis et al. [64] suggest a better response of women and their families with the psychosocial approach, suggesting that psychosocial treatment must take gender into account [65].

As for the doses of medication, some authors have found that men receive a larger amount of antipsychotics, considering that this may reflect a more severe psychopathology or that these patients are more reluctant to receive other treatments such as psychotherapy or social skills training [21]. On the other hand, it can be considered that the best treatment in women may be related to a better outcome. The thought that women in Western culture are more receptive to help and have a more positive attitude to taking medication than men may also help to explain this [66]. It is also well accepted that women have greater access to the network and social support [67], which may be associated with improved adherence.

27.5 Effects of Estrogens and Estrogen as a Treatment

It is common to refer to affective disorders when looking for gender differences in mental illness, leaving schizophrenia aside. However, when talking about schizophrenia, there are interesting differences that lead us to consider the estrogens as protective elements or even as coadjuvants in its treatment.

What are the effects of estrogens that can make a difference in the clinical expression of schizophrenia in women? They can be summarized in the following points:

- Neural organization during neurodevelopment: these effects take place preferably before brain maturation. The sexual brain differentiation extends from the prenatal period to puberty. Estrogens facilitate the fact that during early maturation, women mature faster than men (in the brains of the latter it was found that neural connections and the axonal and lateralization of brain functions occur later). This can cause male brains to be more vulnerable to pre-/perinatal damage associated with structural alterations in schizophrenia associated with negative symptoms and early onset [59].
- Neuronal growth and synapse formation, neurons at Wernicke area have longer dendrites in women than in men [68], not forgetting that there are gender differences in areas such as suprachiasmatic and paraventricular nuclei [69, 70].

- Modulation of neurotransmitters: 17B estradiol decreases the sensitivity of D2 receptors in neonatal rats [71], modifies dopaminergic mechanism-dependent behavior, modifies the total mRNA, and also increases D2 receptor cDNA [71] and the maximum expression of 5HT2A receptor binding [72]. There are other data suggesting the effect of estrogen on serotonergic and glutamatergic systems [73].
- Interaction with neural growth factors and other neurotrophins: mainly with increased BDNF expression. Another direct protective factor derived by estrogen exposure is increasing intracellular cAMP CREB phosphorylation (factor transcription) [73]. Furthermore, the 17B estradiol protects cells from apoptosis, improves the fluidity of the membrane by its action on neuronal ionic canals and by increasing the expression of apoprotein-E.
- Antioxidant effect [74, 75]: it has been shown that concentrations of 17B estradiol protect cells from death caused by amyloid beta.
- Affect mature brain neuronal activator: modulation of neuronal hyper: from the beginning of the fertile period, the circulation of sex hormones (usually excitatory) requires compensating for neurophysiological changes to enhance the action of inhibitory systems in the brain that counteract the action of these endocrine systems. The failure of this system favors the appearance of the first episode of schizophrenia. All this focuses on two structures: the amygdala and the hippocampus.
- Moreover, a significant participation of estrogens in dopaminergic, serotonergic, and glutamatergic systems possibly gives them properties similar to those of atypical antipsychotic drugs [76–78].

27.6 Estrogen as a Treatment

Sex differences in the incidence, onset, and course of schizophrenia have led to the hypothesis that estrogens play a protective role in the pathophysiology of this disorder [79].

Moreover, and supporting the above life cycle, studies have also demonstrated that women are more susceptible to a first episode or relapse of psychosis in two periods of hormonal changes, characterized by a decrease in estrogen levels such as postpartum [80] and during the menopause [81, 82].

Several studies have found that estrogen has significant positive effects on the central nervous system above and beyond their primary endocrine and reproductive functions, to the extent that it has been considered a factor of a "psychoprotective nature," as already mentioned, being able to modulate multiple neurotransmitter systems, including dopaminergic, serotonergic, and glutamatergic pathways [79]. Estrogens can also be used in the treatment of schyzophrenia because of their anti-inflammatory properties as shown by [83].

Numerous open studies have indicated that adding estrogen to antipsychotic treatment showed a significantly greater effect on psychotic symptoms

[84]. Hormone replacement therapy appears to reduce the intensity of negative symptoms in the postmenopausal period [33].

Double-blind studies have also been conducted that have compared estrogen vs placebo added to usual treatment groups showing a better response in the control of psychotic symptoms [35, 85] and the general psychopathology score and Positive and Negative Syndrome Scale (PANSS) score. A recent meta-analysis has shown that estrogens given for a few weeks have a positive effect in improving psychotic symptoms in women.

First intervention trials with estrogen substitution for neuroleptic therapy have demonstrated antipsychotic effects [27].

27.7 Are There Differences in the Dopaminergic System Associated with Sex?

In recent years researchers have described numerous differences in the structure and brain function in patients with schizophrenia associated with gender. Parellada and collaborators have explored this aspect by determining postsynaptic D2 receptors in the striatal SPECT region and on the other, differences in presynaptic dopamine transporter. In conclusion, we found no sex differences in the density of postsynaptic D2 receptors, although there were differences in presynaptic dopamine transporter. All this makes it clear that further neuroimaging study should be carried out to evaluate the dopaminergic system: the extra-estriatal and mesolimbic D2/D3 receptor system, the different D2 receptor subtypes, and other systems involved in the pathogenesis of schizophrenia.

27.8 Physical Health and Metabolic Complications

There have also been concerns about gender differences in relation to physical health and metabolic complications in psychosis.

Atypical and older antipsychotics are very useful drugs, but they can be associated with hyperprolactinemia and related disorders. These endocrine aspects are particularly significant. Women have greater metabolic and endocrine-induced antipsychotic side effects. In fact, every woman exposed to atypical antipsychotics is at risk of developing hyperprolactinemia-related problems, particularly young women [86, 87]. Previous studies have consistently reported a higher prevalence of hyperprolactinemia in women receiving antipsychotics, and cross-sectional studies in the USA and UK have estimated hyperprolactinemia prevalence rates of up to 42 % in men and 75 % in women with schizophrenia who were receiving conventional antipsychotics or risperidone [85]. It is known that hyperprolactinemia is associated with a number of physical health problems in men and women, particularly endocrine and immunological system changes, as well as growth hormone alterations.

Hyperprolactinemia affects long-term health in women. Menstrual irregularities have been found in up to 48 % of women receiving antipsychotic treatment. Reduced bone mineral density has been demonstrated in 57 % of men and 32 % of women treated with prolactin-raising antipsychotics for over 10 years [88].

Although sexual dysfunction appears to be inherent to the illness in patients with schizophrenia, it is also frequently reported during antipsychotic treatment, with interesting gender differences. More than 50 % of men and 30 % of women have been shown to experience sexual dysfunction during conventional antipsychotic treatment [89, 90].

A Spanish national cross-sectional study in 733 patients diagnosed with schizophrenia on treatment with second-generation antipsychotics and admitted to short-stay hospital units detected different cardiovascular risk factors in women than in men. Men were treated for hypertension (OR = 25.34, $p < 0.03$) and women for diabetes (OR = 0.02, $p < 0.03$) [91].

Metabolic syndrome is associated with the development of coronary heart disease and diabetes mellitus. A higher presence of metabolic syndrome has been detected in women. In a Turkish sample, Boke et al. found that 61.4 % of women, but only 22.4 % of men, had metabolic syndrome [92].

The prevalence of metabolic syndrome in 1,460 US patients from the Clinical Antipsychotic Trials of Intervention Effectiveness (CATIE) showed important gender differences. In women, depending on the criteria used, it was 51.6 % (NCEP) or 54.2 % (AHA), compared with 36.0 % (NCEP; $p = 0.0002$) or 36.6 % (AHA; $p = 0.0003$) for men. 73.4 % of all women (including nonfasting subjects) met the waist circumference criterion compared with 36.6 % of men. In a logistic regression model with age, race, and ethnicity as covariates, CATIE men were 138 % more likely to have metabolic syndrome than a general population-matched sample (NHANES), and CATIE women, 251 % more likely than their general-population counterparts. Even when controlling for differences in body mass index, CATIE men were still 85 % more likely to have MS than the NHANES male sample and CATIE women, and 137 % more likely to have MS than women in NHANES [4].

Individuals with nonaffective psychosis appear to have an increased prevalence of abnormal glucose tolerance prior to antipsychotic treatment, but this predisposition also appears not to be gender-sensitive [93]. Similarly, a large community study in Ontario (Canada) with 1,123 schizophrenic outpatients failed to detect gender differences in dysglycemia.

Regarding metabolic and endocrine-induced antipsychotic side effects, women had a higher prevalence of symptoms. Hyperprolactinemia and diabetes are more present in women, while hypertension is more prevalent in men with schizophrenia.

27.9 Treatment Effects

Women in general are more vulnerable to the adverse effects because of the pharmacokinetics of each sex [35, 94]. It has been found that women have a higher free drug concentration, improved dopaminergic blockade by estrogen, increased storage of antipsychotics in adipose tissue given the characteristics of the female body, increased prevalence of immune reactions, resulting in an increased risk of drug interactions owing to the presence of comorbidity and treatment for other diseases. In all this lies the importance of not giving higher doses than is absolutely necessary [95].

Antipsychotic drugs can cause drowsiness in both men and women, affecting their academic performance and driving skills, but the women are even more affected when mothers need to remain vigilant in caring for their babies [96].

Men and women differ in the incidence of specific side effects compared with antipsychotics. Thus, QTc interval prolongation is a major risk posed by women, especially older women [97]. Hyperprolactinemia is a problem present in women with subsequent gynecomastia, galactorrhea, amenorrhea, and increased risk of osteoporosis and breast cancer [98].

It is important to consider that antipsychotic drugs generate a series of conditions that may increase the risk of breast cancer presentation such as obesity, elevated prolactin levels, and states of hyperglycemia. Furthermore, these women have low parity, mammographic controls do little to detect disease, they are less likely than other mothers to breastfeed, have frequent conditions of social disadvantage, higher levels of smoking and alcohol consumption, and lower levels of physical activity levels than other women [99].

27.10 Tardive Dyskinesia

Is this the most distinctive condition in relation to gender differences regarding side effects?

Women of childbearing age have less tardive dyskinesia than men of the same age [100]; there was a lower risk among women until beyond the menopause. Thus, after the age of 70 years, tardive dyskinesia is more common in women with a ratio of 49.1 % compared with 24 % of men, relating to the falling estrogen trigger.

This side effect is also correlated with age, occurring in 20–24 % of patients taking antipsychotic medication [101]. While for a time it was suggested that it was less common in women, recent studies show that patients with tardive dyskinesia have comparable gender ratios, are younger, and have a reduced exposure to neuroleptics. It seems that gender is correlated with the risk of tardive dyskinesia in terms of older women being at a higher risk of tardive dyskinesia, while the risk in men increases if they are young.

Conclusions

- The prognosis of schizophrenic disease is worse for male patients. This is because they have an earlier onset of the illness, worse premorbid adjustment, more negative symptoms, more substance abuse comorbidity, and greater cognitive impairment.
- Women have better social functioning; they are more often married and have children. However, this can be a risk factor too, as we have seen in previous chapters. They are better at mentalizing, not just cognitively but also with regard to social abilities.

References

1. Ochoa S, Usall J, Cobo J, Labad X, Kulkarni J. Gender differences in schizophrenia and first-episode psychosis: a comprehensive literature review. Schizophr Res Treatment. 2012;2012: 916198. doi:10.1155/2012/916198. Epub 2012 Apr 8.
2. Aleman A, Kahn RS, Selten JP. Sex differences in the risk of schizophrenia: evidence from meta-analysis. Arch Gen Psychiatry. 2003;60(6):565–71.
3. Zhang XY, da Chen C, Xiu MH, Yang FD, Haile CN, Kosten TA, Kosten TR. Gender differences in never-medicated first-episode schizophrenia and medicated chronic schizophrenia patients. J Clin Psychiatry. 2012;73(7):1025–33. doi:10.4088/JCP.11m07422.
4. McEvoy JP, Meyer JM, Goff DC, Nasrallah HA, Davis SM, Sullivan L, Meltzer HY, Hsiao J, Scott Stroup T, Lieberman JA. Prevalence of the metabolic syndrome in patients with schizophrenia: baseline results from the clinical antipsychotic trials of intervention effectiveness (CATIE) schizophrenia trial and comparison with national estimates from NHANESIII. Schizophr Res. 2005;80(1):19–32. Epub 2005 Aug 30.
5. Chan RC, Chen EY, Cheung EF, Chen RY, Cheung HK. The components of executive functioning in a cohort of patients with chronic schizophrenia: a multiple single-case study design. Schizophr Res. 2006;81(2–3):173–89. Epub 2005 Sep 26.
6. Usall J, Busquets E, Araya S, Ochoa S, Gost A. Gender differences in schizophrenia. A literature review. Actas Esp Psiquiatr. 2000;28(3):178–85.
7. Häfner H, Maurer K, Löffler W, Fätkenheuer B, an der Heiden W, Riecher-Rössler A, Behrens S, Gattaz WF. The epidemiology of early schizophrenia. Influence of age and gender on onset and early course. Br J Psychiatry Suppl. 1994;23:29–38.
8. Kirov G, Jones PB, Harvey I, Lewis SW, Toone BK, Rifkin L, Sham P, Murray RM. Do obstetric complications cause the earlier age at onset in male than female schizophrenics? Schizophr Res. 1996;20(1–2):117–24.
9. Verdoux H, Bourgeois M. A comparative study of obstetric history in schizophrenics, bipolar patients and normal subjects. Schizophr Res. 1993;9(1):67–9.
10. Forsyth JK, Ellman LM, Tanskanen A, Mustonen U, Huttunen MO, Suvisaari J, Cannon TD. Genetic risk for schizophrenia, obstetric complications, and adolescent school outcome: evidence for gene-environment interaction. Schizophr Bull. 2013;39(5):1067–76. doi:10.1093/schbul/sbs098. Epub 2012 Sep 1.
11. Preti A, Cardascia L, Zen T, Marchetti M, Favaretto G, Miotto P. Risk for obstetric complications and schizophrenia. Psychiatry Res. 2000;96(2):127–39.
12. Goldstein JM, Faraone SV, Chen WJ, Tolomiczencko GS, Tsuang MT. Sex differences in the familial transmission of schizophrenia. Br J Psychiatry. 1990;156:819–26.
13. Pulver AE, Liang KY. Estimating effects of proband characteristics on familial risk. The association between age at onset and familial risk in the Maryland schizophrenia sample. Genet Epidemiol. 1991;8(5):339–50.

14. Maier W, Lichtermann D, Minges J, Heun R, Halmayer J. The impact of gender and age at onset on the familial aggregation of schizophrenia. Eur Arch Psychiatry Clin Neurosci. 1993;242(5):279–85.
15. González-Pinto A, Vega P, Ibáñez B, Mosquera F, Barbeito S, Gutiérrez M, Ruiz de Azúa S, Ruiz I, Vieta EJ. Impact of cannabis and other drugs on age at onset of psychosis. J Clin Psychiatry. 2008;69(8):1210–6.
16. Foti DJ, Kotov R, Guey LT, Bromet EJ. Cannabis use and the course of schizophrenia: 10-year follow-up after first hospitalization. Am J Psychiatry. 2010;167(8):987–93.
17. Barnes TRE, Mutsatsa SH, Hutton SB, Watt HC, Joyce EM. Comorbid substance use and age at onset of schizophrenia. Br J Psychiatry. 2006;188:237–42.
18. Rodríguez-Jiménez R, Aragüés M, Jiménez-Arriero MA, et al. Dual diagnosis in psychiatric in patients: prevalence and general characteristics. Invest Clin. 2008;49(2):195–205.
19. Galderisi S, Bucci P, Üçok A, Peuskens J. No gender differences in social outcome in patients suffering from schizophrenia. Eur Psychiatry. 2012;27(6):406–8.
20. Arendt M, Rosenberg R, Foldager L, Perto G, Munk-Jørgensen P. Cannabis-induced psychosis and subsequent schizophrenia-spectrum disorders: follow-up study of 535 incident cases. Br J Psychiatry. 2005;187:510–5.
21. Thorup A, Albert N, Bertelsen M, et al. Gender differences in first-episode psychosis at 5-year follow-up—two different courses of disease? Results from the OPUS study at 5-year follow-up. Eur Psychiatry. 2014;29(1):44–51.
22. González-Pinto A, Alberich S, Ruiz de Azúa S, Martínez-Cengotitabengoa M, Fernández M, Gutiérrez M, Saenz M, Besga A, Galdós P, de Leon J. Psychosis and smoking cessation: difficulties in quitting associated with sex and substance abuse. Psychiatry Res. 2012; 195(1–2):45–50.
23. Salokangas RK. Prognostic implications of the sex of schizophrenic patients. Br J Psychiatry. 1983;142:145–51.
24. Shtasel DL, Gur RE, Gallacher F, Heimberg C, Gur RC. Gender differences in the clinical expression of schizophrenia. Schizophr Res. 1992;7(3):225–31.
25. Tang YL, Gillespie CF, Epstein MP, Mao PX, Jiang F, Chen Q, Cai ZJ, Mitchell PB. Gender differences in 542 Chinese inpatients with schizophrenia. Schizophr Res. 2007;97(1–3): 88–96. Epub 2007 Jul 12.
26. Allen DN, Strauss GP, Barchard KA, Vertinski M, Carpenter WT, Buchanan RW. Differences in developmental changes in academic and social premorbid adjustment between males and females with schizophrenia. Schizophr Res. 2013;146(1–3):132–7. doi:10.1016/j.schres.2013.01.032. Epub 2013 Mar 13.
27. Häfner H. Gender differences in schizophrenia. Psychoneuroendocrinology. 2003;28 Suppl 2:17–54.
28. Krysta K, Murawiec S, Klasik A, Wiglusz MS, Krupka-Matuszczyk I. Sex-specific differences in cognitive functioning among schizophrenic patients. Psychiatr Danub. 2013; 25 Suppl 2:244–6.
29. Halari R, Mehrotra R, Sharma T, Ng V, Kumari V. Cognitive impairment but preservation of sexual dimorphism in cognitive abilities in chronic schizophrenia. Psychiatry Res. 2006; 141(2):129–39. Epub 2006 Jan 19.
30. Abu-Akel A, Bo S. Superior mentalizing abilities of female patients with schizophrenia. Psychiatry Res. 2013;210(3):794–9.
31. Moriarty PJ, Lieber D, Bennett A, White L, Parrella M, Harvey PD, Davis KL. Gender differences in poor outcome patients with lifelong schizophrenia. Schizophr Bull. 2001; 27(1):103–13.
32. Riecher-Rössler A, Häfner H, Stumbaum M, Maurer K, Schmidt R. Can estradiol modulate schizophrenic symptomatology? Schizophr Bull. 1994;20(1):203–14.
33. Lindamer LA, Buse DC, Lohr JB, Jeste DV. Hormone replacement therapy in postmenopausal women with schizophrenia: positive effect on negative symptoms? Biol Psychiatry. 2001; 49(1):47–51.

34. Kulkarni J, Riedel A, de Castella AR, Fitzgerald PB, Rolfe TJ, Taffe J, Burger H. Estrogen a potential treatment for schizophrenia. Schizophr Res. 2001;48(1):137–44.
35. Rao ML, Kölsch H. Effects of estrogen on brain development and neuroprotection–implications for negative symptoms in schizophrenia. Psychoneuroendocrinology. 2003; 28 Suppl 2:83–96.
36. Keenan PA, Ezzat WH, Ginsburg K, Moore GJ. Prefrontal cortex as the site of estrogen's effect on cognition. Psychoneuroendocrinology. 2001;26(6):577–90.
37. Krysta K, Murawiec S, Klasik A, Wiglusz MS, Krupka-Matuszczyk I. Sex-specific differences in cognitive functioning among schizophrenic patients. Psychiatr Danub. 2013; 25 Suppl 2:S244–6.
38. Myin-Germeys I, Krabbendam L, Delespaul PA, van Os J. Sex differences in emotional reactivity to daily life stress in psychosis. J Clin Psychiatry. 2004;65(6):805–9.
39. Ochoa S, Usall J, Haro JM, Araya S, Autonell J, Busquets E, Gost A. Grupo Nedes. Comparative study of the needs of patients with schizophrenia by gender [Article in Spanish]. Actas Esp Psiquiatr. 2001;29(3):165–71.
40. Kao YC, Liu YP. Effects of age of onset on clinical characteristics in schizophrenia. BMC Psychiatry. 2010;10:63. doi:10.1186/1471-244X-10-63.
41. Angermeyer MC, Kühn L, Goldstein JM. Gender and the course of schizophrenia: differences in treated outcomes. Schizophr Bull. 1990;16(2):293–307.
42. Uggerby P, Nielsen RE, Correll CU, Nielsen J. Characteristics and predictors of long-term institutionalization in patients with schizophrenia. Schizophr Res. 2011;131(1–3):120–6. doi:10.1016/j.schres.2011.03.001. Epub 2011 Apr 1.
43. Opjordsmoen S. Long-term clinical outcome of schizophrenia with special reference to gender differences. Acta Psychiatr Scand. 1991;83(4):307–13.
44. Ram R, Bromet EJ, Eaton WW, Pato C, Schwartz JE. The natural course of schizophrenia: a review of first-admission studies. Schizophr Bull. 1992;18(2):185–207. Review.
45. Andreasen NC, Ehrhardt JC, Swayze VW, Alliger RJ, Yuh WT, Cohen G, Ziebell S. Magnetic resonance imaging of the brain in schizophrenia. The pathophysiologic significance of structural abnormalities. Arch Gen Psychiatry. 1990;47(1):35–44.
46. Nopoulos P, Laum M, Andreasen NC. Sex differences in brain morphology in schizophrenia. Am J Psychiatry. 1997;154:1648–54.
47. Gur RE, Mozley PD, Shtasel DL, Cannon TD, Gallacher F, Turetsky B, Grossman R, Gur RC. Clinical subtypes of schizophrenia: differences in brain and CSF volume. Am J Psychiatry. 1994;151(3):343–50.
48. Lewine RRJ, Gulley LR, Risch SC, Jewart R, Houpt JL. Sexual dimorphism, brain morphology and schizophrenia. Schizophr Bull. 1990;16:195–204.
49. Raine A, Harrison GN, Reynolds GP, Sheard C, Cooper JE, Medley I. Structural and functional characteristics of the corpus callosum in schizophrenics, psychiatric controls and normal controls. A magnetic resonance imaging and neuropsychological evaluation. Arch Gen Psychiatry. 1990;47(11):1060–4.
50. Ward KE, Friedman L, Wise A, Schulz SC. Meta-analysis of brain and cranial size in schizophrenia. Schizophr Res. 1996;22:197–213.
51. Haijma SV, Van Haren N, Cahn W, et al. Brain volumes in schizophrenia: a meta-analysis in over 18.000 subjects. Schizophr Bull. 2013;39(5):1129–38.
52. Gruner P, Christopher C, Robinson DG. Pituitary volume in first episode schizophrenia. Psychiatry Res. 2012;203:100–2.
53. Romo-Nava F, Hoogenboom WS, Pelavin PE. Pituitary volume in schizophrenia spectrum disorders. Schizophr Res. 2013;146:301–7.
54. Cowell PE, Kostianovsky DJ, Gur RC, Turetsky BI, Gur RE. Sex differences in neuroanatomical and clinical correlations in schizophrenia. Am J Psychiatry. 1996;153(6):799–805.
55. Malla AK, Tarhar J, Norman RMG, Assis L. Computed tomographic findings in schizophrenia: relation with symptom dimensions and sex differences. J Psychiatry Neurosci. 1999;24(2): 131–8.

56. Seeman MV. Interaction of sex, age, and neuroleptic dose. Compr Psychiatry. 1983;24(2): 125–8.
57. Galderisi S, Bucci P, Üçok A, Peuskens J. No gender differences in social outcome in patients suffering from schizophrenia. Eur Psychiatry. 2012;27(6):406–8. doi:10 1016/j.eurpsy.2011. 01.011 (Epub ahead of print).
58. Gattaz WF, Vogel P, Riecher-Rössler A, Soddu G. Influence of the menstrual cycle phase on the therapeutic response in schizophrenia. Biol Psychiatry. 1994;36(2):137–9.
59. Seeman MV, Lang M. The role of estrogens in schizophrenia gender differences. Schizophr Bull. 1990;16(2) 185–94.
60. Lane HY, Chang YC, Chang WH, Lin SK, Tseng YT, Jann MW. Effects of gender and age on plasma levels of clozapine and its metabolites: analyzed by critical statistics. J Clin Psychiatry. 1999;60(1):36–40.
61. Gur RC, Gur RE, Obrist WD, Hungerbuhler JP, Younkin D, Rosen AD, Skolnick BE, Reivich M. Sex and handedness differences in cerebral blood flow during rest and cognitive activity. Science. 1982;217(4560):659–61.
62. Seeman MV. Neuroleptic expressed prescription for men and women. Soc Pharmacol. 1989; 3:219–36.
63. Haas GL, Glick ID, Clarkin JF, Spencer JH, Lewis AB. Gender and schizophrenia outcome: a clinical trial of an inpatient family intervention. Schizophr Bull. 1990;16(2):277–92.
64. Davis JA, Goldstein MJ, Nuechterlein KH. Gender differences in family attitudes about schizophrenia. Psychol Med. 1996;26(4):689–96.
65. Riecher-Rössler A, Häfner H. Gender aspects in schizophrenia: bridging the border between social and biological psychiatry. Acta Psychiatr Scand Suppl. 2000;407:58–62.
66. Galdas PM, Cheater F, Marshall P. Men and health help-seeking behaviour: literature review. J Adv Nurs. 2005;49:616–23.
67. Gayer-Anderson C, Morgan C. Social networks, support and early psychosis: a systematic review. Epidemiol Psychiatr Sci. 2013;22(2):131–46.
68. Supprian T, Kalus P. Sexual dimorphism of the human brain–a review of the literature. Fortschr Neurol Psychiatr. 1996;64(10):382–9.
69. Saugstad LF. The maturational theory of brain development and cerebral excitability in the multifactorially inherited manic-depressive psychosis and schizophrenia. Int J Psychophysiol. 1994;18(3):189–203. discussion 187-8.
70. Downhill Jr JE, Buchsbaum MS, Wei T, Spiegel-Cohen J, Hazlett EA, Haznedar MM, Silverman J, Siever LJ. Shape and size of the corpus callosum in schizophrenia and schizotypal personality disorder. Schizophr Res. 2000;42(3):193–208.
71. Häfner H, an der Heiden W, Hambrecht M, Riecher-Rössler A, Maurer K, Löffler W, Fätkenheuer B. A chapter in systematic schizophrenia research the search for causal explanations for sex differences in age of onset. Nervenarzt. 1993;64(11):706–16. Review. German.
72. Leung A, Chue P. Sex differences in schizophrenia, a review of the literature. Acta Psychiatr Scand Suppl. 2000;401:3–38.
73. Haus-Seuffert P, Meisterernst M. Mechanisms of transcriptional activation of cAMP-responsive element-binding protein CREB. Mol Cell Biochem. 2000;212(1–2):5–9.
74. Kölsch H, Lütjohann D, Tulke A, Björkhem I, Rao ML. The neurotoxic effect of 24-hydroxycholesterol on SH-SY5Y human neuroblastoma cells. Brain Res. 1999;818(1): 171–5.
75. Kölsch H, Ludwig M, Lütjohann D, Rao ML. Neurotoxicity of 24-hydroxycholesterol, an important cholesterol elimination product of the brain, may be prevented by vitamin E and estradiol-17beta. J Neural Transm. 2001;108(4):475–88.
76. Hughes ZA, Liu F, Marquis K, Muniz L, Pangalos MN, Ring RH, Whiteside GJ, Brandon NJ. Estrogen receptor neurobiology and its potential for translation into broad spectrum therapeutics for CNS disorders. Curr Mol Pharmacol. 2009;2:215–36.

77. Taylor GT, Maloney S, Dearborn J, et al. Hormones in the mentally disturbed brain: steroids and peptides in the development and treatment of psychopathology. Cent Nerv Syst Agents Med Chem. 2009;9(4):331–60.
78. Kulkarni J, Hayes E, Gavrilidis E. Hormones and schizophrenia. Curr Opin Psychiatry. 2012; 25:89–95.
79. Kulkarni J, Gavrilidis E, Worsley R, Hayes E. Role of estrogen treatment in the management of schizophrenia. CNS Drugs. 2012;26(7):549–57.
80. Kendell RE, Chalmers JC, Platz C. Epidemiology of puerperal psychoses. Br J Psychiatry. 1987;150:662–73.
81. Riecher-Rossler A, Seeman MV. Oestrogens and schizophrenia: introduction. Arch Womens Ment Health. 2002;5(3):91–2.
82. Seeman MV. Psychopathology in women and men: focus on female hormones. Am J Psychiatry. 1997;154(12):1641–7.
83. Sommer IE, van Westrhenen R, Begemann MJ, de Witte LD, Leucht S, Kahn RS. Efficacy of anti-inflammatory agents to improve symptoms in patients with schizophrenia: an update. Schizophr Bull. 2014;40(1):181–91.
84. Kulkarni J, de Castella A, Smith D, Taffe J, Keks N, Copolov D. A clinical trial of the effects of estrogen in acutely psychotic women. Schizoph Res. 1996;20(3):247–52.
85. Kinon BJ, Gilmore JA, Liu H, Halbreich UM. Prevalence of hyperprolactinemia in schizophrenic patients treated with conventional antipsychotic medications or risperidone. Psychoneuroendocrinology. 2003;28 Suppl 2:55–68.
86. O'Keane V. Review antipsychotic-induced hyperprolactinaemia, hypogonadism and osteoporosis in the treatment of schizophrenia. J Psychopharmacol. 2008;22(2 Suppl):70–5.
87. Dursun SM, Wildgust HJ, Strickland P, Goodwin GM, Citrome L, Lean M. The emerging physical health challenges of antipsychotic associated hyperprolactinaemia in patients with serious mental illness. J Psychopharmacol. 2008;22(2 Suppl):3–5.
88. Meaney AM, Smith S, Howes OD, O'Brien M, Murray RM, O'Keane V. Effects of long-term prolactin-raising antipsychotic medication on bone mineral density in patients with schizophrenia. Br J Psychiatry. 2004;184:503–8.
89. Montejo AL. Review prolactin awareness: an essential consideration for physical health in schizophrenia. Eur Neuropsychopharmacol. 2008;18 Suppl 2:S108–14.
90. Ghadirian AM, Chouinard G, Annable L. Sexual dysfunction and plasma prolactin levels in neuroleptic-treated schizophrenic outpatients. J Nerv Ment Dis. 1982;170(8):463–7.
91. Bobes J, Arango C, Aranda P, Carmena R, Garcia-Garcia M, Rejas J, CLAMORS Study Collaborative Group. Cardiovascular and metabolic risk in outpatients with schizophrenia treated with antipsychotics: results of the CLAMORS Study. Schizophr Res. 2007;90(1–3): 162–73.
92. Boke O, Aker S, Sarisoy G, Saricicek EB, Sahin AR. Prevalence of metabolic syndrome among inpatients with schizophrenia. Int J Psychiatry Med. 2008;38(1):103–12.
93. Fernandez-Egea E, Bernardo M, Donner T, Conget I, Parellada E, Justicia A, Esmatjes E, Garcia-Rizo C, Kirkpatrick B. Metabolic profile of antipsychotic-naive individuals with non-affective psychosis. Br J Psychiatry. 2009;194(5):434–8.
94. Seeman MV. Women and psychosis. Womens Health. 2012;8(2):215–24.
95. Seeman MV. Secondary effects of antipsychotics: women at greater risk than men. Schizophr Bull. 2009;35(5):937–48.
96. Seeman MV. Antipsychotic-induced somnolence in mothers with schizophrenia. Psychiatr Q. 2012;83(1):83–9. doi:10.1007/s11126-011-9185-z (Epub ahead of print).
97. Vieweg WV, Wood MA, Fernandez A, Beatty-Brooks M, Hasnain M, Pandurangi AK. - Pro-arrhythmic risk with antipsychotic and antidepressant drugs: implications in the elderly. Drugs Aging. 2009;26(12):997–1012.
98. Yasui-Furukori N, Saito M, Nakagami T, et al. Gender-specific prolactin response to antipsychotic treatments with risperidone and olanzapine and its relationship to drug

concentrations in patients with acutely exacerbated schizophrenia. Prog Neuropsychopharmacol Biol Psychiatry. 2010;34(3):537–40.
99. Seeman MV. Preventing breast cancer in schizophrenia. Acta Psychiatr Scand. 2011;123(2): 107–17.
100. VanOs J, Walsh E, van Horn E, Tattan T, Bale R, Thompson SG. Tardive dyskinesia in psychosis: are women really more at risk? UK700 Group. Acta Psychiatr Scand. 1999;99(4): 288–93.
101. Os V, et al. Tardive dyskinesia: who is at risk? Acta Psychiatr Scand. 1997;96(3):206–16.
102. Fink G, Sumner E, McQueen JK, Wilson H, Rosie R. Sex steroid control of mood, mental state and memory. Clin Exp Pharmacol Physiol. 1998;25(10):764–75. Review.
103. Akhondzadeh S, Nejatisafa AA, Amini H, Mohammadi MR, Larijani B, Kashani L, Raisi F, Kamalipour A. Adjunctive estrogen treatment in women with chronic schizophrenia: a double-blind, randomized, and placebo-controlled trial. Prog Neuropsychopharmacol Biol Psychiatry. 2003;27(6):1007–12.
104. Smith S. Gender differences in antipsychotic prescribing. Int Rev Psychiatry. 2010;22(5): 472–84. doi:10.3109/09540261.2010.515965. Review.

Gender Differences in Bipolar Disorder 28

Saioa López-Zurbano, Ana González-Pinto, and Purificación López

Abstract

The main objective of this chapter is to summarize the clinical differences found in the literature between men and women suffering from bipolar disorder. The secondary objective is to analyze the treatment and how there are gender differences in the adherence to medication. Briefly, we could say that in men the manic component predominates, both at onset and throughout their lifetime, and that they usually have comorbid drug abuse. On the other hand, women usually tend to have a predominance of depression; they have a depressive polarity both at onset and during their lifetime and experience more mixed mania episodes. Furthermore, in women onset often occurs at an older age, comorbidity of physical pathological conditions is common, and adherence to medication is greater than in men.

We cannot forget that women can experience two very important periods: pregnancy and postpartum. Both can be critical periods for the disorder, and a relapse or recurrence at either stage can have serious consequences not just for the woman but also for her baby. Because the effect of medication on the fetus

S. López-Zurbano (✉)
Alava University Hospital, Vitoria, Spain
e-mail: saioadoc@gmail.com

A. González-Pinto
Alava University Hospital, Vitoria, Spain

University of the Basque Country UPV/EHU, Guipúzcoa, Spain

CIBERSAM, Barcelona, Spain
e-mail: anamaria.gonzalezpintoarrillaga@osakidetza.net

P. López
Alava University Hospital, Vitoria, Spain

University of the Basque Country UPV/EHU, Guipúzcoa, Spain
e-mail: MARIAPURIFICACION.LOPEZPENA@osakidetza.net

M. Sáenz-Herrero (ed.), *Psychopathology in Women*,
DOI 10.1007/978-3-319-05870-2_28

still remains unclear, it makes it even more difficult to set the treatment during these periods.

28.1 Introduction

Bipolar disorder is a lifelong serious mental disorder that causes extreme dysregulation in mood, energy, and functioning. It affects approximately 1.3 % of the general population, and both genders are equally at risk of developing the illness. The onset of bipolar disorder usually occurs in adolescence or early adulthood, but it can appear during other periods in a life time, such as childhood or later adulthood. It can be a difficult disease to live with because it affects familial relationships, social aspects, and employment, causing a general worsening in the quality of life of the patient.

The clinical course of bipolar disorder is characterized by the occurrence of one or more manic or mixed episodes, and often individuals also have recurrent episodes of major depression. Manic episodes are periods of abnormally and persistently elevated, irritable, or expansive mood during which the person may have the following symptoms: inflated self-esteem or grandiosity; flight of ideas or subjective experience of racing thoughts; decreased need for sleep; feeling more talkative than usual or feeling pressure to keep talking; distractibility; psychomotor agitation; or excessive involvement in pleasurable activities that can be the cause of painful consequences [1]. The most important symptoms associated with major depressive episodes are the presence of a depressed mood most of the day, significant weight loss (when not dieting) or weight gain, insomnia or hypersomnia, fatigue or loss of energy, markedly diminished interest or pleasure in (almost) all activities, psychomotor agitation or retardation, feelings of worthlessness or excessive or inappropriate guilt, diminished ability to think or concentrate, indecisiveness, and recurrent thoughts of death [1]. Usually, a person with bipolar disorder only has some of these symptoms; it is very uncommon that they all manifest at the same time.

There are two types of diagnosis: bipolar I disorder and bipolar II disorder. Bipolar I disorder is characterized by recurrent episodes of mania and depression, whereas bipolar II disorder is defined as recurrent episodes of depression and hypomania [1].

Many aspects of bipolar disorder have been investigated in several studies, including diagnosis, course of illness, psychiatric and physical comorbidity, suicide attempts, rapid cycling, and mixed states [2]. However, the role gender could play in all those aspects still remains unclear. In this chapter, we review all the information currently available on the matter.

Table 28.1 Gender differences in bipolar disorder

Characteristics	Women	Men
More common episode	Depressive	Manic
Onset episode	Depressive	Manic
Age of onset	Older	Younger
Mixed episodes	More frequent	Less frequent
Seasonal episodes	More frequent	Less frequent
Rapid cycling	More frequent	Less frequent
Physical comorbidity	More frequent (thyroid diseases)	Less frequent
Psychiatric comorbidity	Eating disorder, anxiety disorders	Drug abuse

28.2 Gender Differences in Bipolar Disorder

Most studies show that the prevalence of bipolar I disorder is the same for both genders, whereas there are more women than men with bipolar II disorder [3–5]. Traditional epidemiological studies give prevalence rates of 0.4–1.6 % for bipolar I disorder and 0.5–1.9 % for bipolar II disorder [1]. As the bipolarity spectrum is being extended and the newer entity of bipolar II disorder is even more prevalent in the general population, the affected population is about 5 % [6].

28.3 Course and Clinical Characteristics of Illness

The biggest gender differences are seen for bipolar I disorder, especially when we refer to clinical features, course of illness, and comorbidity (Table 28.1) [7]. In women, the disease is characterized by a predominance of depression [8, 9]: this means that the polarity at the onset [10] and during a lifetime is depressive. Studies show that women spend more time in the depressed phase, with longer hospitalization for this reason [5, 11]. They also have more depression symptoms in manic phases; thus, they are more likely to experience mixed mania [4, 8]. This way, women also experience more suicidal ideation and more suicide attempts (whereas men make fewer attempts, but they are more violent) [7, 8, 12]. They also have a higher probability of experiencing mood instability [8], seasonal episodes, and rapid cycling [4, 11]. On the other hand, men tend to have a predominance of manic components: their temperament is hyperthymic and the onset of the illness is usually with a manic episode [7, 8, 10, 11]. The disorder begins at a younger age in men, with an earlier first hospitalization [5]. This may explain why men are more often single [8].

Women are more often hospitalized than men and take more antidepressive and sedative/hypnotic treatments [8, 11, 12], which can be explained with different reasons. First of all, women seek more treatment, probably because of their depressive polarity, as it is described how bipolar patients ask for help during depressive phases. Second, women being more frequently married and having feminine gender behavioral expectations, it is likely that their relatives bring women to health care facilities more easily [13]. Third, men (as we will see later in the chapter) have a higher rate of substance abuse comorbidity; therefore, they can be misdiagnosed with mania. Finally, as women experience more suicide attempts and they have more mixed mania episodes, they are more usually hospitalized to prevent the risk of suicide [8].

28.3.1 Bipolar Depression in Women and Misdiagnosis

Gender differences in unipolar depression have been studied in detail, and, cultural studies included, the results of these investigations confirm that the risk of a major depressive episode throughout life is two times higher in women [1, 14, 15]. This same trend, with smaller differences, is also observed in bipolar disorder [4, 7, 8]. As we have already explained, the illness in women is more usually characterized by the predominance of depression symptoms. Depressive polarity is more common at the onset of the disorder and during a lifetime [7, 11]; they have a greater number of temperaments with depressive propensities such as mood instability and cyclothymic temperament, and have more depressive subsyndromal symptoms [8].

The clinical characteristics of bipolar depression in women are different from those in men with regard to both bipolar I and bipolar II disorders. They more commonly suffer from psychotic [7] and atypical symptoms (such as hypersomnia, increased appetite or incongruent psychotic symptoms) [8, 10, 16]. This, connected with the fact that the first signs of the disorder in women are often depressive, can explain both why they are later diagnosed [7, 17] and why they take more antidepressants and benzodiazepines than men [12].

28.3.2 Misdiagnosis

Precise establishment of a proper diagnosis by the first manifestations of bipolar depression is one of the biggest challenges in psychiatry these days. The depressive phase of bipolar disorder is many times indistinguishable from that of unipolar depression, especially if familial and personal history is not taken into account. The misdiagnosis often leads to the prescription of only antidepressants and in high doses [4], as often happens in bipolar women [17], and this causes the destabilization of the course of the disorder. This incorrect prescription can provoke switches to mania/hypomania, increases the number of episodes with occurrence of rapid cycles or the development of mixed states [18]. It is estimated that it takes about 9.6 years from the onset of symptoms to the formal diagnosis of bipolar disorder

[17]. Moreover, it has been observed that this delay is longer in patients with a younger age at onset, especially when they do not show psychotic symptoms or social dysfunction during the first episode [19].

According to Hirschfeld [20] more than a third of bipolar patients seek professional help during the first year after the onset of symptoms. Unfortunately, 69 % are misdiagnosed and often receive the diagnosis of unipolar depression. Those who are misdiagnosed usually consult four therapists before receiving the correct diagnosis, and over a third of those have to wait for 10 years. This delay in the diagnosis and in the prescription of the correct treatment often brings significant psychosocial problems, such as conflicts with family and friends, professional or academic problems, alcohol and substance abuse, with the corresponding worsening of patients' quality of life.

28.3.3 Suicide Risk

Together with all this, one of the most serious consequences associated with the misdiagnosis in bipolar patients is the increased suicide risk. The risk is higher during the first 5 years after the affective symptoms emerge [21]. In fact, about 40 % of bipolar patients attempt suicide at 8.6 $\pm$ 6.6 years after the onset of affective symptoms. The suicide rate in the bipolar population ranges from 10 to 20 % [22]. There is evidence that bipolar depressed patients attempt suicide earlier than unipolar patients during a specific episode. However, the patients with the highest risk of suicide are those experiencing mixed symptoms. This is because they combine the hopelessness of depression and the anxiety and impulsivity of mania. Some authors report that patients with bipolar II disorder make more suicide attempts than bipolar I and unipolar patients, although there is some controversy about this [22]. The clinical variables most associated with an increased risk of suicide are: the presence of severe depressive episodes, drug use, a family background of affective disorders, younger age at onset, and the presence of mixed symptoms. We should pay special attention if there are behavior disorders or a history of suicidal behavior comorbidity [23]. Studies show that women tend to attempt suicide more frequently and more times than men, but men's attempts are more violent (Table 28.2) [7, 8].

Table 28.2 Factors associated with suicidal risks (adapted from Undurraga et al. [22] and López et al. [23])

Risk factors	Suicidal acts	Suicidal ideation
More mixed episodes	✓	✓
Female sex	✓	
Predominantly depressed	✓	✓
Latency to bipolar diagnosis	✓	
Melancholic at any time		✓
Hospitalization for depression	✓	

28.3.4 Rapid Cycling in Women

Rapid cycling is one of the clinical patterns collected nowadays in the Diagnostic and Statistical Manual of Mental Disorders text revision [1] for bipolar disorder. The main characteristic of rapid cycling bipolar disorder is the occurrence of four or more mood episodes during the previous 12 months. Episodes can occur in any combination and order. They have to meet the diagnostic criteria (symptoms and duration) for a major depressive, manic, mixed or hypomanic episode, and can be delimited by a remission or by a change in polarity. The only exception in a rapid cycling bipolar disorder is that episodes occur more often than in a nonrapid cycling pattern. It appears that rapid cycling is a temporary evolution form in bipolar disorder; it occurs temporarily.

Typically, rapid cycling and mood fluctuation have been associated with the female gender, but there has always been controversy about this. Early in the pre-pharmacological age Falret (1794–1870) referred to the higher prevalence of women in hospitalized patients with a diagnosis of circular insanity. However, Perris [24] pointed out that it was understandable why there was a larger proportion of women in hospitals, explaining that for families it was easier to take care of a sick man than a sick woman.

A meta-analysis of published studies about rapid cycling in the 1990s showed that the proportion of women included in the study reached 74 %; thus, the female/male ratio was 3:1. They established that the risk of developing rapid cycling in women was 29.6 % compared with 15.5 % in men. To Coryell [25], female gender is a strong predictor for rapid cycling. Different explanations have been proposed [26], including hypothyroidism, the effect of gonadal steroids, and antidepressant use. Hypothyroidism is common in bipolar patients, as it is a common secondary effect of lithium salts [8]. Thyroid abnormalities are more common in women in the general population, which may also explain the differences in the bipolar population.

Women's hormonal fluctuation throughout the reproductive cycle has been suggested to be an etiological factor of mood dysregulation in women [27]. Rasgon's group [28] showed that a majority of bipolar women have a significant mood change during at least one menstrual cycle and that women receiving oral contraception had fewer symptoms of depression. However, more studies need to be carried out, because short cycles also occur in postmenopausal women when there is not a hormonal explanation.

What seems clear is that some rapid cycling is iatrogenic. We know that women take more antidepressive and sedative/hypnotic treatments than men [12], and that they appear to be more sensitive to polypharmacy. Thus, this could be one reason for the higher prevalence of rapid cycling in women. In a study by Altshuler [29] of the 9 patients referred by suffering by rapid cycling due to antidepressants, 8 were women.

However, the higher prevalence of rapid cycling in women still remains unclear. Some current studies confirm this [4, 11, 26, 28], but others do not [8, 30]. Nevertheless, according to an international general population study, rapid cycling is associated with more severe depressive symptoms, greater impairment from depressive symptoms, and more anxiety disorders [30], which are linked to female gender. Thus, it is likely that in the bipolar population, especially during the first phases of the disease, when misdiagnosis is so frequent, women receive more antidepressants with the corresponding risk of developing rapid cycling.

28.3.5 Mania in Women

We have already mentioned that men tend to have a more hypomanic temperament and (hypo) manic polarity when suffering from bipolar disorder and that the onset usually occurs with a manic episode. Nevertheless, women also experience manic episodes, and differences can be observed between genders.

Women tend to achieve higher severity scores on scales (e.g., the Young Mania Rating Scale [YMRS]), which is due to the higher prevalence of psychotic symptoms in these patients [13, 31]. Psychotic features tend to be incongruent in women [8], with more overall delusions and more paranoid and reference delusions. They also experience more hallucinations per patient.

As women's polarity is often depressive, they usually experience more depressive symptoms; mood lability, depressed mood, greater guilt, higher suicide and anxiety scores, even in mania episodes. This leads to the fact that women experience more mixed manias [8, 13, 31]. Some theories explain that they can be mediated by the predominance of anxiety symptoms in the female sex. Men, on the other hand, experience higher motor activity, grandiosity, and contact [13]. They are more likely to report "behavioural problems" and "being unable to hold a conversation" [10].

28.3.6 Comorbid Conditions

In psychiatric comorbidity, women tend to have more comorbid eating [10], anxiety, especially phobias [4, 8, 11], and axis II disorders [7]. Even though the relation between bipolar disorder and anxiety is particularly complex (one leads to the other and vice versa), some studies on this particular subject have been carried out [12]. As anxiety disorders are more common in women in the general population, the same is expected to happen in the bipolar population, which is confirmed in most studies. Bipolar women suffer more frequently than men from panic disorder, obsessive compulsive disorder, and specific phobia [12]. Bipolar women suffering from panic disorder spend fewer years at school and are more frequently treated with antidepressants [12]. Some studies show that panic disorder and obsessive compulsive disorder aggregate in families; thus, it is possible that women with familial bipolar disorder might be more likely to experience comorbid anxiety disorders.

It is also known that even social phobias are equally prevalent among female and male populations; women suffering bipolar disorder and social phobia are four times more prone to have comorbid alcohol abuse [12]. Comorbid drug abuse is more common in men with bipolar disorder (alcohol, cocaine, cannabis) [8, 10, 12], and other studies also find pathological gambling and conduct disorder [8].

Patients with bipolar disorder have a greater comorbidity of physical pathological conditions, as the disease and its treatment increase the risk of cardiovascular, metabolic, and endocrine diseases [32]. Women suffer higher comorbidity of thyroid disease, obesity or being overweight [4, 8]. Lifetime prevalence of thyroid disease (excluding thyroid cancer) is four to ten times higher in women, which links with the fact that bipolar disorder treatment (lithium salts) increases the risk of thyroid diseases itself. Women with thyroid diseases and bipolar disorder are more likely to have eating disorders, which may explain the more frequent obesity among women. Bipolar men are more prone to suffer from neurological cancer disorders, which may be due to the higher comorbidity with substance abuse [8]. However, there are no gender differences in the risk of experiencing cardiovascular diseases [8].

28.4 Treatment of Bipolar Disorder

Medication for the treatment of bipolar disorder includes lithium, anticonvulsants, and atypical antipsychotics, which are used both for acute episodes and for long-term maintenance treatment. These drugs are often combined with benzodiazepines when there are coexisting symptoms of anxiety or insomnia.

The treatment of bipolar disorder is complex and must be individualized for each patient. This gets even more difficult when the patient is a woman, because there is always the possibility of a pregnancy. The drugs mentioned above all interact with oral contraceptives, increase the risk of endocrine pathological conditions (hypothyroidism), and can be harmful to the fetus [33].

28.4.1 Treatments and Hormones in Women

Medications and doses used in common clinical practice are similar for both women and men. This is because there have not been enough investigations into the different metabolic, endocrine, and social effects that treatment has in each gender; thus, clinicians tend to treat men and women the same way.

28.4.2 Reproductive Axis

Studies reflect that bipolar women have reproductive dysfunctions, even prior to treatment. These can aggravate with the treatment, which is confirmed by the fact that bipolar women taking medication have higher rates of long menstrual cycles [9] than non-bipolar patients. Some medications habitually used in bipolar disorder can diminish reproductive hormone blood levels and consequently alter the hypothalamic–pituitary–gonadal (HPG) axis and reproductive function [33]. They also interfere with contraceptive medications and induce other menstrual abnormalities such as polycystic ovary syndrome.

Estrogens seem to be related to depressive symptoms, as there is an increased risk of depressive symptoms in the premenstrual, postpartum, and perimenopausal periods. The hypothesis is that its effects on the serotonergic system, brain-derived neurotrophic factor, and protein kinase C might increase that risk [34].

Hormonal differences have also been proposed for explaining the differences between genders in the response to anxiety. All steroids, progesterone metabolites included, act as gamma aminobutyric acid A (GABA-A)/benzodiazepine receptor agonists, whose activation has an anxiolytic effect, and they up-regulate the GABA-A/benzodiazepine receptors. Thus, it is likely that the cyclic withdrawal of estrogens and progestins induces an anxiolysis withdrawal, provoking anxiety states in women [13].

28.4.3 Endrocrine Secondary Effects

As we have mentioned before, it is known that women, particularly those in treatment with lithium, are at a higher risk of hypothyroidism [8]. Besides, many of the psychotropic medications used in the treatment of this disorder are associated with insulin resistance, weight gain, and dyslipidemia. This can provoke a dysregulation of the neuroendocrine system in women with bipolar disorder, which can also cause non-adherence [33].

The information we have nowadays about the reproductive and metabolic function in women with bipolar disorder shows a vulnerability, increased by medication, of later-life cardiovascular disease and diabetes, among other morbidities.

28.4.4 Response to Medication

The response to medication may also be different, as is shown by the different prevalence of secondary effects; for example, in lithium treatment it is more common for men to experience tremor and women to gain weight and suffer hypothyroidism [35].

28.4.5 Adherence to Treatment

Adherence to medication for the treatment of bipolar disorder has been a topic of interest in last few years as a potentially modifiable factor for improving patient outcomes. Good medication adherence is necessary to prevent recurrence of affective episodes, which are associated with cumulative increases in morbidity risks, treatment nonresponse, full syndromal recurrence, and suicide [23, 36]. Non-adherence to medication in bipolar disorder is estimated to range from 12 to 64 %, and studies with longer follow-up intervals have higher rates of non-adherence [37]. Lithium, the gold standard treatment in bipolar disorder, has a high rate of discontinuation as shown in a 6-year follow-up study, where the median adherence time to treatment was only 76 days [38].

Factors affecting the ability of a person with bipolar disorder to take their medication as prescribed or to understand other treatments include [39]:

(1) Demographic factors: such as male gender, youth, early onset of the illness, single status, and lower level of education [37, 39, 41].
(2) Clinical factors, which include substance abuse, previous episodes of psychotic mania, greater affective morbidity, hospitalization, comorbid obsessive compulsive disorder [39, 40].
(3) Treatment-related factors, such as the treatment's adverse effects (especially those involving cognitive and autonomic functioning) or regimen complexity [39].
(4) Psychological factors, including poor insight, distrust of clinician or medications, denial of illness [39].

28.4.6 Gender Differences in Adherence to Treatment and Factors Associated with Non-adherence

Although men have been described to be less adherent than women [42], there are few specific studies on bipolar disorder patients showing gender differences in adherence to treatment. Substance abuse is associated with non-adherence, as patients use it as self-medication. Some studies find that all kinds of drug abuse lead to non-adherence [40], but others only find this link with alcohol abuse [39]. Nevertheless, men have higher drug abuse comorbidity than women, including alcohol abuse, with rates of 82 % compared with 68.8 % in women [7].

Another factor related to treatment non-adherence in bipolar disorder is the subjective experience of illness [43]. Some researchers have demonstrated that a good illness experience can be a primary and effective motivator for patients to keep to their treatment plan, whereas a poor subjective experience of illness often leads to lowered treatment adherence. Experience of illness is a multifactorial outcome that includes the level of social support, experience of positive or negative effects of medications, and perceived stigma. Studies have found gender differences in these factors: women are concerned about weight gain, the possible negative side effects of medication, and want more social support than men [44, 45]. Kriegshauser et al. [43] did not find any differences between men and women in self-stigmatizing attitudes, perception of stigma, and in perceived weight gain. However, they did find that women had more concern than men about weight gain and perceived higher quality relationships than men. This should be taken into account when prescribing a treatment, as women are more likely to have the secondary effect of weight gain, and when undergoing psychotherapy, to include their social network.

28.5 Special Considerations During Pregnancy and the Postpartum Period

The management of bipolar disorder in women during pregnancy, childbirth, and the postpartum period needs special consideration and is currently an important source for investigation. This is because the knowledge about morbidity risks and the optimal treatment is very limited, which can lead to significant consequences both for the patient and for the fetus/newborn.

For hundreds of years the strong association between psychotic and major affective episodes in the puerperal period has been known [46]. Epidemiological studies show contradictory results about pregnancy being a risk or a protective factor for affective illness [47]. What evidence reveals is the importance of maintaining the mood stabilizer during pregnancy, because the discontinuation of maintenance treatment, especially if it is abrupt, increases the risk of early depressive or mixed states [48].

The risk of a mood relapse is the same for bipolar disorders I and II [47]. The most prevalent relapse during pregnancy is major depression, and it seems that the highest risk is during the first trimester and that it declines in the later trimester [47]. This may be because of treatment discontinuation just before or at the beginning of pregnancy, which may contribute to those early relapses. The factors associated with affective episodes in pregnancy were: younger age at onset, previous postpartum episodes, fewer years of illness, fewer children, and single status [47]. Therefore, during pregnancy, there is a need to balance the teratogenic and adverse effects of medication against the consequences of a relapse in the mother's illness for both the mother and the child.

With regard to the postpartum period, some studies have reported that between 20 and 30 % of women with bipolar disorder have a postpartum affective episode, predominantly of the depressive type, within 1 month of childbirth [47, 49]. Other studies have reported that between 9 and 20 % of women have hypomanic symptoms after delivery [49, 50]. Hypomanic symptoms are harder to diagnose because they may be confused with the normal joyfulness experienced by mothers after delivery.

If bipolar disorder begins in the postpartum period and with a depressive phase, misdiagnosis with unipolar disorder can be a common problem. Sharma et al. explain that more than half of the patients seen with a diagnosis of postpartum depression are later diagnosed as having bipolar disorder [49, 51]. This misdiagnosis can lead to delays in the prescription of appropriate pharmacological treatment. Moreover, unsuitable treatment with antidepressants can precipitate mania or a mixed state and, in the worst cases, psychiatric hospitalization.

Table 28.3 Recommendation for treatment during pregnancy and breast feeding (adapted from Medrano et al. [55])

– Whenever possible, try to avoid the use of drugs during the first trimester of pregnancy, especially during weeks 3rd and 11th
– Doses fragmentation is preferable in order to avoid high plasma peaks, as it is supposed to provoke less impact on the fetus than once-daily
– The doses should be as low as possible, but effective. It should be considered that, toward the end of pregnancy a higher dose is often required, as the distribution volume increases
– One single drug rather than several should be used with these patients. The addition of medications theoretically provokes more side effects and interactions, and there are even fewer studies on the use of several psychotropic drugs in pregnancy
– The most recent drugs should be avoided, because they have fewer exposed cases, and therefore more unpredictable effects

28.6 Treatment During Pregnancy

Some authors recommend suspending pharmacological treatment during the first trimester of pregnancy and even during the 2–3 weeks before conception, proposing that this would avoid teratogenic effects of treatment on the fetus [52]. However, stopping the medical treatment during gestation can have deleterious effects for both mother and fetus, such as interference with activities of daily living, including taking care of a child [53], inadequate nutrition, increased alcohol or tobacco use, exposure to other medications or natural remedies (herbal, homeopathy), problems in the family environment, and deficits in mother–infant bonding [54]. Therefore, there is information about the consequences of relapses during pregnancy, but not about taking bipolar disorder medication during that period; the few studies available on this subject are limited and have reported conflicting results.

Nevertheless, there are some recommendations that should be taken into account (Table 28.3). It is important to discuss with the patient and her family the potential risks of the treatment weighed against the risks of a mood relapse (for her and for the baby), in order to decide on the best medication. Both the mother's psychopathological and physical states and the fetus' physical state must be monitored throughout gestation. The treatment should be with the minimum, but always effective, doses. We should try to avoid polytherapy, new drugs, and the use of medication during the first trimester to mitigate any teratogenic side effects.

28.6.1 Mood Stabilizers

Studies show that patients who use lithium during pregnancy have a congenital malformation occurrence rate of 4–12 %, whereas the untreated population has an estimated rate of malformation of 2–4 % [56]. Relatively recent updates on the risk of fetal structural malformations associated with lithium exposure suggest that this medication is not a significant human teratogen [57]. Thus, the "historical" fear of cardiac Ebstein's anomaly in lithium-exposed children should be reduced [58]. Lithium is associated with a higher risk of neonatal complications, such as lower Apgar scores, longer hospital stays, and central nervous system and neuromuscular adverse reactions, which are directly related to the level of the drug in serum [58]. Other adverse effects that have been anecdotally reported are premature birth, diabetes insipidus, thyroid dysfunction, and polyhydramnios [59].

Antiepileptic drugs, except for lamotrigine, are the medications that show the worst reproductive safety profile [58].

Valproate is estimated to have a rate of 11.3 % of birth defects in newborns of epileptic women treated with valproate monotherapy [60]. The risk of fetal malformations seems to be dose-dependent and they include epicanthic folds, medial eyebrow deficiency, a long thin upper lip, a thick lower lip, cardiac malformations, hypospadias, an infraorbital groove, a flat nasal bridge, a short nose with anteverted nares, a small downturned mouth, and spina bifida [59]. The risk of valproate-induced birth defects seems to rise when it is combined with other drugs, especially with lamotrigine or carbamazepine [61].

Carbamazepine has been thought to be very teratogenic, but recent investigations show that the birth malformation rate with carbamazepine is similar to that of the general population [55]. We must remember that this risk rises when combined with valproic acid [61]. Carbamazepine-induced malformations are epicanthic folds, an orofacial cleft, cardiac malformations, a short nose with hypoplastic nares, a long philtrum, upward slanting palpebral fissures, and spina bifida [58].

Lamotrigine is the antiepileptic that we have more experience of during pregnancy. It is a safe drug in pregnant women, except for its risk of cleft lip or palate [62].

To sum up, the monitoring of mood stabilizers in serum is recommendable during pregnancy, always taking into account the physiological changes that women's bodies experience during gestation, such as a bigger distribution volume, glomerular filtration alterations, or increased frequency of urination [55, 58].

28.6.2 Antipsychotics

Research into the risk of malformations in children exposed to antipsychotic medication is limited, and it is summarized in Table 28.4. Information from retrospective and prospective studies finds that antipsychotics are not associated with a higher risk of major malformations. Clozapine is commonly used during pregnancy, because different studies show a low risk of complications or congenital anomalies [63, 64]. There are anecdotal reports of neonatal convulsions, floppy baby, and gestational diabetes, although the cause–effect relation is doubtful [55]. Studies show risperidone to be a safe drug in pregnancy [65]. Quetiapine and aripiprazole seem to be safe too, but the information available is sparse [5, 4, 58]. Olanzapine-exposed children showed a tendency toward higher rates of hospitalization in neonatal intensive care units and higher birth weight [58].

Table 28.4 Antipsychotics during pregnancy (adapted from Medrano et al. [55])

Antipsychotic drug	Risks
Phenothiazines	– Contradictory data – Possible slightly increased risk of malformation – Possible increased risk of neonatal toxicity in exposed lactants – Avoid in pregnancy
Haloperidol	– It is considered safe during the first trimester – Risk of neonatal extrapyramidal symptoms
Risperidone	– No risk data for the first quarter – Risk of neonatal extrapyramidal symptoms
Olanzapine	– No teratogenic risk data – Increased risk of being overweight and gestational diabetes – Higher rate of admission in neonatal intensive care unit
Clozapine	– No teratogenic risk data – Increased risk of being overweight and gestational diabetes
Others	Scarce information on quetiapine, amisulpride, aripiprazole, and ziprasidone

28.6.3 Antidepressants

In the selective serotonin reuptake inhibitors (SSRI) group, paroxetine, fluoxetine, sertraline, and citalopram seem to increase the risk of fetal cardiac abnormalities. Paroxetine also seems to spread the risk of hypospadias. Escitalopram, for the moment, appears to be a safe medication [58]. However, the arbitrariness of the findings and the limitation of the studies render these results inconsistent [66].

In the serotonin/norepinephrine reuptake inhibitors (SNRI) group, the most frequently studied drug has been venlafaxine, with the finding that it does not increase the risk of malformation. There are no studies available on duloxetine [58].

28.6.4 Electroconvulsive Therapy

Electroconvulsive therapy (ECT) is often the treatment of choice for depression during pregnancy as it is recommended by the American Psychiatric Association Task Force on ECT [67]. It has been reported to be a safe and effective option in pregnant women [67]. The few studies that describe ECT in pregnant women report secondary effects of vaginal bleeding and premature uterine contractions, although child development after delivery was normal. It is essential to have proper coordination with obstetric and anesthetic services. Anesthetics used during ECT cross the placenta and fetal blood–brain barrier, but they are not a serious threat owing to the brevity of exposure.

28.7 Treatment During Breast Feeding

During the postpartum period, medication is needed in bipolar women because they are at an increased risk of affective episodes, which if severe, can unusually lead to suicide or infanticide [69].

In lactation, the aim of the treatment is to minimize infant exposure and adverse effects while maintaining optimal maternal mental health. The mood stabilizers valproate and carbamazepine are considered suitable during lactation, whereas lamotrigine should be used with caution and lithium use is not recommended [55, 58]. There are no solid determinations about the risks or benefits of most antipsychotic drugs in breastfeeding, but clozapine and olanzapine should be considered contraindicated during breastfeeding, although further long-term data studies are required [55].

Electroconvulsive therapy can be used safely during breastfeeding if care is taken not to breastfeed the child too soon after the session so that the anesthetics, muscle relaxants, and anticholinergics are not ingested by the infant.

28.8 Discussion

There is a predominance of depression in women: the polarity at onset and throughout a lifetime is depressive. They spend more time in a depressed phase, and have more depression symptoms during manic phases; thus, they are more likely to experience mixed mania.

Women have a higher probability of experiencing mood instability, seasonal episodes, and rapid cycling. They experience more suicidal ideation and more suicide attempts (whereas men make fewer attempts, but they are more violent).

Depressed bipolar women more commonly suffer from psychotic and atypical symptoms (such as hypersomnia, increased appetite or incongruent psychotic symptoms).

Women are more likely to be misdiagnosed with unipolar depression and they take more antidepressants and benzodiazepines than men. As women's polarity is often depressive, they usually experience more depressive symptoms: mood lability, depressed mood, greater guilt, suicide and anxiety scores, even in mania episodes. Thus, women experience more mixed manias. When manic, psychotic features tend to be incongruent, with more overall delusions and more paranoid and reference delusions. They also experience more hallucinations per patient.

Women tend to have more comorbid eating, anxiety, especially phobias, and axis II disorders. They suffer more frequently than men from panic disorder, obsessive compulsive disorder, and specific phobias. Even social phobia is equally prevalent among female and male populations; women suffering from bipolar disorder and social phobia are four times more prone to having comorbid alcohol abuse. The female gender suffers a higher comorbidity of thyroid disease, obesity or being overweight.

Women are considered to be more adherent to treatment, but they are concerned about weight gain, the possible negative side effects of medication, and want more social support than men.

Pregnancy and especially the postpartum period are risk factors for mood disorder relapse, and depressive relapses are more frequent. It is contraindicated to stop treatment abruptly if pregnant, so there should be a balance between treatment-provoked risk factors against the deleterious effects of an affective relapse.

In conclusion, there is a requirement for more research on gender differences in bipolar disorder. Moreover, a better understanding of treatment in women with bipolar disorder during pregnancy and lactation is needed to improve outcomes for both the mother and her child.

References

1. American Psychiatric Association. Diagnostic and statistical manual of mental disorders. 4th ed. Washington, DC: American Psychiatric Press; 1994.
2. González-Pinto A, Gutierrez M, Mosquera F, et al. First episode in bipolar disorder: misdiagnosis and psychotic symptoms. J Affect Disord. 1998;50(1):41–4.
3. Hendrick V, Altsuler LL, Gitlin MJ, Delrahim S, Hammen C. Gender and bipolar illness. J Clin Psychiatry. 2000;61(5):393–6.
4. Arnold LM. Gender differences in bipolar disorder. Psychiatr Clin North Am. 2003;26(3):595–620.
5. Popovic D, Torrent C, Goikolea JM, Cruz N, Sánchez-Moreno J, González-Pinto A, Vieta E. Clinical implications of predominant polarity and the polarity index in bipolar disorder: a naturalistic study. Acta Psychiatr Scand. 2013. doi:10.1111/acps.12179. [pubmed in process].
6. Ketter TA. Diagnostic features, prevalence and impact of bipolar disorder. J Clin Psychiatry. 2010;71:e14.
7. Nivoli AM, Pacchiarotti I, Rosa AR, Popovic D, Murru A, Valenti M, Bonnin CM, Grande I, Sanchez-Moreno J, Vieta E, Colom F. Gender differences in a cohort study of 604 bipolar patients: the role of predominant polarity. J Affect Disord. 2011;133(3):443–9. doi:10.1016/j.jad.2011.04.055. Epub 2011 May 26.
8. Azorin JM, Belzeaux R, Kaladjian A, Adida M, Hantouche E, Lancrenon S, Fakra E. Risks associated with gender differences in bipolar I disorder. J Affect Disord. 2013;151(3):1033–40. doi:10.1016/j.jad.2013.08.031. pii: S0165-0327[13]00665-4, Epub ahead of print.
9. Rasgon N, Bauer M, Glenn T, Elman S, Whybrow PC. Menstrual cycle related mood changes in women with bipolar disorder. Bipolar Disord. 2003;5(1):48–52.
10. Kawa I, Carter JD, Joyce PR, et al. Gender differences in bipolar disorder: age at onset, course, comorbidity, and symptom presentation. Bipolar Disord. 2005;7(2):119–25.
11. Altshuler LL, Kupka RW, Hellemann G, Frye MA, Sugar CA, McElroy SL, Nolen WA, Grunze H, Leverich GS, Keck PE, Zermeno M, Post RM, Suppes T. Gender and depressive symptoms in 711 patients with bipolar disorder evaluated prospectively in the Stanley Foundation bipolar treatment outcome network. Am J Psychiatry. 2010;167(6):708–15. doi:10.1176/appi.ajp.2009.09010105. Epub 2010 Mar 15.
12. Saunders EF, Fitzgerald KD, Zhang P, McInnis MG. Clinical features of bipolar disorder comorbid with anxiety disorders differ between men and women. Depress Anxiety. 2012;29(8):739–46. doi:10.1002/da.21932. Epub 2012 Mar 27.

13. Bhattacharya A, Khess CR, Munda SK, Bakhla AK, Praharaj SK, Kumar M. Sex difference in symptomatology of manic episode. Compr Psychiatry. 2011;52(3):288–92. doi:10.1016/j.comppsych.2010.06.010. Epub 2010 Aug 13.
14. Freeman MP, Smith KW, Freeman SA, McElroy SL, Kmetz GE, Wright R, Keck Jr PE. The impact of reproductive events on the course of bipolar disorder in women. J Clin Psychiatry. 2002;63(4):284–7.
15. Payne JL. The role of estrogen in mood disorders in women. Int Rev Psychiatry. 2003;15(3):280–90.
16. Benazzi F. Gender differences in bipolar II and unipolar depressed outpatients: a 557-case study. Ann Clin Psychiatry. 1999;11(2):55–9.
17. Drancourt N, Etain B, Lajnef M, Henry C, Raust A, Cochet B, Mathieu F, Gard S, Mbailara K, Zanouy L, Kahn JP, Cohen RF, Wajsbrot-Elgrabli O, Leboyer M, Scott J, Bellivier F. Duration of untreated bipolar disorder: missed opportunities on the long road to optimal treatment. Acta Psychiatr Scand. 2013;127:136–44. doi:10.1111/j.1600-0447.2012.01917.x.
18. Hirschfeld RM, Vornik LA. Recognition and diagnosis of bipolar disorder. J Clin Psychiatry. 2004;65 suppl 15:5–9.
19. Goldberg JF, Ernst CL. Features associated with the delayed initiation of mood stabilizers at illness onset in bipolar disorder. J Clin Psychiatry. 2002;63(11):985–91.
20. Hirschfeld RM, Lewis L, Vornik LA. Perceptions and impact of bipolar disorder: how far have we really come? Results of the national depressive and manic-depressive association 2000 survey of individuals with bipolar disorder. J Clin Psychiatry. 2003;64(2):161–74.
21. González-Pinto A, Aldama A, González C, Mosquera F, Arrasate M, Vieta E. Predictors of suicide in first-episode affective and nonaffective psychotic inpatients: five-year follow-up of patients from a catchment area in Vitoria, Spain. J Clin Psychiatry. 2007;68:242–7.
22. Undurraga J, Baldessarini RJ, Valenti M, Pacchiarotti I, Vieta E. Suicidal risk factors in bipolar I and II disorder patients. J Clin Psychiatry. 2012;73(6):778–82.
23. López P, Mosquera F, de León J, et al. Suicide attempts in bipolar patients. J Clin Psychiatry. 2001;62(12):963–6.
24. Perris C. A study of bipolar (manic-depressive) and unipolar recurrent depressive psychoses. Introduction. Acta Psychiatr Scand Suppl. 1966;194:9–14.
25. Coryell W, Endicott J, Keller M. Rapidly cycling affective disorder. Demographics, diagnosis, family history, and course. Arch Gen Psychiatry. 1992;49(2):126–31.
26. Rasgon N, Baue M, Grof P, Gyulai L, Elman S, Glenn T, Whybrow PC. Sex-specific self-reported mood changes by patients with bipolar disorder. J Psychiatr Res. 2005;39(1):77–83.
27. Freeman MP, Smith KW, Freeman SA, McElroy SL, Kmetz GE, Wright R, Keck Jr PE. The impact of reproductive events on the course of bipolar disorder in women. J Clin Psychiatry. 2002;63(4):284–7.
28. Burt VK, Rasgon N. Special considerations in treating bipolar disorder in women. Bipolar Disord. 2004;6(1):2–13.
29. Altshuler LL, Post RM, Leverich GS, Mikalauskas K, Rosoff A, Ackerman L. Antidepressant-induced mania and cycle acceleration: a controversy revisited. Am J Psychiatry. 1995;152(8):1130–8.
30. Lee S, Tsang A, Kessler RC, Jin R, Sampson N, Andrade L, Karam EG, Mora ME, Merikangas K, Nakane Y, Popovici DG, Posada-Villa J, Sagar R, Wells JE, Zarkov Z, Petukhova M. Rapid-cycling bipolar disorder: cross-national community study. Br J Psychiatry. 2010;196(3):217–25. doi:10.1192/bjp.bp.109.067843.
31. Bräunig P, Sarkar R, Effenberger S, Schoofs N, Krüger S. Gender differences in psychotic bipolar mania. Gend Med. 2009;6(2):356–61. doi:10.1016/j.genm.2009.07.004.
32. Ketter TA. Diagnostic features, prevalence, and impact of bipolar disorder. J Clin Psychiatry. 2010;71(6):14. doi:10.4088/JCP.8125tx11c.
33. Kenna HA, Jiang B, Rasgon NL. Reproductive and metabolic abnormalities associated with bipolar disorder and its treatment. Harv Rev Psychiatry. 2009;17(2):138–46. doi:10.1080/10673220902899722.

34. Payne JL. The role of estrogen in mood disorders in women. Int Rev Psychiatry. 2003;15(3):280–90.
35. Henry C. Lithium side-effects and predictors of hypothyroidism in patients with bipolar disorder: sex differences. J Psychiatry Neurosci. 2002;27:104–7.
36. González-Pinto A, Mosquera F, Alonso M, et al. Suicidal risk in bipolar I disorder patients and adherence to long-term lithium treatment. Bipolar Disord. 2006;8(5 Pt 2):618–24.
37. Colom F, Vieta E, Martínez-Arán A, Reinares M, Benabarre A, Gasto C. Clinical factors associated with treatment noncompliance in euthymic bipolar patients. J Clin Psychiatry. 2000;61:549–55.
38. Johnson RE, McFarland BH. Lithium use and discontinuation in a health maintenance organization. Am J Psychiatry. 1996;153:993–100.
39. Baldessarini RJ, Perry R, Pike J. Factors associated with treatment nonadherence among US bipolar disorder patients. Hum Psychopharmacol. 2008;23(2):95–105.
40. Lang K, Korn J, Muser Choi JC, Abouzaid S, Menzin J. Predictors of medication nonadherence and hospitalization in Medicaid patients with bipolar I disorder given long-acting or oral antipsychotics. J Med Econ. 2011;14(2):217–26.
41. González-Pinto A, Aldama A, Pinto AG, et al. Dimensions of mania: differences between mixed and pure episodes. Eur Psychiatry. 2004;19(5):307–10.
42. Vega P, Alonso M, Alberich S, et al. Why do bipolar men not comply with treatment? The Spanish CIBERSAM data. Eur J Psychiatry. 2009;23:63–9.
43. Kriegshauser K, Sajatovic M, Jenkins JH, et al. Gender differences in subjective experience and treatment of bipolar disorder. J Nerv Ment Dis. 2010;198(5):370–2.
44. Leskela U, Merlartin T, Rytsälä H, Sokero P, Lestelä-Mielonen P, Isometsä E. The influence of major depressive disorder on objective and subjective social support: a prospective study. J Nerv Ment Dis. 2008;196:876–83.
45. Franzoi SL, Koehler V. Age and gender differences in body attitudes: a comparison of young and elderly adults. Int J Aging Hum Dev. 1998;47:1–10.
46. Trede K, Baldessarini RJ, Viguera AC, Bottero A. Treatise on insanity in pregnant, post-partum, and lactating women (1858) by Louis-Victor Marcé: a commentary. Harv Rev Psychiatry. 2009;17(2):157–65. doi:10.1080/10673220902891802.
47. Viguera AC, Tondo L, Koukopoulos AE, Reginaldi D, Lepri B, Baldessarini RJ. Episodes of mood disorders in 2,252 pregnancies and postpartum periods. Am J Psychiatry. 2011;168(11):117985. doi:10.1176/appi.ajp.2011.11010148. Epub 2011 Jul 28.
48. Viguera AC, Whitfield T, Baldessarini RJ, Newport DJ, Stowe Z, Reminick A, Zurick A, Cohen LS. Risk of recurrence in women with bipolar disorder during pregnancy: prospective study of mood stabilizer discontinuation. Am J Psychiatry. 2007;164(12):1817–24. quiz 1923.
49. Sharma V, Burt VK, Ritchie HL. Bipolar II postpartum depression: detection, diagnosis and treatment. Am J Psychiatry. 2009;166(11):1217–21.
50. Heron J, Haque S, Ovebode F, Craddock N, Jones I. A longitudinal study of hypomania and depression symptoms in pregnancy and the postpartum period. Bipolar Disord. 2009;11(4):410–7.
51. Sharma V, Khan M, Corpse C, Sharma P. Missed bipolarity and psychiatric comorbidity in women with postpartum depression. Bipolar Disord. 2008;10:742–7.
52. Álamo C, Alonso Z, Álvarez I, et al. Manejo de psicofámacos en situaciones vitales específicas. In: Salazar M, Peralta C, Pastor FJ, editors. Manual de Psicofarmacología. Madrid: Editorial Médica Panamericana; 2011. p. 87–92.
53. Einarson A, Boskovic R. Use and safety of antipsychotic drugs during pregnancy. J Psychiatr Pract. 2009;15(3):183–92.
54. ACOG Committee on Practice Bulletins—Obstetrics. ACOG Practice Bulletin: clinical management guidelines for obstetrician-gynecologists number 92, April 2008 [replaces Practice Bulletin number 87, November 2007]. Use of psychiatric medications during pregnancy and lactation. Obstet Gynecol. 2008;111(4):1001–20.

55. Medrano J, Zardoya MJ, Pacheco L. In: Medrano J, editor. Uso de Psicofármacos en el Embarazo y Lactancia. Badalona: Euromedicine Ediciones Médicas SL, 2009. p. 47–58
56. Cohen LS, Friedman JM, Jefferson JW, Johnson EM, Weiner ML. A reevaluation of risk of in utero exposure to lithium. JAMA. 1994;271(2):146–50.
57. Yacobi S, Ornoy A. Is lithium a real teratogen? What can we conclude from the prospective versus retrospective studies? A review. Isr J Psychiatry Relat Sci. 2008;45(2):95–106.
58. Gentile S. Drug treatment for mood disorders in pregnancy. Curr Opin Psychiatry. 2011;24(1): 34–40. doi:10.1097/YCO.0b013e3283413451. Review.
59. Gentile S. Prophylactic treatment of bipolar disorder in pregnancy and breastfeeding: focus on emerging mood stabilizers. Bipolar Disord. 2006;8:207–20.
60. Mawer G, Briggs M, Baker GA, Bromley R, Coyle H, Eatock J, Kerr L, Kini U, Kuzmyshcheva L, Lucas SB, Wyatt L, Clayton-Smith J, Liverpool & Manchester Neurodevelopment Group. Pregnancy with epilepsy: obstetric and neonatal outcome of a controlled study. Seizure. 2010;19(2):112–9. doi:10.1016/j.seizure.2009.11.008. Epub 2009 Dec 24.
61. Holmes LB, Mittendorf R, Shen A, Smith CR, Hernandez-Diaz S. Fetal effects of anticonvulsant polytherapies: different risks from different drug combinations. Arch Neurol. 2011;68 (10):1275–81. doi:10.1001/archneurol.2011.133. Epub ahead of print.
62. Holmes LB, Wyszynski DF, Baldwin EJ, Habecker E, Glassman LH, Smith CR. Increased risk for non-syndromic cleft palate among infants exposed to lamotrigine during pregnancy [Abstract]. Birth Defects Res A Clin Mol Teratol. 2006;76:318.
63. Sethi S. Clozapine in pregnancy. Indian J Psychiatry. 2006;48(3):196–7.
64. Duran A, Ugur MM, Turan S, Emul M. Clozapine use in two women with schizophrenia during pregnancy. J Psychopharmacol. 2008;22(1):111–3.
65. Coppola L, Russo LJ, Kwarta Jr RF, et al. Evaluating the postmarketing experience of risperidone use during pregnancy: pregnancy and neonatal outcomes. Drug Saf. 2007;30: 247–94.
66. Gentile S, Bellantuono C. Selective serotonin reuptake inhibitor exposure during early pregnancy and the risk of fetal major malformations: focus on paroxetine. J Clin Psychiatry. 2009;70:414–22.
67. Rasmussen K. The practice of electroconvulsive therapy: recommendations for treatment, training, and privileging (2nd edition). J ECT. 2002;18(1):58–9.
68. Rabheru K. The use of electroconvulsive therapy in special patient populations. Can J Psychiatry. 2001;46(8):710–9.
69. Yonkers KA, Vigod S, Ross LE. Diagnosis, pathophysiology, and management of mood disorders in pregnant and postpartum women. Obstet Gynecol. 2011;117(4):961–77.

Mixed Forms in Bipolar Disorder and Relation to Gender

29

Ana González-Pinto, Ana Isabel Cano, Saioa López-Zurbano, and Purificación López

Abstract

Mixed states describe the simultaneous presence of manic and depressive symptoms in the same patient. This phenomenon is more prevalent in women. Activation, thinking, and mood are combined in a strange form, and it is possible that some of these dimensions are increased from the euthymic period, whereas others are decreased. The presentation of irritable mood is quite common, along with rapid thinking, suicidal ideas, anxiety, helplessness, and sexual disinhibition. Sometimes there are variations in the clinical presentation on the same day.

There are some depressive symptoms present in the mixed states that are more relevant for diagnosis: depressed mood, guilt, suicidal ideation, anhedonia, and fatigue. Irritable mood and psychotic symptoms are also frequently present in mixed states. One aspect that is relevant for the prognosis of mixed states is the earlier age at onset. The younger age at onset, and the delay in the diagnosis, explain some, but not all, of the differences in prognosis of this severe disease. These patients are also at a higher risk of drug and alcohol abuse.

Currently, the DSM-5 has partially included this aspect and has considered the diagnosis of mixed symptoms as a specifier of mania, hypomania, bipolar

A. González-Pinto (✉)
University of the Basque Country UPV/EHU, Guipúzcoa, Spain

Alava University Hospital, Vitoria, Spain

CIBERSAM, Barcelona, Spain
e-mail: anamaria.gonzalezpintoarrillaga@osakidetza.net

A.I. Cano • S. López-Zurbano
Alava University Hospital, Vitoria, Spain

P. López
University of the Basque Country UPV/EHU, Guipúzcoa, Spain

Alava University Hospital, Vitoria, Spain
e-mail: MARIAPURIFICACION.LOPEZPENA@osakidetza.net

M. Sáenz-Herrero (ed.), *Psychopathology in Women*,
DOI 10.1007/978-3-319-05870-2_29

depression, andunipolar depression. The special follow-up of those patients with unipolar major depression and three manic symptoms is currently diagnosed as major depression with mixed symptoms. A careful follow-up should be made in those patients to consider a bipolar disorder in the future.

29.1 Historical Evolution of the Concept of Mixed States

Mixed states or mixed episodes have been recognized since ancient times. Aretaeus de Cappadocia described violent anger in melancholic patients. In 1759 the Spanish doctor Andrés Piquer [1] described the symptoms of a mixed episode, referring to the last phase of the illness of King Ferdinand VI: "Sometimes affections are dominating and sometimes the opposite." According to González-Pinto [2], in the early nineteenth century (1818) Heinroth called these clinical presentations "mixtures" (*Mischungen*) [3]. Probably one of the most important authors in the history of the concept of mixed states was the German psychiatrist Weygandt (1899) [4], who described: "Manic stupor, agitated melancholia and unproductive mania." Kraepelin's description of mixed states in the same year, 1899, is based on this monograph [5]. Both psychiatrists were the first to suggest the existence of mixed episodes in the context of manic depressive insanity. Finally, Kraepelin was the one who focused attention on mixed episodes, and the one who developed the concept up to the present day. An entire chapter was included in his book *Manic - Depressive Insanity and Paranoia* [6]. Kraepelin conceptualized mixed forms, sometimes as clinical states and sometimes as transitional phenomena, between the two major forms of the disease. "Some morbid symptoms fade quickly, others more slowly, while other phenomena, in a developing state, start to emerge."

The author classifies them into six different types depending on the various combinations of manic and depressive symptoms considering mood, activity, and thought: depression with flight of ideas, agitated depression, manic stupor, unproductive mania, depressive or anxious mania, and inhibited mania [6] (Table 29.1).

29.2 Psychopathology of Mixed Mania in Women

As stated by Kraepelin, mixed episodes are characterized by the presence of different combinations of opposite directions in mood, motor activation, and thinking. Mood is frequently irritable, but sometimes it is depressed. Infrequently euphoria is present, and in these cases motor activity or thinking are inhibited. The most frequent presentations of mixed episodes in women are characterized by irritability and anxiety. Negative self-evaluation, suicide, dysphoria, psychic and somatic anxiety, social withdrawal, indecisiveness, worry, self-reproach, phobia, fatigue, discouragement, dullness of thought, loss of interest, depersonalization, panic, feelings of inadequacy, and ruminations are also frequent symptoms associated with irritable mood.

Table 29.1 Kraepelin classification of mixed states

	Humor	Activity	Thinking
Depression With flight of ideas	Depression Hopelessness, anxiety, sadness, lability	Motor delay Show interest in the environment, but remain virtually silent and rigid	Ideofugal Frequently without flight of ideas and delusional fears, flight of ideas can only be recognized when they write
Excited or agitated depression	Anxiety Tearful, irritable, self-accusations	Hyperactivity They run back and forth. Throwing objects. Weeping and wailing, monotonous cries	Inhibited. Extraordinary poverty of thought; delusional interpretations
Manic stupor	Euphoria Content, laugh without cause, seductive, erotic	Gross motor delay Inaccessible, can reach the trance, unexpectedly show hostility and immediately return to the inaccessibility	Inhibited Only occasionally are isolated delusions, usually well-oriented
Mania with poverty of thought	Euphoria	Hyperactivity Grinning, dancing, and throwing things. Impulsivity that sometimes explodes into violence	Inhibited Perception slow and inadequate with difficulty thinking. Large fluctuations
Depressive or anxious mania	Anxiety Despair, anxious	Hyperactivity Great agitation without awareness of increased activity	Ideofugal Distractible, no goal. The thoughts themselves are imposed
Inhibited mania	Euphoria. Exultant, irritable, distractible with a tendency to joke	Motor delay Apparently inhibited, great internal tension that could explode into violence	Ideofugal Jocular conversation with racing ideas and numerous associations for assonance

An important issue in recognizing mixed episodes is to consider not only the actual clinical presentation, but to observe the changes present over 24 h, or over a few days. Mood changes sometimes from one pole to the opposite, and lability is present in combination with anxiety. Women with mixed states are tearful, and it is important to consider this symptom as a part of the disease.

In relation to activity it is more usual to see motor hyperactivity, although when there is euphoria the patient can be inhibited. It is possible to see mixed cases with depression and inhibition, but with accelerated thinking and flight of ideas.

The most frequent presentation of thinking in mixed states in women is with rapid thinking and flight of ideas. These symptoms are accompanied by distractibility and absence of goal. As the clinical presentations are broad, following Kraepelin's descriptions and modern ones, there are some patients with slow thinking, generally accompanied by psychomotor inhibition and euphoria or irritability.

The presence of delusions is common, especially at younger ages. Mood congruent and mood incongruent symptoms are possible in the clinical presentations of mixed mania. It is important to ask patients about delusions, as some of them do not talk about their ideas. Patients with mixed states are usually more conscious about having a mental illness than other bipolar patients. Nevertheless, they do not capture exactly what is wrong, with a bad insight in the first stages of the disease.

29.2.1 Categorical Conceptualizations of Mixed Mania

The first categorical description of mixed states corresponds to the Research Diagnostic Criteria (RDC) [7], establishing two presenting options for these pictures. In the first, the manic and depressive symptoms coexist simultaneously in the same period, while in the second, the manic and depressive episodes occur without interruption.

For the first time in diagnostic manuals, the DSM-III-R recognized mixed states as a subtype of bipolar disorder, which appeared subclassified as mixed bipolar disorder, manic or depressive episode according to the clinical presentation today. Mixed bipolar disorder was defined according to two criteria: (a) the current or most recent episode included full symptoms of manic episodes and major depressive episodes (requiring a minimum of 2 weeks for depressive symptoms), both symptomatologies rapidly alternating; (b) predominant depressive symptoms lasting at least 1 complete day. Like the DSM-III-R, the ICD-9 did not provide empirically derived criteria for mixed state, but refers to the criteria for mania and depression in a further vague and ambiguous definition: "Manic-depressive psychosis, circular type, mixed: affective psychosis in which both manic and depressive symptoms are present at the same time."

In DSM-IV, and DSM-IV-TR [8] diagnostic criteria for mixed episodes were more restrictive for better differential diagnosis with rapid cycling. It constituted a different diagnostic category with manic and depressive episodes, and DSM-IV provided descriptions of the course and prognosis for this condition, which were not considered before. However, it continues without providing specific diagnostic criteria, and still requires the presence of a full depressive episode with a manic episode, with the only change that the temporal criteria for the depressive episode is reduced to only 1 week. ICD-10 [9] also insists on the simultaneous presence of manic and depressive symptoms for the diagnosis of mixed episodes, but only refers to it and there is no complete clinical description.

Some symptoms may be particularly relevant to describing depressive mixed states. In fact, Cassidy et al. [10] found that only five (depressed mood, guilt, suicidal ideation, anhedonia, and fatigue) of the nine depressive symptoms of the DSM-III-R had predictive value for the diagnosis of mixed mania. Following these two perspectives of mixed states, there are two types of definitions described: intermediate and broad definitions [11].

The *intermediate categorical definition* proposal includes mainly Bauer's [12] definition according to his great impact, and was also adopted by the Cincinnati

Table 29.2 Diagnostic criteria for dysphoric mania [14]

(a) A full manic episode according to DSM-III-R
(b) Simultaneous presence of at least three of the following depressive symptoms:
1. Depressed mood
2. Markedly diminished interest or pleasure in all or most activities
3. Substantial weight gain or increased appetite
4. Hypersomnia
5. Psychomotor retardation
6. Fatigue or loss of energy
7. Feelings of failure or excessive or inappropriate guilt
8. Feelings of inadequacy or hopelessness
(c) Recurrent thoughts of death, recurrent suicidal ideation or a specific plan for committing suicide

group [13]. This group, conducted by MacElroy, adopted the term "dysphoric mania" to refer to Kraepelin's anxious mania in 1992 (Table 29.2) [14]. They propose a diagnosis from the DSM-III-R criteria for mania plus two substantial depressive symptoms, defined as one that, from the clinical point of view, does not overlap with manic symptoms.

On the other hand, the *broad categorical definitions* describe mixed mania as any manic episode accompanied by minimal depressive symptoms.

In conclusion, the most accepted definition of mixed mania by most of the current research requires a full manic episode with coexisting depressive symptoms. The fact that the theories proposed by Akiskal [15, 16] and Perugi [17] have had a great impact, and that the Cincinnati group's [14] definition has become a paradigm, determines which are the most relevant depressive symptoms at the time of establishing this diagnosis.

29.2.2 Dimensional Conceptualizations of Mixed Mania

In recent decades a new classification for symptomatology has begun, from a dimensional perspective. It is used in research to find consistent symptom clusters. This dimensional approach can identify different subtypes or dimensions of symptoms that can lead to very heterogeneous diagnostic categories, making the diagnosis more difficult, but that can correlate with etiological and prognostic variables very accurately (Table 29.3).

Precisely manic factorial studies have empirically tested Kraepelin's observations: different dimensions have been identified and combine to make distinct manic subtypes. Arguably, this line of research started in 1998 with the work of Cassidy et al. [18]. In general, almost all dimensional studies of mania have focused on confirming the mixed anxiety–depressive subtype equivalent to the DSM and ICD definition for mixed episodes.

Table 29.3 Dimensions of depressive mania

	Scales	Symptoms	N
Cassidy et al. [18]	SMS	Depressed mood, anxiety, guilt, suicide, emotional lability	237
Dilsaver et al. [21]	SADS	Negative self-evaluation, suicide, dysphoria, psychic and somatic anxiety, social withdrawal, indecisiveness, worry, self-reproach, phobia, fatigue, discouragement, dullness of thought, loss of interest, depersonalization, panic, agitation	105
Swan et al. [22]	SADS and MSRS	Self-reproach, negative evaluation, worry, despair, suicide, dysphoria, psychic and somatic anxiety	162
Rossi et al. [23]	Bech-Rafaelsen Mania and Melancholia	Mental retardation, psychic anxiety, suicide, depressed mood, blame	124
Hantouche et al. [24]	MVAS-BP	Neglect, worry, feelings of inadequacy	104
Sato et al. [19]	AMDP	Depressed mood, feelings of guilt, rumination, suicide, delirium of guilt, feelings of impoverishment, anxiety	576
Akiskal et al. [25]	MSRS	Appearance depression, feelings of depression, impulsivity	104
González-Pinto et al. [20]	YMRS and HDRS-21	Depressed mood, suicide, guilt, obsessive symptoms, psychic anxiety	103

Thus, the manic-depressive anxious Kraepelin type would be defined by the combination of purely manic dimensions (hedonism activation, dysphoria, psychosis) with a depressed mood dimension. In most studies [16, 18–21] this depressive dimension has a bimodal distribution; it appears in some manic patients, but not in others, which also empirically confirms the categorical separation of pure and mixed manic subtypes. Regarding the symptoms that constitute the depressive dimension, most of the clinical identifying research finds coincidences between depressed mood and psychic anxiety using different scales for evaluation. Specifically, the group of Dr. Gónzalez-Pinto [11] propose that "depressive dimension of acute mania consists of the following five items of the Hamilton Depression Rating Scale [HDRS-21]: depressed mood, suicidal ideation, guilt, obsessive–compulsive symptoms, and psychic anxiety."

It is also noted that authors such as Sato et al. [19] found a factor of "depressive inhibition" independent from "depressed mood," which supports the Kraepelin classification of mixed states. Kraepelin described three mixed subtypes with depressive inhibition; however, this syndrome has aroused little interest among researchers.

Below are some of the dimensional models of major mania.

(a) **Model "paranoid-destructive/euphoric-grandiose" (Murphy and Beigel, 1974)** [26].
In 1974, Murphy and Beigel analyzed factorially the Manic State Rating Scale (MSRS) and they identified two subtypes of mania: "paranoid–destructive" and "euphoric–grandiose." Although this typology was widely accepted and efforts were made for it to be confirmed, it had limited success.

(b) **Three-dimensional models of mania (Double, 1990)** [27].
Double tried to replicate the results obtained by Beigel and Murphy with the completion of two separate factor analyses from the MSRS and the Young Manic Rating Scale and yielded two three-factor solutions. The YMRS identified: "thought disorder, aggressive behavior and hyperactivity and mood elevation and vegetative symptoms," and from the MSRS: "speech motor disorder, aggression and mood unrealistic expansiveness."

(c) **Model of five dimensions: the dimension of dysphoric mania (Cassidy et al., 1998)** [18].
In 1998 Cassidy published an interesting study that analyzed the dimensions of mania in a large sample of bipolar I patients with manic and mixed episodes. He used his own scale: the Scale for Manic States (SMS). The relevance of this work lies mainly in that it was a dimensionally focused study of mania and mixed states in an attempt to clarify their nature, providing statistical support, and their relationship with pure mania. It identifies five independent clinical dimensions; one of them, the "dysphoria factor," represents depressive symptoms during mania and has a bimodal distribution, which confirms that dysphoric mania is a subtype of mania within the overall mania. This model represents the starting point for the study of the patients with mixed manic dimensions, since it analyzes and presents, for the first time, the presence of a depressive dimension in mania.

(d) **Model of longitudinal dimensions (Serreti et al., 1999)** [28].
Serreti et al. tried to validate the results obtained by Cassidy, but the dimensional study of mania was from a longitudinal approach. They use a selection of 16 of the 38 items of the Operational Criteria Checklist for Psychotic Illness and identify three factors of mania ("physical arousal and motor," "psychosis," and "irritability") consistent with those described by Cassidy, except that Serreti does not identify a clinical depression dimension.

(e) **Dimensional model (Dilsaver et al., 1999)** [21]**: the depressive dimension.**
Dilsaver et al. revise the dimensional study of mania along the lines proposed by Cassidy et al., and identify a solution of four factors, which includes a depressive dimension. For factor analysis they use a selection of 37 items of the Schedule for Affective Disorders and Schizophrenia (SADS), which includes an explicit evaluation of depressive symptoms.

(f) **Five-component model: symptoms of depressive dimension (Gonzalez-Pinto et al., 2003)** [16].
One of the most recently proposed models has been developed by the research group of Dr. Gonzalez-Pinto. Using two standardized scales commonly used in clinical practice to quantify the affective symptoms, it has managed to replicate

the model initially proposed by Cassidy et al. From the Hamilton Depression Rating Scale [HRSD-21] and the YMRS, it has identified five component solutions that include a "depressive dimension" with a composition almost identical to the dysphoric factor by Cassidy et al. In addition, further work has shown the need to assess depressive symptoms in all manic depressive disorders since the dimension appears in pure mania patients diagnosed with DSM-IV-TR. Thus, virtually all clinical studies of manic dimension have focused on anxious depressive mixed subtype; it confirmed that it would be the equivalent to the definition of the DSM and ICD for mixed episodes. Thus, Kraepelin's anxious depressive mania was defined by the combination of purely manic dimensions (hedonism activation, dysphoria and psychosis), with depressed mood dimension. In most of the work, this depressive dimension presents a bimodal behavior: it appears in some manic patients but not in others, so that it also confirms empirically the categorical separation of pure manic and mixed subtypes. For symptoms that make up the depressive dimension, most research identifies that clinical symptomatology coincides with depressive mood and mental anxiety using different scales for evaluation.

29.3 Contributions and Mixed Episodes: New Approach in DSM-5

29.3.1 Mixed Features Specifier

In the fifth edition of the DSM [29], diagnosis of mixed episode is replaced by "mixed characteristic specification," which can be applied to episodes of major depression, hypomania or mania. The change reflects the ways in which the mixed characteristic can interact with depression, mania or hypomania symptoms. This can lead to benefits in the diagnosis and in patient care.

In DSM-IV [8], a diagnosis of mixed episodes required that the individual fulfilled all the criteria for a major depressive episode simultaneously with an episode of mania.

During the review of the latest research, the working research group of mood disorders in DSM-5 acknowledged that people rarely meet the full criteria for the two types of episodes at the same time. To be diagnosed with the new specifier in the case of major depression, the new DSM-5 [29] requires the presence of at least three symptoms of mania/hypomania that do not overlap with symptoms of major depression. In the case of mania or hypomania, the specifier requires the presence of at least three symptoms of depression linked with the episode of mania/hypomania.

29.3.2 Using Specifiers

If an individual is predominantly manic or hypomanic, depressive symptoms, and also the specification of mixed characteristics may be considered. Depressive symptoms can include depressed mood, diminished interest or pleasure, physical and emotional lability retardation, fatigue or loss of energy, and recurrent thoughts of death. At least three of these symptoms must be present nearly every day during the last week of a manic episode or during the last 4 days of a hypomanic episode.

Moreover, if an individual is predominantly depressive with some of the manic or hypomanic symptoms, mixed features specifier can be also considered. These manic or hypomanic symptoms may include elevated mood, higher self-esteem, decreased need for sleep, and increased energy or goal-directed activities. At least three of these symptoms must be present nearly every day for the last 2 weeks of major depressive episode.

29.3.3 Improvement in Diagnosis and Care

The specifier will allow doctors to diagnose more accurately their patients who may be suffering from comorbid symptoms of depression and mania/hypomania, and give them better treatment to the extent of their behaviors. This is especially important, since many patients with mixed characteristics, have a poor response to lithium or are destabilized when taking antidepressants [30, 31]. In addition, an early identification of these behaviors could allow doctors to recognize people with unipolar disorder who are at an increased risk of progression to bipolar disorder [32].

29.3.4 Mixed Forms in Women

Regardless of the type of definition used for diagnosis, mixed episodes are more common among women [33], although the differences are often more striking when using conventional categorical and stringent criteria. Current studies find that 67 % [34] of women who present a first bipolar mixed episode is diagnosed according to ICD-10 criteria, and González-Pinto [35] indicates similar rates [62 %] when the diagnosis is established using the DSM-IV. In 2010 Diflorio and Jones [36] performed a systematic review between January 1980 and 2010 on gender differences in bipolar disorder, manic depression, and mania. The search included an extensive database and it excluded studies with fewer than 20 subjects and survival studies. In this review, we found that a number of studies focused on mixed episodes, and found that most of these episodes are more frequent in women with bipolar disorder [55].

Clinical studies on the manic dimension, report the association of female gender with the depressive dimension [37], hovering around 66 % in the study by Cassidy [38] and 60 % in the work of Sato et al. [19].

In conclusion, both mixed and dysphoric mania defined in terms of diagnostic criteria or intermediate depressive manic dimension, appear more often in women compared with men with a ratio of 60/40 [39] and in some studies, up to 70/30. This difference is not present if we consider depressive mixed states.

The female predominance of depressive symptoms during mania could be related to the increased susceptibility of women to depression in general (The risk of a depressive episode throughout life is twice as high in women) [40, 41]. Theories that attempt to explain these discrepancies are mainly based on constitutional rate differences associated with endocrine, genetic or temperamental factors.

29.3.5 Hormonal Factors

29.3.5.1 Reproductive Life Cycle and Depression

The influence of the reproductive life cycle on women and its link to the affective state have been studied in-depth. Virtually all of the reproductive cycle events are associated in some women with an anxious–depressive clinical picture. There is a clinical description of premenstrual syndrome and premenstrual dysphoric disorder [42], postnatal blues and postpartum depression [43], of oral contraceptive dysphoria [44], and perimenopausal depression [45].

The relationship between emotional disorders and the hormonal cycle [41, 46] has also been investigated in women diagnosed with bipolar disorder, especially in order to set some special considerations with regard to drug therapy at critical moments. Although bipolar women describe striking mood swings during the menstrual cycle [42], studies have not been able to establish a consistent pattern between the hormonal cycle phase and the direction of mood changes, probably because of the phenotypic heterogeneity of bipolar disorder, the small size of the samples or the interference with medication. Although more studies are needed to investigate systematically the variations in manic phenomenology associated with the effect of gonadal hormones, mood disturbances are described as being the main changes related to depressive symptoms [47].

With regard to pregnancy and the postpartum period [41], although pregnancy traditionally has been considered to be a protective factor against relapse, this assumption is being challenged by new research. What we have found repeatedly is that the postpartum period is a high risk of mental disorder [48]. The risk of first hospitalization for bipolar disorder is multiplied by 7 during the first months after birth. Compared with women with no psychiatric history, women with bipolar disorder are at an increased risk of developing postpartum psychosis [47]. There are also studies indicating that 67 % of bipolar patients presented a relapse postpartum, almost certainly the depressive type, and in all cases, this returned to with successive deliveries [49]. That is, periods of intense hormonal fluctuations are associated with a risk of affective dysregulation, primarily depression, in women diagnosed with bipolar disorder.

29.3.5.2 Thyroid Dysfunction and Depression

The women have a high prevalence of thyroid dysfunction related to a greater vulnerability to developing autoimmune abnormalities. In fact, in 1995 Whybrow

[50] indicated that the prevalence of thyroid disease throughout life was 4–10 times greater in women.

Thyroid disorders, on the other hand, have been linked to an increased risk of psychiatric disorders, mainly anxiety and affective disorders [51, 52]. Regarding the latter, an association was described between mania and hyperthyroidism, between depression and hypothyroidism, and even between hypothyroidism and rapid cycling bipolar disorder.

The influence of thyroid hormones in the clinical expression of the pictures and their relationship to manic gender of patients have been extensively studied. We compared thyroid function in pure and mixed manic patients and found mild abnormalities (increased TSH and decreased thyroxine) in the mixed group, but could not objectify differences between thyroid function in men and women with mixed episodes [2].

29.3.5.3 Genetic Factors

Classical bipolar disorder research authors have begun to study the high comorbidity detected between this disorder and anxiety disorders, which is between 30 and 51 % [53]. The anxiety disorders are associated with bipolar panic disorder (with or without agoraphobia), social phobia, and, less often, OCD [53].

These comorbid conditions are associated with an earlier age at onset of bipolar disorder, a rapid cyclization, poorer response to lithium treatment, and higher levels of drug use [54]. Furthermore, it was observed that suicide rates are duplicated in bipolar patients who have had at least one GAD throughout life, except in the case of obsessive compulsive disorders [55, 56].

One of the plausible reasons to explain this association is that bipolar and anxiety disorders may share a biological or genetic risk, a thesis supported by the relatively high rates of affective disorders in patients with anxiety disorder, and because they all respond well to drug treatment. Specifically, Mackinnon et al. [53] considered that the risk of panic disorder in families of patients with bipolar disorder is an inherited trait. Going one step further, Rotondo et al. [57] argue that comorbid panic disorder identifies a genetic subtype of bipolar disorder and suggests the vulnerability to these symptoms associated with certain polymorphisms in catechol O-methyltransferase (COMT Met 158) and in serotonin transporter (5-HTTLPR). However, it has also been suggested that comorbidity between the two disoders could refer to a predisposition to manic mixed episodes, where depressive mood appears with an intense anxious component. The depressive dimension described by González-Pinto's group [11] includes obsessive symptoms and psychic anxiety. Additional comorbid conditions are associated with a more torpid evolution of bipolar disorder and an increased risk of suicide [55].

Therefore, perhaps the greatest prevalence of mixed mania in women is also associated with a higher genetic predisposition to anxiety that becomes more severe forms of bipolar disorder.

29.3.5.4 Characterological or Temperamental Factors

Akiskal in 1992 develops a theory about the nature of mixed states [58]. He considers that these pictures would be a result of an opposition between temperament and current affective state, rather than the superposition of two different affective states (Table 29.4). This research study describes three kinds of mixed bipolar disorders:

- Type I: depressive and manic temperament. It is developed on the basis of a depressive temperament and is usually accompanied by psychotic symptoms, sometimes incongruent with the mood. Therefore, this type is often confused with schizoaffective disorder, and even acute polymorphic psychotic disorder or *delusional bouffée*.
- Type II: cyclothymic temperament and major depression. Overall, this second type is not accompanied by psychotic symptoms. This combination produces symptoms such as mood lability, irritability, flight of ideas, sexual impulsivity, and substance abuse. According to Akiskal, the risk of these misdiagnosed depressions provokes a borderline personality diagnosis.
- Type III: hyperthymic temperament and major depression, which is often refractory to treatment with antidepressants.

Akiskal's theory has had a major impact. In addition, it was found that women present depressive temperaments more frequently than men, making them more vulnerable to depressive and mixed mania episodes [37].

Recently, Akiskal's team has attempted to validate this hypothesis by studying the relationship between the dimensions of manic affective temperaments and gender [60]. The starting point of this work is the consideration that the opposition between the affective state and temperament is a further evidence of the central dysregulation that characterizes mania and that mixed mania cannot be defined solely on a clinical basis (DSM, ICD), but also dimensionally con a temperament basis. It is confirmed that women have higher scores on the depressive dimension of mania [61] and it seems that there is a high correlation between this dimension and depressive temperament.

Table 29.4 Affective temperaments (based on the criteria established by Akiskal and Mallya in 1987) [59]

Depressive temperament	Hyperthymic temperament
• Sad, pessimistic, unable to enjoy	• Irritable, happy, optimistic or exuberant
• Standing, passive or indecisive	• Self-confident, great
• Skeptical, hypercritical or complainant	• Full of plans, reckless, impulsive
• Tendency to worry	• Talkative
• Self-disciplined	• Outgoing
• Self-critical	• Very involved
• Feelings of inadequacy and guilt	• Promiscuous

Therefore, from this approach, we are back with a variable trait, a depressive temperament, which provides more data to support the hypothesis that female predisposition to mixed mania is associated with an increased vulnerability to depression.

29.3.5.5 Depression: Male Equivalents

As has been presented previously, among other gender-related differences in the phenomenology of manic consumption, is the increase of drug use in men [40]. Overall, comorbid substance is very high in patients with a diagnosis of bipolar disorder (38 % for alcohol, 25 % for other substances).

Perhaps the differences in drug use between men and women could be explained if we consider the increased consumption of drugs as a depressive equivalent in men. A high comorbidity is detected between harmful consumption substances and major depression in men [62]. It is also seen that substance abuse is a risk multiplied by 7 with regard to suicide and 87 % of suicides take place in alcohol-dependent men, compared with 13 % of women. More details are obtained for research on affective disorders and suicide in the Amish population (remember that this religious community of Swiss origin has banned alcohol and drugs, and is a very homogeneous population culturally and genetically). A classic study [63] found that 71 % of the mentally ill in the community had a major affective disorder and that the incidence and prevalence of unipolar disorders were identical for men and women. Depression rates were multiplied by 3 and this was related to his doctrine of non-hostility and teetotalism. Based on these observations, Walinder and Rutz [64] propose a “male depressive syndrome” characterized by low tolerance for frustration, acting out behavior, poor impulse control, and substance abuse.

Already in 1976, Himmelhoch [65] considered that “abuse of alcohol and other substances, including organic factors may be necessary for the development of mixed mania in men.”

29.4 Discussion

Faced with the same disease, women have some specific characteristics, i.e., they have a greater vulnerability to mixed mania and depression. In fact, depressive symptoms associated with mania in women appear from a depressive trait or temperament under which it could underlie a genetic or constitutional correlate linked to hormonal factors. In short women are more vulnerable to depression in general.

Substance use is significantly higher among men than among women with acute mania and this fact can be understood as the expression of the male of depressed mood. Perhaps, in this sense, it might be enlightening to study the temperament of manic patients who have comorbid toxicity.

Finally, the differences between men and women regarding depressive symptoms are so striking, as the data apparently reveal, or a part of these differences could be explained by the way we value depressive symptoms. The means of communication with our patients is primarily language and is valued by the clinical response to their complaints, which give information on how they are emotionally. In this sense we are more able to assess depression in women. From the cognitive point of view women are more verbal than men, with higher yields in visuospatial tasks [66]. In fact one of the issues debated in neuropsychological research is the extent to which language is more cerebrally bilaterally represented in women.

Women are "designed" to express verbally, men are ontogenetically oriented toward fighting action. From the point of view of the evolution of the species, women have developed a more passive role occupied with housework and care, primarily parenting, while men have developed a more active role in fighting, attacking, being charged with providing food, fulfilling the basic needs of the family, to ensure their survival. The woman asks and the man provides. Women are ontogenetically determined to express their needs (or complaints), and men are determined to solve them by acting (or are determined just to act). Women are verbal, as indeed neuropsychological studies demonstrated, indicating a predominance of verbal hemisphere (dominant/left) in women versus emotional hemisphere dominance in men. Women are evolutionarily more prepared than men to verbally express our emotions and also ask for assistance. It seems that for men is much more difficult to recognize and, above all, to express their affective states and tend to resolve unpleasant emotions by acting, drinking, fighting, taking action or simply denying them. Is our psychopathology a female psychopathology? Are the pain and discomfort of men sufficiently recognized by psychiatry? Why when a man loses his job does he begin to abuse alcohol or is more irritable with his family? He is a bad person, or perhaps he is depressed?

References

1. Perez J, Baldessarini RJ, Cruz N, Salvatore P, Vieta E. Andres Piquer-Arrufat [1711–1772]: contributions of an eighteenth-century Spanish physician to the concept of manic-depressive illness. Harv Rev Psychiatry. 2011;19(2):68–77.
2. Gonzalez-Pinto A, Aldama A, Mosquera F, Gonzalez Gomez C. Epidemiology, diagnosis and management of mixed mania. CNS Drugs. 2007;21(8):611–26.
3. Heinroth JCA. Lehrbuch der Störungen des Seelenlebens Oder der Seelenstörungen und Ihre Behandlung vRSaE. Leipzig, Germany: F. W. Vogel; 1918.
4. Marneros A. Origin and development of concepts of bipolar mixed states. J Affect Disord. 2001;67(1):229–40.
5. Kraepelin E. Psychiatrie. Ein Lehrbuch für Studierende und Ärzte, Klinische Psychiatrie. Leipzig, Germany: Verlag von Johann Ambrsius Barth; 1899.
6. Kraepelin E. Manic depressive insanity and paranoia. J Nerv Ment Dis. 1921;53(4):350.
7. Spitzer RL, Endicott J, Robins E. Research diagnostic criteria: rationale and reliability. Arch Gen Psychiatry. 1978;35(6):773.
8. American Psychiatric Association. Diagnostic and statistical manual of mental disorders: DSM-IV-TR®. Washington, DC: American Psychiatric Association, ; 2000.
9. World Health Organization. The ICD-10 classification of mental and behavioural disorders: clinical descriptions and diagnostic guidelines. Geneva: World Health Organization; 1992.
10. Cassidy F, Carroll BJ. The clinical epidemiology of pure and mixed manic episodes. Bipolar Disord. 2001;3(1):35–40.

11. Gonzalez-Pinto A, Aldama A, Pinto AG, Mosquera F, Perez de Heredia JL, Ballesteros J, et al. Dimensions of mania: differences between mixed and pure episodes. Eur Psychiatry. 2004;19(5):307–10.
12. Bauer MS, Whybrow PC. Rapid cycling bipolar affective disorder. II. Treatment of refractory rapid cycling with high-dose levothyroxine: a preliminary study. Arch Gen Psychiatry. 1990;47(5):435–40.
13. McElroy SL, Strakowski SM, Keck Jr PE, Tugrul KL, West SA, Lonczak HS. Differences and similarities in mixed and pure mania. Compr Psychiatry. 1995;36(3):187–94.
14. McElroy SL, Keck Jr PE, Pope Jr HG, Hudson JI, Faedda GL, Swann AC. Clinical and research implications of the diagnosis of dysphoric or mixed mania or hypomania. Am J Psychiatry. 1992;149(12):1633–44.
15. Akiskal HS, Benazzi F. Toward a clinical delineation of dysphoric hypomania—operational and conceptual dilemmas. Bipolar Disord. 2005;7(5):456–64.
16. Hantouche EG, Akiskal HS, Azorin JM, Chatenet-Duchene L, Lancrenon S. Clinical and psychometric characterization of depression in mixed mania: a report from the French National Cohort of 1090 manic patients. J Affect Disord. 2006;96(3):225–32.
17. Perugi G, Micheli C, Akiskal HS, Madaro D, Socci C, Quilici C, et al. Polarity of the first episode, clinical characteristics, and course of manic depressive illness: a systematic retrospective investigation of 320 bipolar I patients. Compr Psychiatry. 2000;41(1):13–8.
18. Cassidy F, Murry E, Forest K, Carroll BJ. Signs and symptoms of mania in pure and mixed episodes. J Affect Disord. 1998;50(2–3):187–201.
19. Sato T, Bottlender R, Kleindienst N, Moller HJ. Syndromes and phenomenological subtypes underlying acute mania: a factor analytic study of 576 manic patients. Am J Psychiatry. 2002;159(6):968–74.
20. Gonzalez-Pinto A, Ballesteros J, Aldama A, Perez de Heredia JL, Gutierrez M, Mosquera F, et al. Principal components of mania. J Affect Disord. 2003;76(1–3):95–102.
21. Dilsaver SC, Chen YR, Shoaib AM, Swann AC. Phenomenology of mania: evidence for distinct depressed, dysphoric, and euphoric presentations. Am J Psychiatry. 1999;156(3):426–30.
22. Swann AC, Janicak PL, Calabrese JR, Bowden CL, Dilsaver SC, Morris DD, et al. Structure of mania: depressive, irritable, and psychotic clusters with different retrospectively-assessed course patterns of illness in randomized clinical trial participants. J Affect Disord. 2001;67(1–3):123–32.
23. Rossi A, Daneluzzo E, Arduini L, Di Domenico M, Pollice R, Petruzzi C. A factor analysis of signs and symptoms of the manic episode with Bech-Rafaelsen Mania and Melancholia Scales. J Affect Disord. 2001;64(2–3):267–70.
24. Hantouche EG, Allilaire JP, Bourgeois ML, Azorin JM, Sechter D, Chatenet-Duchene L, et al. The feasibility of self-assessment of dysphoric mania in the French national EPIMAN study. J Affect Disord. 2001;67(1–3):97–103.
25. Akiskal HS, Azorin JM, Hantouche EG. Proposed multidimensional structure of mania: beyond the euphoric-dysphoric dichotomy. J Affect Disord. 2003;73(1–2):7–18.
26. Murphy DL, Beigel A, Weingartner H, Bunney Jr WE. The quantitation of manic behavior. Mod Probl Pharmacopsychiatry. 1974;7:203–20.
27. Double DB. The factor structure of manic rating scales. J Affect Disord. 1990;18(2):113–9.
28. Serretti A, Rietschel M, Lattuada E, Krauss H, Held T, Nothen MM, et al. Factor analysis of mania. Arch Gen Psychiatry. 1999;56(7):671–2.
29. American Psychiatry Association. Mixed Features Specifier. www.psychiatry.org wDo.
30. Vieta E. Bipolar mixed states and their treatment Expert Rev. Neurother. 2005; 5:63–68.
31. Muralidharan K, Ali M, Silveira LE, Bond DJ, Fountoulakis KN, Lam RW, et al. Efficacy of second generation antipsychotics in treating acute mixed episodes in bipolar disorder: a meta-analysis of placebo-controlled trials. J Affect Disord. 2013;150(2):408–14.
32. Hirschfeld RM. Bipolar spectrum disorder: improving its recognition and diagnosis. J Clin Psychiatry. 2001;62 Suppl 14:5–9.

33. Kawa I, Carter JD, Joyce PR, Doughty CJ, Frampton CM, Wells JE, et al. Gender differences in bipolar disorder: age of onset, course, comorbidity, and symptom presentation. Bipolar Disord. 2005;7(2):119–25.
34. Dell'Osso L, Placidi GF, Nassi R, Freer P, Cassano GB, Akiskal HS. The manic-depressive mixed state: familial, temperamental and psychopathologic characteristics in 108 female inpatients. Eur Arch Psychiatry Clin Neurosci. 1991;240(4–5):234–9.
35. Gonzalez-Pinto A, Barbeito S, Alonso M, Alberich S, Haidar MK, Vieta E, et al. Poor long-term prognosis in mixed bipolar patients: 10-year outcomes in the Vitoria prospective naturalistic study in Spain. J Clin Psychiatry. 2011;72(5):671–6.
36. Diflorio A, Jones I. Is sex important? Gender differences in bipolar disorder. Int Rev Psychiatry. 2010;22(5):437–52.
37. Nivoli AM, Pacchiarotti I, Rosa AR, Popovic D, Murru A, Valenti M, et al. Gender differences in a cohort study of 604 bipolar patients: the role of predominant polarity. J Affect Disord. 2011;133(3):443–9.
38. Cassidy F, Yatham LN, Berk M, Grof P. Pure and mixed manic subtypes: a review of diagnostic classification and validation. Bipolar Disord. 2008;10(1 Pt 2):131–43.
39. Benazzi F. Delineation of the clinical picture of dysphoric/mixed hypomania. Prog Neuropsychopharmacol Biol Psychiatry. 2007;31(4):944–51.
40. Azorin JM, Belzeaux R, Kaladjian A, Adida M, Hantouche E, Lancrenon S, et al. Risks associated with gender differences in bipolar I disorder. J Affect Disord. 2013;151(3): 1033–40.
41. Payne JL. The role of estrogen in mood disorders in women. Int Rev Psychiatry. 2003;15(3): 280–90.
42. Teatero ML, Mazmanian D, Sharma V. Effects of the menstrual cycle on bipolar disorder. Bipolar Disord. 2014;16(1):22–36.
43. Vliegen N, Casalin S, Luyten P. The course of postpartum depression: a review of longitudinal studies. Harv Rev Psychiatry. 2014;22(1):1–22.
44. Gupta N, O'Brien R, Jacobsen LJ, Davis A, Zuckerman A, Supran S, et al. Mood changes in adolescents using depot-medroxyprogesterone acetate for contraception: a prospective study. J Pediatr Adolesc Gynecol. 2001;14(2):71–6.
45. Gibbs Z, Lee S, Kulkarni J. Factors associated with depression during the perimenopausal transition. Womens Health Issues. 2013;23(5):e301–7.
46. Freeman MP, Gelenberg AJ. Bipolar disorder in women: reproductive events and treatment considerations. Acta Psychiatr Scand. 2005;112(2):88–96.
47. Di Florio A, Forty L, Gordon-Smith K, Heron J, Jones L, Craddock N, et al. Perinatal episodes across the mood disorder spectrum. JAMA Psychiatry. 2013;70(2):168–75.
48. Vesga-Lopez O, Blanco C, Keyes K, Olfson M, Grant BF, Hasin DS. Psychiatric disorders in pregnant and postpartum women in the United States. Arch Gen Psychiatry. 2008;65(7): 805–15.
49. Freeman MP, Smith KW, Freeman SA, McElroy SL, Kmetz GE, Wright R, et al. The impact of reproductive events on the course of bipolar disorder in women. J Clin Psychiatry. 2002;63(4): 284–7.
50. Gottschalk A, Bauer MS, Whybrow PC. Evidence of chaotic mood variation in bipolar disorder. Arch Gen Psychiatry. 1995;52(11):947–59.
51. van de Ven AC, Muntjewerff JW, Netea-Maier RT, de Vegt F, Ross HA, Sweep FC, et al. Association between thyroid function, thyroid autoimmunity, and state and trait factors of depression. Acta Psychiatr Scand. 2012;126(5):377–84.
52. Ibach B, Poljansky S, Marienhagen J, Sommer M, Manner P, Hajak G. Contrasting metabolic impairment in frontotemporal degeneration and early onset Alzheimer's disease. Neuroimage. 2004;23(2):739–43.
53. MacKinnon DF, Zandi PP, Cooper J, Potash JB, Simpson SG, Gershon E, et al. Comorbid bipolar disorder and panic disorder in families with a high prevalence of bipolar disorder. Am J Psychiatry. 2002;159(1):30–5.

54. Saunders EF, Fitzgerald KD, Zhang P, McInnis MG. Clinical features of bipolar disorder comorbid with anxiety disorders differ between men and women. Depress Anxiety. 2012; 29(8):739–46.
55. Hawton K, Sutton L, Haw C, Sinclair J, Harriss L. Suicide and attempted suicide in bipolar disorder: a systematic review of risk factors. J Clin Psychiatry. 2005;66(6):693–704.
56. Lopez P, Mosquera F, de Leon J, Gutierrez M, Ezcurra J, Ramirez F, et al. Suicide attempts in bipolar patients. J Clin Psychiatry. 2001;62(12):963–6.
57. Rotondo A, Mazzanti C, Dell'Osso L, Rucci P, Sullivan P, Bouanani S, et al. Catechol o-methyltransferase, serotonin transporter, and tryptophan hydroxylase gene polymorphisms in bipolar disorder patients with and without comorbid panic disorder. Am J Psychiatry. 2002; 159(1):23–9.
58. Akiskal HS. The distinctive mixed states of bipolar I, II, and III. Clin Neuropharmacol. 1992;15(Suppl 1 Pt A):632A–3.
59. Akiskal HS, Mallya G. Criteria for the "soft" bipolar spectrum: treatment implications. Psychopharmacol Bull. 1987;23(1):68–73.
60. Akiskal HS, Hantouche EG, Bourgeois ML, Azorin JM, Sechter D, Allilaire JF, et al. Gender, temperament, and the clinical picture in dysphoric mixed mania: findings from a French national study [EPIMAN]. J Affect Disord. 1998;50(2–3):175–86.
61. Altshuler LL, Kupka RW, Hellemann G, Frye MA, Sugar CA, McElroy SL, et al. Gender and depressive symptoms in 711 patients with bipolar disorder evaluated prospectively in the Stanley Foundation bipolar treatment outcome network. Am J Psychiatry. 2010;167(6): 708–15.
62. Kendler KS, Gardner CO. Sex Differences in the Pathways to Major Depression: A Study of Opposite-Sex Twin Pairs. The American journal of psychiatry. 2014.
63. Egeland JA. Bipolarity: the iceberg of affective disorders? Compr Psychiatry. 1983;24(4): 337–44.
64. Rutz W, Walinder J, von Knorring L, Pihlgren H, Rihmer Z. [Is depression in men under-treated? High frequency of sudden, unexpected suicides]. Lakartidningen. 1995;92[42]: 3893-4, 9-900.
65. Hasin D, Carpenter KM, McCloud S, Smith M, Grant BF. The alcohol use disorder and associated disabilities interview schedule [AUDADIS]: reliability of alcohol and drug modules in a clinical sample. Drug Alcohol Depend. 1997;44(2–3):133–41.
66. Sommer IE, Aleman A, Bouma A, Kahn RS. Do women really have more bilateral language representation than men? A meta-analysis of functional imaging studies. Brain. 2004;127(8): 1845–52.

Gender Differences in Personality Disorders

30

Eva Garnica de Cos

Abstract

Personality disorder is an enduring pattern of inner experience and behavior that deviates markedly from the expectations of the individual's culture, is pervasive and inflexible, has an onset in adolescence or early adulthood, is stable over time, and leads to distress or impairment. There has been a growing awareness of the importance of gender in medical treatment and research, and gender bias with regard to the criteria for personality disorders has been controversial. We summarize what some of the literature considers about sex differences and also take a look at gender bias, sometimes proved by studies, with regard to some of the diagnoses.

30.1 Introduction

Personality disorders (PDs) in the Diagnostic and Statistical Manual of Mental Disorders, 5th edition (DSM-5) [1] have the same criteria as those in the DSM-IV-TR (4th edition, text revision). With any ongoing review process, especially one with this degree of complexity, different points of view emerge, and an effort was made to accommodate them. Thus, PDs are included in both section II (diagnostic criteria and codes) and section III (emerging measures and models). This preserves continuity with current clinical practice, while also introducing a new approach that aims to address the numerous shortcomings of the current approach to PDs.

The material in section II represents an update of the text with the same criteria as those found in the DSM-IV-TR, whereas section III includes the proposed research model for PD diagnosis and conceptualization developed by the DSM-5 work group. For example, the typical patient criteria to be met for a specific PD

E.G. de Cos (✉)
Zamudio Hospital, Vizcaya, Spain
e-mail: evamaria.garnicadecos@osakidetza.net

M. Sáenz-Herrero (ed.), *Psychopathology in Women*,
DOI 10.1007/978-3-319-05870-2_30

frequently overlap with criteria for other PDs. Similarly, other specified or unspecified PDs are often the correct (but mostly uninformative) diagnosis, in the sense that patients do not tend to present with patterns of symptoms that correspond with only one PD [1].

In the alternative DSM-5 model, PDs are characterized by impairments in personality functioning and pathological personality traits. The specific PD diagnoses that may be derived from this model include antisocial, avoidant, borderline, narcissistic, obsessive compulsive, and schizotypal PDs. This approach also includes a diagnosis of PD trait specified that can be made when a PD is considered present, but the criteria for a specific disorder are not met [1].

A diagnosis of a PD requires two determinations: an assessment of the level of impairment in personality functioning and an evaluation of pathological traits. These criteria are relatively inflexible and pervasive across a broad range of personal and social situations that are relatively stable over time, with onsets that can be traced back to at least adolescence or early adulthood, that are not better explained by another mental health disorder, that are not attributable to the effects of a substance or another medical condition, and that are not better understood as normal for an individual's developmental stage or sociocultural environment.

Disturbances in self- and interpersonal functioning constitute the core of personality psychopathology and in this alternative diagnostic model they are evaluated on a continuum. Self-functioning involves identity (the experience of oneself as unique, with clear boundaries between oneself and others; the stability of self-esteem and accuracy of self-appraisal; the capacity for, and ability to regulate, a range of emotional experience) and self-direction (the pursuit of coherent and meaningful short-term and life goals; utilization of constructive and pro-social internal standards of behavior; ability to self-reflect productively).

Interpersonal functioning involves empathy (comprehension and appreciation of others' experiences and motivations; tolerance of differing perspectives; understanding the effects of one's own behavior on others) and intimacy (depth and duration of connection with others; desire and capacity for closeness; mutuality of regard reflected in interpersonal behavior.

Impairment in personality functioning predicts the presence of a PD, and the severity of impairment predicts whether an individual has more than one PD or one of the more typically severe PDs.

In the alternative DSM-5 model for PD, histrionic PD is left out of the classification. The clinical utility of the DSM-5 section III personality trait model (organized into five broad domains: negative, affectivity, detachment, antagonism, disinhibition, and psychoticism) domains adds value to the others in predicting important antecedent (e.g., family history, history of child abuse), concurrent (e.g., functional impairment, medication use), and predictive (e.g., hospitalization, suicide attempts) variables [1].

Gender differences are variations that result from biological sex as well as an individual's self-representation that includes the psychological, behavioral, and social consequences of one's perceived gender. Gender bias with regard to criteria for PDs has been controversial and widely debated [2, 3].

Judgments about personality functioning must take into account the individual's ethnic, cultural, and social background. PDs should not be confused with problems associated with acculturation following immigration or with the expression of habits, customs or religious and political values professed by the individual's culture of origin. It is useful for the clinician, especially when evaluating someone from a different background, to obtain additional information from informants who are familiar with the person's cultural background [1].

Gender differences are variations that result from biological as well as the individual's self-representations, the social, behavioral, and social consequences of one's perceived gender. The term gender difference is used more commonly in research than sex differences.

30.2 Epidemiological Data

The DSM-IV-TR does suggest that some PDs might be more common in men: antisocial, narcissistic, obsessive–compulsive, paranoid, schizotypal, and schizoid. They also suggest that borderline, histrionic, and dependent PDs might be more frequent in women [4]. Avoidant PD seems to be similar in both genders (and this also may be the case for schizotypal PD). Borderline PD (BPD) is diagnosed predominantly (about 75 %) in women according to the DSM-5 [1].

In clinical settings, histrionic PD has been diagnosed more frequently in women. In contrast, some studies using structured assessments report similar prevalence rates among men and women [1].

Norms for interpersonal behavior, personal appearance, and emotional expressiveness vary widely across cultures, genders, and age groups. Before considering the various traits (e.g., emotion, seductiveness, dramatic interpersonal style, novelty seeking, sociability, charm, impressionability, a tendency to somatization) to be evidence of histrionic PD, it is important to evaluate whether they cause clinically significant impairment or distress [1].

Other PDs may be confused with histrionic PD because they have certain features in common. It is therefore important to distinguish among these disorders based on differences in their characteristic features. However, if an individual has personality features that meet criteria for one or more PDs in addition to histrionic PD, all can be diagnosed.

Many individuals may display histrionic personality traits. Only when these traits are inflexible, maladaptive, persistent, and cause significant functional impairment or subjective distress do they constitute a PD.

Certain PDs are diagnosed more frequently in men. Others (e.g., borderline, histrionic, and dependent PDs) are diagnosed more frequently in women. Although these differences in prevalence probably reflect real gender differences in the presence of such patterns, clinicians must be cautious not to overdiagnose or underdiagnose certain PDs in women or in men because of social stereotypes of gender roles and behaviors. However, many studies have been carried out to try to be more accurate and to search for gender biases in these results. Also, some authors have tried to explain why these biases occur.

Ford and Widiger [5] tried to investigate whether the differences found in antisocial PD (more frequent in men) and histrionic PD (more frequent in women) represent actual differences between men and women, or the influence of stereotyping and sex biases on clinical diagnosis. They proved that there is a tendency for therapists to perceive men as antisocial personalities and women as hysterical personalities even when the patients have identical features. They interviewed 354 psychologists, giving them case histories or individual behaviors, either informing them if the case was a woman or a man, or not informing about this characteristic at all. Using this method they found that subjects failed more often to diagnose histrionic PD in male than in female patients; and for the antisocial PD, subjects failed more often to make a correct diagnosis in female than in male patients and, even more remarkable, even antisocial female patients were significantly more likely to be diagnosed with histrionic PD than with antisocial PD. Another interesting clue they gave us is that these biases have a higher influence on the global PD diagnosis than on each individual criterion, which were more accurately diagnosed correctly.

Regarding antisocial PD, other research has been carried out. It is interesting to know that it has been demonstrated that these women suffer from more frequent childhood emotional neglect and sex abuse, parent-related adverse events during childhood, and adverse events during adulthood. It is remarkable that women with antisocial PD present less violent antisocial behaviors and higher rates of aggressiveness and irritability, as well as higher rates of victimization, greater impairment, and lower social support [6].

Another interesting investigation was carried out by Jane et al. [3] including a nonclinical sample of 599 military men and women, and a college student sample. They found that 26 % of the military sample and 18 % of the college sample qualified for a diagnosis of at least one PD (obsessive compulsive being the most common) and there were no significant gender differences in the distribution of specific PD diagnoses. However, they did find that three of the items that have potential gender bias were from the criterion set for antisocial PD. They found that those criteria were more likely to be endorsed by men than women, even when both genders were at the same level of antisocial pathology. They think that the current antisocial criteria do not adequately reflect how the construct is expressed in women. They found similar biases for paranoid PD, which was more frequently diagnosed in men, but in general, their results suggested that there could be relatively little systematic gender bias in the diagnostic criteria for PDs.

Klonsky et al. [7] made another remarkable investigation to find out whether or not Kaplan's argumentation about dependent and histrionic PDs representing exaggerations of traditional feminine behaviors was accurate or not. They examined whether college students with greater masculinity or femininity were more likely to exhibit symptoms of the DSM-IV PDs. Data were collected from 665 students and they found PDs in 27 % of men and 20 % of women. Men more frequently had an antisocial PD, narcissistic, paranoid, and schizoid PD. Women more frequently had a dependent PD. The rest of the PDs were similar in both men and women. They found positive correlations between masculinity and antisocial PD, narcissistic and histrionic PD, and negative correlations between masculinity and avoidant, schizotypal, and schizoid PD. They also found positive correlations between femininity and dependent, histrionic PD, and narcissistic PD, and negative correlations with schizotypal and schizoid PD. It is interesting that feminine-acting men exhibited the highest levels of personality pathology, and that this same pattern was not as evident for women. An explanation for this difference could be that in today's society, it may still be more acceptable for women than for men to behave contrary to their expected role (although this may have changed over the last few years and can change in the future). They also remark that BPDs are not more often found in women, and this is consistent with the literature, which finds this disorder to be more frequently found in women only when clinical samples are studied (not in the general population).

With regard to BPD many investigations have been made. Years ago it was said that BPD was far more frequent in women, as remarked in the DSM-IV-TR [4], but more recent research has proved this disorder to be equally prevalent in men and women [8, 9]. This difference may be due to traditional settings for prevalence studies (psychiatric settings) that do not accurately reflect general population disorders. If we take a closer look at gender differences in BPD patients, we find some interesting data: regarding personality traits, men are characterized by explosive temperaments as well as high levels of novelty seeking and harm avoidance, whereas women with BPD are characterized by high levels of harm avoidance but not novelty seeking. With regard to Axis I comorbidity, substance abuse is consistently more common in men [2, 8–11], while eating disorders are more common in women [8, 9]. Women also suffer from more anxiety, mood disorders, and post-traumatic stress disorders (PTSDs) [8], although an important piece of research did not find this PTSD difference between men and women with BPD [9]. Antisocial PD is more frequently associated in these patients (looking at Axis II) when they are men [8, 9]. Looking at self-harm behavior, most studies support that the notion that it is more frequent in women [12], but this difference is not always found [8].

It is not easy to find clinical research that is based on hospital in-patients with PDs; most research is carried out in the general population, or in clinical outpatients. We are currently participating in this kind of research in three acute psychiatric units in three different hospitals in the north of Spain (not yet published). It has been a 3-year follow-up study in which we took a look at gender differences in this population. Three hundred and ninety-three inpatients were interviewed using the DSM-IV-TR International Personality Disorder Examination (IPDE) in order to find out if any PDs were present in these patients, and to search for gender differences. As expected, PDs were more often found in women (41.27 %) than in men (31.4 %). Women also had a higher association of several PDs. In women, the results were that the most common PD was borderline (21.7 %), and they were more often than men diagnosed with borderline, schizotypal, histrionic, and dependent PD. As a second associated PD, they were diagnosed with dependent, avoidant, and antisocial PD; and in the third place they also scored positive for schizoid, dependent, and obsessive compulsive PD. On the other hand, men were most frequently diagnosed with borderline (7.4 %) and antisocial PD (5.9 %). They scored higher than women for paranoid, schizoid, narcissistic, antisocial, avoidant, and obsessive compulsive PDs. As a second PD, men scored positive for borderline, antisocial, and avoidant PDs, and as a third PD, they scored positive for BPD. Most of these findings are similar to those found in literature.

In our clinical research, these PD inpatients also had gender differences with regard to other associated diagnoses: men had more substance abuse problems and any psychotic syndrome, while women had more associated affective or neurotic disorders. We also found that women had more frequently undergone previous suicidal attempts, and a higher number of them, which is often reflected in the literature (although men commit suicide more frequently than women). We also found that women had a higher treatment adherence, despite the poor results found in improving their mental health.

After this initial research, we followed up these patients, and again we found some remarkable gender differences: women had longer admissions (and readmissions), more frequent readmissions, they went more often to emergency rooms, and they underwent more suicide attempts. We found that men were more often involuntarily admitted and they also escaped more often from psychiatric units.

To conclude, it has been demonstrated that some gender prevalence differences in PDs vary hugely from one study to another; thus, this is still a matter that should be investigated in more depth.

30.3 Treatment Approaches

As happens with other mental disorders, women more frequently seek treatment [13], and this difference is even more remarkable when affective or anxiety disorders appear in these PD patients. This difference changes when any drug abuse disorder is present [2, 8, 10], probably because of cultural influences (women endorse stigmatization as a reason for not seeking treatment) [10]. It is also remarkable that women are more likely to utilize pharmacotherapy and psychotherapy services, while men with PD disorders are more likely to be found in prisons (they often act more aggressively) and in hospitals (they do not seek help until their illnesses are severe) [8]. Much more research is needed to determine whether gender is an influence on receiving adequate and appropriate mental health treatment. In the medical literature biological sex and gender are often used synonymously.

30.4 Discussion

It is interesting to take a look at why these gender differences, and sometimes biases, are observed, and some authors have focused on this aspect. Some explanations of these findings may be based on evolution, history, and biology. For example, they all give us a wider vision of why gender roles are so important to receiving a PD diagnosis or another, depending on our gender. Masculinity and femininity are what men's and women's personalities are supposed to be like, what they are supposed to think or how they are supposed to act; thus, biological and cultural influences are very important in personality traits and therefore to understanding personality disorders and their gender biases.

Personality traits are of course influenced by hormones and other biological factors that are present while a fetus is still growing in his or her mother's uterus. Depending on our genetically determined sex, some of our behaviors and ways of perceiving and thinking are heavily biased: men are most likely to express their emotional states by aggressive behaviors, for example, because of testosterone and many other factors, while women prefer verbal expression [14], and this may explain some of the differences in PD prevalence. Our brains are different to some extent, and therefore we act and behave differently. These biological and cultural differences are based on and modified by evolution, and its way of selecting what is more useful for humans (and every species), because it helps our survival.

Some authors, such as Klonsky [7], have investigated the link between gender role and PDs, finding a close relationship between what people find to be "masculine" or "feminine," and some personality traits and PDs. The similarities between "femininity" and depression have also been remarked upon, for example, dependency, passivity, lack of assertiveness, need for emotional support, low self-esteem, etc. [15]. Looking at these kinds of differences, we might say that the more "feminine" a woman is, the more likely she is to endorse criteria for some PDs or some related affective disorders (and we can also find the opposite explanation for men: they are less likely to suffer from depression, for example, if they fit in with typically masculine traits). We can even find some psychoanalytically based explanations as to why women's and men's personalities and ways of behaving and thinking are different, and as a result, tend to show a higher prevalence in one or other PD [16]. But, most important of all, we must not forget that what our culture thinks about what a woman (or a man) is supposed to be, how she is supposed to behave, think, etc., is changing with history and political and social changes, and it has to be noted that medical thinking has always been influenced by these changes over the years [17].

The question is: what is reality and who defines it? To explore the role of culture and ethnicity future research is needed. We must be much more critical with what we read about personality traits and disorders and their gender differences [18] and notice that we are influenced by the many inputs we receive every day, some of which we are not aware of at all.

References

1. American Psychiatric Association. Diagnostic and statistical manual of mental disorders. 5th ed. Arlington, VA: American Psychiatric Association; 2013.
2. Back SE, Contini R, Brady KT. Substance abuse in women: does gender matter? Psychiatr Times. 2006;24(1):48.
3. Jane JS, Oltmanns TF, South SC, Turkheimer E. Gender bias in diagnostic criteria for personality disorders: an item response theory analysis. J Abnorm Psychol. 2007;116(1): 166–75.
4. American Psychiatric Association. Diagnostic and statistical manual of mental disorders (4th edn, text rev.). 2000; Washington, DC.
5. Ford MR, Widiger TA. Sex bias in the diagnosis of histrionic and antisocial personality disorders. J Consult Clin Psychol. 1989;57(2):301–5.
6. Alegria AA, Blanco C, Petry NM, Liu SM, Grant B, Hasin D. Sex differences in antisocial personality disorder: results from the national epidemiological survey on alcohol and related conditions. Personal Disord. 2013;4(3):214–22.
7. Klonsky ED, Jane JS, Turkheimer E, Oltmanns TF. Gender role and personality disorders. J Personal Disord. 2002;16(5):464–76.
8. Sansone RA, Sansone LA. Gender patterns in borderline personality disorder. Innov Clin Neurosci. 2011;8(5):16–20.
9. Zlotnick C, Rothschild L, Zimmerman M. The role of gender in the clinical presentation of patients with borderline personality disorder. J Personal Disord. 2002;16(3):277–82.
10. Khan S, Okuda M, Hasin DS, Secades-Villa R, Keyes K, Lin K, et al. Gender differences in lifetime alcohol dependence: results from the national epidemiological survey on alcohol and related conditions. J Clin Psychiatry. 2008;69(10):1606–16.
11. Ramsay R, Welch S, Youard E. Needs of women patients with mental illness. Adv Psychiatr Treat. 2001;7:85–92.
12. Monnin J, Thiemard E, Vandel P, Nicolier M, Tio G, Courtet P, et al. Sociodemographic and psychopathological risk factors in repeated suicide attempts: gender differences in a prospective study. J Affect Disord. 2012;136:35–43.
13. Montero I, Aparicio D, Gómez-Beneyto M, Moreno-Küstner B, Reneses B, Usall J, et al. Género y salud mental en un mundo cambiante. Gac Sanit. 2004;18 Suppl 1:175–81.
14. García E. Neuropsicología y género. Rev Asoc Esp Neuropsiq. 2003;23(86):2175–86.
15. Dio Bleichmar E. La depresión en la mujer. Rev Asoc Esp Neuropsiq. 1991;11(39):283–7.
16. González de Chávez A. Mujer: cultura, identidad y salud mental. Rev Asoc Esp Neuropsiq. 1992;12(40):9–29.
17. Diéguez A. Psiquiatría y género: el naciente discurso médico-psiquiátrico en España y el estatuto social de la mujer. Rev Asoc Esp Neuropsiq. 1999;19(72):637–52.
18. Hill TD, Needman BL. Rethinking gender and mental health: a critical analysis of three propositions. Soc Sci Med. 2013;92:83–91.

31 Borderline Personality Spectrum

Olatz Napal

> *"En lo hondo no hay raíces*
> *hay lo arrancado."*
> *Hugo Mújica*

Abstract

People who receive a diagnosis of borderline personality disorder (BPD) find themselves "*at the border*" in several ways. They display behaviors that society deems inexplicably mad, and they frequently do so in a way that places them at variance with the Western binary stereotype—masculine and feminine—that is, on the border between so-called masculine and feminine behavior. They teeter on the edge of social acceptability.

It is not by chance that this diagnosis is more frequent in women and homosexual, transsexual, transgendered people, and so on, in a society in which the concept of the universal "*subject*" has been built from the masculine model. Anyone outside of its margins is considered the "*other*" and can be labeled unhealthy in a society where the difference has been medicalized.

The feminization of the borderline category is argued by several theories that suggest the BPD category as a contemporary successor to hysteria, showing that, like hysteria, this diagnosis has expanded into an overinclusive and diffuse category. Another aspect exposed is the large number of patients with BPD with histories of trauma (physical, sexual, etc.) and how sometimes the symptoms that seem to be grouped under the label of BPD represent patterns of adaptation to trauma.

The body becomes a "speaking body" (following Foucault's idea); thus, we consider it essential to address the self-injuries experience, not as a sign of specific diagnosis, but as a way of being in the world and in between the world (body in suffering). Finally, we present some of the current theories that

O. Napal (✉)
Alava University Hospital, Vitoria, Spain
e-mail: olatz.napalfernandez@osakidetza.net

M. Sáenz-Herrero (ed.), *Psychopathology in Women*,
DOI 10.1007/978-3-319-05870-2_31

denounce the dominant social norms and the inextricable links of power and their influence in the construction of our identity.

31.1 Introduction

The term "*borderline*" was first used in 1938 by analyst Adolph Stern [1] to describe patients who appeared more severely disturbed than the neurotics who Freud felt were suitable for psychoanalysis, yet who did not show signs of outright psychosis, placing them "*on the border line between neurosis and psychosis*." These patients appeared to be more profoundly disturbed than those suffering neurotic symptoms, but they could not be classified as psychotic. Stern felt that these patients showed signs of regressing to an early narcissistic state in which they had withdrawn libidinal energy from the outside world and turned it upon themselves. Thus, these patients showed evidence of pre-oedipal conflicts having to do with the earliest acquisition of a self, rather than the oedipal conflicts of neurotic patients.

In contemporary psychiatry, the borderline diagnosis appeared in the DSM-III (APA 1980, revisited in 1987), where it was defined as a personality disorder, characterized by a "pervasive pattern of instability of self-image, interpersonal relationships, and mood, beginning in early adulthood and present in a variety of contexts" [2]. A central feature of BPD is the appearance of an identity disturbance that is manifested by several life issues such as self-image, sexual orientation, long-term goals of career choice, types of friends or lovers to have, etc.The person often experiences this instability of self-image as chronic feelings of emptiness or boredom.

Roth and Fonagy [3] offer this definition of BPD:

> The essential feature of this disorder is a pervasive pattern of instability of self-image, interpersonal relationships and mood. The person's sense of identity is profoundly uncertain. Interpersonal relationships are unstable and intense, fluctuating between the extremes of idealization and devaluation. There is often a terror of being alone, with great efforts made to avoid real or imagined abandonment. Affect is extremely unstable, with marked shifts from baseline mood to depression and anxiety usually lasting a few hours. Inappropriate anger and impulsive behavior are common, and often this behavior is self-harming. Suicidal threats and self-mutilation are common in more severe forms of this disorder.

Kernberg's contribution in BPD can be summarized in two trends: (a) the construction of the borderline condition as a defensive ego or personality type, the borderline personality organization; and (b) providing a theory of the roots of the disorder in early childhood and infancy (the pre-oedipal period), describing this period, based on object relations theory, as the source of the borderline patient's unstable self.

For Kernberg the major difference between the neurotic and the borderline patient is the borderline patient's lack of a clear sense of identity. The neurotic patient is able to provide a verbal description of the self; borderline patients are not able to provide a coherent portrait of themselves; their descriptions are contradictory, incomplete, and the behavior is inconsistent. One essential symptom is "*splitting*," in which one holds two contradictory perceptions of the self or others as

Table 31.1 Borderline personality disorder criteria according the DSM-5 [6]

Borderline personality disorder
(A) Significant impairments in **personality functioning** manifested by: 1. Impairments in **self-functioning** (a or b): (a) **Identity**: markedly impoverished, poorly developed, or unstable self-image, often associated with excessive self-criticism; chronic feelings of emptiness; dissociative states under stress. (b) **Self-direction**: instability in goals, aspirations, values, or career plans AND 2. Impairments in **interpersonal functioning** (a or b): (a) **Empathy**: compromised ability to recognize the feelings and needs of others associated with interpersonal hypersensitivity (i.e., prone to feeling slighted or insulted); perceptions of others selectively biased toward negative attributes or vulnerabilities. (b) **Intimacy**: intense, unstable, and conflicted close relationships, marked by mistrust, neediness, and anxious preoccupation with real or imagined abandonment; close relationships often viewed in extremes of idealization and devaluation and alternating between over-involvement and withdrawal.
(B) Pathological **personality traits** in the following domains: 1. **Negative affectivity**, characterized by: (a) **Emotional lability**: unstable emotional experiences and frequent mood changes; emotions that are easily aroused, intense, and/or out of proportion to events and circumstances. (b) **Anxiousness**: intense feelings of nervousness, tenseness, or panic, often in reaction to interpersonal stresses; worry about the negative effects of past unpleasant experiences and future negative possibilities; feeling fearful, apprehensive, or threatened by uncertainty; fears of falling apart or losing control. (c) **Separation insecurity**: fears of rejection by—and/or separation from—significant others, associated with fears of excessive dependency and complete loss of autonomy. (d) **Depressivity**: frequent feelings of being down, miserable, and/or hopeless; difficulty recovering from such moods; pessimism about the future; pervasive shame; feeling of inferior self-worth; thoughts of suicide and suicidal behavior. 2. **Disinhibition**, characterized by: (a) **Impulsivity**: acting on the spur of the moment in response to immediate stimuli; acting on a momentary basis without a plan or consideration of outcomes; difficulty establishing or following plans; a sense of urgency and self-harming behavior under emotional distress. (b) **Risk-taking**: engagement in dangerous, risky, and potentially self-damaging activities, unnecessarily and without regard to consequences; lack of concern for one's limitations and denial of the reality of personal danger.
(C) The impairments in personality functioning and the individual's personality trait expression are relatively stable across time and consistent across situations.
(D) The impairments in personality functioning and the individual's personality trait expression are not better understood as normative for the individual's developmental stage or socio-cultural environment.
(E) The impairments in personality functioning and the individual's personality trait expression are not solely due to the direct physiological effects of a substance (e.g., a drug of abuse, medication) or a general medical condition.

being either all good or all bad, and is unable to integrate them into a coherent total image. The patient vacillates from one image to the other.

Borderline personality organization is characterized by "*immature*" ego defense mechanisms, which include "*splitting*" as well as "*magical thinking*" or superstitions, feelings of omnipotence, phobias, obsessive compulsive behavior, projection of one's unpleasant characteristics onto others, and "*projective identification,*" in which the person perceives and identifies with the projected characteristics. This borderland pathological ego structure, for Kernberg, is rooted in the person's earliest childhood, and the object relations theory gives the mother a pivotal role in determining the shape of the infant's personality during this period [4, 5].

In 2013 the new edition of the DSM-V appeared, whose criteria are shown in Table 31.1 [6].

Throughout its short history, BPD has been a controversial diagnosis [3], criticized for its weighted construction, its inconsistent and unclear meaning, and its uneven, stigmatizing, and punitive application [7]. Studies cite BPD rates of approximately 0.4–1.8 % among community samples [8, 9] and 10–25 % among clinical samples [10, 11]. BPD is more often diagnosed in women, which estimates that approximately two thirds to three quarters of those diagnosed with BPD are women [12, 13].

The basis of diagnostic prevalence alone (75 % of those diagnosed with BPD are women) invites us to consider the possibility that it might be a gendered diagnosis. Dana Becker [14] argues that the borderline diagnosis has been "feminized" and that BPD has become a new "female malady" for the late twentieth century.

One of the main features on the borderline is the patient's unstable, fragmented or missing self. People deemed borderline are not only placed "on the borders," at the edges of sanity; they are also placed at the very margins of selfhood [15]. Their selves are described as "empty" [16], "dead" [17], "unstable" or "split" among "part-selves" [18], as containing a "defect in the organizing structure of the self" [19]; such patients manifest a "blurring of ego boundaries" (confusion between one's own thoughts and feelings and those of others) [20].

Butler critiques the pre-social conceptions of identity and subjecthood and argues about the inseparability of gender and identity. They cannot be separated; to speak of "*selves*" necessarily draws one into a consideration of gender. Butler calls into question the neutrality and universality of the notion of "*self.*" Her analysis (a part of the feminist critique of the gendered quality of self) has shown how conceptions of the self or subject are conflated with conceptions of masculine subjectivity, reflecting the experiences, desires, and illusions of this masculine position [21]. Some authors refer to women having been constructed as "*other,*" over-determined by their feminine position in the gender binaries of patriarchal logic [22–24].

Within this binary logic of the self and the other and of masculine and feminine, the status of feminine identity is unstable, marked by paradox and contradiction. Women are in a representational and experiential double bind, between the traditional essentialist feminine identity, on the one hand, and the psychologically defined norm or ideal of healthy, normal selfhood, on the other. Ambiguity and confusion surround this double bind [15].

Men are in the minority of patients receiving the diagnosis of BPD; 25–30 % of those diagnosed are males [14]. One of the explanations offered for the low numbers of men diagnosed as borderline is that men showing similar traits to borderline women tend to be diagnosed as sociopathic, or as having antisocial personality disorder [25]. According to this view, some male patients may express the same confusion and uncertainty or instability and rage as women, but tend to direct their rage toward others, rather than toward themselves (according to Bourdieu's theory in *The Male Domination*). They become involved with the legal system, rather than the mental health system. 25 % of patients with antisocial personality disorder also fulfill the criteria for BPD. Looking for this fact, Gunderson and Zanarini write: "Sex bias probably prejudices clinicians to overlook the antisocial features of female patients and the dependent, needy (borderline) features of male patients" [26], but other authors disagree with this argument, reporting that antisocial personality disorder does not include the fluctuating emotions described in BPD, and consider that the male equivalent of borderlines may be as close to narcissistic as to antisocial personality disorders [25].

It is important to draw attention to the fact that a high proportion of people who receive the diagnosis of borderline are said to be gay, lesbian, transsexual, transgender, etc. The question is whether these people express similar kinds of identity "*disturbances*" that are said to be characteristic of the borderline patient; or whether this pattern is an outcome of clinicians perceiving and labeling. Some men may escape the label of borderline because most of their expressions of borderline-like behaviors are viewed as appropriate to the masculine gender role, so there are no signs of pathology. Some papers found that men in the general population reported more borderline characteristics than normal women. "It is interesting to speculate that clinicians may consider these characteristics as more congruent with male sex roles and may find them more tolerable in men. Conversely, in women these traits may be seen as less appropriate to sex role, and therefore women may be more likely to be labeled as having borderline personality disorder" [27]. Men who are diagnosed as borderline are those who deviate from the masculine gender stereotype [15].

31.2 Gender and Madness: A Historical View

Tracing the history of the modern concept of madness back to the pre-modern discourse of witchcraft, some authors describe how this discourse positioned as "witch" and "outsider" the woman whose deviant behavior threatened social norms [14, 28]. A woman positioned in this way could be punished for her deviancy, and the threat that she posed to social norms could be controlled and neutralized. In the movement from this pre-modern, religious world view to the current scientific (rational paradigm of modernism), Foucault described the emergence of a scientifically determined and controlled concept of insanity [29]. This reflects the change from "witchcraft" as the primary discourse applied to women's deviancy, to the appearance of the concept of "*hysteria*" in the nineteenth century. Hysteria became the signifier par excellence that positioned women as pathological and irrational in the last two centuries.

In her historical study of women and madness Elaine Showalter has shown the symbolic association of madness with femininity in the history of Western society, which the author attributes to "a cultural tradition that represents woman as madness and that uses images of the female body...to stand for irrationality in general" [30]. The neurologist Mitchell described the hysteria like "the nosological limbo of all unnamed female maladies. It was also called *mysteria*" [31].

Showalter argued that hysteria is not, therefore, an individual pathology, hysteria was a response to powerlessness arising from a contradictory expectation about feminine behavior. Chesler coined the term "double bind" to describe the processes by which women can be pathologized both for conforming to, and for failing to conform to, expectations of feminine passivity [32]. Women labeled "hysterical" were, on the one hand, unable to meet social norms and on the other, unable to release themselves from the force of these norms, since the norms had been internalized. Hysteria undermined the norm of female refinement in two ways: directly, through the "fits" or unseemly emotional outbursts to which hysterical individuals were prone, and second, through debilitating physical symptoms that rendered the individual helpless, in a caricature of feminine delicacy [33].

"The more women became hysterical, the more doctors became punitive toward the disease; and at the same time, they began to see the disease everywhere...until they were diagnosing every independent act by a woman as 'hysterical'" [30]. Hysteria became an epidemic, with women accepting their "*illness*" and at the same time "finding a way to rebel against an intolerable social role" [14]. "Sickness became not only a way of life but also a means of rebellion, and 'medical treatment,' which had always had strong overtones of coercion, revealed itself as frankly and brutally repressive" [30].

There has been an increasing recognition that the label "*borderline*" may function in the same way that "*hysteria*" did in the late nineteenth and early twentieth century as a label for women. According to Jimenez, "the similarities between the diagnoses of BPD and hysteria are striking. Both diagnoses delimit appropriate behavior for women and many of the criteria are stereotypically feminine" [34]. Several authors have made reference to this association [14]. "Borderline disorder is a more aggressive version of hysteria, the distinction is the inclusion of anger and other 'aggressive' characteristics in BPD, such shoplifting, reckless driving and substance abuse. 'If the hysteric was a damaged woman, the borderline woman is a dangerous one'" [34]. According to a social construction model, BPD (like witchcraft and hysteria) is constructed as a deviation, in this case from the concepts of rationality and individuality [35].

The gendered consequences of the psychiatric preoccupation with "rationality" have been well explored in feminist theory: women are "typically situated on the side of irrationality, silence, nature and body, while men are situated on the side of reason, discourse, culture and mind," says Showalter [30], along the same lines of argument as Bourdieu [24]. The consequences of this approach are evident in the psychiatric response to "*borderline symptoms*": the BPD diagnostic depends upon a psychiatrist judging whether emotions are appropriate/healthy with reference to the norm of "rationality." Both anger and fear of abandonment can be judged to be inappropriate, as opposed to being understandable in the context of a person's history of being violated or abandoned [35].

In the case of BPD, the diagnoses can be applied to women who fail to live up to their gender role because they express anger and aggression. Jimenez argues that "this successor to hysteria, in depicting the borderline patient as a 'demanding, aggressive and angry woman,' and in highlighting as one of its features 'promiscuity' in sexuality, is reflective of contemporary moral judgments of normal female behavior" [34]. At the same time, the diagnoses is also given to women who conform "too easily," by internalizing anger and expressing this through self-focused behavior such as self-injury [35]. Wirth-Cauchon discusses how "women diagnosed with BPD are representing society's contradictions about femininity, with the double-bind of being denigrated for both emotionality and rationality, for active sexuality and for passive servicing of men" [15].

These contradictions are also held in the therapeutic space, as we can see for example in Samuels, who writes that the borderline patient can create a fascination because the "'*ecstasy*' of a madness that maintains a grasp on '*reality*': intense affect, depersonalization; impulsive behavior, sometimes against the self, brief psychotic experiences; disturbed personal relationships, sometimes exceedingly intimate and sometimes distant. This could be the profile of a saint" [36].

On the other hand, the language describing mental disorder may be pejorative, as it frequently is in definitions of BPD [37, 38]; this lays "the groundwork for a view of patients that is critical of women rather than compassionate toward them" [14].

31.3 Social Causation of Distress: Trauma

The document *Women's Mental Health: Into the Mainstream Strategic Development of Mental Health Care for Women* [39] acknowledges that many women with a diagnosis of BPD have a history of trauma. At least 70 % have been sexually abused as children [40]. Some studies say that 88 % of people diagnosed with BPD had experienced abuse: for 80 % this was childhood abuse; for 70 % this was early sexual abuse [41], this can lead us to think childhood sexual abuse is a powerful example of the social causation of distress with relation to BPD. However, the history of societal responses to childhood sexual abuse is a history of denial and distortion, and we can also find this in psychiatry's denial of the etiological relevance of abuse, trauma, and oppression for psychological distress [35]. Freud chose to conceal revelations of childhood sexual abuse by women with the diagnosis of hysteria, by presenting them as memories of fantasies, rather than memories of actual experiences [42]. In consequence, the result was that the extent and impact of childhood sexual abuse was silenced for a century, and continues to be.

As a result of this, some authors consider the diagnosis of BPD a powerful new manifestation of this tendency to deny the extent and impact of childhood sexual abuse, neglect or emotional abuse [35]. Some papers describe how the "symptoms" that define BPD can be better understood as adaptive reactions to early relational traumas. They suggest that it is much more helpful to understand people's behavior as an attempt to ensure "some measure of mastery, control and alliance with others, in the face of trauma, helplessness and inner vulnerability" than as the result of "a disorder of the personality, that is, solely an internal deficit" [43–45].

The symptoms of post-traumatic stress disorder (PTSD) overlap considerably with symptoms of BPD, and focus on unstable emotions, behavior, and relationships [25]. Herman considers that the BPD behaviors are a form of adaptation to trauma, with the most prominent aspect being the "disturbance in identity and relationship." Borderline is the most prominent psychiatric diagnosis (with somatization disorder and multiple personality disorder) given to people suffering from childhood trauma. The symptoms were attributed in the last century to hysteria. Given the range of responses to trauma, Herman argues that even the category of PTSD is too narrowly defined, focusing on singular events such as combat, disaster and rape, thus missing the more complex picture of prolonged abuse. She proposes a new category to encompass the spectrum of conditions related to trauma: "complex post-traumatic stress disorder" [46]. This author criticized Otto Kernberg because he minimized the importance of sexual abuse to the appearance of some of the symptoms of the borderline disorders. For Herman, the borderline's relations to other people can often be understood as strategies of adaptation held over from past relations with abusive caretakers:

> Why would a child fail to integrate idealized or terrifying images of his/her caretakers? The reason would have to be either constitutional or adaptive. Splitting is adaptive. Children must preserve some sense of connection at any cost, in this case by walling off the image of the abusive figure from the positive one. I think they do so in a state-dependent way, flipping between modes of affection and terror that accurately reflect their environments. They grow up constantly scanning their interpersonal environments to see if they're safe, reading subtleties of expression, posture, gesture, and so forth, in an almost uncanny way. However, if you ignore the original reason for this behavior, it looks perverse, incomprehensible, and ultimately pathological [25].

For Herman, trauma provides comprehensibility to the symptoms expressed by people diagnosed as borderline. The patient's instability becomes understood as a response to an external event, rather being rooted in a character or personality disorder. With the label "borderline personality disorder" there is a risk of losing narrative comprehensibility, placing the patient's symptoms within a scientific–medical framework of character pathology.

Yet, while sexual and physical abuse are major factors, they do not fully account for the predominance of women diagnosed as borderline, since not all borderline individuals have histories of childhood abuse, and abuse has occurred in 20–40 % of women diagnosed as borderline [14].

Sexual abuse is more prevalent in women than in men. However, the fact that men show a greater reluctance and difficulty to relate these experiences may have an influence on the lower ratio of men, as (in terms of Bourdieu's *habitus*) they would not "live up to what society has imposed on them as men," but quite the opposite, they would be the "dominated" within the "masculine dominance," needless to say, if the authorship of such abuse belonged to women.

31.4 People on the Borders

Western representational systems stand in a precarious and unstable place in relation to the humanist ideal of a generic, neutral, universal "*subject*" [47]. Some authors consider than women are represented as "other" to this ideal of the universal subject.

Lévi-Strauss showed that in cultures built on gift exchange, women (and other valuable gifts as food, words, names, tools, powers, etc.) [48] are the most precious gifts within the basic exchange in marriage. The exchange takes place between kin groups. For Lévi-Strauss women become central as an exchange to the foundation of culture. A woman in this exchange assumes the status of gift, object, and not that of a subject who exchanges. Thus, women are located in the interstices of social exchange, serving as the medium of exchange between subjects. The position of a woman functions as (according to Butler) "a relational term between groups of men; she does not have an identity, she reflects masculine identity precisely through being the site of its absence" [21].

This ambiguous position is a "stress point" in the cultural logic, a place where meaning is mobile and shifting, thus revealing the instability of the cultural order. Jane Gallop comments on this dual status of women as both subject and object [49]. According to Bourdieu, who describes the hierarchical relation through the oppositional binarism (outside/inside; public/private; objective/subjective; culture/nature; political/emotional; etc.) [24] the identity is defined through difference.

Susan Bordo analyzes Descartes' stance, in which the senses of the body are ignored in favor of pure objective reason, resulting in the Cartesian experience of the self as inwardness ("I think, therefore I am") and the sense of distance from the "not-I" [50]. Women become apprehended as part of the denied separate world, "she is the 'Other'," in de Beauvoir's words [22], but for Irigaray the female sex is not a "lack" or an "other" that immanently and negatively defines the subject in its masculinity. On the contrary, the female sex eludes the very requirements of representation, for she is neither "other" nor the "lack" [21], the feminine is not a negatively defined derivative or opposite of masculinity, but another version of the same masculine image. Women are defined as the derivative of the subject.

Kristeva developed the concept of the "*abject*" to denominate that which is excluded from the body in order to demarcate it as a bounded and homogeneous entity. Butler describes the "*abject*" as "that which has been expelled from the body, as excrement, literally rendered '*Other*.' The construction of the '*not-me*' as the abject establishes the boundaries of the body which are also the first contours of the subject" [21]. Butler applies the concept of "*abjection*" to bring to the foreground society's exclusion of certain social identities in order to maintain the illusion of the dominant boundaries and coherence, self-identical subject [51], "'it is at once setting of a boundary, and also the repeated inculcation of a norm'; and such instances of social boundary marking 'contribute to that field of discourse and power that orchestrates, delimits and sustains that which qualifies as 'the human'" [21].

Grosz argues that "*the Abject's* location is in the borderline between inner and outer, self and not-self, that is threatening, because it remains irreducible to either subject/object, or inside/outside. The *abject* necessarily partakes of both polarized terms but cannot be clearly identified with either. The borderline states, functions and positions are considered as danger, sites of possible pollution or contamination. That which is marginal is always located as a site of danger and vulnerability" [52].

31.5 The Description of BPD

"Do I contradict myself? Very well, then I contradict myself, I am large, I contain multitudes."—Walt Whitman

BPD is said to be defined by instability: "it not only causes instability, but also symbolizes it" [25], instability in mood, self-image, relationships, and feeling of emptiness or rage.

One diagnostic criterion for BPD pertains to a disturbance in "*identity*." Indeed, some authors have argued that identity disturbance, along with unstable relationships, are at the core of "*borderline pathology*" [53].

In DSM-III, identity disturbance was operationalized as an "uncertainty about several issues such as self-image, gender identity, long-term goals or career choice, friendship patterns, values, and loyalties." In DSM-III-R, it was described as an "uncertainty about at least two of the following: self-image, sexual orientation, long-term goals or career choice, type of friends desired, [or] preferred values." In the DSM-IV TR, it was simply characterized as a "markedly and persistently unstable self-image or sense of self." In the DSM-5 it is characterized by a markedly impoverished, poorly developed, or unstable self-image, often associated with excessive self-criticism; chronic feelings of emptiness; dissociative states under stress [6].

31.5.1 Fragmented Selves

Showalter says that the conception of a female subjectivity split between outward appearance of the body as an object and inner subjecthood is important in the analysis of borderline narratives [30]. She interprets this split as an exaggeration of women's "*normal*" state, citing the art historian John Berger, who maintains that a woman's psyche is divided in two by virtue of her need to be simultaneously both actor and observer. He says of the woman:

> She is almost continually accompanied by her own image of herself. Whilst she is walking across a room or whilst she is weeping at the death of her father, she can scarcely avoid watching herself walking or weeping. From earliest childhood she has been taught and persuaded to survey herself continually. And so she comes to consider the *surveyor* and the *surveyed* within her as the two constituent yet always distinct elements of her identity as a woman [54].

Wirth-Cauchon refers to how Showalter sees poet Sylvia Plath's autobiographical fiction *The Bell Jar* as expressing in complex ways these conflicts and splits, and notes that the heroine in the novel, Esther, is "split between the feminine and creative selves." Esther believes that "motherhood and writing are incompatible. Esther's sense of an absolute division between her creativity and her femininity is the basis of her schizophrenia." "The analysis of madness as an exaggeration of the cultural double binds of feminine identity to analyze the fragmented self depicted in the borderline narratives" [15].

In accordance with this author (Wirth-Cauchon) we will use the same classification/description for these fragmented selves.

31.5.1.1 Mask Self

The themes of artificiality and superficiality frequently appear in the borderline case narratives. The patient expresses feelings of artificiality or falsity often accompanied by sensations of emptiness and numbness. "This is described as a superficial, surface mask or person that is a kind of empty adaptation to the surroundings" [15].

Sometimes these patients try to have with the other a closer relation, relying not on others to give them a "setting and pulse," but on fragmentary feeling sensations to "anchor" their identities. The "false self" is created to alienate the horror of feelings of inner emptiness or deadness. Sometimes, the physical feeling (pleasant or unpleasant) can become a kind of anchor point to the external world, providing a reference to "some" existence in the experience of a large internal void.

"As If" Personality

Helene Deutsch described a group of women patients who appear to exhibit a superficiality and inner emptiness in their personalities. The "*as if*" personality. Such persons appear to be "normal"; yet, on closer observation, lack warmth or depth: "It is like the performance of an actor who is technically well trained but who lacks the necessary spark to make his impersonations true to life." The "*as if*" personality shows a "completely passive attitude to the environment with a highly plastic readiness to pick up signals from the outer world and to mold oneself and one's behavior accordingly" [55]. In the place of a personality, there is only imitation of others, identification with the environment that facilitates "good adaptation" to the world without depth or inner life. Deutsch says that "if it is a woman, she seems to be the quintessence of feminine devotion, imparted by her passivity and readiness for identification. The lack of real warmth brings such an emptiness and dullness to the emotional atmosphere that the man as a rule precipitously breaks off the relationship" [55]. She continues: "All their experiences can be based on identifications and… so many identifications that their conduct can appear erratic. They can be considered 'crazy' by those who know them" [56].

Deutsch believes that the "*as if*" personalities represented a phase leading up to the onset of schizophrenia, they are not accepted forms of neurosis, and they are too well adjusted to reality to be called psychotic.

Hoch and Polatin used the concept "*pseudoneurotic schizophrenia*" to refer some patients who showed a deeper level of anxiety and a wider variety of symptoms than the neurotic. Like Deutsch's, their patients were predominantly women. They describe patients whose symptoms include "*ambivalence*," which is "not localized, but it is diffuse and widespread involving the patient's aims, the social adaptation and sexual adjustment"; "polymorphous anxiety"; and a combination of the symptoms of neurosis that they call "*pan-neurosis*" [57].

31.5.1.2 Lost Self

Yalom (in a work co-authored with his patient "Ginny Elkin") [58] edited a jointly produced book, with both Yalom and Elkin writing the post-session reports. It was an agreement between them, and Elkin wrote the sessions as payment for therapy. Yalom wrote:

> Because of her ego boundary blurring, her autism, her dream life, the inaccessibility of affect, most clinicians would affix to her a label of 'schizoid' or, perhaps, 'borderline'... in the group therapy sessions she's ethereal...a haughty but self-conscious amusement at the whole proceedings...never fully her energies, alternated between being someone who was extraordinary sensitive and reactive to others, to someone who simply was not there at all [58].

Elkin wrote:

> ...although I did occasional "great" work, I like nothing better than to be a human sundial, a curled up outdoor nap[...]my qualifications dripped like Dali's watch, as I was tempted toward everything and nothing...I react to someone rather than act first, they put me in a place, set my borders and limits...I know my problem has something to do with suspension of action and feeling...I just shop a lot of attitudes and feelings without buying any...I only pose, a model for my shadow, a shadow for my silhouette.

In this case, we can see the mutable meaning of the borderline label, simultaneously close to, and different from, psychosis. The patient also seems like a marginal presence that refuses to be integrated within the group, being inaccessible and placing herself out of the bounds of normality, without being declared psychotic. She is unable to get a fix on her desires and looks like she is passively watching life pass by, she is unfocused, and passively responds to the needs of others [15].

31.5.1.3 Repressed Self

Flax argues that, in some cases, the "*core self*" is split between an outward false self that conforms to the feminine role, and a repressed, autonomous self for which expression is "forbidden" in contemporary Western culture. The borderline patient's symptoms are expressions of confusions and contradictions faced by women as each of these parts of the self fight for expression [15]. Jane Flax describes this duality of self in women thus:

> My clinical experience and reading convince me that the repressed is gendered in the sense that women in our culture tend to repress distinctive aspects of the self which are bound up with autonomy and aggression. One dimension of what is repressed is women's non-object related ambition and interest in exerting various sorts of mastery: interpersonal,

> intellectual, or creative. Both men's and women's sense of gender and the self partially grow out of and are dependent upon the repression of women's desire and ambition. Both genders maintain an active interest in forestalling or prohibiting the return of this repressed material [18].

In accordance with that, Wirth-Cauchon says that the construction of the self as feminine creates a double bind. On the one hand, they must suppress their "non-feminine" aspects: autonomy and aggression. On the other hand, they must disavow their feminine embodiment: "In order to be valuable persons worthy of self esteem, women must control the body and access to it. The world of thought and action is the world of men; to enter it women must leave their distinctively female bodies and sexuality '*outside*'. One cannot be both a sexual, embodied woman and an esteemed thinker and effective actor in the world" [15].

Flax argues that "in women, '*social self*' predominates at the cost of the 'mutilation or denial of the other selves, sometimes, the social self is the part of the self that women are usually praised for—it strives to satisfy the needs of others it is capable of empathy; it desperately wants and needs interpersonal interactions… and one of the 'repressed selves can be the '*sexual self*'" [18]. Flax pays attention to cultural prohibitions and repressions and their psychic and bodily costs for women (Bourdieu's *habitus*).

31.5.1.4 Double Self

On the opposite side, we can find the alternate personality who, continuing with the "*sexual self*," for example, can sometimes perform the self described previously (more passive, reclusive, etc.) and at other times emerges like a alternate personality, seductive, dark, hypersensual, reproducing the cultural split between passive femininity and "forbidden" sexual autonomy, "the bitch" (with another voice, more authoritative, forceful). Yalom described the case of Marge in *Therapeutic Monogamy* [59] that illustrates an alternate personality with the previously mentioned features and where the split self can be understood as the embodiment or personification, in exaggerated form, of the dual image of women in Western perception, a duality that makes the passive and subordinate self irreconcilable with the powerful, hypersensual and sexual, and self-assertive self. Those aspects are split off and embodied in another person.

We can consider this as a rebellion of the self against the imposition from the socio-cultural environment (Bourdieu's *habitus*) of the dichotomist identity of women. The ultimate revenge would be the re-appropriation of hyperfemininity and the experience, in an integrated manner, of the female body "in evidence," the empowerment of the *"perra" ("bitch")* [60].

31.5.1.5 Interrupted Self

Sometimes the patients give descriptions of depersonalization, numbness, and emptiness. Susanna Kaysen, a woman who was hospitalized for nearly 2 years in McLean Psychiatric Hospital, describes some of the perceptions that contextualize on "the ever-shifting borderline that like all boundaries beckons and asks to be crossed." Kaysen's memoir uses spatial metaphors to describe the blurred border between sanity and madness, naming the area of madness the "parallel universe": "There are so many of them: worlds of the insane, the criminal, the crippled, the dying, perhaps of the dead as well. These worlds exist alongside this world and resemble it, but are not in it" [61]. She slips through one of the "perforations in the membrane between here and there."

She also narrates an altered perception of herself and her own body, describing a profound alienation from her body and fight against a sense that she does not exist as a flesh-and-blood person. She bites and scratches the body (the hand) to "try to get to the bottom of this; I wanted to see that my hand was a normal human hand, with bones" [61].

Susanna describes her emptiness like a response to her inability to fit into the narrow roles society offers white middle-class privileged girls. The feelings of inadequacy (unfitness) mixed with her resistance to these roles. She describes her madness as a form of resistance:

> As far as I could see, life demanded skills I didn't have. The result was chronic emptiness and boredom. . .Emptiness and boredom: what an understatement. What I felt was complete desolation. Desolation, despair and depression. . .
>
> My ambition was to negate. The world, whether dense or hollow, provokes only my negations. When I was supposed to be awake, I was asleep; when I was supposed to speak, I was silent; when a pleasure offered itself to me, I avoided it. My hunger, my thirst, my loneliness and boredom and fear were all weapons aimed at my enemy, the world. . .All my integrity seemed to lie in saying "NO," it was a very big NO—the biggest NO this side of suicide [61].

31.6 At the Border: Dependency and Fear of Abandonment, Anger, and Regulation of Emotion

> *Locura es la lógica estúpida de la vigilia que insiste en*
> *Que la identidad se sostiene a lo largo del tiempo y las desdichas.*
> *Como si yo, sin vos, fuera la misma persona*—Ana María Shua [62].

Many of the symptoms listed in the BPD diagnosis are indices of the difficulties that some individuals have in meeting their dependency needs and expressing their anger. Those are related to the difficulty in tolerating aloneness, engaging in self-destructive behavior, and proneness to outbursts of rage. Many BPD symptoms are severe manifestations of the problems commonly reported by "normal" women [14].

31.6.1 Dependency and the Fear of Abandonment

The term *dependent* has been used in a variety of ways: "to describe a need state (longing, oral needs), an affective state (feelings of helplessness, neediness), and even a personality trait (passive-dependent). A fixation at the oral or dependent stage signifies a failure on the adult's part to have attained maturity" [63]. Westkott points out, "ironically, female dependency is the developmental consequence of the historically created adult male dependence on women's physical and emotional caretaking" [64].

Becker said that in a society in which many women are encouraged "to suppress anger and placate those on whom they depend, it is not difficult to mistake social learning for intrapsychic phenomena and thereby to end up equating 'over-dependency' with mental illness" [14], with the same significance as the *habitus* of Bourdieu.

Stiver [63] differentiates dependency from the boundary confusions and fear of loss of self experienced by those whose wish to merge with another, which results from a lack of a cohesive self. The trend toward merger occurs not because of a failure to separate, but because of an inability to remain connected with others while asserting a distinct sense of self [65]. "This constitutes, therefore, a failure of connectedness and not a failure of autonomy. Even if people define themselves in relation to others, they must have some sense of the 'part' they are in the relation to the 'whole' in order to achieve interdependence in relationships" [14].

> The ability to make themselves known through the assertion of their needs is difficult for individuals who feel themselves to be the most unworthy and the boundary between assertiveness and aggression may be particularly ill-defined for women who do not feel that they have the right to make demands to others, creating a predicament potentially fraught with anxiety and guilt [66].

Sometimes, the dependent patients believe that they are worthless and they experience this sense of worthlessness as a hatred of their body, as the damping down of real feeling, and as a dislike of those characteristics that form their sense of their true self. Despite what they see as their real self, they compose another, idealized, self, made up of stereotypical and abstract feminine (or masculine) characteristics. In this way they have unwittingly achieved the internalization of culturally prescribed notions of femininity [14].

Karen Horney [67] said that a dependent woman literally lives "in the eyes of others," concerned with how others respond to her and judge her, "watching others, watch her." If she exists only in the eyes of others, she finds it difficult to be alone; she only has a self if she is interacting with others. For her, "being alone means both the loss of identity and the proof of being despicable, she may seek out the company of others with a compulsiveness that disregards their needs for privacy" (p. 160). Their vulnerability to criticism, disinterest from others or to disagreement makes any of these feel like an extreme attack. Because she is dependent on those who might mean her harm, her ability to discern harmful or abusive conditions is compromised, and she deals with such conditions by alternating between accusing the other and accusing herself [67].

31.6.2 Anger

Golpeando la puerta
De la casa vacía
No para que me abran
Para escucharme llamado—Hugo Mújica

Adolescent girls soon discover that expressing anger may expose them to criticism and isolation. The experience of anger itself can bring with it a sense of separateness, difference, and aloneness [68]. Depending upon the strength of the inhibition against its direct expression, anger can take forms that range along a continuum, one pole of which is self-destructive behavior [64]. The suppression of anger results in both frustration and inaction, producing a sense of weakness and a lack of self-esteem, further contributing to a sense of unworthiness and inferiority that, in turn, generates more anger. Women often report feeling filled with unwarranted, irrational anger, and although this description does not relay an accurate picture of their psychological situation, it is one "that the external world—so called 'reality'—is only too ready to confirm, because any anger is 'too much anger in women'. Indeed, the risk of expressing can appear grave and disorganizing. All this can end in a kind of self-fulfilling prophecy" [69].

"Too much is made of '*borderline*' anger and hostility, even though other emotions—sadness, anxiety, panic, shame, guilt, humiliation, and fear—are present for '*borderline*' women in great measure" [37]. Whether much of what is considered "*borderline*" *behavior* is seen to be associated with anger seems to depend on who is doing the observing. "Inferring anger and aggression from 'borderline' behavior rather than desperation and fear may well be related to the clinician" [37]. Many women (and some men also) tend to express anxiety as a secondary elaboration of suppressed anger. When they are confronting situations that are genuinely angering, they experience acute anxiety because they are not able to permit themselves to express the anger directly or because the suppression of anger has become so automatic that they cannot feel the anger at all [14].

We can see, in fact, that often women (or people around them) feel the necessity to justify their anger by attributing it to hormones in the premenstrual period, trying to accord the cause an external factor, biological because they do not feel within their rights to be able to express this as their own genuine emotion.

Macaulay points out that the psychoanalytical and psychodynamic schools have long endorsed a view of angry women being women who have "identity problems, are rejecting their proper sex role, are being poisoned by bottled-up anger, or are being destroyed by aggression turned inward—or all of these at once" [70].

31.6.3 Regulation of Emotion

In Linehan's view, BPD is in the main, a disorder of emotional dysregulation, and most borderline behaviors stem either from attempts to regulate intense emotion or are the results of affecting dysregulation. "Emotional dysregulation is both the problem the individual is trying to solve and the source of additional problems" [37]. Linehan's theory of the etiology of BPD symptoms rests upon biological as well as social learning foundations; however, some authors defend that social learning, in itself can help to create emotional vulnerability. Adaptation is a continuously transforming experience; faults of adaptation at one point affect how the individual adapts to the next phase.

31.7 The Body Talks

Nichter proposed the concept "*idiom of distress*" in 1981 to refer to "socially and culturally resonant means of experiencing and expressing distress in local worlds." "Idioms of distress communicate experiential states that lie on a trajectory from the mildly stressful to depths of suffering that render individuals and groups incapable of functioning as productive members of society" [71].

The symptoms of each of the diseases (hysteria, anorexia and bulimia, and BPD) becomes, in itself, a text converted in a body. It attributes to the body an increased meaning in relation to the ideals that are projected onto women, with a social, economic and political meaning (also emotional) that varies depending on the rules that determine the construction of gender in each historical period. In her analysis of "*female maladies*" such hysteria, agoraphobia, and anorexia, Bordo suggests that the symptoms of these disorders may be read as "literalizations" of women's social situation, the symptoms of these female maladies are politically symbolic: loss of mobility, loss of voice, inability to leave the home, feeding others while starving herself, taking up space, and whittling down the space one's body takes up, all have symbolic meaning, all have political meaning within the varying rules governing the historical construction of gender. Bordo argues that these women can be viewed as unconsciously protesting against the constraints of gender roles through their bodies, rather than through verbal articulation. Their bodily symptoms, therefore, can be read as signs of women's subjectivity and social position [50]. Romanyshyn provides a perspective for an interpretive reading of symptoms as signs of culturally excluded meanings; symptoms are carriers that the dominant culture would deny or repress. "A symptom as a way of ignoring or forgetting something is also a way of preserving or remembering it" [72].

Describing the feminine disorders such as post-traumatic stress disorder, anorexia/bulimia, and BPD, Griggers reads them as exaggerated signs of a more widespread social dysfunction. The author focuses in particular on dissociation, a common symptom in BPD. For Griggers dissociation in women signifies not simply individual women's suppressed memories, but the suppression and denial of historical memories of a circulating social violence. The symptomatic resurfacing of these memories in the form of numbness, states of depersonalization, or self-mutilation is frequently managed through psychopharmacology that aids in viewing such symptomatic memories as only individual rather than social in origin. Griggers' cultural analysis helps to reconnect these individual women's symptoms to their social sources [73].

The symptoms that come to be commonly grouped together under the borderline label—fragmented or unstable identity, feelings of emptiness or numbness, depersonalization, self-mutilation—may be meaningfully understood as exaggerated or extreme forms of some of the cultural contradictions of gender in late modern society, as fault lines of a cultural order in which the contradictions are visible at the moment of breakdown of the feminine subject.

People may find their "efforts to be heard and truly listened to intensely frustrating when the other person seems emotionally impervious. The result is often an escalation of intense feelings with increased loss of focus and diffusion of intense affective expression" [63].

31.7.1 Self-Destructiveness[1]

31.7.1.1 Self-Injury

Es quitar costra
Tras costra sobre nunca
Sangrar
Es rasguñar espejos
Con las uñas mordidas
¿por qué creerme más mi sangre
Que mis dedos?—Hugo Mújica

> How do you feel? Alive. Real. Calm. Satisfied. You smear the blood around. It's sick, but the blood feels real, feels human, feels good! At the same time, you feel the pain, you deserve the pain. You tell some people. They say you are manipulative, attention seeking. You believe it. Only serves to make you feel worse. Some people think you're sick, you're weird. One or two may understand, but they're still wary, still shocked by it. Some think you are suicidal. You're not [74].

The anthropological theory of the body discussed the self-injury from two theoretical frameworks:

(a) *Outside-in* theories (the body in the context of the culture): interpreting the symbolic meaning of the self-injury into the paradigm within the body as a metaphor for the paradigm in which the body is the metaphor of the *body–self–social*
(b) *Inside-out* theories (the body as a subject perceived): incorporating the emotional dimension (phenomenological) [75]

The self-injuries are related to three concepts:

(a) The embodied self
(b) Embodied emotions

[1] To compliment the information in this section we recommend the reader to consult the chapter *Life Instinct and Gender* (Chap. 13).

(c) Objectified body

Many people diagnosed as having BPD drink too much, shop too much, have eating problems, and/or engage in sexually promiscuous behavior; these behaviors are more likely to be viewed as variants of "normal" behaviors, whereas cutting, burning one's skin, or trying to kill oneself are not [14].

Self-injurious behavior (SIB) may take the form of self-mutilation through cutting, burning, or other; risk-taking behavior that could lead to self-harm; impulsivity in the form of substance or food abuse; or suicide attempts, etc., the different forms of self-injury, chronic self-mutilation is unarguably the behavior most readily recognized as "borderline," even though it is by no means restricted to the borderline patient [76].

Self-injurious behavior can become a central means by which borderline clients give expression to separation/abandonment conflicts [77] and relieve the cumulative tensions arising from the struggle for expression of anger and other emotional needs [76, 78]. Cutting the body may be conceived of literally as making an opening through which anger, tensions, anxiety, and a sense of badness can escape. These emotions, "often accompanied by feelings of powerlessness," affect an individual's sense of "stability and well-being and may create the sensation of an impending bodily explosion" [76].

Frequently, we find that the BPD's behavior is interpreted as "*manipulative*" and "*attention-getting*"; the patient him-/herself does not perceive it that way. The sense that many borderline patients have that their pain is worse than anyone else's may well be justified. The individual believes that no one cares about knowing the trouble, as no one has cared in the past; and, on the other hand, the patients believe that no one can ever know the trouble because no one has ever felt anything like the pain that they have experienced.

"For women at the border—and we also include here some men (on all gay people), transsexuals, intersexuals, etc., the sense that no one can comprehend the extent and intensity of her suffering is an understandable consequence of the sense of never having *been known*. The patients are saying to those around them, *not* 'I want you to suffer as I have suffered', but 'it is through my pain you shall know me'" [14].

31.7.1.2 Suicide

Susanna Kaysen describes how the lack of place and position in the society/life and her feelings of desolation led to a suicide attempt prior to her hospitalization. She explains her act as a war between aspects of herself. She took 50 aspirin and passed out in a supermarket in front of the meat counter and she describes her subjectivity like the meat at the meat counter [15]: "Bruised, bleeding, and imprisoned in a tight wrapping. I wanted to get rid of a certain aspect of my character. I was performing a kind of self-abortion with those aspirin." After having her stomach pumped, she feels she has succeeded, if only temporarily: "I felt good, I wasn't dead, yet something was dead" [61]. She tried to kill the fragmented side of the self whose existence is unbearable.

Van der Kolk considers that suicide attempts by "*borderlines*" may well be guided by interpersonal communications, whereas cutting primarily serves to regulate interwork emotional states [79]. According to Linehan, parasuicidal behaviors constitute an attempt, albeit a maladaptive one, to gain control over unbearably painful, overwhelming negative effects. From the point of view of patients: "Suicidal behavior is a reflection of serious at times frantic suicide ideation and ambivalence over whether to continue life or not. Although the patients' communication of extreme ideas or enactment of extreme behaviors may be accompanied by the desire to be rescued by the persons they are communicating with, this does not necessarily mean that they are acting in this manner in order to get help. Function does not prove intention" [37].

31.8 Reflection

Dana Becker argues that the borderline diagnosis has been "feminized" and that BPD became a new "female malady" for the late twentieth century [14]. We would like to add that today it is not only a feminized diagnosis, but someone who plays at the edges of the neutral, universal "*subject*" is at risk of being labeled.

As we have already mentioned in the text, in Western representational systems the humanistic vision of identity stands as a "generic, neutral, universal '*Subject*'" [47], based on a "masculine-type" construction. Many authors believe that women are represented as "*Other*" to this ideal of the universal subject. But not only the women are represented in this other, but anyone who does not meet or identify with that ideal of "*subject*."

There is a crucial debate about the intersection of the criticism of the obligatory heterosexuality and the rules on the able-bodied and "*ableism*" [80]. Ableism is based on the belief that some capacities are inherently more valuable, and those who possess them are "better" than the other; it is also based on the fact that there are a few bodies *able to* and others do not, some people who have functional disability and others who lack it. Ableism remarks that this division is sharp [81]. This ableism is composed of a medicalized notion of the "normal body" and a normative pattern of beauty that is central in our western society. Many voices draw attention to the parallels of critical theories on the functional diversity (*crip* theory) and its equivalent on sexuality (*queer* theory) that served to understand that sexuality or the functional diversity issues are not natural, or biological, but extremely rooted in cultural values, and are a product of specific historical moments.

Crip theory emerges after a long struggle against the injustices experienced by people who are regarded as "second-class" or located on the margins. *Crip* is a colloquial expression that is used to designate a person who has a disability and may not use any of its members. *Crip* is used also for designating someone who presents an significant limitation in a particular area. *Queer* theory is based on the concept of gender as a social construction, cultural and historic manufacturing that would not be determined by a truth or a substrate either natural or ontological.

The nexus between these theories is that both show that there are subjects with functional diversity and/or with non-normative sexualities that have a historical legacy of pathologization, subjects who need medical or legal monitoring and need the recognition of society to be accepted as "*people*." They also have a historical path by which they have been considered "sinful subjects," demonic or defective, comparable to the conception of witchcraft in women to which we have already referred in the text.

We consider the contributions of the *queer* and *crip* theories to be interesting, because they appear to look at the more dominant social norms, denouncing the inextricable links of power they subjected people to, and not so much in the "acceptation" of the subjects who break these rules (voluntarily or involuntarily). Their goal is not seeking to be accepted or assimilated by a mainstream society, the goal is posing serious challenges to the notions of normality or tolerance, which we consider essential in terms of gender aspects (and others also).

The DSM-5 says that to diagnose BPD, it is necessary to fulfill the "impairment in identity" criteria. If my identity is not in keeping with the "ideal and universal subject," if I feel myself on the margin, who am I? Where is my essence? Added to this "singing out of tune" are the confusion and the feeling of emptiness. At the same time we call into question the diagnosis of gender dysphoria or gender identity disorder. The need for people on the fringes is given by this need to benefit in a society where difference is institutionally rejected.

The diagnosis of BPD itself offers etiological closure, severing the causal link with trauma and abuse. The patients are now distressed (and "*difficult*") *because they have BPD*, rather than the behaviors associated with BPD being the result of oppression and abuse. Words such as "disorder" have the power to obstruct further understanding and can in themselves shape thought and practice. Diagnosing BPD positions the diagnosed as "other" in their distress and the recognition of the role of context difficult. Thus, the rapid rise in the diagnostic prevalence of BPD represents sometimes a shift from a limited recognition of the extent and impact of the trauma associated with sexual or physical abuse, to a widespread acceptance of an individualizing and pathologizing model of mental distress that conceals sexual abuse by focusing on categorizing, blaming, and "treating" the survivors. If we continue to define distress as symptoms of psychiatric illness rather than as a "realistic response to an unacceptable reality," we continue to deny the agency of people who have already been abused and silenced; we also deny ourselves the possibility of constructing a more acceptable life/reality. "Me and a gun and a man On my back But I haven't seen Barbados So I must get out of this" sings the artist Tori Amos, describing an episode in which she was raped. There have been admirers, but also much negative criticism of her exposure, accused of being indecent by making it public.

It is possible that the rise of new technologies and the possibility of living "alternative lives" online is not by chance. The aseptic space of the virtual world offers the possibility of living other identities expropriated from real life, claiming a space that has been denied.

The survival instinct warns us that we cannot be satisfied with a simple definition or with a limited vision of our individuality—de Lauretis [82].

References

1. Stern A. Psychoanalytic investigation of and therapy in the border line group of neuroses. Psychoanal Q. 1938;7:467–89.
2. APA. Diagnostic and statistical manual of mental disorders. 3rd ed. Washington, DC: American Psychiatric Association; 1987. Revised edition.
3. Roth A, Fonagy P. What works for whom? A critical review of psychotherapy research. London: Guildford; 1996.
4. Kernberg O. In: Wirth-Cauchon, editor. Women and the borderline personality disorder: Symptoms and stories. New Brunswick, NJ: Rutgers University Press; 2003.
5. Kernberg O. Borderline conditions and pathological narcissism. New York: Jason Aronson; 1975 (5º ed 2012).
6. APA. Diagnostic and statistical manual of mental disorders. 5th ed. Arlington, VA: American Psychiatric Association; 2013.
7. Lewis G, Appleby L. Personality disorder: The patients psychiatrists dislike. Br J Psychiatry. 1988;153:44–9.
8. Torgensen S, Kringlen E, Cramer V. The prevalence of personality disorders in a community sample. Arch Gen Psychiatry. 2001;58:590–6.
9. Johnson DM, Shea MT, Yen S, Battle CL, Zlotnick C, Sanislow CA, Grilo CM, Skodol AE, Bender DS, McGlashan TH, Gunderson JG, Zanarini MC. Gender differences in borderline personality disorder: Findings from the collaborative longitudinal personality disorders study. Compr Psychiatry. 2003;44(4):284–92.
10. APA. Diagnostic and statistical manual of mental disorders. 4th ed. Washington, DC: American Psychiatric Association; 1994.
11. Gunderson JG, Zanarini MC. Current overview of the borderline diagnosis. J Clin Psychiatry. 1991;42:1015–102.
12. Zanarini MC, Williams AA, Lewis RE, Reich RB, Vera SC, Marino MF. Reported pathological childhood experiences associated with the development of borderline personality disorder. Am J Psychiatry. 1997;154:1101–6.
13. Zanarini MC, Frankenburg FR, Reich DB, Marino MF, Haynes MC, Gunderson JG. Violence in the lives of adult borderline patients. J Nerv Ment Dis. 1999;187:65–71.
14. Becker D. Through the looking glass: Women and borderline personality disorder. Boulder, CO: Westview; 1997.
15. Wirth-Cauchon J. Women and the borderline personality disorder: Symptoms and stories. New Brunswick, NJ: Rutgers University Press; 2003.
16. Singer M. The experience of emptiness in narcissistic and borderline states: II. The struggle for a sense of self and the potential for suicide. Int Rev Psychoanal. 1977;4:471–9.
17. Schwartz-Salant N. The dead self in borderline personality disorders. In: Levin DM, editor. Pathologies of the modern self: Postmodern studies on narcissism, schizophrenia and depression. New York: New York University Press; 1987.
18. Flax J. Re-membering the selves: Is the repressed gendered? Mich Q Rev. 1986;26:92–110.
19. Ross M. The borderline diathesis. Int Rev Psychoanal. 1976;3:305–21.
20. Boyer BL. Working with a borderline patient. Psychoanal Q. 1977;46:386–424.
21. Butler J. Gender trouble: Feminism and the subversion of identity. New York: Routledge; 1990.
22. Beauvoir S. The second sex. New York: Vintage; 1989 (Trans. E.M. Parshley).
23. Cixous H, Clément C. The newly born woman. Minneapolis, MN: University of Minnesota Press; 1986 (Trans. B. Wing).

24. Bourdieu P. La domination masculine. París: Ëditions du Seuil; 1998 (7ª edición, Editorial Anagrama Barcelona, 2012).
25. Cauwels J. Imbroglio: Rising to the challenges of borderline personality disorder. New York: WW Norton; 1992.
26. Gunderson JG, Zanarini MC. Current overview of the borderline diagnosis. J Clin Psychiatry. 1987;48:5–11.
27. Henry KA, Cohen CI. The role of labeling processes in diagnosing borderline personality disorder. Am J Psychiatry. 1983;140(11):1527–9.
28. Sazsz T. The myth of mental illness. London: Paladin; 1972.
29. Foucault M. Madness and civilization – A history of insanity in the age of reason. London: Tavistock; 1967.
30. Showalter E. The female malady: Women, madness and English culture 1830–1980. New York: Penguin; 1985.
31. Mitchell SW. Rest in nervous disease (quoted in Strouse), 1980; p. 112.
32. Chesler P. Women and madness. 2nd ed. New York: Harcourt Brace Jovanich; 1989.
33. Hale Jr NG. Freud and the Americans: The beginnings of psychoanalysis in the United States, 1876–1917. New York: Oxford University Press; 1971.
34. Jimenez MA. Gender and psychiatry: Psychiatric conceptions of mental disorders in women, 1960–1994. Affilia. 1997;12(2):154–75.
35. Saw C, Proctor G. Women at the margins: A critique of the diagnosis of borderline personality disorder. Fem Psychol. 2005;15:483. doi:10.1177/0959-353505057620.
36. Samuels A. Gender and the borderline. In: Schwartz-Salant N, Stein M, editors. The borderline personality in analysis. Wilmette, III: Chiron; 1988.
37. Linehan M. Cognitive-behavioral treatment of borderline personality disorder. New York: Guilford Press; 1993.
38. Reiser DE, Levenson H. Abuses of the borderline diagnosis: A clinical problem with teaching opportunities. Am J Psychiatry. 1984;141(12):1528–32.
39. Department of Health. Women's mental health: Into the mainstream strategic development of mental health care for women. London: Department of Health; 2002.
40. Meichenbaum D. Treating post traumatic stress disorder: A handbook and practice manual for therapy. Chichester: Wiley; 1994.
41. Castillo H. You don't know what it's like. Mental Health Care. 2000;4(2):42–23, 53–58.
42. Masson J. The assault of truth: Freud's suppression of the seduction theory. Harmondsworth: Penguin; 1985.
43. Warner S, Wilkins T. Diagnosing distress and reproducing disorder: Women, child sexual abuse and borderline personality disorder. In: Reavey P, Warner S, editors. New feminist stories of childhood sexual abuse. London: Routledge; 2003. p. 167–86.
44. Wilkins TM, Warner S. Understanding the therapeutic relationship- women diagnosed as borderline personality disordered. Br J Forensic Pract. 2000;2(3):30–7.
45. Wilkins TM, Warner S. Women in special hospitals: Understanding the presenting behavior of women diagnosed with borderline personality disorder. J Psychiatr Ment Health Nurs. 2001;8: 289–97.
46. Herman J. Trauma and recovery. New York: Basic Books; 1992.
47. Sass L. The self and its vicissitudes: An archaeological study of the psychoanalytic avant-garde. Soc Res. 1988;55(4):551–607.
48. Rubin G. The traffic in women: Notes on the political economy of sex. In: Reiter RR, editor. Toward and anthropology of women. New York: Monthly Review Press; 1975.
49. Gallop J. Reading Lacan. Ithaca, NY: Cornell University Press; 1985.
50. Bordo S. Unbearable weight: Feminism, Western culture and the body. Berkeley, CA: University of California Press; 1997.
51. Herman A. The better angels of capitalism: Rhetoric, narrative and moral identity among men of the upper class. Boulder, CO: Westview Press; 1999.

52. Grosz E. Volatile bodies: Toward a corporeal feminism. Bloomington, IN: Indiana University Press; 1994.
53. Devita Singh MA, McMain S, Zucker KJ. Gender identity and sexual orientation in women with borderline personality disorder. J Sex Med. 2010;8(2):447–54.
54. Berger J. Ways of seeing. In: Showalter E, editor. The female malady: Women, madness and English culture 1830-1980. New York: Penguin; 1985. p. 212.
55. Deutsch H. Some forms of emotional disturbance and their relationship to schizophrenia. In: Stone MH, editor. Essential papers on borderline disorders: One hundred years at the border. New York: New York University Press; 1942.
56. Deutsch in Stone MH. Essential papers on borderline disorders: One hundred years at the border. New York: New York University Press, 1986.
57. Hoch P, Pollatin P. Pseudoneurotic forms of schizophrenia. Psychiatry Q. 1949;23:248–76.
58. Yalom ID, Elkin G. Every day gets a little closer: A twice-told therapy. New York: Basic Books; 1974.
59. Yalom ID. Therapeutic monogamy. In: Love's executioner and other tales of psychotherapy. New York: McGraw Hill; 1989.
60. Ziga I. Devenir perra. 1st ed. España: Melusina; 2009.
61. Kaysen S. Girl, interrupted. New York: Turtle Bay Books; 1993.
62. Shua AM. La muerte como efecto secundario. Buenos Aires: Editorial Sudamericana; 1997. p. 43.
63. Stiver IP. The meanings of dependency in female-male relationships. In: Jordan JV, Kaplan AG, Miller JB, Stiver IP, Surrey JL, editors. Women's growth in connection. New York: Guilford; 1991. p. 143–61.
64. Westkott M. The feminist legacy of Karen Horney. New Haven, CT: Yale University Press; 1986.
65. Gilligan C. In a different voice. Cambridge, MA: Harvard University Press; 1982.
66. Kirsch B. Status and verbal power assertion: Does gender of popularity better predict directive use? In: Franks V, Rothblum ED, editors. The stereotyping of women: Its effects on mental health. New York: Springer; 1983.
67. Horney K. The neurotic personality of our time. New York: WW Norton; 1937.
68. Lerner HG. Internal prohibitions against female anger. In: Lerner HG, editor. Women in therapy. Northvale, NJ: Jason Aronson; 1988. p. 59–75 (Reprinted from American Journal of Psychoanalysis 1980;40(2):137–48).
69. Miller JB. The construction of anger in women and men. In: Jordan JV, Kaplan AG, Miller JB, Stiver IP, Surrey JL, editors. Women's growth in connection. New York: Guilford; 1991. p. 181–96.
70. Macaulay J. Adding gender to aggression research: Incremental or revolutionary change? In: O'Leary VE, Unger RK, Wallston BS, editors. Women, gender and social psychology. Hillsdale, NJ: Lawrence Erlbaum; 1985. p. 191–224.
71. Nichter M. Idioms of distress: Alternatives in the expression of psychosocial distress: A case study from South India. Cult Med Psychiatry. 1981;5(5):379–408.
72. Romanyshyn R. Technology as dream and symptom. New York: Routledge; 1989.
73. Griggers C. Becoming woman. Minneapolis, MN: University of Minnesota Press; 1997.
74. Strong M. A bright red scream: Self-mutilation and the language of pain. New York: Viking Press; 1998.
75. Casadó ML. Antropología de las autolesiones corporals: cuerpo, identidad, género y emociones. Editorial Académica Española: OmniScriptum GmbH& Co. Alemania; 2013.
76. Favazza AR. Bodies under siege. Baltimore, MD: Johns Hopkins University Press; 1987.
77. Perry JC, Cooper SH. A preliminary report on defenses and conflicts in borderline personality disorder. J Am Psychoanal Assoc. 1986;34:863–93.
78. Waites E. Trauma and survival: Post-traumatic and dissociative disorders in women. New York: Norton; 1993.

79. van der Kolk BA, Perry JC, Herman JL. Childhood origins of self-destructive behavior. Am J Psychiatry. 1991;148:1665–71.
80. Peers D, Brittain M, Mcruer R. Crip excess, art and politics: A conversation with Robert Mcruer. Rev Educ Pedagogy Cult Stud. 2012;34(3–4):148–55.
81. Toboso M, Guzmán F. Cuerpos, capacidades, exigencias funcionales… y otros lechos de Procusto. Política y Sociedad. 2010;47(1):67–83.
82. De Lauretis, T. Diferencia e indiferencia sexual, Diferencias. Etapas de un camino a través del feminism. Cuadernos inacabados, nº 35, horas y Horas, Madrid, 2000.

Pathological Gambling: Clinical Gender Differences

32

Itxaso González-Ortega, Enrique Echeburúa, Paz de Corral, and Rocío Polo-López

Abstract

Little is known about gender-related differences among pathological gamblers in clinical samples because available data on the etiology and treatment of pathological gambling have involved predominantly male patients. However, significant gender differences in the clinical presentation of pathological gambling exist. Female gamblers are older than men and more likely to be divorced or widowed and to have a lower annual income. Women became more dependent on bingo and men on slot machines. Gambling motivation and the course of illness for the two sexes are also different. Female gamblers are more anxious and have poorer self-esteem than male gamblers and are more affected by depressive symptoms; in turn, men are more impulsive and greater sensation seekers than women and are more affected by drug/alcohol abuse. Among female gamblers, 70 % reported being victims of intimate partner violence. There are no gender differences with regard to the motivation for treatment. Future research should examine gambling behaviors and psychological functioning and suggest treatment approaches to address specific goals according to these gender-related differences.

I. González-Ortega (✉)
Department of Psychiatry, Alava University Hospital, Vitoria, Spain

CIBERSAM, Madrid, Spain

University of the Basque Country, San Sebastián, Guipúzcoa, Spain
e-mail: ITXASO.GONZALEZORTEGA@osakidetza.net

E. Echeburúa
CIBERSAM, Madrid, Spain

University of the Basque Country, San Sebastián, Guipúzcoa, Spain

P. de Corral • R. Polo-López
University of the Basque Country, San Sebastián, Guipúzcoa, Spain

M. Sáenz-Herrero (ed.), *Psychopathology in Women*,
DOI 10.1007/978-3-319-05870-2_32

32.1 Introduction

Over the past several decades, there has been a significant increase in the availability of legalized gambling in developed countries. The increasing availability of internet gambling through the uncontrolled presence of slot machines in bars and entertainment venues, along with the abundant supply of bingo, casinos, and more traditional games (football pools, sweepstakes, coupons, horse racing, etc.) has led to a considerable increase in pathological gambling [1].

Pathological gambling is characterized by loss of control over the game and by the establishment of a relationship of dependence. Gambling addiction is often accompanied by other disorders, such as alcohol abuse [2], depression [3], or personality disorders [4]. It is not, therefore, a single or isolated problem, but a serious disorder that interferes negatively with the quality of life and emotional well-being of those affected and the people around them [5]. In fact, this condition is considered a serious public health problem [6].

For a long time it was considered that pathological gambling, like other addictions, affects men more [7]. In fact, epidemiological studies conducted in the general population show that the disorder is much more common in men than in women (ratio of 7:3). Women constitute 30 % of all gamblers, but only 10–15 % of those attending treatment centers seek therapeutic help; thus, they are much more reluctant to recognize the problem. There is a double social moral in the gambling of women. Excessive gambling is tolerated in men in the early stages; however, women are classified quickly as vicious, leading to a greater concealment of the problem and therefore greater resistance to seeking therapeutic help [8]. Therefore, pathological gambling is not just a problem for men. In fact, helplessness against this onslaught of games of chance particularly affects teenagers and more psychologically vulnerable people. For many women and teens recreational game play has gone from a hobby to an addiction, with many additional problems: debts, school failure, family crises, problems with the law, etc. [9].

The psychological process that leads both sexes to acquire gambling behavior and the subsequent onset of pathological gambling is similar. That is, gamblers of both sexes are characterized by an emotional dependence on gambling, a loss of control, and a negative interference in the normal functioning of daily life [10], but they adopt differential profiles by gender. Differences in pathological gambling in women relative to men are manifested both in sociodemographic and gambling variables—that is, the gambling types involved, the motivation for gambling, and the acquisition and development of the disorder—as well as in the psychopathological and personality factors and the impact everyday life. The attitude toward treatment and therapeutic needs is also different in each case.

32.2 Differential Clinical Profile of Pathological Gambling in Men and Women

32.2.1 Sociodemographic Characteristics

Men and women gamblers differ in their sociodemographic profile. Overall, female gamblers were older than men [11, 12]. The most common age range for women is 46–65 years, that is, most are middle-aged women [12, 13]. By contrast, men are younger [12–14], around 38 years old, on average, predominantly within the range of 31–45 years and younger 30 [1]. In terms of marital status, both men and women are mainly married. However, women are more likely to be divorced or widowed and men to be single [11–13]. When the educational levels of gamblers are compared, there are no differences in terms of gender. Most men and women have had a primary education [12, 14]. Occupationally, most men and women are active. However, there is a higher percentage of women who remain in prolonged low work compared with men [11, 12, 14], with a lower socioeconomic status than male gamblers [11, 12]. Finally, familial support, however, is stronger in women than in men. Although female gamblers may be socially isolated more often than men, one reason for this controversial finding may be that the family in Spain is a powerful network and women have stronger bonds with relatives than men.

32.2.2 Gambling Variables

Gambling measures also reflect a wide range of gender-related differences.

32.2.2.1 Types of Gambling

There are differences in the types of gambling chosen by men and women gamblers. Slot machines were the most popular gambling method for both women and men pathological gamblers. Men tend to engage in types of gambling that involve strategy or competition and especially those involving high sensation seeking, and they are more dependent on slot machine gambling. Women, however, have problems with nonstrategic types of gambling, i.e., passive and less interpersonal and interactive gambling. Considering the characteristics of women gamblers, in addition to some cultural factors (bingo being socially acceptable in Spain for women), the bingo atmosphere has been described as more suitable for them than other gambling options (comfortable social situation and optimal strategy for escaping from problems and isolation) [14–18]. When women request the casinos and bingos prohibit them from entering, the risk of addiction on slot machines, however, increases, slot machines being the first choice for gambling and the bingo, the second option.

32.2.2.2 Motivation for Gambling

The diversity in terms of gender is also reflected in the differences in motivations for gambling. Whereas male gamblers were motivated to easily make money through gambling and were influenced by peer pressure, women were more motivated to gamble in order to cope with loneliness and to escape from unpleasant emotions, such as negative mood [12, 14]. Even gambling may be used to regulate any kind of negative emotional states associated with life events, dissatisfaction, and frustrations [19]. An alternative explanation is that problem gambling may exacerbate depressive symptoms more severely in women than men [20]. The findings of some studies highlight a stronger relationship between depressed mood and gambling pathology in women compared with men [11]. The nature of this relationship (problem gambling and depression) remains incompletely understood. More research is needed to identify gender-specific factors in this area.

32.2.2.3 Course of Illness

Regarding the course of illness, there are some significant aspect differentials between men and women gamblers. As occurs in other addictive behaviors (alcohol, smoking, etc.), women have a later age at onset of both gambling and the disorder. Men are more frequently early-onset gamblers and thus are more quickly affected by pathological gambling than women. However, women, even though they begin to gamble later than men, they become dependent on gambling more quickly than men [12, 14]. The explanation for this issue is controversial. Several studies have justified these findings from socio-cultural aspects [21] to psychopathological [22] or even neurobiological factors [23].

In terms of pathological gambling severity, there were no differences between men and women. Likewise, many pathological gamblers accumulated large debts, but no major differences by gender were found (58.8 % in men versus 42 % in women) [12, 13].

32.2.2.4 Predictors of Pathological Gambling Severity

Although certain predictors of pathological gambling are common to both men and women, there are gender differences in terms of pathological gambling severity. Specifically, depression is a predictor of pathological gambling severity in men [23–26]. There is no common consensus on whether patients suffer from depression before or after their gambling problem. It has been suggested that gambling can serve to enhance mood [27]. However, other authors have argued that depression arises as result of gambling-related problems [28], which would explain the higher incidence of depressive symptoms, suicidal ideation, and suicide attempts in this group [29, 30].

For female gamblers, duration of gambling disorder is a predictor of pathological gambling (PG) severity [26]. Early-onset gamblers had participated in gambling activities for a greater number of years, which may be associated with the development of psychiatric problems over the course of their lifetimes [31]. The development of disorder in women is faster when they have to cope with adverse life circumstances, such as loneliness or problems with the partner or children. Thus, PG usually appears in women in middle age or late life, controlled by negative reinforcement (avoidance of emotional distress and escape from everyday frustrations). A faster progression to PG also occurs when women lack self-management, communication, and problem-solving skills or when they have few resources to cope with psychological stress situations, most of all if the social support is low and the use of leisure time is unsatisfactory [12, 32].

With regard to gender differences in more severe pathological gamblers, female gamblers were older than male gamblers and started gambling later in life, but became dependent on gambling more quickly. This difference in the progress of the disorder (the telescoping effect) has also been found in other studies related to gambling [15, 33–36], but it is not so clear in the case of alcohol dependence [37]. The explanation of the telescoping effect is controversial. Several studies have justified these findings on the basis of socio-cultural [21], psychopathological [22] or even neurobiological factors [23].

Family support was also associated with female gamblers in the more severe subgroup [26]. Although female gamblers may fall into social isolation more often than men, one reason for this controversial finding may be that, as already mentioned, the family in Spain is a strong network and that women bond better with relatives than men [12].

In turn, alcohol abuse is associated with the subgroup of severe male gamblers [26]. Alcohol abuse is a common comorbid problem related to PG, and numerous studies have reported that there is a more frequent comorbid problem in male gamblers than in female ones [24, 34, 35, 38–40]. In fact, there is more genetic vulnerability to alcohol dependence and gambling in men [41], which is related to impulsivity in male gamblers. Impulsive behavior leads them to gambling more, and to having higher financial losses and more legal problems related to gambling [36, 42].

Finally, although in general low self-esteem is more likely to be associated with female gamblers [34, 36, 43], in the subgroup of more severe gamblers this variable is associated with men [26].

32.2.3 Personality Variables

Regarding personality variables, both men and women show a high level of impulsivity. However, as far as the difference between the genders is concerned, women are more anxious and suffered from a poorer self-esteem than male gamblers. Men, by contrast, are more impulsive and higher sensation seekers than women [12]. The high level of sensation seeking in men [44] may facilitate the initial contact and persistence with the gambling [43]. Moreover, the high level of anxiety/trait in women may be related to avoidance/exhaustive behaviors and anticipatory concern about a possible danger. The low self-esteem is also associated with a low level of autonomy and self-control, including skills such as responsibility for their own decisions, the availability of coping resources, self-esteem, and efficacy [36].

32.2.4 Psychopathological Variables

Pathological gamblers have a remarkable history of several other psychiatric disorders (51.5 %), which are likely to be key factors in developing harmful patterns of gambling. This fact affected women (60.8 %) more than men (40.4 %) [12].

Specifically, women have a higher level of depressive symptoms [11, 12, 14]. In fact, women show a greater history of suicide attempts than men, depression, with the risk of suicide, being the most common comorbid disorder in female gamblers, especially when gambling involves a phase of deterioration, which happens in the phases of loss, despair, and surrender [34].

The relationship between depression and pathological gambling in women can be explained by three factors [45] (a) is a disorder that occurs at higher rates among women in the general population and, therefore, also between pathological women players, (b) sometimes the gambling is the "escape" from the daily problems that are not seen out and (c) the gambling can serve as a trigger to overcome a depressed mood. However, this excessive gambling will cause other, more serious problems in the future, maintaining and even worsening depression and provoking the problem of pathological gambling. Depression in women is also more common when there is intimate partner violence or when the patient feels overwhelmed by family responsibilities (children's education, precarious economic situation, rejection of the couple, etc.), which entails greater feelings of loneliness and adaptive difficulties [46].

Therefore, depression in women may be a predisposing factor for gambling, suggesting that women with depressive symptoms may be involved in gambling, accentuating the depression with the unfavorable impact of gambling [11]. Thus, a vicious circle that is very hard to get out of is created. In men, however, depression may be secondary to gambling, linked to negative consequences of any kind [46].

It has also been suggested that women gamblers have a higher level of anxiety compared with men [11, 14, 40]. This would reinforce the idea that women gambling to escape their negative emotions, developing pathological gambling in an attempt to relieve anxiety–depressive symptoms [14].

On the other hand, men abuse alcohol and other drugs more than women do [12, 39, 47, 48]. However, there are conflicting results. Some studies indicate that both men and women gamblers show similar rates with respect to the abuse of tobacco, alcohol, and other drugs [49, 50]. Other studies, however, argue that the comorbidity between pathological gambling and abuse of alcohol and other drugs is associated with women [15, 51].

32.3 Impact of Pathological Gambling

Regarding the impact of pathological gambling, both in men and in women gamblers, pathological gambling has a number of negative consequences in different areas of life (personal, family, social, labor, economic, and legal). However, these problems manifest differently in men and women.

Personally, pathological gambling is often accompanied with other psychiatric comorbidity, such as alcohol and drug use in men and depression in women. For women gamblers, the suffering caused by financial losses and the insecurity of the addiction being discovered generate a state of irritability, nervousness, and emotional instability. The lies and delusions related to the gambling also accentuate the feeling of worthlessness and impair the self-esteem of women gamblers, facilitating the emergence of a depressed mood, which sometimes exists, but in others, it is a result of personal degradation and the family and social rejection experienced by women because of the addiction [46].

Regarding the negative impact on the family, and more specifically in the relationship, in the case of the woman gamblers the reaction of the husband or partner is much more intransigent than when he is having problems with the gambling [52]. In this context, there is intimate partner violence in 70 % of women gamblers (especially among women who are in situations of prolonged lows and/or jubilation) [12]. Gambling may be a way of escaping from a violent relationship, but that intimate partner violence may be also related to domestic conflict caused or exacerbated by financial or other stressors directly associated with gambling activities. All these findings highlight the importance of routinely screening gambling patients for anger and intimate partner violence and disrupted behavior in children, and the need to develop public policy, prevention and treatment programs to address these problems [53].

On the other hand, the negative social stigma, accentuated in the case of women, contributes to greater social isolation, which is the result of the attempt of women to hide their reality to other people and the social rejection of people around [46]. However, women have more family support than men (92 % of cases). This may be due to the skewed ideas of women with regard to the availability of perceived support and actual support. Another explanation may be also related to the fact that women may have the support of other significant family-level people (brothers, sons, uncles, etc.), and the support of the partner.

Moreover, the emotional consequences associated with gambling problems manifest as feelings of guilt, shame or fear. In this sense, both men and women report feelings of guilt for playing that reach a very high percentage (92.3 % and 96.1 % respectively) [12]; unlike other studies, which have found that these feelings are more pronounced in the case of women [54].

Finally, with regard to the consequences at the working level, there is a higher percentage of women who remain in a state of prolonged low (19 %) compared with men (6 %). Moreover, both men and women experience a variety of financial problems and high rates of gambling-related debt. 58.4 % of the gamblers of both sexes show significant debts [12].

32.4 Motivation for Treatment

As is well-known [55], many pathological gamblers do not seek treatment. Motivating pathological gamblers to enter and adhere to treatment is difficult. Even though pathological gamblers decide to seek treatment, they are not uniformly committed to change. In fact, the dropout rates during assessment were six times higher than those of a clinical control of non-addict treatment-seeker patients [12].

Some studies indicate that women gamblers come to less frequently than men to treatment centers seeking therapeutic help [56] and are therefore less likely to receive treatment for a gambling problem [57]. However, the percentage of pathological women gamblers in the population is greater than in treatment centers [58]. This is especially problematic, as women experience a greater negative impact as a result of pathological gambling compared with men [16].

This pattern of behavior is far from what usually happens in mental health centers with other psychiatric disorders [59] or primary care services [60], where prevalence rates are higher in women, which means that, in general, they seek therapeutic help further and faster than men. However, some studies have found that it is more likely that female gamblers (32 %) seek therapeutic help compared with men (13 %) [61]. This finding is consistent with other studies in which the rate of therapeutic help finding is also higher among women than among men [17, 39].

Crisp et al. [62], found that the proportion of men and women attending treatment centers is similar. However, women were more likely to complete treatment and resolve the gambling problem. In the study conducted by Echeburúa et al. [12], however, there were no gender-related differences among drop-outs.

High rates of treatment seeking among women may be explained by the fact that women, unlike men, although they initially hide the problem, once they recognize it, they believe that professional help is needed [63]. Moreover, women have a more positive attitude toward mental health in general, as well as a greater willingness to seek therapy. They therefore tend to show comfort when talking about problems with a professional and do not feel embarrassed about the need to seek help [64].

Women often perform gambling behavior in secret. The negative social stigma, particularly marked in women, helps to hide problem recognition and delay seeking therapeutic help. Generally, the female gambler is seeks treatment alone. Unlike male gamblers, who are usually accompanied by some of their close relatives (spouse or mother), the woman attends by herself and has an active collaboration in the treatment of a spouse or adult children [65]. Usually, women tend to seek treatment after having a very serious episode of gambling and come very emotionally affected to the centers [66]. It is often the deterioration of the family relationship that is the critical variable that determines seeking of therapeutic help. In contrast to male gamblers, who adopt a more egocentric, arrogant and denying attitude, women gamblers, once they have taken the first step toward seeking help, they are more aware of what has happened and show great shame [45].

Generally, most pathological gamblers seek help when they have health or psychological problems or face financial ruin, rather than being motivated by the gradual recognition of the problem behavior. Major depression and the inability to pay bills or to return money loans are the main sources of their problems and the critical factor for change. The main obstacles to seeking therapeutic help are psychological factors such as denial of the problem or embarrassment and the belief that they will finally be able to gain control by themselves, or they will be able to make more money out of their difficulties [67].

These impediments hinder the seeking of therapeutic help in women more than in men, making them initially more reluctant to resort to assistive devices [68]. Personal and interpersonal variables can interfere with access to treatment seeking in female gamblers. The influence of his intimate partner, the stage of recovery, the feelings of shame, guilt and fear, among other things, may give rise to denial that a problem exists, delaying an opportunity of going for treatment [54]. Not knowing what help is available or believing that her problem is simply financial can also lead women to feel ashamed and that they have to cope alone with the countless financial problems. Moreover, the socio-environmental factors, such as lack of social or family support, lack of financial resources, the negative social stigma, and the lack of specialized training by professionals, can also hinder or delay therapy seeking for women [69]. In response to these limitations, there is a need to increase the visibility in terms of problem gambling, especially in women, and to increase treatment services and specialized personnel in the area of pathological gambling [54].

32.5 Conclusions

There are relevant gender-related differences in demographics, gambling measures, psychological functioning, and motivation for treatment in pathological gamblers, which may be taken into account when planning an effective intervention (Table 32.1).

These findings suggest that gender carries factors determining distinct pathogenetic mechanisms in pathological gambling. There are many explanations for gender playing patterns. Among the explanations put forth are: genetics [70], social norms [36], motivations [71], impulsivity [72], and finances [73]. It is important, however, not merely to explain gender differences about prejudices with regard to the way men and women "are." Such gross generalizations are unlikely to maintain any predictive power over time as gender roles change [18].

Treatment of pathological gambling must address the gender differences that relate to gambling behavior. Currently, treatment programs for PG are primarily designed for men [74] and are not adjusted to the specific characteristics of women gamblers [75]. The need to establish an empathic relationship and adapt the therapy to their specific problems and requirements is critical to successful treatment [8].

Table 32.1 Gender differences among pathological gamblers [12]

	Women	Men
Socio-demographic factors		
Age	46–55	31–45
Marital status	Married	Single
Educational level	Primary studies	
Employment status	Prolonged low	Active
Socioeconomic level	Lower	Medium
Personality variables	Anxiety Self-esteem	Sensation seeking
Psychopathological variables	Depression	Alcohol and other drugs abuse
Gambling variables		
Types of gambling	Bingo	Gambling machines
Motivation for gambling	Loneliness/escape	Social pressure Winnings
Course of illness	Late onset Faster progression	Early onset Slower progression
Predictors of pathological gambling severity	Duration of the disorder	Depression

32.6 Future Challenges

The main challenge for the future in the field of pathological gambling is to develop treatment programs specifically geared toward the different needs of men and women gamblers. The treatment oriented toward women gamblers should focus on the gambling, in addition to other related pathological deficits experienced by women gamblers, such as depression, loneliness, low self-esteem or couples therapy. It is very important to design interventions that promote a new lifestyle that gives them more social reinforcement, greater economic autonomy, incorporation into the workforce, and higher professional qualifications, which all help these women to overcome their social isolation [76].

Considering the most pronounced impact in the case of women in the family and couples, treatment should also include assessment and counseling on gender violence and guidelines for the education of children, as well as social skills and problem-solving training [56].

Moreover, support groups for women gamblers represent an important aspect of treatment because women addicted to gambling often do not have family/social support and experience social isolation [69].

A key aspect is also to design motivational strategies to attract women to treatment centers. Having early detection instruments (for application, e.g., in the field of primary care centers or social services), given the presence of somatic symptoms in women gamblers, is fundamental.

Finally, a suggested line of research is to develop intervention programs for accompanying women gamblers (couples, daughters or mothers), so that efforts to attract treatment to patients or to act as co-therapists are as effective as possible [46].

References

1. Labrador FJ, Becoña E. Conductas adictivas. Teoría, evaluación y tratamiento. In: Graña JL, coordinador. Juego patológico: Aspectos epidemiológicos y teorías explicativas. Madrid: Debate; 1994. p. 495–520.
2. Kessler RC, Hwang I, LaBrie R, Petukhova M, Sampson NA, Winters KC, Shaffer HJ. DSM-IV pathological gambling in the National Comorbidity Survey Replication. Psychol Med. 2008;38: 1351–60.
3. Kim SW, Grant JE, Eckert ED, Faris PL, Hartman BK. Pathological gambling and mood disorders: Clinical associations and treatment implications. J Affect Disord. 2006;92:109–16.
4. Echeburúa E, Fernández-Montalvo J. Are there more personality disorders in treatment-seekers pathological gamblers than in other kind of patients? A comparative study between the IPDE and the MCMI. Int J Clin Health Psychol. 2008;8:53–64.
5. Fernández-Montalvo J, Echeburúa E. Pathological gambling and personality disorders: An exploratory study with the IPDE. J Person Disord. 2004;18:500–5.
6. Muñoz-Molina Y. Meta-análisis sobre juego patológico. 1997–2007. Revista de Salud Pública. 2008;10:150–9.
7. Potenza M, Steinberg M, McLaughlin S, Wu R, Rounsaville B, O'Malley S. Gender-related differences in the characteristics of problem gamblers using a gambling helpline. Am J Psychiatry. 2001;158:1500–5.
8. Corral P. Ludopatía y mujer. Mente y cerebro. 2007;22:2–7.
9. Becoña E, Míguez M, Vázquez F. El juego problema en los estudiantes de enseñanza secundaria de 14 y más años de Galicia. Psicothema. 2001;13:551–6.
10. Echeburúa E, Báez C. Enfoques terepeúticos en el tratamiento psicológico del juego patológico. Revista Española de Terapia del Comportamiento. 1991;8:127–46.
11. Desai RA, Potenza MN. Gender differences in the associations between past-year gambling problems and psychiatric disorders. Social Psychiatry Psychiatr Epidemiol. 2008;43:173–83.
12. Echeburúa E, González-Ortega I, de Corral P, Polo-López R. Clinical gender differences among adult pathological gamblers seeking treatment. J Gambl Stud. 2011;27:215–27.
13. Weiss L, Petry N. Psychometric properties of the Inventory of Gambling Situations with a focus on gender and age differences. J Nerv Ment Dis. 2008;196:321–8.
14. Granero R, Penelo E, Martínez-Giménez R, Alvarez-Moya EM, Aymamí N, Bueno B, et al. Sex differences among treatment-seeking adult pathologic gamblers. Compr Psychiatry. 2009;50:173–80.
15. Potenza MN, Steinberg MA, Wu R, Rounsaville BJ, O'Malley SS. Characteristics of older adult problem gamblers calling a gambling helpline. J Gambl Stud. 2006;22:241–54.
16. Grant J, Von Kim S. Gender differences in pathological gamblers seeking medication treatment. Compr Psychiatry. 2002;43:56–62.
17. Crisp BR, Thomas SA, Jackson AC, Smith S, Borrell J, Ho W, et al. Not the same: A comparison of female and male clients seeking treatment from problem gambling counselling services. J Gambl Stud. 2004;22:81–99.
18. LaPlante DA, Nelson SE, LaBrie RA, Shaffer HJ. Men & women playing games: Gender and the gambling preferences of Iowa gambling treatment program participants. J Gambl Stud. 2006;22:65–80.
19. Scannell ED, Quirk MM, Smith K, Maddern R, Dickerson M. Females' coping styles and control over poker machine gambling. J Gambl Stud. 2000;16:417–32.

20. Lesieur HR, Blume SB. When lady luck loses: Women and compulsive gambling. In: Van Den Bergh N, editor. Feminist perspectives on addictions. New York: Springer; 1991. p. 181–97.
21. Cunningham-Williams RM, Cottler LB, Comptom WM, Spitznagel EL. Taking chances: Problem gamblers and mental health disorders: Results from the St. Louis epidemiologic catchment area study. Am J Public Health. 1998;88:1093–6.
22. Lynch WJ, Maciejewski PK, Potenza MN. Psychiatric correlates of gambling in adolescents and young adults grouped by age at gambling. Arch Gen Psychiatry. 2004;61:1116–22.
23. Potenza MN, Xian H, Shah K, Scherrer JF, Eisen SA. Shared genetic contributions to pathological gambling and major depression in men. Arch Gen Psychiatry. 2005;62:1015–21.
24. Ibáñez A, Blanco C, Donahue E, et al. Psychiatric comorbidity in pathological gamblers seeking treatment. Am J Psychiatry. 2001;158:1733–5.
25. Beck AT, Steer RA. Manual for the Beck depression inventory. San Antonio: Psychological Corporation; 1993.
26. González-Ortega I, Echeburúa E, de Corral P, Polo-López R, Alberich S. Predictors of pathological gambling severity taking gender differences into account. Eur Addict Res. 2013;19:146–54.
27. Roy A, Custer R, Lorenz V, Linnoila M. Depressed pathological gamblers. Acta Psychiatr Scand. 1988;77:163–5.
28. McCormick RA, Taber JI. Attributional style in pathological gamblers in treatment. J Abnorm Psychol. 1988;297:368–70.
29. Lesieur HR. The chase. Career of the compulsive gambler. Cambridge: Schenkman Books; 1984.
30. Taber JT, McCormick RA, Ramirez LF. The prevalence and impact of major life stressors among pathological gamblers. Int J Addict. 1987;22:71–9.
31. Burge AN, Alesia N. Age of gambling initiation and severity of psychiatric, family/social, and substance abuse problems among treatment-seeking pathological gamblers. UCHC Graduate School Masters Theses. Paper 2. 2005.
32. Echeburúa E, González-Ortega I, Corral P, Polo-López R. Pathological gamblers and a non-psychiatric control group taking gender differences into account. Span J Psychol. 2013; 16(e2):1–9.
33. Grant JE, Kim SW, Odlaug BL, Buchanan SN, Potenza MN. Late-onset pathological gambling: Clinical correlates and gender differences. J Psychiatr Res. 2009;43:380–7.
34. Ibáñez A, Blanco C, Moreryra P, Saiz J. Gender differences in pathological gambling. J Clin Psychiatry. 2003;64:295–301.
35. Tavares H, Martins SS, Lobo DS, Silveira CM, Gentil V, Hodgins D. Factors at play in faster progression for female pathological gamblers: An exploratory analysis. J Clin Psychiatry. 2003;64:433–8.
36. Ladd GT, Petry NM. Gender differences among pathological gamblers seeking treatment. Exp Clin Psychopharmacol. 2002;10:302–9.
37. Keyes KM, Martins SS, Blanco C, Hasin DS. Telescoping and gender differences in alcohol dependence: New evidence from two national surveys. Am J Psychiatry. 2010;167:969–76.
38. Welte JW, Barnes GM, Wieczorek WF, Tidwell M, Parker J. Alcohol and gambling pathology among US adults: Prevalence, demographic patterns, and comorbidity. J Stud Alcohol. 2001; 62:706–12.
39. Blanco C, Hasin DS, Petry N, Stinson FS, Grant BF. Sex differences in subclinical and DSM-IV pathological gambling: Results from the National epidemiologic survey on alcohol and related conditions. Psychol Med. 2006;36:943–53.
40. Wenzel HG, Dahl AA. Female pathological gamblers – A critical review of the clinical findings. Int J Ment Health Addict. 2009;7:190–202.
41. Slutske WS, Eisen S, True WR, Lyons MJ, Goldberg J, Tsuang M. Common genetic vulnerability for pathological gambling and alcohol dependence in men. Arch Gen Psychiatry. 2000; 57:666–74.

42. Nelson SE, LaPlante DA, LaBrie RA, Shaffer HJ. The proxy effect: Gender and gambling problem trajectories of Iowa Gambling Treatment Program participants. J Gambl Stud. 2006; 22:221–40.
43. Álvarez-Moya EM, Jiménez-Murcia S, Granero R, Vallejo J, Krug I, Bulik CM, et al. Comparison of personality risk factors in bulimia nervosa and pathological gambling. Compr Psychiatry. 2007;48:452–7.
44. Blaszczynski A, Steel Z, McConaghy N. Impulsivity in pathological gambling: The antisocial impulsivity. Addiction. 1997;92:75–87.
45. Becoña E. Características de la mujer jugadora patológica. Revista de Psicopatología y Psicología Clínica. 1997;2:21–34.
46. Corral P, Echeburúa E, Irureta M. Perfil psicopatológico diferencial de las mujeres ludópatas: implicaciones para el tratamiento. Análisis y Modificación de Conducta. 2005;31:539–56.
47. Dannon PN, Lowengrub K, Aizer A, Kotler M. Pathological gambling: Comorbid psychiatric diagnoses in patients and their families. Isr J Psychiatry Relat Sci. 2006;43:88–92.
48. Desai RA, Maciejewski PK, Pantalon MV, Potenza MN. Gender differences among recreational gamblers: Association with the frequency of alcohol use. Psychol Addict Behav. 2006; 20:145–53.
49. Grant JE, Potenza MN. Tobacco use and pathological gambling. Ann Clin Psychiatry. 2005; 17:237–41.
50. Martins SS, Tavares H, da Silva Lobo DS, Galett AM, Gentil V. Pathological gambling, gender, and risk-taking behaviors. Addiction. 2004;29:1231–5.
51. Petry NM, Stinson FS, Grant BF. Comorbidity of DSM-IV pathological gambling and other psychiatric disorders: Results from the National Epidemiologic Survey on Alcohol and Related Conditions. J Clin Psychiatry. 2005;66:564–74.
52. Custer RL, Milt H. When luck runs out. New York: Facts on File Pub; 1985.
53. Picó-Alfonso MA, Echeburuúa E, Martínez M. Personality disorder symptoms in women as a result of chronic intimate male partner violence. J Fam Violence. 2008;23:577–88.
54. Piquette-Tomei N, Dwyer SC, Norman E, McCaslin E, Burnet J. Women problem gamblers want more. Saskatchewan Notes (Canadian Centre for Policy Alternatives–SK). 2007;6:1–4.
55. Hodgins DC, Currie SR, El-Guebaly N. Motivational enhancement and self-help treatments for problem gambling. J Consult Clin Psychol. 2001;69:50–7.
56. Ciarrocchi J. Counseling problem gamblers: A self regulated manual for individual and family therapists. San Diego, CA: Academic Press; 2002.
57. Urbanoski KA, Rush BR. Characteristics of people seeking treatment for problem gambling in Ontario: Trends from 1998 to 2002. J Gambl Stud. 2006;16:1–21.
58. Echeburúa E, Báez C, Fernández-Montalvo J, Páez D. El Cuestionario de Juego de Soath Oaks (SOGS): validación española. Análisis y Modificación de Conducta. 1994;20:769–91.
59. Wang PS, Lane M, Olfson M, Pincus HA, Wells KB, Kessler RC. Twelve-month use of mental health services in the United States: Results from the National Comorbidity Survey replication. Arch Gen Psychiatry. 2005;62:629–40.
60. Smith JA, Braunack-Mayer A, Wittert G. What do we know about men's help-seeking and health service use? Med J Aust. 2006;184:81–3.
61. Pulford J, Bellringer M, Abbott M, Clarke D, Hodgins D, Williams J. Barriers to helpseeking for a gambling problem: The experiences of gamblers who have sought specialist assistance and the perceptions of those who have not. J Gambl Stud. 2009;25:33–48.
62. Crisp B, Thomas S, Jackson A, Thomason N, Smith S, Borrel J, et al. Sex differences in the treatment needs and outcomes of problem gamblers. Res Soc Work Practice. 2000;10:229–42.
63. Kessler RC, Brown RL, Broman CL. Sex differences in psychiatric help-seeking: Evidence from four large-scale surveys. J Health Soc Behav. 1981;22:49–64.
64. Mojtabai R. Americans' attitudes toward mental health treatment-seeking: 1990–2003. Psychiatr Serv. 2007;58:642–51.

65. Arbinaga F. La mujer con problemas en los juegos de apuesta: una aproximación desde los estudios epidemiológicos realizados en nuestro país y el análisis de nuevos datos sobre un grupo de mujeres en Punta Umbría (Huelva). Psicologemas. 2001;15:133–52.
66. Echeburúa E. Nuevas fronteras en el estudio del juego patológico. Madrid: Fundación Ramón Areces; 2006.
67. Evans L, Delfabbro P. Motivators for change and barriers to help-seeking in Australian problem gamblers. J Gambl Stud. 2005;21:133–55.
68. Rush B, Moxam RS, Urbanoski KA. Characteristics of people seeking help from specialized programs for the treatment of problem gambling in Ontario. J Gambl Issues. 2002;6:1–21.
69. Boughton R, Brewstern J. Voices of women who gamble in Ontario: A survey of women's gambling, barriers to treatment and treatment service needs. Toronto: Ontario Ministry of Health and Long-Term Care; 2002.
70. Winters KC, Rich T. A twin study of adult gambling behavior. J Gambl Stud. 1998;14:213–25.
71. Trevorrow K, Moore S. The association between loneliness, social isolation and women's electronic gaming machine gambling. J Gambl Stud. 1998;14:263–84.
72. Langewisch MW, Frisch G. Gambling behaviour and pathology in relation to impulsivity, sensation seeking, and risk behaviour in male of college students. J Gambl Stud. 1998;14:245–62.
73. Hing N, Breen H. Profiling lady luck: An empirical study of gambling and problem gambling amongst female club members. J Gambl Stud. 2001;17:47–69.
74. American Psychological Association. Guidelines for psychological practice with girls and women. Am Psychol. 2007;62:949–79.
75. Tavares H, Zilberman ML, Beites FJ, Gentil V. Gender differences in gambling progression. J Gambl Stud. 2001;17:151–9.
76. Llinares MC, Santos P, Albiach C, Camacho I, Palau C. Diferencias de sexo en adictos a las máquinas tragaperras. Adicciones. 2006;18:371–6.

Somatoform and Factitious Disorders 33

Julia García-Albea, Pedro García-Parajuá, and Marta Navas

Abstract

Gender seems to be a core issue in the diagnosis and treatment of somatomorphic disorders. It is well known that the categorization of these disorders has caused some controversy. On the one hand, this controversy shows the limitation of the mind–body dual model that underlies Western medical thinking, in some way overlooking that pain and corporal awareness are not divided from the subjective experience of the self. This group of mental disorders has suffered several modifications, as shown in the different editions of the *Diagnostic and Statistical Manual of Mental Diseases* (DSM), although its validity and gender neutrality is still inconclusive. First in this chapter, we analyze gender perspective related to somatization and in particular the somatoform disorder classification. Second, we describe somatoform disorders as in the classic terminology, considering the new definition proposed in the latest edition of the DSM. Nevertheless, it is not clear whether these new diagnostic criteria for somatoform disorders have reached gender neutrality.

33.1 Introduction

The somatomorphic disorder group represents one of the groups that has changed the most in their classification system for mental illnesses [1, 2]. This chapter includes somatization disorder, hypochondriac disorder, conversion disorder, and

J. García-Albea (✉)
University Clinic Hospital, Madrid, Spain
e-mail: Jul16598@yahoo.es

P. García-Parajuá
Clinical University Hospital Puerta de Hierro, Madrid, Spain

M. Navas
Department of Psychiatry, Infanta Leonor Hospital, Madrid, Spain

M. Sáenz-Herrero (ed.), *Psychopathology in Women*,
DOI 10.1007/978-3-319-05870-2_33

factitious disorder, bearing in mind their appellation and categorization in the *Diagnostic and Statistical Manual of Mental Diseases, fifth edition* (DSM-V). Dysmorphic body disorder is also included, even though it has been relocated in the new edition of the DSM to the group of disorders related to obsessive compulsive disorder. What these disorders have in common is the presence of physical symptoms with no medical explanation (also known as somatic symptoms), concerns for these symptoms, and illness behavior including medical consultation and sanitary resource consumption.

Symptoms with no medical explanation (or somatization) or the excessive concern for the symptoms frequently present a clinical problem that accounts for half of all primary consultations [3]. However, categorization of these disorders has caused some controversy. On the one hand, this argument shows the limitation of the mind–body dual model that underlies Western medical thinking, in some way overlooking the idea that pain and corporal awareness are not divided from the subjective experience of the self [4]. On the other hand, from the beginning of the proposal as a psychiatric diagnosis, a great variability in expressions and frequency has been observed, depending on the cultural and social group. In Western culture, except for hypochondriac and dysmorphic body disorders, it has come to attention that there is a high prevalence of women with disorders compared with men. Beyond specific sexual somatic symptoms, these differences clearly question gender disorder neutrality.

33.2 Gender and Somatization

The term "gender," introduced in the 1950s by Money, is not equivalent to "sex." However, it is very frequent that medical literature uses gender and sex as interchangable [5]. Gender refers to the self-representation of people as man or woman and psychosocial representations of living like a man or a woman. It includes biological, psychological, and social aspects as well as their complexities; thus, it is actually a distinctive feature. A person's sex is genetically determined at the moment of conception and is not a question of choice. However, the way a man or a woman lives in the gender assigned can diverge in many different directions [6]. Gender can affect virtually all aspects in psychopathology, including the prevalence of mental illness, symptom expression, the course of the illness, the different ways patients search for help, and the response to treatment.

In this way, gender is the result of a complex process of interaction between genome and environment, interaction that takes place during the different phases of development and peaks with the expression of a particular phenotype, which includes the individual's conduct characteristics [7]. Gender is an assigned identity that includes conduct within its diverse forms of expression, which is precisely one of the key elements in the configuration of psychiatric diagnoses. Women, on the other hand, are more exposed to adverse environmental circumstances, which can be conducive to specific clinical patterns.

Based on the reproductive capacity of women, sexual division was established within human activities, as well as demands and expectations of society, regarding the subjects by sex. According to the dominant interpretation of sexual difference, because women have the capacity for pregnancy, parenting, and looking after the household, they are considered as tasks specifically for them. According to this notion, women are conceived as a "beings for others" [8]. The psyche of women is then influenced by symbolic and material prodigality; this assignment builds a symbolic and material space whose referent is the household, the private space.

If we go back to a more psychoanalytical perspective as a way of a woman expressing her somatic symptoms compared with men, we find that there is an early attachment of women to their mother, which establishes the sense of herself based on the connection and fusion with each other. In women, attachment is carried over to the husband; this fact can originate a higher level of responsibility that women show in marriage commitments and they are more affected by damage to family ties.

All these factors create a feminine identity generally characterized by subjectivity, subordination, fear, weakness, and dependence. This is translated into body expression with discomfort, showing somatization, pain, and conversion, and displeasure for not agreeing with what has been imposed for years, the inability to rebel against or deny the wish for a domestic life of motherhood.

Although men have been provided with greater possibilities of self-realization and enjoy sexual and professional advantages, this can imply certain health risks. Males build their identity in opposition to the feminine; the first reference with whom they interact is their mother and through her they enter the symbolic world.

Male behavior supposed as essential is configured through defensive maneuvers, which include aggressiveness, competitiveness, independence, and attachment to external reality. This set of attributes also includes more security, decisiveness, domain and protective with the weak, more physical strength, "adventurous spirit," less responsibility for family commitments, and more experimentation [9, 10].

Although it is being modified, women's social recognition is still restricted to the domestic and family ambience. The male identifying process is modulated by social demands, which include economic success and public recognition. The feminine character, delimited by a greater internalization of women and the devaluation of their concerns by themselves, can lead them easily to failure and sadness, and with this would come somatizations, which are so often associated with a low mood [11]. Social and employment situations for women in Europe have been modified very significantly in the last few years, as well as coexistence, because of demographic and sanitary changes that have occurred (increase in chronic diseases and life expectancy). This new scenery has led institutions to implement diverse public policies around them, so-called family and work conciliation [12].

Historical data leave no doubt: three quarters of caring is done by families, and within them, a similar proportion by adult women [13]. Nowadays, caring is an absolutely gendered task and it is an activity that is not well seen or socially recognized. It is assumed that women for the virtue of being, have the abilities and knowledge needed to be a caregiver; additionally, this task remains private so it makes it difficult to be recognized. Also, the highly affective and moral burden of the caregiver's job makes it even more difficult to have the right to complain and there are high chances of developing somatic patterns as the only method of expression.

33.2.1 Gender Differences in Somatic Disorder Classification

Almost from the beginning of the proposal as a somatomorphic disorder diagnosis, somatic disorder in particular; the gender issue has been present as a subject of debate.

Except for hypochondria and body dysmorphic disorder, the somatomorphic disorders (under the new name, somatic symptom disorder) have a prevalence that is ten times higher in women.

Neutral gender diagnostic criteria for men and women are identical, assuming they are equally valid for both sexes. This option is used in almost all sets of DSM-IV TR diagnostic criteria, except for a few. The problem with this option occurs when there is a gender slant when a diagnosis is applied wrongly, more frequently to one sex or the other. The huge difficulty in developing criteria with gender neutrality with a similar validity arises in the DSM-5.

One of the clearest examples is found in the somatomorphic disorders. Diagnostic criteria contemplated in the DSM-III included 37 somatic symptoms organized into seven different categories, one of which was called "reproductive symptoms of women" and included painful, irregular, and intense bleeding during menstruation and intense vomiting during pregnancy. These criteria cannot be considered with gender neutrality because they can only be used for somatic disorder diagnoses for women. Surely, they cannot be equally applied to men and neither are they valid for disorder diagnosing in men. The DSM-II points out that somatic disorder "is usually not diagnosed in men," but this rate differential in sexual prevalence could be partially due to the lack of diagnostic criteria with gender neutrality.

After the DSM-III was published, Cloninger et al. [14] pointed out that the diagnostic threshold should have been reduced to approximately 8 of the 37 diagnostic criteria, in order to equate the somatic disorder prevalence (according to the DSM-III criteria) in men and women. However, it is not made clear if the use of a set of criteria that establishes an equal prevalence in men and women would be valid for a disorder that may actually be more frequent in women than in men [15].

In the DSM-IV contemplation of exclusive symptoms in women persist (menstrual irregularity, excessive hemorrhage during menstruation, and vomiting throughout pregnancy), although in this case they are compensated by specific male symptoms (erectile dysfunction or ejaculation) under the "sexual symptom" requirement. Nonetheless, we still do not know if symptom example inclusions of men compensates for the feminine clinical pattern. Additionally, if aforementioned specific symptoms in women are important and valid clinical symptoms in respect of women's somatic disorders, eliminating them in order to reach "gender neutrality" could be problematic.

Another core issue is if women somatize more than men [16]. And if so, why? Indeed, women present more somatic symptoms and more intense symptoms than men. The previous editions of the DSM have supported the diagnosis in itself of somatic symptoms and symptom number and also the illness behavior toward themselves. The DSM-5, on the contrary, abandons this approach and highlights the psychological component of physical sensations (feelings, thoughts, and behaviors). Despite the changes, some factors that contribute to the gender differences in somatic symptoms and the illness behavior have not yet been considered. Below are a number of factors related to somatization, which could contribute to gender differences [17–19]:

- Etiological factors:
  - History of sexual abuse during childhood and/or current sexual abuse, in both cases incidence is higher in women.
  - Biological differences: differences in nociception, and autonomous physiological response to pain.
- Assessment and appraisal of corporal sensations:
  - Tendency in women toward a higher somatic awareness.
  - Women have greater recall of prior symptoms.
- Social roles:
  - Greater stoicism in men.
  - Greater recognition of discomfort in women.
- Comorbidity with other psychiatric disorders:
  - Association of anxiety and depression, both more frequent in women.
- Bias in gender:
  - Gender bias in research.
  - Gender bias in clinical practice.

33.3 Somatomorphic Disorders (Somatic Symptom Disorders)

The term somatization, beyond the definition used in different DSM editions, has been classically used to describe a subconscious process through which an individual expresses its emotional discomfort through somatic complaints, in the absence of clinical findings, which would allow an organic cause of the pattern to be postulated. Somatizations, from the psychopathology point of view, establish the common denominator of a group of disorders, included in the current nosological classifications of the CIE-10 [20] and the DSM, under the denomination of somatomorphic disorders.

It is a heterogeneous group of disorders that have not been entirely validated and that have an imprecise nosological location. In this group we find the following disorders: hypochondriac, conversion and body dysmorphic disorder, and somatization. In fact, the new DSM-5 edition proposes a new denomination for the majority of them (Table 33.1).

Table 33.1 Changes in the denomination and location of the somatoform disorders in the last two editions of the DSM

DSM-IV	DSM-5
Somatomorphic disorders – Somatization disorder – Undifferentiated somatoform disorder – Pain disorder – Hypochondriasis disorder	Somatic symptom and related disorders – Somatic symptom disorder – Illness anxiety disorder
Conversion disorder	Conversion disorder (functional neurological symptom disorder)
Body dysmorphic disorder	
	Psychological factors affecting other medical conditions
Factitious disorder	Factitious disorder

Factors that increase risks of suffering unexplainable somatic symptoms—with the exception of the hypochondriac disorder—include being a woman, young, different race from white, low cultural level, and low level of income [21].

33.3.1 Historical Evolution

The existence of patients, women in most of the cases, with multiple and recurrent physical complaints for which it is impossible to find an organic explanation, and are therefore interpreted as a mental illness, have a long history.

In 1859 Paul Briquet, in his work *Traite Clinique et Therapeutique de L'Hysté rie*, described a psychopathological pattern suffered by young women, characterized by sexual complaints and pain symptoms. This syndrome was understood to be a type of hysteria that appeared at an early age and was stable throughout time [22]. There is a certain unanimity in the scientific literature in designating Steckel as the author who coined the term somatization [23, 24], who granted a similar meaning to Freud's conversion concept. Steckel (1943) defined the term as "the process in which a psychological disorder can produce corporal disorders" [24].

In the 1960s more than 60 symptoms were listed, belonging to more than ten categories, of which at least 25 are needed to diagnose de Briquet syndrome [14, 25]. In the DSM-III, the term somatization disorder is used for the first time, substituting the de Briquet syndrome and the somatomorphic disorders category is included. Somatomorphic disorder is defined as a chronic disorder, although it is fluctuating, polysymptomatic, that begins before the age of 30 years, and occurs primarily in women.

The DSM-III R proposes seven symptoms that could be considered almost pathognomic [26]. These authors indicate that the presence of two or more symptoms of this group of seven (dysmenorrhea, feeling a lump in one's throat, vomiting, breathing problems, rectal, mouth or genitalia burning, pain in the extremities, and amnesia) give an accurate diagnosis.

In the DSM-IV [1] for the somatization disorder the symptoms have to be specified, with at least four pain symptoms being necessary, two gastrointestinal, one sexual symptom, and one neurological symptom. Another highlight in the DSM-IV is the necessity of these symptoms to provoke an important deterioration in crucial activities the person does or that lead this person to search for medical care.

The somatization disorder is not included in the CIE until the last version. It does not specify the number of symptoms that the patient must suffer, but it does say that they must be multiple and variable, there must not exist a medical explanation that justifies the clinical and that the patient must show a persistent negative attitude to accepting medical explanations. This disorder provokes a deterioration of personal, professional, and social behavior.

The DSM-5 recently published proposes a change in the somatomorphic disorder diagnosis to somatic symptoms and related disorders. It defines them more as a somatic symptom, which generates distress and anxiety and/or ends up disturbing everyday life. This must be associated with thoughts, feelings or behaviors involving symptoms or health conditions. It becomes chronic after 6 months.

Somatization, hypochondria, pain, and somatomorphic undifferentiated disorders are deleted from the DSM-5. Somatization and somatomorphic undifferentiated disorders are combined to become somatic disorder symptoms, which does not need a specific number of somatic symptoms. In the DSM-5, people with chronic pain can be diagnosed as having a disorder of somatic symptoms with predominant pain or as psychological factors, which affect other medical conditions. Finally, it proposes the predominance of somatic symptoms, anxious or painful; hypochondria is renamed anxiety disorder owing to illness and conversion disorder becoming neurological function disorder.

33.3.2 Need for Change DSM IV–DSM 5

Next are listed some of the possible reasons why the somatomorphic disorders have been modified in the DSM-5 [27].

- In the DSM IV the only common characteristic of the somatomorphic disorders is the presence of somatic symptoms, which are not referable to medical illness. There are multiple coincidences with psychiatric disorders that are defined equally because of the presence of somatic symptoms, such as depression and anxiety; thus, there is a clear disposition to errors of diagnosis.
- Many of the somatomorphic disorders cannot be extrapolated to other cultures that conceive mind and body in a less dual way: for example, the Chinese classification excludes somatomorphic disorders.
- The exclusion of medical illness as essential criteria to diagnose a somatomorphic disorder also leads to errors, because it is not made clear if the

"somatic functional symptoms," such as irritable bowel, chronic fatigue or fibromyalgia would also be excluded from the diagnosis.

- In general, many of the diagnostic subcategories included within somatomorphic disorders lack validity as an independent disease and would be included with better criteria under other disorders. The clearest example is the dysmorphic body disorder, included under somatomorphic disorders, which would require relocation toward obsessive disorders.
- The terminology is unacceptable for patients, as far as somatic symptoms with no medical explanation are considered, and "mental," in other words products of the mind, are not "real."

33.3.2.1 Disorders with a Predominance of Somatic Symptoms

Somatization Disorder The term somatization has been used to refer to a wide variety of clinical phenomena. From a more traditional view it could be defined as the inability to express emotional distress, the somatic symptoms being a "distress idiom." Another point of view would define somatization as somatic complaints in the presence of an anxiety disorder or an underlying depression. The third view presents somatization as the presence of somatic symptoms that do not have a clear medical explanation. Each of the three ways used to define somatization may identify different groups of patients. Several studies indicate varying prevalence rates, from 0.2 % to 2 % in women and less than 0.2 % in men. Individuals with somatization disorder are usually young women, who describe their symptoms in a striking and exaggerated way. They tell of multiple, relevant, somatic complaints that affect various systems. The majority of individuals with this disorder report the presence of nausea and bloating. The disease is diagnosed before the age of 25, and the first symptoms can start to occur during adolescence; in women menstrual irregularities constitute one of the signs that manifest it more promptly. Sexual symptoms are often associated with marital conflict. The reasons why these patients are often seen in mental health facilities are because of the presence of significant symptoms of anxiety and depression. There is a positive correlation between depression and somatic symptoms [28], constituting in certain studies up to 85 % [29]. From this close relationship the term "masked depression" arises, which explains the manifestation of a depressive disorder primarily by physical symptoms, which are more intense and severe than the psychic symptoms [30]. In the work of Kirmayer and Robins [31], only 21 % of the patients presenting an anxious or depressive disorder communicate mental symptoms to their general physician.

Disorders related to substance abuse are frequently associated with somatization disorder, as are histrionic personality, and limited and antisocial disorders. It is important to differentiate between somatization disorder and simulation and factitious disorders. In the latter, unlike with somatization, the patient exerts control of his symptoms either by faking them or by self-inducing them.

Pain Disorder Pain is defined by the International Association for the study of Pain (IASP) as "an unpleasant sensation and emotional experience, associated with a present or potential damage in tissues," and it is a subjective experience only recognized by the patient who can be believed or not by the treating physician. Pain disorder is defined in the CIE as "a persistent pain without a clear medical explanation"; it differs from the DSM definition, which believes that "psychological factors play an important role in the onset, severity, exacerbation or the persistence of pain." It is more frequent in women with a ratio of 2 to 1.This disorder can appear at any age. Women seem to experience certain types of chronic pain, such as headaches and musculoskeletal pain, more frequently than men. The pain may seriously alter several aspects of daily life. Unemployment, disability, and family problems have been frequently observed among individuals who suffer from chronic forms of pain disorder.

Dependence or abuse of iatrogenic opiates and/or benzodiazepines may occur; therefore, the use of these drugs should be avoided. Individuals suffering from pain associated with severe depression or related to a terminal illness, primarily cancer, are at an increased risk of suicide. Patients with recurrent acute pain or chronic pain are convinced that somewhere there is a health professional who has the healing method for their pain. There is no voluntary control of the symptoms and it is often difficult to find a psychological factor in the psychogenesis of pain. Comorbidity with anxiety and depression as well as with conversion disorders is very common.

Conversion Disorder It is historically referred to as hysterical neurosis of conversion. The essential characteristic of conversion disorder is the presence of symptoms or deficits that affect the motor or sensory functions and which suggest a neurological disorder or any other medical illness. Conversion symptoms are related to voluntary or sensory motor activity, and therefore are called "pseudo-neurological." Typical motor symptoms are disturbances of coordination and balance, paralysis or localized muscle weakness, localized hoarseness, difficulty swallowing, sensation of a lump in the throat, and urinary retention. The sensory type symptoms tend to be loss of touch and painful sensitivity, diplopia, blindness, deafness, and hallucinations. Crisis or seizures may also occur. The less medical knowledge the patient has, the more implausible are his referring symptoms. Individuals with symptoms of conversion may manifest *la belle indifference* (a relative lack of concern about the nature or the implications of the symptoms) or present attitudes of a dramatic or histrionic type. Owing to the easy suggestibility of these individuals, their symptoms may be modified or may disappear according to external stimuli; however, it must be kept in mind that this is not specific to conversion disorder and that it can occur in different medical diseases. It is common for symptoms to appear after a situation of extreme psychosocial stress.

Other Clinical Pictures Various specific somatic syndromes have been described that are defined by somatic symptoms; these are part of entities such as fibromyalgia, irritable bowel syndrome or chronic fatigue syndrome. Most of these syndromes occur more frequently in women than in men [32]. Primary care studies have found that several of these syndromes are associated with symptoms of anxiety and depression [33].

33.3.2.2 Disorders with Predominant Cognitive Symptoms

Hypochondria The essential feature of hypochondriasis is worry and fear of suffering, or the conviction of having a serious illness, from the erroneous interpretation of one or more signs or somatic symptoms. It usually starts between the ages of 20 and 30, being somewhat more frequent in women and having a chronic evolution. The fact that it is more frequent in women may have to do with the high proportion of women being treated in the medical facilities.

The physical examinations and different tests that these patients undergo because of the etiology of their symptoms are negative. Despite these negative results, patients are persistent in their belief and are alarmed when there is any indicative sign of possible illness, constantly observing their bodies. Often, patients tend to present their clinical history in a very detailed and extensive manner. The presence of "medical pilgrimages" (doctor shopping) and the deterioration of the patient–physician relationship, with frustration and anger on both sides, are frequent. Sometimes these patients believe that they do not receive appropriate care and refuse to be sent to mental health centers. People suffering from this disorder may be alarmed when reading or hearing about diseases, with the news that someone has been ill or even by observing what is happening in their own body. Being concerned about the disease often becomes the individual's central feature of self-perception, in a repeated conversation subject, and in response to a stressful situation. It is important to differentiate between hypochondriasis and apprehensive people. In hypochondriasis discomfort is significant, affecting employment, social life, or other important areas in the person's life. Rates of psychiatric comorbidity of hypochondria are high, up to 80 %, including anxious disorders, depressive disorders, and personality disorders [34, 35]. In the latter case, many authors argue that hypochondria is really a pattern of dysfunctional personality with a tendency to interpret somatic sensations [36].

Dysmorphic Body Disorder Dysmorphic body disorder consists of repeated and persistent concerns about an imagined or exaggerated defect in the physical appearance, which causes significant discomfort or is associated with a severe deterioration of the patient.

The nuclear phenomenology of this disorder is not related to somatomorphic disorders; however, in previous DSM editions it was included because of relatively superficial matters, such as corporality and the tendency of people who suffer body dysmorphic disorder to consult physicians and surgeons. The DSM-5 relocates body dysmorphic disorder to the obsessive–compulsive disorder and related disorders chapter.

Currently, concerns with beauty, physical appearance, and body image have become elements that generate huge consumption and in an industry that moves billions of Euros a year. Great importance has been granted to beauty since the body image is closely related to one's professional and personal satisfaction. Women become their body's slaves since this is the vehicle to achieving success. On many occasions they undergo aggressive (surgical, cosmetic, dermatological, capillary, etc.) treatments repeatedly and with irrational demands [37]. These treatments may worsen the disorder, causing the emergence of new and more intense concerns, which, in turn, lead to new therapeutic procedures without success; therefore, these people can have "synthetic" noses, ears, breasts, and hips that are still not to their liking. The current prevalence rate of the disorder is between 1 % and 2 % of the general population [38, 39]. The incidence is similar in both sexes, although women tend to go more frequently to the surgeon and men to the psychiatrist. The age of the patients varies between 15 and 40 years old and there is an over-representation of single people and others without partners [40]. The most common symptoms refer to imaginary defects of little importance on the face or head, such as hair thinning, acne, wrinkles, scars, vascular signs, paleness or redness of the skin, swelling, facial asymmetry or disproportion, and excess hair on the face [41]. These individuals may also be concerned about the shape, size or other aspects of their nose, eyes, eyelids, eyebrows, ears, mouth, lips, teeth, jaw, chin, cheeks, and head. However, other parts of the body can be of equal concern (genitals, breasts, buttocks, abdomen, arms, hands, legs, hips, shoulders, spine, large areas of the body, and even the entire body).

Differences in the genders' clinical manifestations have been found [42], women being more prone to focusing on hips and weight, scratching their skin, hiding behind make-up, and men worrying more about hair loss, their build, and their genitals. People with this disorder, who stubbornly adhere to an appreciation not shared by the majority of people, are afraid that others will realize the alleged physical defect, showing feelings of guilt and shame, constantly worrying, feeling overvalued or delusional, avoiding social situations and showing their bodies, they have rituals, and they request repeated medical and cosmetic treatments [43]. The avoidance of their usual activities can lead to extreme social isolation. In some cases individuals leave their house only at night (when they cannot be seen) or remain in it for a long time, sometimes even years. Dysmorphic body disorder may be associated with a major depressive disorder, a delusional disorder, social phobia, and an obsessive compulsive disorder [44, 45].

33.4 Factitious Disorders

Factitious disorders are characterized by a voluntary production or faking of physical or psychological symptoms repeatedly and consistently in the absence of disorder, disease, or somatic or mental incapacity and without justifying this behavior with the presence of external incentives (or of secondary gain). In factitious disorders the production of diseases or injury is intentional and conscious, but the real motivation is unconscious and often involves the need to become "patients" and thus be cared for by the health team.

However, it should be acknowledged, that the presence of factitious signs or symptoms does not imply the absence of real disorders. In fact, factitious disorders are related to serious personality disorders. Factitious disorders are more frequent in middle-aged women, except for Münchausen syndrome, which is typical in men. Confusion with denominations exists. Often, Münchausen syndrome appears to be synonymous with factitious disorder, which is incorrect. Münchausen syndrome is a subtype of factitious disorders, the most common and serious, and is characterized by the predominant production of physical signs and symptoms in middle-aged men, who are often unemployed, unmarried, and uprooted from their families, often wandering from hospital to hospital or from city to city, sometimes with a history of psychotic behavior and of toxic abuse, multi-systemic complaints, and a history of voluntary medical discharges [46]. Factitious disorders occur in women (in a 3:1 ratio compared with men), at between 20 and 40 years of age; they usually develop a profession in the healthcare area (around 50 %), with greater family rooting and with no pilgrimage behavior, complaints centered on a single system, a minor history of hospitalizations, and they have personalities with immature, dependent, hypochondriac, and passive traits.

Münchausen Syndrome by Proxy In this variant of Münchausen syndrome, described for the first time by the pediatrician Roy Meadow in 1977, it is the parent or caregiver who is the one simulating or deliberately generating symptoms or signs of disease in a dependent child, thus causing tests and unnecessary and potentially harmful treatments, making the child a mere victim. The Münchausen syndrome by proxy (MSbP) is a particular form of child abuse, the severity of which lies in its high morbidity and mortality, difficult diagnosis, and subsequent management.

The majority of people who suffer from this syndrome are young married women. They present themselves to others as mothers concerned about their children's well-being and being dedicated to them, but when they are alone with the children they show little interest in them and hardly acknowledge them. They have an intense need to get involved with medical personnel and hospitals and use their children to obtain these contacts. While in the hospital they get actively involved in their child's care, they do not leave the hospital, and they tend to establish good relations with the staff. They are often found to be more dedicated to establishing relationships with doctors and nurses or offering their support to other mothers of hospitalized children than taking care of their own children. They enjoy being part of an environment whose main objective is the care of sick children. There they feel heard and part of something. They rarely receive visits from the outside, including from the children's fathers, whom are barely involved in their child's health and often remain absent. They appear to have no relationships with the exception of those formed in the hospital. It is not strange to hear them tell stories of accidents such as fires in their home, robberies, etc., often outlandish or exaggerated, in a very dramatic way. Many authors [47] argue that in one third of the mothers there is a history of factitious disorders.

Often these mothers have medical knowledge and sometimes practice professions related to medicine or caring for the sick. They tend to relate to others in a superficial way and have few social skills, except when referring to medical topics.

They demand more tests or specific interventions in their children and can get angry when they do not get their way, demanding that the doctor practice a specific test or procedure that he or she does not consider necessary. They are associated with personality disorders, primarily with the histrionic and borderline, and they also commonly have eating disorders [48]. The approach is highly complicated and should be multidisciplinary, since the child must be separated from the mother, but with the risk that if she feels she has been discovered, she could run away with the child. The mother usually does not cooperate and with regard to the child, tracking should be carried out, since he or she runs the risk of suffering a factitious disorder in adulthood [47].

Conclusions

The latest DSM-5 classification represents a substantial change in these somatomorphic disorders, especially with regard to the somatization disorder and hypochondriasis. These new categories, beyond clinical utility, continue to be non-entirely validated.

Gender issues concerning the somatization phenomenon itself continue to be unsatisfactorily solved. Although the new "somatic symptom disorder" and "illness anxiety medical disorder" convey a more neutral vision of the gender issue than the previous diagnostic categories, there is still a clinical and categorical challenge.

References

1. American Psychiatric Association. Diagnostic and statistical manual of mental disorders (DSM-IV). 4th ed. Washington, DC: American Psychiatric Publishing; 1994.
2. American Psychiatric Association. Diagnostic and statistical manual of mental disorders (DSM-V). 5th ed. Washington, DC: American Psychiatric Publishing; 2013.
3. Schappert SM. National Ambulatory Medical Care Survey: 1991 summary. Adv Data. 1993;230:1–16.
4. Sims A. Symptoms in the mind. An introduction to descriptive psychopathology. 3rd ed. Oxford (UK): Elsevier; 2003.
5. Ristvedt SL. The evolution of gender. JAMA Psychiatry. 2014;71(1):13–4.
6. Gaviria Arbeláez SL, Alarcon RD. Psicopatología y genéro: visión longitudinal e histórica a través del DSM. Revista Colombiana de Psiquiatría. 2010;39(2):389–404.
7. Narrow WE, First MB, Sirovatka PJ, Regier DA, editors. Age and gender considerations in psychiatric diagnosis: A research agenda for DSM-5. Washington, DC: American Psychiatric Publishing; 2007.

8. Lagarde M. Antropología de los cautiverios: Madresposa, monjas, putas, presas y locas. México: Universidad Nacional Autónoma de México; 1992.
9. Badinter E. XY La identidad masculina. Madrid: Alianza Editorial; 1992.
10. Quintanar J. lo Masculino en la edad de la latencia. México: Instituo de Investigación en Psicología Clínica y Social, AC; 1987.
11. Granados JA, Ortiz L. Patrones de daños a la salud mental: psicopatología y diferencias de género. Salud Mental (México). 2003;26(1):42–50.
12. Esteban ML. Cuidado y salud: costes en la salud de las mujeres y beneficios socials. En: Congreso Internacional Sare 2003. Cuidar cuesta: costes y beneficios del cuidado. Instituto vasco de la Mujer y Comunidad Europea/Fondo Social Europeo; 2004. p. 63–84.
13. Durán MA. Costes invisibles de la enfermedad. Bilbao: Fundación BBV; 1999.
14. Cloninger CR, Martin RL, Guze SB, Clayton PJ. A prospective follow-up and family study of somatization in men and woman. Am J Psychiatry. 1986;143:873–8.
15. Widiger TA, Spitzer RL. Criticisms of DSM-III-R. Am J Psychiatry. 1989;146(4):566–7.
16. Wool CA, Barsky AJ. Do women somatize more than men? Gender differences in somatization. Psychosomatics. 1994;35:445–52.
17. Barsky AJ, Peekna HM, Borus JF. Somatic symptom reporting in women and men. J Gen Intern Med. 2001;16(4):266–75.
18. Gijsbers van Wijk CM, Huisman H, Kolk AM. Gender differences in physical symptoms and illness behavior. A health diary study. Soc Sci Med. 1999;49(8):1061–74.
19. Paras ML, Murad MH, Chen LP, Goranson EN, Sattler AL, Colbenson KM, et al. Sexual abuse and lifetime diagnosis of somatic disorders: A systematic review and meta-analysis. JAMA. 2009;302(5):550–61.
20. Organización Mundial de la Salud (OMS). Criterios diagnósticos y de investigación de los trastornos mentales y del comportamiento (CIE-10). Madrid: Meditor; 1993.
21. Barsky AJ, Wyshak G, Klerman GL, Latham KS. The prevalence of hypochondriasis in medical outpatients. Soc Psychiatry Psychiatr Epidemiol. 1990;25(2):89–94.
22. Simon GE, Gureje O. Stability of somatization disorder and somatization symptoms among primary care patients. Arch Gen Psychiatry. 1999;56(1):90–5.
23. Chorot P, Matínez P. Trastornos somatoformes. In: Belloch A, Sandín B, Ramos F, editors. Manual de Psicopatología, col 2. Madrid: McGraw Hill; 1995. p. 225–66.
24. García CJ. Usted no tiene nada. La somatización. Barcelona: Océano; 1999.
25. Guze SB, Perley MJ. Observation on the natural history of hysteria. Am J Psychiatry. 1963;119:960–5.
26. Othmer E, DeSouza C. A screening test for somatization disorder (hysteria). Am J Psychiatry. 1985;142(10):1146–9.
27. Mayou R, Kirmayer LJ, Simon G, Kroenke K, Sharpe M. Somatoform disorders: Time for a new approach in DSM-5. Am J Psychiatry. 2005;162:847–55.
28. Martin RL, Yutzy SH. Trastornos de somatización. In: Hales RE, Yudofsky SC, Talbott JP, editors. Tratado de psiquiatría. 2nd ed. Áncora: Barcelona; 1996. p. 350–96.
29. García-Campayo JJ, Sanz-Carrillo C, Perez-Echeverria MJ, Campos R, Lobo A. Screening of somatization disorder: Validation of the Spanish version of the Othmer and DeSouza test. Acta Psychiatr Scand. 1996;94(6):411–5.
30. Hällström PM. Depressive disorders among somatizing patients in primary health care. Acta Psychiatr Scand. 1998;98:187–92.
31. Kirmayer LJ, Robbins JM. Patients who somatize in primary care: A longitudinal study of cognitive and social characteristics. Psychol Med. 1996;26:937–51.
32. Wolfe F, Ross K, Anderson J, Russell I. Aspects of fibromyalgia in the general population: Sex, pain threshold, and fibromyalgia symptoms. J Rheumatol. 1995;22:151–6.
33. Pawlikowska T, Chalder T, Hirsch S, Wallace P, Wright D, Wessely S. Population-based study of fatigue and psychological distress. BMJ. 1994;308:763–6.
34. Barsky AJ, Wyshak G, Klerman GL. Psychiatric comorbidity in DSM-III R hypochondriasis. Arch Gen Psychiatry. 1992;49:101–8.

35. Kellner R, Abbott P, Winslow WW, Pathak D. Anxiety, depression, and somatization in DSM-III hypochondriasis. Psychosomatics. 1989;30(1):57–64.
36. Tyrer P, Fowler-Dixon R, Ferguson B, Kelemen A. A plea for the diagnosis of hypochondriacal personality disorder. J Psychosom Res. 1990;34(6):637–42.
37. Hollander E, Cohen LJ, Simeon D. Body dysmorphic disorder. Psychiatr Ann. 1993;23:359–64.
38. Hollander E, Wong C. Body dysmorphic disorder, pathological gambling and sexual compulsions. J Clin Psychiatry. 1995;56:7–12.
39. Hollander E, Aronowitz BR. Comorbid social anxiety and body dysmorphic disorder. Managing the complicated patient. J Clin Psychiatry. 1999;60:27–31.
40. Phillips KA. Body dysmorphic disorder clinical aspects and treatment strategies. Bull Menninger Clin. 1998;62:33–48.
41. Phillips KA, McElroy SL. Insight, overvalued ideation, and delusional thinking in body dysmorphic disorder: Theoretical and treatment implications. J Nerv Ment Dis. 1993;181:699–702.
42. Phillips KA, Diaz S. Gender differences in body dysmorphic disorder. J Nerv Ment Dis. 1997;185:570–7.
43. Neziroglu R, Yaryura-Tobias JA. A review of cognitive behavioral and pharmacological treatment of body dysmorphic disorder. Behav Modif. 1997;21:324–40.
44. Hollander E, Neville D, Frenkel M, Josephson S, Liebowitz MR. Body dysmorphic disorder. Diagnostic issues and related disorders. Psychosomatics. 1992;33(2):156–65.
45. Vitiello B, De Leon J. Dysmorphophobia misdiagnosed as obsessive-compulsive disorder. Psychosomatics. 1990;31:220–2.
46. Reich P, Gottfried LA. Factitious disorders in a teaching hospital. Ann Intern Med. 1983;99(2):240–7.
47. Cordess C, Cox M. Forensic psychotherapy: Crime, psychodynamics & the offender patient. London: Jessica Kingsley; 1995.
48. Rosenberg DA. Web of deceit: A literature review of Munchausen syndrome by proxy. Child Abuse Negl. 1987;11(4):547–63.

Printed by Printforce, the Netherlands